MEDICAL MANAGEMENT OF THE CARDIAC SURGICAL PATIENT

MEDICAL MANAGEMENT OF THE CARDIAC SURGICAL PATIENT

Edited by
RICHARD J. GRAY, M.D.
Director, Surgical Cardiology
Cedars-Sinai Medical Center
Los Angeles, California

JACK M. MATLOFF, M.D.
Director, Thoracic and Cardiovascular Surgery
Cedars-Sinai Medical Center
Los Angeles, California

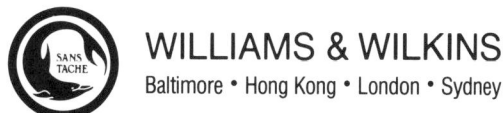

WILLIAMS & WILKINS
Baltimore • Hong Kong • London • Sydney

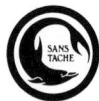

Editor: Michael Fisher
Associate Editor: Carol Eckhart
Copy Editor: Thomas Lehr
Designer: Bets Ltd.
Cover Design: Richard Gray/Lance LaForteza
Illustration Planner: Lorraine Wrzosek
Production Coordinator: Barbara J. Felton

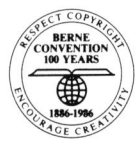
Accurate indications, adverse reactions, and dosage schedules for drugs are provided in this book, but it is possible that they may change. The reader is urged to review the package information data of the manufacturers of the medications mentioned.

Printed in the United States of America

Library of Congress Cataloging-in-Publication Data

Medical management of the cardiac surgical patient / edited by Richard J. Gray, Jack M. Matloff.
    p.   cm.
    Includes index.
    ISBN 0-683-03437-5
    1. Heart—Surgery. 2. Postoperative care. I. Gray, Richard J. (Richard James), 1943–
II. Matloff, Jack M.
    [DNLM: 1. Heart Surgery. 2. Postoperative Care.]
RD598.M464   1990
617′.412—dc19   89-5373
                                          CIP

                           90 91 92 93 94
1   2   3   4   5   6   7   8   9   10

To our parents, James E. and Lorraine E. Gray and Hyman and Ruth Matloff, who valued, above all material things, the importance of rational thought and a love of learning. They attempted both by word and by deed to impart those traits in us to better serve those in need. We hope that they would have felt that their efforts were rewarded.

Foreword

More than three decades ago, I was privileged to participate in, literally, the beginnings of open-heart surgery. The pioneering work of Clarence Crafoord in Sweden and Robert Gross in the United States had demonstrated the feasibility of surgical correction of coarctation of the aorta and patent ductus arteriosus, respectively. Harken and Bailey had demonstrated the feasibility of closed mitral valvotomy for mitral stenosis. In England, Brock applied the same principle to the management of pulmonary and aortic stenosis, while Henry Swan and John Kirklin repaired atrial septal defects by way of an atrial well. However, in 1952, a series of tragic results in young adult patients with pulmonary stenosis and severe subpulmonary hypertrophy convinced Kirklin—others were of like mind—that temporary total cardiopulmonary bypass was absolutely essential for the successful surgical management of heart disease. Human cross-circulation, atraumatic pumps, and screen and bubble oxygenators were developed and refined. Simple and then complex congenital cardiac malformations underwent reconstruction and abnormal valves were replaced. But the basic substrate of patients undergoing these procedures was that of a healthy myocardium. The patients were young, even those with serious valve diseases. "Medical management" of these patients consisted of establishing an accurate diagnosis and the need of surgical intervention and overseeing the hospital stay with all of its details; these were the responsibilities of the cardiac surgeon. In these early—one hesitates to say pioneering—days, hospital mortality rates, which would necessitate the continuation or suspension of a surgical program, were considered evidence of superior practice. As in the surgical tradition of the times, the speed and dexterity of the operation was considered to be the primary determinant of outcome. Indeed, I well remember the pragmatic Kirklin stating that outcome was determined fundamentally in the operating room. Postoperatively, cardiologists were allowed to visit their patients, comment on arrhythmias and digitalis dosage, and then leave.

This text by Dr. Richard Gray and his colleagues results from the changes in both knowledge and clinical practice over these last three decades and defines an area of specialized skills to be acquired by some, but not by all, cardiologists—namely, the medical management of the postoperative cardiac surgical patient. The substrate of patients presenting today is completely different. Cardiac surgery services are offered in every large and many small hospitals across the country. The number of patients undergoing cardiac surgery has increased a hundredfold since 1960. Surgery for congenital malformations—once dominant—now accounts for but a few percent of patients. Surgical treatment of coronary artery disease has dominated the last decade and a half. Almost by definition, these patients seldom have healthy myocardium. Active myocardial ischemia is, in fact, a physiologic indicator for surgical revascularization; today, the majority of coronary artery disease patients also have greater or lesser degrees of permanent myocardial damage. The patients are in their sixth or seventh decade and, not infrequently, in their ninth. Disease of other organs characterizes a significant proportion of cardiac surgical patients today. Thus, the challenges have shifted from the technical skill and speed of the operating surgeon—fundamental as that remains—to support systems provided by many colleagues with differing skills, including the clinical or invasive cardiologist, anesthesiologist, intensivist, and others in relevant medical subspecialties. Indeed, it is because the substrate of the concurrent cardiac surgical patients exhibits inherently heterogeneous challenges in intra- and postoperative management that this substantive change in responsibilities has taken place. Individual patients demonstrate disorders of renal, pulmonary, and hepatic function in association with coronary disease and each may require uniquely different perioperative and later support. The fact that the average cardiac surgical patient is older, sicker, and possibly being treated with a "reoperation" places equal burdens on the anesthesiologist and those responsible for postoperative management, as well as the operating surgeon.

At Cedars-Sinai Medical Center, a "surgical cardiology" service has been in existence for close to two decades. Our surgical practice has reflected the needs of an older community with a propensity for atherosclerosis. An appropriate division of labor has placed substantive responsibility for the care of the postsurgical patient in the hands of trained and experienced cardiologists for postoperative matters that are essentially nonoperative. These include recovery from hypothermia and anesthesia; management of low-output syndrome; and detection and treatment of cardiac arrhythmias, pulmonary and renal insufficiency, disorders of the central nervous system, nonsurgical bleeding, and the like. Not only does this free the surgeon for appropriate consultative and intraoperative functions and the management of operatively derived complications, but allows the formulation of a logical and effective application of the best skills in the most relevant situations. For the medical and surgical specialists involved in postoperative care, this book provides a comprehensive guide to the medical aspects of surgical treatment of patients with heart disease. For the general cardiologist and internist who must deal with day-to-day practice, it focuses the issues on continued attention to the medical needs of this challenging group of patients.

H.J.C. Swan, M.D., Ph.D., F.A.C.C., M.A.C.P.

Preface

During the past three decades, cardiac surgery has resulted in successful management of some of the most serious and prevalent cardiac diseases. For this reason, recommendations in favor of heart surgery are made to ever-increasing numbers of patients. In recent years, however, the character of these patients has changed significantly, evolving toward greater age and much greater acuity and complexity of disease. This is due to dramatic changes in the medical and surgical management of cardiac diseases, growth of the elderly segment of the population, and gradually changing attitudes toward aggressive medical care of the elderly. Unfortunately, great strides in the success of cardiac surgery have brought with them enormous potential for often unique complications. Even the normally convalescing patient will exhibit unusual features that may be puzzling, especially to the medical subspecialists who are bearing an increasing role in postoperative care. Thus, the many individuals caring for these patients must be ever vigilant in the practice of their respective arts.

The purpose of this book is to educate the many medical and surgical subspecialty physicians, as well as critical care nurses, in the management of adult patients before and after various types of open-heart surgery. Although coronary bypass procedures predominate in the United States, this book also addresses the special problems faced by patients undergoing valve procedures and is generally applicable to other procedures such as arrhythmia surgery as well. Senior medical students, physicians in training, and practitioners interested in the fields of cardiac

surgery, cardiology, pulmonology, nephrology, infectious disease, general surgery, neurology, and general internal medicine will find areas of interest within this book. Chapters specific to the needs of liaison and critical care nurses have also been included. These include specific nursing care guidelines and protocols.

The material is presented at a level intended not only for the student physician and physician in training, but for the practitioner as well. The physiologic principles and, in many cases, the research bases of disease concepts are presented for greater understanding. Details of therapy are also presented of course, including, where indicated, medication dosage and duration.

The organization of the book parallels the course taken by a patient through the process of an operation and also parallels the history of cardiac surgery. Section 1 reviews the past experience with open-heart surgery, discusses the current indications for coronary bypass and valve procedures, and elaborates on one of the most important new trends, namely cardiac surgery in the elderly. Section 2 includes two chapters on preoperative workup, one for physicians and one for liaison nurses. Section 3 begins with a discussion of the technical aspects of open-heart surgery, including cardiopulmonary bypass and the techniques of coronary bypass. The remainder of this section addresses important concepts in anesthesia and hemodynamic monitoring. Section 4 outlines the expected course in an uncomplicated patient and highlights important and frequently occurring complications encountered by the patient from the time of his or her emergence from the operating room until hospital discharge. Section 5 describes problems in management during the period from hospital discharge through the first six postoperative weeks. Finally, Section 6 describes a systematic approach to the management of cardiac surgical patients months or even years after their operations. The last chapter describes trends in cardiac surgery and challenges for the future.

Contributors

Timothy M. Bateman, M.D.
Consulting Cardiologist
Mid America Heart Institute
St. Luke's Hospital
Associate Clinical Professor of Medicine
University of Missouri
Kansas City, Missouri

Herman Bernstein, M.D.
Cardiac Anesthesiologist
Cedars-Sinai Medical Center
Los Angeles, California

Carlos Blanche, M.D.
Surgical Associate, Thoracic and Cardiovascular
Surgery
Cedars-Sinai Medical Center
Los Angeles, California

John Bussell, M.D.
Cardiovascular Anesthesiologist
Cedars-Sinai Medical Center
Los Angeles, California

Aurelio Chaux, M.D.
Codirector, Thoracic and Cardiovascular Surgery
Cedars-Sinai Medical Center
Los Angeles, California

Lawrence S. C. Czer, M.D.
Associate Director, Surgical Cardiology
Cedars-Sinai Medical Center
Assistant Professor of Medicine
University of California, Los Angeles
School of Medicine
Los Angeles, California

James E. Dalen, M.D., M.P.H.
Vice Prevost for Medical Affairs
Dean, College of Medicine
The University of Arizona Health Sciences Center
Tucson, Arizona

Arnold S. Friedman, M.D.
Cardiovascular Anesthesiologist
Cedars-Sinai Medical Center
Los Angeles, California

Dennis Goldfinger, M.D.
Director of Blood Bank
Cedars-Sinai Medical Center
Los Angeles, California

Leo A. Gordon, M.D., F.A.C.S.
Attending Surgeon
Cedars-Sinai Medical Center
Los Angeles, California

Richard J. Gray, M.D.
Director, Surgical Cardiology
Cedars-Sinai Medical Center
Adjunct Associate Professor of Medicine
University of California, Los Angeles School of
Medicine
Los Angeles, California

Erroll L. Hackner, M.D.
Coordinator, Cardiac Anesthesiology
Cedars-Sinai Medical Center
Clinical Assistant Professor, Anesthesiology
University of California, Los Angeles
Los Angeles, California

Steven S. Khan, M.D.
Associate Cardiologist, Cedars-Sinai Medical
Center
Assistant Professor of Medicine
University of California, Los Angeles

Cynthia Kristensen, M.D.
Assistant Professor
Department of Medicine/Nephrology
University of Texas Health Science Center
San Antonio, Texas

Myles Edwin Lee, M.D.
Director of Cardiac Surgery
Centinel Hospital
Inglewood, California

Robert E. Lee, R.N., M.S.N., C.C.R.N., C.N.A.
Director, Perioperative Nursing
Mt. Zion Hospital and Medical Center
President, Lee & Associates
San Francisco, California

Daniel A. MacKay
Senior Perfusionist
Cedars-Sinai Medical Center
Los Angeles, California

William J. Mandel, M.D.
Director, Clinical Electrophysiology
Cedars-Sinai Medical Center
Adjunct Professor of Medicine
University of California, Los Angeles School of
Medicine
Los Angeles, California

Jack M. Matloff, M.D.
Director, Thoracic and Cardiovascular Surgery
Cedars-Sinai Medical Center
Los Angeles, California

Emerson A. Moffitt, M.D.
Professor of Anesthesia
Victoria General Hospital
Halifax, Nova Scotia
Canada

Rachel Ramos, R.N., M.S.N., C.C.R.N.
Clinical Nurse Specialist
Hartford Hospital
Hartford, Connecticut

Domenica L. Rocey, R.N.
Cardiac Surgical Liaison Nurse
Cedars-Sinai Medical Center
Los Angeles, California

Virginia Rurycz, R.N.
Cardiac Surgical Liaison Nurse
Cedars-Sinai Medical Center
Los Angeles, California

Dhun H. Sethna, M.D.
Director, Cardiac Anesthesia
Desert Hospital
Palm Springs, California

Stephen J. Shapiro, M.D., F.A.C.S
Attending Surgeon
Cedars-Sinai Medical Center
Los Angeles, California

Tsung-Po Tsai, M.D.
Surgical Associate
Thoracic and Cardiovascular Surgery
Cedars-Sinai Medical Center
Los Angeles, California

Stephen J. Uman, M.D.
Attending Physician
Cedars-Sinai Medical Center
Los Angeles, California

Contents

Section 1
AN OVERVIEW OF PAST EXPERIENCE AND FUTURE TRENDS

Chapter 1
A HISTORICAL PERSPECTIVE OF CARDIAC SURGERY

AURELIO CHAUX, M.D.
JACK M. MATLOFF, M.D.

Throughout history, people have been fascinated by the heart, not only because ancient physicians viewed the heart as the seat of the soul (1), but also because it was recognized as "the first to live and the last to die" (2) among the vital organs. The validity of these concepts was based on the all-too-common observation from cardiac trauma, sustained during battles throughout history, that wounds of the heart were almost universally fatal and therefore not deserving of any therapeutic effort (3). The universal acceptance of these "truths" probably was first challenged by Harvey in his Lumleian lecture of 1616 and his De Motu Cordis of 1628 (4), which elucidated the physiologic basis for the circulation and identified the heart as the dynamic driving force for the blood's circulation. Perhaps more importantly, by this work, Harvey established that the scientific method could be applied to the biologic sciences and medicine.

During the 1700s the concept of the inevitability of death after a wound to the heart began to be questioned. Reports of autopsy findings of healed cardiac wounds were appreciated, and in 1882 Block did the first experiments in which inflicted wounds of the heart were controlled by suture techniques (5). Despite Billroth's admonition that "a surgeon who tries to suture a heart wound deserves to lose the esteem of his colleagues" (6), experimental work to elucidate the effects of cardiac tamponade and the potential for surgical correction of heart wounds proceeded. Along the way significant work by Pasteur in bacteriology, Lister in aseptic technique, Morton in anesthesia, and Haldane in respiratory physiology established the environment in which successful cardiac surgery would one day be accomplished. In 1896 Professor Ludwig Rehn reported the first successful case of suture repair of a cardiac wound (7). In the next 10 years Rehn collected 124 cases of cardiac wounds controlled by suture techniques in which 40% of the patients recovered. As Professor H. M. Sherman wrote in 1902, "The road to the heart is only 2 or 3 cm in a direct line, but it has taken surgery nearly 2,400 years to travel it" (8). Cardiac surgery had begun!

During this time other advances were being made which, while not directly related to cardiac surgery, have had important implications for the development of cardiac surgery. These included the appreciation of the importance of negative intrapleural pressure in thoracic operations and the development by Meltzer and Auer of intratracheal tubes to administer anesthesia (9); the development of methods of vascular suture repair; and the use of autologous venous (10) and arterial homografts (11) and heterografts (12). Finally, Von Frey and Gruber constructed the first artificial heart-lung machine in 1885 (13) in which oxygenation of the perfusate could be accomplished without interrupting blood flow.

VALVULAR HEART SURGERY

It is generally conceded that effective cardiac surgical therapy evolved in relation to correction of congenital or birth defects. In fact, the first phase, as we have seen, had its basis in the treatment of cardiac trauma, and this activity ultimately was the arena for the development of valvular heart surgery. While the lessons learned by Dr. Dwight E. Harken (14) during World War II, as he extracted foreign bodies from within and about the heart, were in immediate proximity to the development of effective heart surgery for valvular heart disease, the basic concepts were actually stated as early as 1898, within two years of Rehn's report, by two physicians, Dr. D. W. Samways (15) and Sir Lauder Brunton (16), who pointed out that the pathologic anatomy of mitral stenosis might best be ameliorated by surgery. Other physicians suggested "cardio-pericardiolysis" for adherent pericarditis and even suggested cutting certain cervical sympathetic nerves to control angina pectoris (17). In the years prior to 1920, unsuccessful attempts were made to relieve pulmonary and aortic stenotic lesions and to carry out pulmonary embolectomy; but it was not until 1923 that Doctors Elliott C. Cutler and Samuel A. Levine reported how their laboratory research efforts to develop a valvulotome culminated in the first successful valvulotomy for mitral stenosis (18). Unbeknownst to the Boston surgical establishment, Sir Henry S. Souttar (19) had worked out a more "modern" operation on a stenotic mitral valve in 1925, an experience duplicated some 20 years later by Drs. Dwight Harken in Boston (20), Charles Bailey in Philadelphia (21) and Lord Russell Brock in London (22). Their work ultimately defined the

limits of closed procedures to effect valve repairs, establishing the presence of calcium and the coexistence of regurgitation and stenosis as circumstances that necessitated total valve replacement.

The first total prosthetic valve replacements of the aortic valve for aortic regurgitation were carried out by Dr. Charles Hufnagle (23) in a location remote from the heart in the descending thoracic aorta. This location was necessitated because there was no practical method available at that time to work within the heart. It remained for Dr. C. Walton Lillehei (24), working at the University of Minnesota, to establish the fact that one could work within the heart to correct congenital defects in young children by using a simple mechanical pump to partially substitute for the circulatory function of the child's heart; and by connecting the circulation of the child to the circulation of a parent it was possible to use the parent's lungs to oxygenate the blood, which was then pumped back to the patient by the combined action of the patient's heart and the mechanical pump. The amazing thing is that Dr. Lillehei's team performed 45 such open heart operations with this technique in a 1-year period; all of the patients were severely ill infants with end-stage cardiac disease, and two-thirds of them survived. It is also amazing that all of the parents involved in these cross-circulation experiments survived without complications.

Ultimately, a workable device for diverting blood extracorporeally from the heart for oxygenation was developed and first used by Dr. John Gibbon on May 6, 1953, to successfully close an atrial septal defect (25). The culmination of Dr. and Mrs. Gibbon's more than 30 years of research had converted Gruber's initial organ perfusion device of the 19th century into the most significant cardiac surgical tool of the 20th century. The availability of this technique has done more to stimulate research and development in the diagnosis and therapy of cardiovascular disease than any other technologic innovation in medicine. With this capability as the driving force, improved prosthetic (26–29) and tissue (30, 31) valve substitutes have been developed, and techniques have been developed to revascularize the coronary arteries (32–

34). Presently, there is no acquired cardiac valvular or vascular lesion that cannot be surgically palliated, even if the heart has to be replaced (35).

CONGENITAL HEART DISEASE

At about the time that Cutler and associates were defining their laboratory and clinical experiences with mitral stenosis, Werner Forssmann, a surgical intern working in Germany, reported a technique for introducing a catheter under radiologic control into the right atrium, through a peripheral arm vein (36). Even these experiments, which he carried out on himself, had previously been accomplished in human subjects without the benefit of radiologic control (37). Within the next 10 years, applications of this technique were developed to determine cardiac output, to visualize intracardiac and great vessel anatomy, and to reproducibly measure right heart pressures in the steady state. These advances were recognized in 1956 when Forssmann, Cournand, and Richards were awarded the Nobel Prize in Medicine. Lewis Dexter's work in developing left heart catheterization and Mason Sones' (38) and Melvin Judkins' development of coronary angiography in 1960 are equally deserving of recognition. Amazingly, the development of these diagnostic techniques occurred during the same time frame that the early valvular and congenital surgical experiences evolved.

In 1938, Sanford Levy and Alfred Blalock (39) attempted to develop an experimental model to study atherosclerosis; their approach, which did not prove successful, was to arterialize the pulmonary artery with the subclavian artery. While these experiments did not achieve their purpose, this experimental design later was adapted as an operation for coarctation of the aorta and as a palliative procedure for blue babies with limited pulmonary blood flow.

At the same time, John W. Strieder (40) and Robert E. Gross (41), working separately in Boston, were evolving the methodology to obliterate a patent ductus arteriosus. While further developments were delayed by the Second World War, the experiences with traumatic cardiac and great vessel wounds prepared the way for

further developments after the war. The names of Crafoord (42), Potts (43), Brock (44), and Glenn (45) were associated with these pioneering efforts. Again, the elements of success included a period of preparation in the laboratory, an experience with trauma, appropriate planning for clinical application, a cooperative effort with a cardiologist, and a courageous surgeon. Additionally, when the time was right, more than one surgeon working in different environs came up with similar solutions to a given problem. And finally, there was the inevitable, unrecognized, even "lost" report; in the instance of the patent ductus arteriosus it had been first recommended by Dr. John Munro in 1907 (46).

Through the years innovative approaches to correcting specific defects have been combined with advances in technology so that at the present time virtually all cardiac birth defects, from the simplest to the most complex, can at the least be palliated so that patients who otherwise would not live or would live very limited existences are now able to carry on with normal lives. The ultimate therapy for otherwise uncorrectable congenital heart disease involves heart transplantation in newborn children as developed by Dr. Leonard Bailey at Loma Linda University (47).

CORONARY ARTERY ATHEROSCLEROSIS

As early as 1899, Francois Franck is said to have proposed cutting certain cervical sympathetic nerves to relieve angina pectoris (17); but it was not until the early 1930s that methods to augment coronary flow, rather than to control pain, were suggested. The initial experimental animal studies, carried out by Claude Beck in the United States and Laurence O'Shaughnessy in Great Britain, were based on the rationale defined by nonsurgeons (48) that vascular communications could be demonstrated at the base of the heart between the coronary arteries and surrounding tissues, especially the pericardium. Thus the clinical applications involved trying to create controlled pericarditis (49). Unfortunately, there were no objective means yet available to assess outcomes.

Notable among these early efforts to revascularize the myocardium was the work of Arthur Vineberg (50), who first reported implantation of the internal thoricac artery in 1946, 11 years after Beck's first clinical experience. He, too, was convinced of the appropriateness of the internal mammary artery implant; but it was not until 1960, when coronary angiography, developed by Sones and Judkins (38), became a reality that both diagnosis and evaluation of the results of surgery were placed on an objective basis. What the availability of coronary angiography did, initially, was to establish an anatomic basis for the diagnosis; no longer would patients be labeled as having coronary disease just because they had a clinical syndrome of chest pain that could be interpreted as Heberden's angina pectoris. Secondly, coronary angiography became the means by which the effects of therapy, especially surgical procedures, could be objectively evaluated. In the case of the Vineberg operation such studies demonstrated that there was the potential with such therapy to develop significant collaterals to obstructed coronary arteries from the internal thoracic (mammary) artery implanted in a myocardial tunnel in proximity to the diseased vessel; when such operations were successful, they were very successful. However, what also became apparent was that there was not a reproducible, predictable result for a significant percentage of patients from this operation; seemingly identical patients, operated by the same surgeon on consecutive days having the same procedure, would not have a similar outcome 1 year later. This fact more than any other relegated this procedure to the realm of historic surgical interest only.

A third effect that coronary angiography had was to serve as the stimulus to the development of what ultimately proved to be a highly reliable, reproducible form of therapy to revascularize the myocardium—coronary artery bypass grafting. After initially experimenting with excision of the plaque, exclusion, and patch graft angioplasty, Dr. Rene Favaloro (32), working at the Cleveland Clinic where Sones had done his primary work on coronary angiography, and Dr. Dudley Johnson (33), working in Milwaukee, developed techniques to bypass the offending proximal coronary atherosclerotic plaques. Venous conduits were used to accomplish these bypasses from the base of the aorta to a location distal to the plaque. There was no attempt to excise or endarterectomize the plaques during these early operations, and the native vessel was left intact to be the source of blood flow to the myocardium. In time, the ideal circumstances for the operation were worked out and included (a) a proximal significant (at least 75%) obstruction in one or more of the three major coronary arteries or their primary branches; (b) a near-normal vessel beyond the plaque; (c) distal, viable myocardium subserved by the obstructed vessel; (d) objective evidence of an ischemic effect on that segment of myocardium; and (e) lack of evidence of infarction, either limited or total, in the segment of myocardium affected.

Use of the internal thoracic artery as a conduit was championed by Dr. George Green (34) of New York and popularized by Dr. Floyd Loop and his associates at the Cleveland Clinic; the latter group has established a significant improvement in the duration that such grafts function, associated with increased patient survival. Today free internal thoracic artery grafts appear to function more like in situ internal thoracic artery grafts than venous grafts. With the use of techniques of specific myocardial preservation including hypothermia and hyperkalemic cardioplegic solutions, complete surgical revascularization, regardless of the number of obstructed vessels, can be carried out in a precisely predictable way with operative survival of 98% in elective cases. In cases that are more complicated, such as by age, acuity of presentation, status of ventricular function, or need for an additional mechanical lesion to be addressed, the results are known from widely reported experiences and are equally predictable. Furthermore, while it is apparent that such therapy is palliative, the duration of function of bypass grafts is known in a general, if not precise, way; and current research efforts are being directed at ways in which graft function can be maintained and extended beyond current experience. It is in this latter context that coronary angiography has had its fourth effect; it has become *the* definitive way in which to follow and characterize the course of coronary atherosclerosis.

As with prior cardiac surgical procedures developed for valvular and congenital cardiac lesions, the first bypass operation was done a significant time before Favaloro and Johnson popularized the concept, by Dr. Michael DeBakey and colleagues (51). An autologous saphenous vein bypass from the ascending aorta to the anterior descending coronary artery was performed on November 23, 1964. The patient suffered an asymptomatic anterior myocardial infarction during operation but made an uncomplicated recovery. Seven years after the operation, the graft functioned with normal left ventricular hemodynamics.

The impetus from treating coronary heart disease by surgical techniques of revascularization has led to a plethora of advances in the care of cardiac disease, primarily because so many people were at risk and needed treatment. One can define the ancillary advances (Fig. 1.1) that

FIGURE 1.1
Ancillary advances in cardiac surgical care.

Preoperative Diagnostic Studies

Noninvasive isotopic scans
Echo color flow doppler
Magnetic resonance imaging
Positron emission tomography
Echocardiography

Anesthetic Management

Premedication
Anesthetic drugs
Cardiotonic drugs
Barbiturates for brain protection
Monitoring of blood chemistries

Intraoperative Surgical Techniques

Finer, nonreactive sutures
Optical magnification
Thermal coronary angiograms
Cardioplegic solutions
Reperfusion solutions

Postoperative Care

Respiratory management
Volume replacement
Pharmacologic support
Temporary mechanical circulatory
   support
Cardiac pacing
Education

have resulted in terms of preoperative diagnostic studies, anesthetic management, intraoperative surgical techniques and postoperative care. While these developments occurred in response to the specific needs of cardiac patients, they has an enormous impact on the care of all hospitalized patients, and in particular those with the greatest acuity, regardless of the organ involved.

CARDIAC REPLACEMENT

Since the heart is largely a pump, it is not surprising that recurring attempts to augment or replace cardiac function with devices or transplanted hearts should have been made throughout the period of time over which heart surgery has evolved.

Within a year of Dr. Gibbon's successful use of a heart-lung machine, Drs. Newman and Dennis of the Downstate Medical Center in New York used a pump oxygenator to support the cardiovascular function of a patient in cardiogenic shock (52). Although they and others had rare successes, the use of such devices did not prove efficacious. The seeming validity and simplicity of the concept did, however, lead to the development of the concept of counterpulsation, that is, removal of blood from the arterial circulation during systole to reduce pressure work and its return during diastole to augment pressure and flow (53). This ultimately led to intra-aortic balloon pumping (54) as we know it today as a partial assist technique. While the technique can be very effective, the circumstances for its successful use are dependent on the heart's putting out enough blood so that the balloon can be used to effectively alter patterns of flow.

Attempts to mechanically assist the circulation, in circumstances where cardiac function is so limited as to preclude any effective cardiac output, have evolved through a whole litany of extracorporeal and intrathoracic devices to totally supplant cardiac function. What these experiences have revealed is that while life can be sustained in excess of a year, there is a significant problem with biocompatability, especially in relation to valve function and the interface between the device and recipient tissues. This has led to a high incidence of thromboembolic phenomena and infection. Further, development of appropriate energy sources to drive the devices and the restricted ability of these devices to respond to varying physiologic conditions have proved to be difficult problems to solve. As a result, governmental support for research to develop total artificial hearts has been curtailed. It is to be hoped that developments in materials will allow this effort to be resumed. For the time being, the temporary use of such devices as a bridge to transplantation in otherwise hopeless cases of cardiac failure remains as a legacy to this effort. In part the decision to give up on these efforts has been underscored by the success of transplants.

Heart transplants have been performed in heterotopic and orthotopic positions. Prior to the advent of cardiopulmonary bypass, heterotopic transplants were attempted. Initially, in a series of experiments conducted by Carrel and Guthrie (55) during the 1st decade of this century, such experiments were carried out to define techniques of vascular anastomoses. Along the way, in other transplant models, they described improved survival with autografts as opposed to homografts. In 1933, Mann (56) described variations of the heterotopic technique developed as a model to study physiologic effects of the heart to various pharmacologic interventions. Mann also described a histologic pattern seen in hearts that failed that presaged the findings of rejection, and he theorized that such failures were more likely due to a biologic factor than to the technique of transplantation. Others expanded on these observations in nonfunctioning hearts, until Vladimir Demikhov (57) in 1946 described a series of experiments in which donor hearts could be orthotopically transplanted in such a way that the left ventricle was a functioning chamber. Unfortunately, he ascribed the failure of these transplants to mechanical problems related to the anastomoses rather than to rejection. Subsequently, Reemtsma and others demonstrated that the intrathoracic placement of an ancillary heart could result in at least partial support of the circulation.

As to orthotopic cardiac transplants, Demikhov also developed techniques, independent of the use of cardiopulmonary bypass, hypo-

thermia, or myocardial preservation to accomplish replacement of the heart. These experiments, along with those of Webb and Howard, demonstrated the feasibility of such an approach, even if it was only for brief periods of time. From 1958 to 1960, the technique currently in clinical use evolved (58); it was based on leaving a cuff of right and left atrium with caval and pulmonary venous connections intact in the recipient, and a matching right and left atrial cuff in the donor to facilitate these anastomoses. During the 1960s, exhaustive experimental work was done, largely by Dr. Norman Shumway's group at Stanford, to define the techniques of preservation, the physiologic responses of denervation, the course of rejection, and the methodologies to modify rejection. All of this experimental work eventuated in the first clinical orthotopic cardiac transplantation by Barnard in 1967 (59). Despite a flurry of clinical activity thereafter, the procedure fell into disrepute, primarily because of inability to control rejection. Notwithstanding, the Stanford group continued, almost singlehandedly, with their clinical work until they were able to follow up on Borel's introduction of cyclosporin A in 1970 with a clinical report of improved results in heart transplants (60). Thus, Shumway's continuing, persistent efforts have largely been responsible for the success that orthotopic cardiac transplants enjoy today, a better than 90% 1-year survival and an approximately 70–75% survival at 5 years. This is a remarkable accomplishment when taken in the context of an anticipated 1-year recipient mortality of 100% without a transplant. Furthermore, the experience with cyclosporin in cardiac transplants led to its equally successful use in all other homografts; it is not inappropriate to say that the transplantation of organs generally is where it is today because of the experience with heart transplants.

In the final analysis, this experience with cardiac transplantation brings this historical perspective of heart surgery almost full circle. Today, there is virtually no cardiac lesion that cannot be successfully corrected or palliated, even if it involves total replacement of the heart. What is needed to complete the circle is further refinement of the techniques of myocardial preservation and of immune suppression. When this time arrives, perhaps even before the 100th anniversary of heart surgery, cardiac surgery will have achieved its full potential. The only link that will surpass the capability of cardiac surgery at that time will be our ability to either prevent or control the mechanisms by which cardiac disease occurs; and these steps will almost certainly be accomplished not by surgery but by molecular biologic manipulations.

SUMMARY

In the 96 years since Rehn's first successful cardiac surgical procedure for trauma, the art and capability of cardiac surgical techniques have developed in an unbelievable, virtually exponential manner. Although patients with cardiac illnesses have obviously benefited the most, the stimulus from the experiences to the development of all aspects of medical science has been enormous. In many ways, the history of cardiac surgery is more a reflection of the development of medical science generally than the story of how surgical techniques have evolved in response to the needs of patients with specific cardiac diseases. This statement is only the clinical expression of the fact that history has established, that is, the reality that cardiac surgery is an extremely dependent discipline which can only achieve its ultimate expression in an environment of superb general medical practice.

References

1. Ballance C: Bradshaw lecture on the surgery of the heart. Lancet 1:1, 1920.
2. Pare A: The Works of Ambrose Pare. In Ballance C: Bradshaw lecture on the surgery of the heart. Lancet 1:1, 1920.
3. Fallopius: Opera Omnia Tractatus de Vulneribus in Genere, cap 10. In Beck C: Wounds of the Heart, pp 207–208. (Original work published 1600.) In Johnson SL: The History of Cardiac Surgery, 1896–1955. Baltimore, The Johns Hopkins University Press, 1970.
4. Leake CD: The historical development of cardiovascular physiology. In Hamilton WF, Dow P (eds): Handbook of Physiology, vol 2. Washington, DC, American Physiological Society, 1962.
5. Block J: Verhandlungen der Deutschen Gesellshaft fur Chirurgie. In Beck C: Wounds of the Heart, p 210. (Original work presented at Elften Congress, Berlin, 1882.)
6. Billroth T: Quoted in Nissen R: Billroth and cardiac surgery. Lancet 2:250, 1963.
7. Rehn L: Uber Penetrierende Herzwunden und Herznaht. Arch Klin Chir 55:315, 1897. (Translated in Beck C: Wounds of the Heart, p 211.)
8. Sherman HM: Suture of heart wounds. Boston Med Surg J 146:653, 1902.
9. Meltzer SJ, Auer J: Continuous respiration without respiratory movement. J Exp Med 11:622, 1909.
10. Gluck T: Die moderne chirurgie des circulation apparatus. Berl Klin 70:1, 1898.
11. Guthrie CC: Survival of engrafted tissues. III. Blood Vessels. Heart 2:115, 1910.
12. Carrel A: Ultimate results of aortic transplantation. J Exp Med 15:389, 1912.
13. Galletti PM, Brecher GA: Heart Lung Bypass. New York, Grune & Stratton, 1962.
14. Berry FB: Surgery in World War II, vol 2. Washington, DC, Office of the Surgeon General, Dept of Army, 1965, p xiii.
15. Samways DW: Cardiac peristasis: its nature and effects. Lancet 1:352, 1902.
16. Brunton L: Possibility of treating mitral stenosis by surgical methods. Lancet 1:352, 1902.
17. Franck F: The growth of cardiac surgery: historical notes. In Litwak RS: Cardiovascular Clinics, Cardiac Surgery I. Philadelphia, FA Davis 3:11–12, 1971.
18. Cutler EC, Levine SA: Cardiotomy and valvulotomy for mitral stenosis. Boston Med Surg J 188:1023, 1923.
19. Souttar HS: Surgical treatment of mitral stenosis. Br Med J 2:603, 1925.
20. Harken DE, Ellis LB, Ware PF, et al: The surgical treatment of mitral stenosis. I. Valvuloplasty. N Engl J Med 239:804, 1948.
21. Bailey CP: The surgical treatment of mitral stenosis (mitral commissurotomy). Dis Chest 15:377, 1949.
22. Baker C, Brock RC, Campbell M: Valvotomy for mitral stenosis: report of six successful cases. Br Med J 1:1283, 1950.
23. Hufnagel CA: Aortic plastic valvular prosthesis. Bull Georgetown Med Ctr 4:128, 1951.
24. Lillehei CW, Cohen M, Warden HE, et al: Direct vision intracardiac surgical correction of tetralogy of Fallot, pentalogy of Fallot and pulmonary atresia defects: report of the first 10 cases. Ann Surg 142:418, 1955.

25. Gibbon JH Jr: Application of a mechanical heart and lung apparatus to cardiac surgery. *Minn Med* 37:171, 1954.

26. Harken DE, Soroff HS, Taylor WJ, et al: Partial and complete prostheses in aortic insufficiency. *J Thorac Cardiovasc Surg* 40:744, 1960.

27. Starr A, Edwards ML: Mitral replacement. Clinical experience with a ball-valve prothesis. *Ann Surg* 154:726, 1961.

28. Bjork VO: A new central-flow tilting disc valve prosthesis. One year's clinical experience with 103 patients. *J Thorac Cardiovasc Surg* 60:355, 1970.

29. Chaux A, Gray RJ, Matloff JM, et al: An appreciation of the new St. Jude valvular prosthesis. *J Thorac Cardiovasc Surg* 81:202–211, 1981.

30. Ross D: Homotransplantation of the aortic valve in the subcoronary position. *J Thorac Cardiovasc Surg* 47:713, 1964.

31. Binet SP, Carpentier A, Langlois J, et al: Implantation de valves heterogenes dans le traitement de cardiopathies aortiques. *C R Acad Sci* 261:5733, 1965.

32. Favaloro RG: *Surgical Treatment of Coronary Atherosclerosis.* Baltimore, Williams & Wilkins, 1970.

33. Johnson WD, Lepley D Jr: An aggressive surgical approach to coronary disease. *J Thorac Cardiovasc Surg* 59:128, 1970.

34. Green GE, Stertzer SH, Gordon RB, et al: Anastomosis of the internal mammary artery to the distal left anterior descending coronary artery. *Circulation* 41:11–79, 1970.

35. Lower RR, Dong E Jr, Shumway NE: Long-term survival of cardiac homografts. *Surgery* 58:110, 1965.

36. Forssmann W: Die sondierung des rechten herzens. *Klin Wochenschr* 8:2085, 1929.

37. Bleichroeder F: Intra arterielle therapeutic *Berl Klin Wochenschr* 49:1503, 1912.

38. Sones FM Jr, Shirey EK: Cine coronary arteriography. *Mod Conc Cardiovasc Dis* 31:735, 1962.

39. Levy SE, Blalock A: Experimental observations on the effects of connecting by suture the left main pulmonary artery to the systemic circulation. *J Thorac Surg* 8:525, 1939.

40. Graybiel A, Strieder JW, Boyer NH: Attempt to obliterate patent ductus arteriosus in patient with subacute bacterial endocarditis. *Am Heart J* 15:621, 1938.

41. Gross RE, Hubbard JP: Surgical ligation of patent ductus arteriosus. *JAMA* 112:729, 1939.

42. Crafoord C, Nylin G: Congenital coarctation of the aorta and its surgical treatment. *J Thorac Surg* 14:347, 1945.

43. Potts WJ, Smith S, Gibson S: Anastomosis of the aorta to a pulmonary artery. *JAMA* 132:627, 1946.

44. Brock RC, Campbell M: Infundibular resection or dilation for infundibular stenosis. *Br Heart J* 12:403, 1950.

45. Glenn WWL: Circulatory bypass of the right side of the heart. IV. Shunt between superior vena cava and distal right pulmonary artery—report of clinical application. *N Engl J Med* 259:117, 1958.

46. Munro JC: Ligation of ductus arteriosus. *Ann Surg* 46:335, 1907.

47. Bailey LL, Nehlsen-Cannarella SL, Doroshow RW, et al: Cardiac allotransplantation in newborns as therapy for hypoplastic left heart syndrome. *N Engl J Med* 315:949–951, 1986.

48. Moritz AR, Hudson CL, Orgain ES: Augmentation of extracardiac anastomosis of the coronary arteries through pericardial adhesions. *J Exp Med* 56:927, 1932.

49. Beck CS: Coronary sclerosis and angina pectoris. Treatment by grafting a new blood supply upon the myocardium. *Surg Gynecol Obstet* 64:270, 1937.

50. Vineberg AM: Development of anastomosis between coronary vessels and transplanted internal mammary artery. *Can Med Assoc J* 55:117, 1946.

51. Garrett HE, Dennis EW, DeBakey ME: Aortocoronary bypass with saphenous vein graft. Seven-year follow-up. *JAMA* 223:792–794, 1973.

52. Newman MM, Stuckey JH, Levowitz BS, et al: Complete and partial perfusion of animal and human subjects with the pump-oxygenator, *Surgery* 38:30, 1955.

53. Clauss RH, Birtwell WC, Albertal G, et al: Assisted circulation. I. The arterial counterpulsator. *J Thorac Cardiovasc Surg* 41:447, 1961.

54. Moulopoulos SD, Topaz S, Kolff WJ: Diastolic balloon pumping (with carbon dioxide) in the aorta. Mechanical assistance to the failing circulation. *Am Heart J* 63:669, 1962.

55. Carrell A, Guthrie CC: The transplantation of veins and organs. *Am Med* 110:1101, 1905.

56. Mann FC, Priestley JT, Markowitz J, et al: Transplantation of the intact mammalian heart. *Arch Surg* 26:219–224, 1933.

57. Demikhov VP: *Experimental Transplantation of Vital Organs.* Haigh B (trans), New York, Consultant's Bureau, 1962.

58. Lower RR, Shumway NE: Studies on the orthotopic homotransplantation of the canine heart. *Surg Forum* 11:18, 1960.

59. Barnard CN: The operation: a human heart transplantation. An interim report of the successful operation performed at Groote Schuur Hospital, Capetown, South Africa. *S Afr Med J* 41:1271, 1967.

60. Borel JF: The history of cyclosporin A and its significance. In White DJG: *Cyclosporin A: Proceedings of an International Conference on Cyclosporin A*. New York, Elsevier Biomedical, 1982.

Chapter 2
CURRENT INDICATIONS FOR CORONARY BYPASS AND/OR VALVULAR SURGERY

JACK M. MATLOFF, M.D.

Deviations of cardiac anatomy and function from normal describe a spectrum of pathologic states, the etiology for which may be congenital or acquired. These effects also describe a continuum of clinical manifestations that are dynamic and progressive, at variable rates of change. Thus, with aortic valvular stenosis that begins as congenital aortic stenosis or as a bicuspid valve, the clinical course described can result in severe cardiovascular compromise early in life or be found as an incidental finding at the end of life. Rheumatic heart disease is more variable in its manifestations, extending from an absence of effects to a situation in which every cardiac valve may be involved, either primarily or secondarily. This highly variable degree of valvular involvement, often coexisting with coronary atherosclerosis (coronary artery disease, or CAD), makes one begin to appreciate just how many specific clinical situations may have to be evaluated for therapy at various times and stages of the disease process.

CAD describes a spectrum of changes in individual vessels and in vessel combinations, the effects of which can be multiplied many times by varying patterns of dominance of one or more of the vessels, as compared to a balanced pattern of circulation in which the three vessels con-

tribute equally. With varying degrees of occlusiveness extending from normal to total occlusion, with unpredictable development of collateral circulation between the vessels occurring over time, and with secondary effects occurring to myocardial muscle function and anatomy segmentally and globally, the clinical manifestations of CAD can become almost protean in their expression.

Finally, when on considers additional etiologic changes that may be infectious (viral or bacteriologic), metabolic, neoplastic, traumatic, or idiopathic, it is clear that while general cardiac disease patterns and clinical manifestations can be identified, each clinical picture is an entity unto itself. Thus, evaluations have to be done for each specific case to elucidate the precise anatomic and functional basis for the clinical manifestations at the time the patient is worked up.

Paralleling these variable pathologic and clinical expressions of abnormal cardiac function is a spectrum of therapies that have evolved in response to the varying needs of patients. These extend from no specific therapy to actual cardiac replacement. Furthermore, therapy can be medical or surgical in nature. Ideally, there should be comparable contributions, with the

12

decision for surgical therapy being made based on response or lack of response to medical therapy at a specific time in the course of the disease process. Thus, the issue should be "when" it is appropriate to add surgical therapy to medical therapy, rather than "which" is appropriate in and of itself. A best-case scenario would involve both medical and surgical therapy, with the former being applied before and after surgery. Unfortunately, discussion in the literature more often becomes one of deciding on medical *versus* surgical therapy; and the decision-making process seeks a scientific basis on which to make the choice. Thus, concepts such as "culprit" vessels, degrees of involvement, territories at risk, complete and incomplete revascularization, and incremental risk factors are introduced; and justification rather than rationale becomes the basis for informed consent to therapy.

In the final analysis, it has to be appreciated that with rare exceptions (patent ductus, secundum atrial septal defects, and coarctation of the aorta), the present goal of cardiac surgical therapy is to achieve *long-term palliation* rather than true cure. Nowhere is this more apparent than in the surgical therapy of CAD, in which the best that can be expected is that successful revascularization will prolong life long enough so that the patient will live to have another problem develop. Thus, while prevention is an often-stated and laudable objective of therapy, true prevention continues to be difficult to achieve under any circumstance. Cures and prevention are matters for the future which should be attainable. In this context, it is the cardiovascular specialist's duty to educate patients about risks, outcomes, and long-term expectations of the various forms of therapy available at a given time for a given pathologic situation, so that the patient can understand what the best decision is for himself or herself. In this understanding, quality of life, in terms of symptomatic and functional status, may have to be weighed against chances for survival, both short- and long-term; and exchanges of one or the other may have to be considered. In a way, this educational process is the beginning of any therapy, and it also becomes the foundation for future therapy, since achieving therapeutic goals

depends primarily on the patient's understanding of what is occurring.

In summary, the timing of and indications for any therapeutic intervention have to be based on a combination of considerations. These involve pathologic anatomy, pathophysiology (function), clinical manifestations, and the natural histories of various therapeutic interventions. While there is a subjective element to the evaluation and decision-making process, as much as possible, objective criteria should be the basis for the decisions that are made.

CORONARY ATHEROSCLEROSIS

The indications for surgical therapy in CAD, ideally, should be taken in relation to the effectiveness of medical therapy. Historically, surgical therapy for CAD evolved in response to the perceived need to correct some of the anatomic, ischemic complications of CAD; it has been only 20 years since revascularization for relief of anginal symptoms has become a reality. At the present, the two generic indications for surgical therapy in CAD remain relief of symptoms and correction of the ischemic complications of acute myocardial infarction.

Relief of Symptoms by Coronary Artery Bypass

CAD is most often detected through a variety of circumstances that constitute clinical markers of the disease. These include angina pectoris, the awareness of an arrhythmia, and the occurrence of acute myocardial infarction, sudden death, or otherwise unexplained cardiac symptoms, such as shortness of breath, decreased exercise tolerance, and increasing fatigability. Variable or atypical presentations also include pain patterns that are not classically defined as angina pectoris, including variant or Prinzmetal's angina that occurs spontaneously without provocation at rest or during sleep.

Quite aside from these manifest symptoms, many patients are truly asymptomatic or minimally symptomatic, so that their situation is not defined by clinical manifestations. Absence of pain is common in patients with diabetes mellitus, and silent ischemia is an increasingly documented phenomenon in nondiabetics. Patients such as these may be identified by a change in ECG, through an evaluation for other operable heart disease, or a positive exercise treadmill test (ETT) done for a variety of reasons. The latter include regular medical evaluations, insurance examinations, or the presence of risk factors, especially a family history of CAD.

Thus, CAD may describe a continuum of presentations extending from a truly asymptomatic state to sudden death. Included in the spectrum of angina are the clinical entities of chronic stable angina, unstable angina, acute myocardial infarction, and postinfarction angina. Unfortunately, a relationship between these clinical manifestations and a specific anatomic substrate has never been established, although a constellation of findings may strongly suggest the presence of a left main coronary obstruction, a left main equivalent, or a very proximal lesion in a dominant left anterior descending.

In the *asymptomatic* or *minimally symptomatic* patient, surgical therapy should not be a primary consideration (1); the randomized Coronary Artery Surgery Study (CASS) experience has established that the outcomes of medical and surgical therapy are not different to 5 years. Annual mortality rates for single vessel disease (SVD) and double vessel disease (DVD) are about 1.5% (2). Notwithstanding, each patient should be evaluated in his or her own merits; and if compelling circumstances are documented, such as the occurrence of significant ischemia at low levels of exercise, global left ventricular dysfunction, or the presence of extremely threatening anatomy (left main 50% or more, proximal obstruction 75% or more in a dominant left anterior descending or triple vessel disease, especially with compromised left ventricular function) (Table 2.1), then coronary artery bypass (CAB) should be entertained. The annual morality rate for patients with triple vessel disease (TVD) is increased to 6%, being 4% for those with good ventricular function and 9% for those with compromised left ventricular function. With the advent of percutaneous transluminal coronary angioplasty (PTCA), such invasive therapy may be more appropriate than CAB in carefully delineated situations. This circumstance has resulted in more patients being evaluated by coronary an-

TABLE 2.1

INDICATIONS FOR BYPASS— NO OR MINIMAL SYMPTOMS

Anatomy	SVD[a]	DVD[b]	TVD[c]	Left Main
Normal ventricle	No[d]	No	Yes	Yes
Abnormal ventricle	No[d]	Yes	Yes	Yes

[a]SVD, single vessel disease.
[b]DVD, double vessel disease.
[c]TVD, triple vessel disease.
[d]Would be yes in presence of markedly positive treadmill test.

giography than ever before. Invasive therapy in the asymptomatic patient may prove to be truly prophylactic in the sense that such patients are at a greater risk for a catastrophe, since they do not have the appropriate warning of an impending ischemic event. In patients who have other pathologies that are being considered for surgical therapy, coincident, asymptomatic coronary artery disease should also be corrected.

Chronic stable angina for which medical therapy is no longer effective or is poorly tolerated constituted the original indication for CAB. Data from the Framingham Study (3) conducted during the 1960s, when coronary revascularization surgery evolved, indicated that 25% of men with angina would experience an acute myocardial infarction within 5 years. More recent CASS data indicate that the prognosis progressively worsens with the number of coronary arteries involved, the number of proximal arterial segments diseased, and more compromised left ventricular function (4); these three indices, which account for approximately 85% of prognostic information available, indicate that 6-year survival varies from 16 to 93% depending on the value of these combined indices. Currently, when patients are refractory to medical therapy or when outcome with medical therapy involves more than 1 to 1½% annualized mortality, CAB is recommended. Aside from improved survival, surgical patients achieve better quality of life. Although this recommendation may be considered "soft" by some, the recommendation is unequivocal when a chronic stable anginal pattern begins to progress or becomes unstable, or when there is objective data that indicate the potential for a life-threatening ischemic event. To the extent that such an outcome can be predicted, the occurrence of episodic acute congestive heart failure, for instance, is an ominous change. More reproducible and objective changes may be heralded by high degrees of ischemic manifestations at low levels of exercise, accompanied by indices of acute left ventricular decompensation such as a decrease in blood pressure or a ventricular arrhythmia. In these circumstances, the recommendation for CAB may be made on a more urgent than elective basis.

Unstable angina pectoris is a manifestation of CAD that is sometimes made more difficult to manage because of semantic nuances than because of medical considerations. A variety of terms have been used to define what is unequivocally a progressive phase of the disease; these include crescendo angina, spontaneous angina, progressive angina, acute coronary insufficiency, intermediate syndrome, impending infarction, and preinfarction angina. Our view of this syndrome is that it represents a change in the pathophysiology of the coronary obstruction which is associated with hemorrhage or thrombus formation at the site of an irregular or ulcerated proximal plaque (5) that is likely to result in total coronary occulsion and an acute myocardial infarction if it is not controlled. We have felt that the terms preinfarction angina (6) or impending infarction best represent the course described by that subset of patients that are identified when unstable angina proves to be medically refractory. Whatever the differences in criteria that establish such definitions, the fact remains that these patients are susceptible to medical failure (7) and are at increased risk for an acute ischemic event, including acute myocardial infarction or death (8). Early surgical experiences with patients manifesting unstable angina were widely divergent. Much of this difference is the result of whether the patient is "cooled off" medically or operated directly; in the former, acute infarctions are ruled out, and in the latter they are often identified as having a high incidence of perioperative infarction. Current medical and surgical protocols allow for an appropriate "cooling off" period, but if this cannot be accomplished, CAB can be carried out emergently with excellent results (6, 9). These excellent results are due to improvements in anesthesia and the use of hypothermic, hyperkalemic cardioplegia.

Increasingly, PTCA is also being offered as therapy in this clinical circumstance (10) with apparent good success when applicable. However, there is concern for the adequacy of such therapy when intracoronary thrombus has been identified.

CAB for *acute myocardial infarction* (AMI) has been recommended with varying results in a number of circumstances (Table 2.2), each of which is best discussed in its individual context. Myocardial reperfusion to terminate evolving AMI has been considered an aggressive application aimed at limiting the effects of the infarction, thereby preserving myocardial viability and function and improving survival. The basic assumption of such therapy is that myocardial necrosis is an evolving process that can be limited by early surgical revascularization. While overall excellent results have been reported both early and late (11, 12), it is clear that these results are stratified according to the time from onset of infarction to revascularization, the number of vessels involved, the location of the infarction, whether or not the infarct is transmural, and whether or not cardiogenic shock has occurred. While 1-year survival of 94% is the primary claim for such therapy, postoperative hemodynamic and scintigraphic studies have indicated that significant improvements in ejection fraction, stroke volume, and reduced left ventricular end-diastolic pressure and volume are also attainable (12, 14, 15). Although these results are impressive and demonstrate the

---

TABLE 2.2

INDICATIONS FOR CORONARY ANGIOGRAPHY AND CORONARY ARTERY BYPASS IN AMI

Preinfarction angina, continuing and refractory to medical therapy[a]

Routinely, during first 6 hours of AMI

After thrombolytic therapy, in presence of critical triple vessel disease

Postinfarction agina with multivessel disease

In patients with nonmechanical cardiogenic shock, if stabilized—acute left ventricular aneurysms

In association with mechanical defects
  Ventricular septal defect
  Mitral regurgitation, intermittent and persistent
  Cardiac rupture with tamponade

[a]Represents earliest phase of AMI.

feasibility of surgical reperfusion by revascularization, they have been obtained at considerable cost of personnel and financial resource. It is apparent that time constraints are also of paramount importance, whether based on an arbitrary time scale (4 to 6 hr) or continued signs of evolution. Unfortunately, it is not common that a community and its medical resources can be committed to such a therapeutic effort. Further, such studies have been criticized as being flawed by severe patient-selection bias and for not providing a control group of medically treated patients. Notwithstanding, experience is rapidly being accumulated that suggests that urgent reperfusion, whether achieved chemically with thrombolysis, mechanically with PTCA, or surgically with CAB, is effective primary therapy for AMI. It is also becoming clear that the result will depend on the local experience that evolves with each technique or combination thereof, as well as on specific clinical indications.

Patients with *postinfarction angina pectoris* are better discussed in the context of the nonmechanical complications of AMI that are amenable to CAB.

Congestive heart failure occurring as *acute pulmonary edema* is an unusual manifestation of CAD, but it clearly does occur and is very dramatic in its presentation. When this occurs acutely and is not an exacerbation of a controlled situation of congestive heart failure, it usually represents a global ischemic insult in an otherwise healthy or normally functioning heart. Critical anatomy, such as proximal triple vessel disease or a left main obstruction of over 75%, is often the anatomic substrate. These cases are unequivocally surgical candidates and they carry a sense of urgency. Outcomes are determined as much by the anatomy as they are by the clinical manifestations; the prepump anesthetic management is as much a key to success as is careful myocardial preservation using all forms of specific myocardial protection.

Percutaneous Coronary Angioplasty and Coronary Artery Bypass

PTCA and CAB are both invasive methodologies to achieve coronary revascularization.

While PTCA has been practiced for 10 years, CAB has reached maturity at twice that life span. As yet, it does not seem appropriate to try to draw parallels or contrasts between the two techniques. This is particularly true in regard to the indications for each therapy. Theoretically, they should share common indications, but this is not yet the case. The increased versatility of CAB is offset by the seemingly decreased morbidity experienced by most patients undergoing PTCA. To date, PTCA continues to be regarded as a temporizing therapy, very often accomplished by multiple, staged interventions. In the presence of multiple occlusions, diffuse distal disease, and coincident mechanical lesions, when total revascularization is the goal of therapy PTCA is probably not indicated.

By way of contrast with what has just been presented for CAB, the most common indications for PTCA include severely symptomatic CAD, regardless of medical therapy; objective evidence of marked ischemia, regardless of symptomatic status; "compelling" anatomy involving proximal lesions of a dominant anterior descending or right coronary; and acute myocardial infarction either before, after, or in conjunction with thrombolytic therapy. However, several of these indications are associated with single or double vessel disease, situations in which there has been some resistance to considering CAB. What the availability of PTCA has accomplished is a change in the thinking of cardiologists toward earlier definitive studies with cardiac catherterization and coronary angiography. To the degree that this increasingly aggressive diagnostic and therapeutic attitude identifies patients who can be treated before ischemic complications occur, significant symptomatic improvement as well as enhanced survival of patients with CAD is expected, given the capabilities of CAB and PTCA today.

Notwithstanding this significant change in attitudes toward aggressive therapy of CAD, it must be appreciated that some complications of angioplasty are beyond the capability of the PTCA operator to control. Coronary dissection, perforation, or complete occlusion of the involved coronary can occur in from 5 to 20%

of patients so treated, with mortality rates after subsequent emergency CAB of from 1 or 2 to 12%. Although emergency surgical correction under these conditions may account for only a modest increase in postoperative mortality, morbidity remains considerably higher than for elective bypass, owing to an increased frequency of postoperative ventricular arrhythmias, hypotension, low cardiac output, and perioperative myocardial infarction (16). Thus, these two forms of therapy have to be taken in conjunction with each other for optimal success to be appreciated from a more timely diagnosis and definition of the anatomy.

Correction of Postinfarction Ischemic Complications

A spectrum of ischemic complications can occur after AMI that may necessitate surgical attention. These can occur at various times after infarction and may be of either a nonmechanical or a mechanical nature. Among the *nonmechanical complications* are (*a*) complete heart block; (*b*) acute pump failure with or without congestive heart failure or cardiogenic shock; (*c*) refractory ventricular arrhythmias; and (*d*) continuing or recurrent postinfarction angina. The *mechanical complications* include (*a*) rupture of the ventricular septum; (*b*) rupture of the free wall of the left ventricle; (*c*) mitral regurgitation from papillary muscle dysfunction, rupture of a papillary muscle or chordae tendineae, or mitral annular dilation; and (*d*) acute and chronic left ventricular aneurysm formation. With the possible exceptions of acute pump failure with cardiogenic shock and acute refractory ventricular arrhythmias, each is an indication for surgery.

Of the nonmechanical complications, *heart block* is the easiest to treat. Current pacemaker technology using intravenous electrodes and extracoporeal generators permits control of both atria and ventricles in a variety of modes that virtually achieve normal function.

Postinfarction acute pump failure resulting in congestive heart failure, whether progressing to cardiogenic shock or not, can occur without a mechanical defect and is predicated on the loss of a large volume (up to 40%) of functioning myocardium. The current value of CAB or PTCA in this circumstance rests on the extent to which there is functionally impaired ischemic but viable ("stunned") myocardium that can regain sufficient contractility to improve global ventricular function after revascularization. To the extent that PTCA can be applied most expeditiously to the infarcted vessel, this is the therapy of choice to try to minimize infarct size and recruit the peri-infarction ischemic zone. In patients with multivessel disease who experience AMI with pump failure, interval CAB to restore segments that are ischemic and in jeopardy remote to the AMI may be indicated. At the present time, these considerations are more theoretic than practical since clinical experience is limited. Whether areas of ischemic damage can be diminished by manipulation of the reperfusing medium (17) remains to be seen.

Refractory ventricular arrhythmias may be controlled by reperfusion when there is an ischemic contribution to their occurrence. Experience has indicated that unless the arrhythmia occurs in conjunction with acute ischemia, it is unlikely to be stabilized by revascularization alone, whether by PTCA or CAB. Anecdotal experiences are, however, beginning to emerge in which electrocardiographic ventricular mapping, ventriculotomy through the acute infarction, and freezing of the responsible area during the acute phase have proved to be helpful in control of such ventricular arrhythmias.

Continuing or recurrent angina after AMI may be an indication that infarct extension or reinfarction at a distance is imminent. Revascularization is clearly indicated if coronary angiography reveals significant but bypassable disease. Concern about such procedures within 30 days of AMI has been moderated by improvements in anesthetic management and techniques of myocardial protection. Ventricular function is a more powerful determinant of survival than the interval between AMI and surgery (18). Based on this, one is encouraged to stabilize and temporize, when possible, to a time beyond 1 week, but if this is not possible, then surgical therapy within the 1st month does not carry a significantly increased mortality (19).

Among the mechanical complications of AMI,

postinfarction ventricular septal defects, rupture of the free wall, mitral regurgitation, and acute left ventricular aneurysm formation occur acutely and are associated with high mortality, especially if they cannot be corrected.

Ventricular septal rupture occurs in only 0.5 to 2% of AMI, from as early as 1 to 10 days after infarction (20), but carries a 24% mortality within 24 hr, 46% within 1 week, 75% at 8 weeks, and 95% at 1 year. It accounts for 5% of all postinfarction deaths (20, 21). Medical therapy with afterload reduction (where possible) and inotropes, mechanical ventilation, and intraaortic balloon pumping (IABP), is, at best, temporizing therapy. Traditionally, the timing of surgical therapy has been a function of balancing the technical problem of dealing with unhealed infarcted tissues seen early with the severe cardiac, renal, cerebral, and pulmonary failure when surgery is delayed to allow some fibrosis to occur in the healing infarct margins. Currently an emergent, radical surgical program is advocated that consists of immediately instituting aggressive medical therapy and establishing a definitive diagnosis. The surgery is performed early and is directed at resecting all of the infarcted tissue (septum, right and left ventricular free walls), using a large patch to reconstruct the septum and coronary artery bypass where indicated. Surgical survival of 75% with this approach compares favorably with the results of other reported cases of early surgical therapy (22).

Rupture of the free cardiac wall is estimated to complicate 1.5 to 8% of AMI and is responsible for from 5 to 24% of infarction deaths (23). Because a higher incidence of rupture occurs in elderly female patients with advanced coronary atherosclerosis and because early diagnosis is often difficult, surgical therapy has not been very effective. Since cardiac rupture is almost uniformly fatal, every attempt should be made to rapidly place the patient on cardiopulmonary bypass, carry out infarctectomy, and repair the defect. When successful, such therapy has been reported to be successful with promising long-term prognosis (24). Pseudoaneurysm can result after rupture when there is containment of the resulting hemopericardium by circumferential adhesions between the pericardium and the epicardium. Because there is usually a narrow neck between the aneurysm and the left ventricle, these can be easily repaired in the chronic phase; the existence of pseudoaneurysm, with or without symptoms, is an indication for surgery.

Postinfarction mitral regurgitation may be the most difficult issue for surgeons to address. The pathologic substrate is variable (Table 2.3), ranging from papillary muscle dysfunction to a variety of coincident, nonischemic causes of mitral valve disease. In the past it has been hard to define surgical indications (especially where the regurgitation is less severe), what type of procedure is best, and how the results could be evaluated. The intraoperative use of color flow Doppler (25) has helped to resolve some of these issues; but the fact remains that when mitral regurgitation exists it is a hallmark of far-advanced coronary disease. Coronary revascularization alone is almost never enough to correct mitral regurgitation (26) since papillary muscle dysfunction is usually associated with an infarction of the papillary muscle or adjacent free wall. Repair of the mitral valve by an annuloplasty procedure of the commissures can be very effective in such cases. When rupture of the chordae tendineae or a minor papillary muscle occurs, successful repair has been claimed using a variety of techniques, including insertion of a mitral annuloplasty ring. We have found that such procedures increase operating time suffi-

TABLE 2.3

CAUSES OF MITRAL REGURGITATION ASSOCIATED WITH ISCHEMIC HEART DISEASE

Papillary muscle dysfunction
  Ischemic paralysis
  Infarction
    Tip of the papillary muscle
    Adjacent free wall

Chordae tendineae rupture

Papillary muscle rupture
  Tip of the muscle
  Head of the muscle

Ischemic myocardiopahty with annular dilation

Nonischemic, incidental nitral valve disease
  Rheumatic
  Infective
  Degenerative

ciently so that complete revascularization cannot be done as safely; thus, surgical discretion becomes an important issue. With frank rupture of a papillary muscle, the therapeutic dilemma occurs in relation to the severity of the infarction and the acuity of the ensuring hemodynamic instability. Emergent catheterization and surgery to replace the valve and bypass the obstructed coronaries may well turn out to be the best therapeutic option. Even so, the intermediate follow-up results are limited (27).

Acute left ventricular aneurysm formation and infarct expansion should be considered, conceptually, as a continuous phenomenon. Acute functional aneurysms can occur within the first 24 hr, and the thinning and dilation that characterize the pathologic changes of infarct expansion occur up to 7 days after infarction. Both of these expressions of transmural infarction may be precursors of acute ruputre of the free wall (28) or of aneurysm formation (29) and are associated with a marked increase in mortality (30). While revascularization very early in the course of the infarction to reverse what is initially a functional aneurysm may be beneficial, infarctectomy with or without concurrent coronary artery bypass has not been widely practiced, primarily because those who have tried have had uniformly dismal results.

Among the mechanical complications of coronary atherosclerosis that require surgical consideration, there remains chronic left ventricular aneurysm formation. Such aneurysms do not rupture, although rupture can occur in an adjacent area where a new infarction occurs. The effects of ventricular aneurysms are functional since they place the entire heart at a mechanical disadvantage by splinting adjacent normal myocardium, predisposing to malalignment of papillary muscles with consequent mitral regurgitation and wasting the contractile energy expended by normal myocardium in passive outward (systolic) bulging of the aneurysm. The diagnosis should be considered when a postinfarction patient develops severe heart failure, recurrent angina, recurrent ventricular arrhythmias, or embolic events. Traditionally, these four clinical presentations were the indications for aneurysmectomy. For whatever reason, fewer chronic aneurysms are being seen now. This

may be because of better acute management that limits the extent of infarction, better late therapy of angina and failure, or because surgical thinking based on past experience has changed. At present, when angina is the presenting symptom (most frequent), the tendency is to be conservative about resecting the scar and to focus on the revascularization. It is only when there is intractable failure, often with mitral regurgitation or recurrent medically refractory arrhythmias, that surgical therapy of the aneurysm is pursued. The operation includes resection of the aneurysm combined with coronary artery bypass, since more than 50% have multivessel disease, and mitral valve repair or replacement if the papillary muscles are involved. When sudden death or refractory, recurrent arrhythmias have brought the aneurysm to attention, the surgical results are infinitely better when resection and ablation are directed by preoperative electrophysiologic studies and intraoperative mapping. The use of an automatic, implantable cardioverter defibrillator (AICD) may also be necessary.

Surgical resection and thrombectomy for recurrent peripheral emboli is almost never indicated, since the clinical significance of this occurrence is 2% or less. Although anticoagulant therapy may be recommended, there are no controlled studies documenting the efficacy of any form of therapy directed at the prevention of thromboembolism. Overall, the result of aneurysmectomy in its various expressions is extremely good, with operative mortality for all subsets at less than 5% and with excellent long-term control of symptoms and survival (31).

The "Reality"—Is This the Future?!

Having carefully defined the various manifestations of coronary atherosclerosis and the indications for considering surgical therapy in the context of each of these manifestations, it seems appropriate to place these indications in juxtaposition to what "noncardiac specialists" have considered the indications to be. Table 2.2 is an exact reproduction of the indications for coronary artery bypass as drawn up for use by Utilization Review committees. No further exposition of these is necessary.

VALVULAR HEART DISEASE

The Generic Indications

Discussion of the indications for valvular heart surgery is less complex than for coronary atherosclerosis, since there is a more finite spectrum of manifestations of valvular heart disease and these can be more precisely defined. Patients with valvular heart disease can be staged according to standard New York Heart Association (NYHA) criteria from class I to class IV and are operated for symptoms caused by congestive heart failure, low cardiac output, thromboembolic episodes, or for the consequences of infective endocarditis. In each instance, the ideal time to recommend surgery is when NYHA class III is reached and symptoms are not due to correctable extracardiac factors or promptly relieved by an adjustment of medical therapy.

The risk of mortality and morbidity must be considered in the decision-making process. These data are known and can be considered, for each institution, to be constant for these purposes. In patients with more advanced pathology (class IV), consideration may include projections of longevity and the decision can be made on the basis of relative projected longevity rather than on the basis of relative quality of life.

Occasionally, the primary manifestation will be angina pectoris, as with aortic stenosis; but this usually occurs in relation to coexisting coronary atherosclerosis. When valve disease is found coexisting with coronary disease, the decision about what should or should not be done to the valve is often more difficult to make, since the indications for correcting the valve may not be so clear as the indications for bypass. Color flow doppler done intraoperatively may be extremely valuable in the decision-making process in this situation.

Finally, prophylactic indications may exist as in aortic or mitral regurgitation associated with Marfan's disease (cystic medial necrosis of the aorta) prior to occurrence of an acute dissection, or as in the progressive left ventricular dilation that occurs with mitral or aortic regurgitation. In these instances, while surgery is undertaken to avoid acute, catastrophic complications or to preserve ventricular function, the decision must be made in the context of the operative risks and the relative functional and symptomatic outcome.

Repair or Replacement of the Valve?

Valvular heart surgery began with mitral valvuloplasty, a reparative procedure. As prostheses were developed, the pendulum moved toward a lower threshold for replacement than for repair. However, prostheses are associated with problems that include thromboembolism, parabasilar insufficiency, hemolysis, infection, and wear; and the desire to minimize these has led to a reemphasis on reparative procedures. With repair as a viable choice, the indications for surgical therapy can be liberalized and be recommended in a less compelling clinical status. Thus, repair moderates the need for patients undergoing valve replacement to exchange one set of problems for another.

The ability to carry out a reparative procedure varies according to the valve that is involved and the nature of the pathology. In congenital aortic stenosis, very adequate repairs are possible and, when possible, should be pursued before advanced left ventricular hypertrophy and syncope become clinical realities. These clinical manifestations are usually seen in patients with calculated valve areas of 0.5 cm^2 or less or with peak-to-peak left ventricular-aortic pressure gradients of greater than 55 mm Hg. A gradient of 40 mm Hg or more associated with electrocardiographic strain pattern is also an indication for surgery.

In adults, aortic stenosis has, in the past, been correctable only by excision and valve replacement; but current developments suggest that débridement by ultrasonic techniques may become a reality. This would be a particularly attractive alternative in patients undergoing coronary bypass who have lesser degrees of aortic stenosis.

Aortic insufficiency is not easily or appropriately correctable by reparative procedures, except in rare cases of aortic dissection in which the valve commissures can be resuspended from a graft used to replace a section of the ascending aorta.

The most significant advances have been made in relation to mitral valve repair. We have already discussed mitral annuloplasty in ischemic heart disease. More extensive repairs in rheumatic disease and some degenerative lesions have been pioneered by Carpentier (32). The availability of these procedures has extended the indications for surgical therapy to class II patients with mitral regurgitation. Reconstruction should be attempted in patients who have posterior leaflet prolapse with annular dilation. Localized anterior leaflet redundancy may be amenable to wedge resection. Similarly, elongated chordae may be shortened, and in come cases repair of torn chordae is feasible.

Congentital pulmonary stenosis is correctable by commissurotomy and should be considered when right ventricular hypertrophy, especially if symptomatic, becomes progressive. Pulmonary insufficiency is not a lesion that can be readily repaired.

Tricuspid insufficiency and stenosis are both amenable to repair, except in the most advanced pathologic situations. Therefore, functional tricuspid regurgitation with right ventricular failure due to left heart failure and less often direct rheumatic involvement should be surgically corrected. While medical therapy directed at the contributing lift-sided abnormality may be effective, this response is not predictable, especially in severe tricuspid malfunction. This fact underscores the need for an aggressive approach to tricuspid valve repair.

Valve Replacement for Specific Lesions

Aortic Valve Disease. Once the onset of any of the classic triad symptoms of heart failure, angina, or syncope occurs, surgical consideration is indicated. This is particularly true in patients with pulmonary hypertension in the presence of atrial fibrillation or flutter, which may precipitate pulmonary edema. In symptomatic patients, if the valve area is 0.75 cm^2 or less, if the peak-to-peak left ventricular-aortic pressure difference is 75 mm Hg or more with a normal cardiac output, or if the mean pressure gradient is 50 to 55 mm Hg or more, valve replacement is indicated. In asymptomatic patients who have these hemodynamic findings, valve replacement also should be pursued if there is left ventricular enlargement or hypertrophy. Average operative mortality for isolated aortic

valve replacement should be under 5%; it is higher in patients who are in funcitonal NYHA class IV or are over 75 years of age. Concomitant need for coronary bypass or another valve procedure also increases the risk of surgery.

Patients with symptomatic aortic insufficiency should undergo aortic valve replacement. A marked reduction of physical working capacity defines a subset of patients with increased operative risk and reduced long-term survival (33). In asymptomatic patients who have objective evidence of left ventricular dysfunction, surgery should be undertaken. If left ventricular funciton is normal or mildly impaired, close follow-up with electrocardiography is indicated, since left ventricular functional deterioration and the onset of significant symptoms can occur precipitously. Operation should be considered to prevent irreversible myocardial damage in minimally symptomatic or asymptomatic patients when left ventricular dysfunction and enlargement become a concern (34). The existence of combined aortic stenosis and regurgitation is difficult to evaluate in regard to either of the functional lesions alone. The combination of both preload and afterload lesions compounds the overall effect so that surgery is indicated at an earlier time than may have been appropriate with either lesion alone. While the same symptomatic guidelines pertain as for pure lesion, the hemodynamic ones are less applicable.

Mitral Valve Disease. As we have noted, lesser degrees of pure mitral stenosis without calcification, can be treated with valvuloplasty. Once symptoms are established at class III levels such surgery is indicated. However, with subvalvular stenosis, calcification, any mix of mitral regurgitation, and pulmonary hypertension, mitral valve replacement is indicated. The occurrence of systemic embolization is felt by some to constitute class III status in and of itself. With valve areas of 1.0 cm^2 and less, surgery is indicated regardless of symptomatic status.

The reason that these conditions represent an indication for surgery is that 5-year survival of patients with mitral stenosis and class III status is 62%, and with class IV status it is 15%. The usual causes of death are pulmonary edema, pulmonary hypertension with right heart failure, pulmonary emboli, infective endocarditis, and systemic embolization. Twenty percent of patients will develop peripheral emboli and in one-quarter this is recurrent (35, 36). With appropriate valve replacement, control of the atrial appendage, antimicrobial prophylaxis, and anticoagulation, all of these manifestations can be controlled.

Mitral regurgitation is similar to aortic regurgitation in that the lesion can be well tolerated for many years. Unfortunately, when significant symptoms occur (classes III and IV) left ventricular dysfunction may be advanced and even irreversibly compromised. When repair cannot be carried out, replacement is an excellent alternate surgical therapy. In patients with class II symptoms, increasing ventricular volumes (diastolic minor axis 5 cm or greater) and regurgitant fractions of 40% or more, surgery is indicated. Morgan and coworkers (37) additionally suggest that class II status with 4+ regurgitation and left ventricular ejection fraction of less than 60% constitutes an indication for surgery. As with aortic regurgitation, acute mitral regurgitation is an urgent indication for valve surgery.

Mixed mitral stenosis and insufficiency with class III symptoms dictates mitral valve replacement.

Tricuspid Valve Disease.   The need for tricuspid valve replacement is rare since reparative procedures are so effective. It has been thought that the tricuspid valve was not necessary for survival since total excision has been performed in some patients with endocarditis (38). However, it is now clear that complete removal will eventuate in congestive heart failure (39). Aside from endocarditis, the situations in which tricuspid valve replacement is necessary all represent severe, advanced pathologic conditions; they include trauma, including pacemaker electrode entrapment, corrected transposition, myxoma, carcinoid, and Ebstein's anomaly. The mortality of tricuspid valve replacement is high when associated with aortic or mitral valve disease (40, 41).

Concurrent Valve Replacement and Coronary Atherosclerosis

In patients undergoing consideration for cardiac valve replacement therapy, cardiac cath-

eterization and angiography are prerequisites of the evaluation. In patients with significant coronary risk factors, and in patients over the age of 35 to 44 years, coronary angiography should be performed whenever possible.

When coronary disease is present, it is clearly indicated that concomitant coronary artery bypass be carried out (42, 43). Such therapy increases longevity, as compared to patients having valve replacement and coronary disease that is not bypassed. In patients with aortic valve disease the incidence of postoperative sudden death is significantly diminished. It is clear, therefore, that appropriate therapy necessitates attention to all elements of the pathologic substrate that is defined at catheterization and angiography.

The Special Circumstance of Valvular Infection

Complications of endocarditis such as congestive heart failure resulting from valvular regurgitation in left-sided endocarditis have a poor prognosis on medical therapy alone, especially when the situation is progressive or unresponsive to medical therapy. Mortality has been reported to range from 50 to 80% (44, 45). In this setting an aggressive posture is warranted, involving early valve replacement (46). Valve repair is not considered an option in the presence of infection. In active endocarditis, the mortality may be reduced to 10 to 15%; and when the infection is controlled, mortality approximates that of elective valve replacement. In either instance, parabasilar leaks are more often seen after surgery than in the absence of preoperative infection.

Other major criteria (47) that are indicators for valve replacement include persistent bacteremia despite antibiotic therapy, recurrence of infection despite adequate antibiotic therapy, and a fungal eitology. Recurrent systemic emboli, especially in the presence of documented vegetations, and extravalvular or extravascular infections (valve ring, hepatic, renal, cerebral, or splenic abscesses) also constitute indications for surgery.

Prosthetic valve infection with dehiscence is a particularly ominous occurrence that usually requires reoperation. While the incidence of such endocarditis has been reported to be as high as 4% per patient year (48), the usual reported incidence is 0.5 to 1.5% per patient year. This incidence may be slightly higher in patients with double valve replacement. When reoperation is necessary for early postoperative prosthetic endocarditis, the mortality rate may be as high as 70%. For late endocarditis the operative mortality is considerably less (49). Parabasilar leaks often are the precursor to postoperative endocarditis, whether it occurs early or late. Late onset of a regurgitant murmur may be the first manifestation of prosthetic endocarditis.

Lesser criteria can be defined that become an indication for valve replacement when they occur in multiple combinations of two and three (47). These include compensated congestive heart failure on therapy, persistent fever without other identifiable cause, single embolic events, the presence of any valve vegetation or flail valve leaflets by echocardiography, and a new regurgitant murmur in a prosthesis late after it has been replaced.

Clearly, any cardiac valve infection is a serious occurrence requiring close, continuing scrutiny, increased anticipation for a disaster, and total flexibility about the course of therapy being pursued. With these principles of therapy (and a little luck), a good outcome can be achieved; but the best therapy is to try to avoid the infection in the first place.

Choice of Valve Substitute

The indicators for valve replacement surgery have been carefully defined. Throughout this discussion we have avoided any comment about the type of valve substitute that should be used. While the choice of a specific valve type may be relevant to making a decision about whether valve replacement is indicated, the *need* for surgery should be separated as much as possible for the *choice* of a valve substitute.

There are specific indications for the use of biologic tissue valves as opposed to wholly fabricated prosthetic valves. It is the characteristic of the generic type of valve that needs to be considered. Biologic valves are more biocompatible, having a lesser incidence of thromboembolism and hemolysis associated with their use. They do not ordinarily require anticoagu-

lant therapy. The most widely used biologic valves are porcine xenografts; homografts are not used as extensively. Prosthetic valves are easier to use, are more durable, and give better hydraulic performance for a given annulus size. However, anticoagulants are necessary for life; and should the need arise to discontinue them, the patient with a prosthesis is at greater risk. The most widely used mechanical valve is the St. Jude valve. The Carpentier-Edwards and Hancock are the porcine valves in current use in the United States.

In the final analysis, a decision for one or the other valve should be based on the patient's specific needs and how these are best met by the well-defined characteristics of the various valve substitutes. Where there may be problems with anticoagulation, especially in the elderly, biologic valves are favored. When longevity and functional capacity are major concerns, a mechanical valve is indicated.

REOPERATIONS

The point has been made that most cardiac surgical therapy, especially for acquired disease, is palliative in nature. In coronary disease, bypass does not "cure" the basic disease process; if the operation is effective it will allow the patient to live long enough to experience a recurrence of some manifestation of the same disease. In valvular disease, longevity of the prosthesis is a concern; and especially in valve replacement, the patient exchanges one set of problems for another, albeit less imminent, set of problems. Thus, one must always anticipate the need for reoperation. This is the cornerstone of the follow-up of patients after coronary and valvular surgery.

The indications for a second operation are really not different than those for a first operation; the same considerations are relevant. If there is a difference in the indications between a first and second operation, there may be greater urgency to proceed once the indication is defined. Furthermore, the operative risks of a second operation are greater, even when one considers the fact that techniques are most often improved by the time another operation is needed. However, once the early postoperative period is over, the outcome for survivors may be as good as after the first operation. While most operations can be considered to be primarily palliative, it is clear that they do offer the opportunity for increased longevity for the individual patient.

Considering the number and ages of patients who have been operated by the senior generation of cardiac surgeons, it should be clear that one of the primary indications for cardiac surgery during the lives of the second and third generations of cardiac surgeons will be the need for a reoperation.

SUMMARY

The capabilities of cardiac surgery have grown and been refined by years of operative experience, research, and follow-up such that there is now almost no cardiac disease for which there is not some form of palliative, if not curative, procedure. This even extends to the potential for replacing an irreparably damaged heart with a transplant.

In this environment of expanded capability we must avoid abusing this capability and continue to evaluate each individual case on the basis of its merits. While we have defined the general guidelines that determine how we proceed, we must never lose sight of the fact that the individual has a disease, rather than the disease being an individual. In our therapeutic decision-making for patients, we must continue to be guided by the dictum enunciated by Professor Francis Weld Peabody of Boston: " . . . the secret of the care of the patient is in caring for the patient" (49).

References

1. Cohn PF: Prognosis and treatment of asymptomatic coronary artery disease. *J Am Coll Cardiol* 1:959–964, 1983.
2. Kent KM, Rosing DR, Ewels CJ, et al: Progress of asymptomatic or mildly symptomatic patients with coronary artery disease. *Am J Cardiol* 49:1823–1831, 1982.
3. Kannel WB, Feinleib M: Natural history of angina pectoris in the Framingham Study: prognosis and survival. *Am J Cardiol* 29:154–163, 1972.
4. Ringqvist I, Fisher LD, Mock M, et al: Prognostic value of angiographic indices of coronary artery disease from the coronary artery surgery study (CASS). *J Clin Invest* 71:1854–1866, 1983.
5. Sherman CT, Litvack F, Grundfest W, et al: Coronary angioscopy in patients with unstable angina pectoris. *N Engl J Med* 315:913–919, 1986.
6. Matloff JM, Sustaita H, Chatterjee K, et al: The rationale for surgery in preinfarction angina. *J Thorac Cardiovasc Surg* 69:73–81, 1975.
7. Conti CR: Unstable angina: long-term followup of surgical and medical treatment. In Rafflenbeul W, Lichtlen PR, Balcon R (eds): *Unstable Angina Pectoris*. New York, Thieme-Stratton, 1981, p 180.
8. Bertolasi CA, Tronge JE, Min GA, et al: Clinical spectrum of "unstable angina." *Clin Cardiol* 2:113, 1979.
9. Rankin JS, Newton JR, Califf RM, et al: Clinical characteristics and current management of medically refractory unstable angina. *Ann Surg* 200:457–465, 1984.
10. DeFeyter PJ, Serruys PW, van denBrand M, et al: Emergency coronary angioplasty in refractory unstable angina. *N Engl J Med* 313:342–346, 1985.
11. DeWood MA, Spores J, Berg RJ, et al: Acute myocardial infarction: decade of experience with surgical reperfusion in 701 patients. *Circulation* 68(II):8–16, 1983.
12. Phillips SJ, Kongtahworn C, Skinner JR, et al: Emergency coronary artery reperfusion: a choice therapy for evolving myocardial infarction. Results in 339 patients. *J Thorac Cardiovasc Surg* 86:679–688, 1983.
13. Kirklin JK, Blackstone EH, Zorn GL, et al: Intermediate-term results of coronary artery bypass grafting for acute myocardial infarction. *Circulation* 72(II):175–178, 1985.
14. DeWood MA, Heit J, Spores J, et al: Anterior transmural myocardial infarction: effects of surgical coronary reperfusion on global and regional left ventricular function. *J Am Coll Cardiol* 1(5):1223–1234, 1983.
15. Venhaecke J, Flameng W, Sergeant P, et al: Emergency bypass surgery: late effects on size of infarction and ventricular function. *Circulation* 72(II):179–184, 1985.
16. Murphy DA, Craver JM, Jones EL, et al: Surgical management of acute myocardial ischemia following percutaneous transluminal coronary angioplasty. *J Thorac Cardiovasc Surg* 87:332–339, 1984.

17. Allen BS, Okamoto F, Buckberg GD, et al: Immediate functional recovery after six hours of regional ischemia by careful control of conditions of reperfusion and composition of reperfusate. *J Thorac Cardiovasc Surg* 92:621–635, 1986.

18. Jones EL, Douglas JS, Craver, JM, et al: Results of coronary revascularization in patients with recent myocardial infarction. *J Thorac Cardiovasc Surg* 76:545–551, 1978.

19. Matloff JM, Chaux A, Sustaita H: Unstable angina. Experience with surgical therapy in the subset of patients having preinfarction angina. *Cleve Clin Q* 45(1):184–188, 1978.

20. Fox AC, Glassman E, Isom OW: Surgically remediable complications of myocardial infarction. *Prog Cardiovasc Dis* 21:461–484, 1979.

21. Sanders RJ, Kern WH, Blount SG: Perforation of the interventricular septum complicating myocardial infarction. *Am Heart J* 51:736–748, 1956.

22. Miyamoto A, Lee M, Kass R, et al: Postmyocardial infarction ventricular septal defect. Improved outlook. *J Thorac Cardiovasc Surg* 86:41–46, 1983.

23. Rasmussen S, Leth A, Kjoller E, et al: Cardiac rupture in acute myocardial infarction: a review of 72 consecutive cases. *Acta Med Scand* 205:11–16, 1979.

24. Cobbs BW, Hatcher CR, Robinson PH: Cardiac rupture. Three operations with two long-term survivors. *JAMA* 223:532–535, 1973.

25. Czer LSC, Maurer G, Bolger AF, et al: Intraoperative evaluation of mitral regurgitation by Doppler color flow mapping. *Circulation* 76(III):108–116, 1987.

26. Czer LSC, Maurer G, Bolger A, et al: Ischemic mitral regurgitation: comparative evaluation of revascularization vs. repair by Doppler color flow mapping. *Circulation* 76(IV):389, 1987.

27. Czer LSC, Matloff JM, Gray RJ, et al: Mitral valve replacement with coronary artery disease. In Duran C, Angel WW, Johnson AD, Oury JH (eds): *Recent Progress in Mitral Valve Disease*. Sevenoaks, England, Butterworth, 1984, pp 304–319.

28. Schuster EH, Bulkley BH: Expansion of transmural myocardial infarction: a pathophysiologic factor in cardiac rupture. *Circulation* 60:1532–1538, 1979.

29. Hochman JS, Bulkley BH: Pathogenesis of left ventricular aneurysms: an experimental study in the rat model. *Am J Cardiol* 60:83–88, 1982.

30. Meizlish JL, Berger HJ, Plankey M, et al: Functional left ventricular aneurysm formation after acute anterior transmural myocardial infarction: incidence, natural history and prognostic implications. *N Engl J Med* 311:1001–1006, 1984.

31. Kaushik VS, Matloff JM, Sustaita H, et al: Determinants of improvement after aneurysmectomy with aortocoronary bypass surgery in patients of ischemic heart disease. *Circulation* 51 & 52(II):201, 1975.

32. Perier P, Chauvaud S, Fabiani S, et al: Reconstructive surgery of mitral valve incompetence: ten-year appraisal. *J Thorac Cardiovasc Surg* 79:338–348, 1980.

33. Bonow RO, Borer JS, Rosing DR, et al: Preoperative exercise capacity in symptomatic patients with aortic regurgitation as a predictor of postoperative left ventricular function and long-term prognosis. *Circulation* 62:1280–1290, 1980.

34. Ross J Jr: Afterload mismatch in aortic and mitral valve disease: implications for surgical therapy. *J Am Coll Cardiol* 5:811–826, 1985.

35. Oleson KH: Natural history of 271 patients with mitral stenosis under medical treatment. *Br Heart J* 24:349–357, 1962.

36. Edmunds LH Jr, Addonizio VP Jr, Tepe NA: Valvular heart disease: prosthetic replacement. In Parmley WW, Chatterjee MB (eds). *Cardiology*. Philadelphia, JB Lippincott, 1987, vol 2, p 33-2.

37. Morgan RJ, Davis JT, Fraker TD: Current status of valve prostheses. *Surg Clin North Am* 65:699–720, 1985.

38. Arbulu A, Thomas NW, Wilson RF: Valvulectomy without prosthetic replacement: a life saving operation for tricuspid pseudomonas endocarditis. *J Thorac Cardiovasc Surg* 64:103–107, 1972.

39. Robin E, Belamaric C, Thoms NW, et al: Consequences of total tricuspid valvulectomy without prosthetic replacement in treatment of Pseudomonas endocarditis. *J Thorac Cardiovasc Surg* 68:461–465, 1974.

40. Kochoukos NT, Stephenson LW: Indications for and results of tricuspid valve replacement. *Adv Cardio* 17:199, 1976.

41. Gersh BJ, Schaff HV, Vatterott PJ, et al: Results of triple valve replacement in 91 patients: perioperative morality and long-term follow-up. *Circulation* 72:130–137, 1985.

42. Czer LSC, Gray RJ, Bateman TM, et al: Mitral valve replacement: impact of coronary artery disease and determinants of prognosis after revascularization. *Circulation* 70(I):198–207, 1984.

43. Czer LSC, Gray RJ, Stewart ME, et al: Reduc-

tion in sudden late death by concomitant re-vascularization with aortic valve replacement. *J Thorac Cardiovasc Surg* 95:390–401, 1988.

44. Richardson JV, Karp RB, Kirklin JW, et al: Treatment of infective endocarditis: a 10 year comparative analysis. *Circulation* 58:589–597, 1978.

45. Parrott JC, Hill JD, Kerth WJ, et al: The surgical management of bacterial endocarditis: a review. *Ann Surg* 183:289–292, 1976.

46. Jung JY, Saab SB, Almond CH: The case for early surgical treatment of left sided primary infective endocarditis. *J Thorac Cardiovasc Surg* 70:509–518, 1975.

47. DiNubile MJ: Surgery in active endocarditis. *Ann Intern Med* 96:950–959, 1982.

48. Brais MP, Bedard JP, Goldstein W, et al: Ionescu-Shiley pericardial xenografts. Follow-up of up to six years. *Ann Thorac Surg* 39:105–111, 1985.

49. Peabody F: The care of the patient. *JAMA* 88(12):877, 1927.

Chapter 3
CARDIAC SURGERY IN THE ELDERLY

TSUNG-PO TSAI, M.D.
JACK M. MATLOFF, M.D.

Older persons constituted 11% of the U.S. population in 1981, and with yearly increases it is anticipated that they will constitute 21% of the population by 2040. Cardiovascular disease accounts for 40% of deaths in individuals over 75 years old (1). Seventy-two percent of cardiovascular deaths in the United States occur in patients over 65 years of age (2). This concurrence of facts has resulted in a growing cohort of patients over age 65 that are being considered for cardiac surgical therapy.

In the United States the average life expectancy for females aged 70 is an additional 14.8 years, while that for males is 11.1 (3), and the average life expectancy for females aged 80 is an additional 7 years, while that for males is 6.2 years (4).

Age has been stated as an incremental risk factor or a contraindication for any form of surgical therapy (5, 6) because the aging process is felt to be associated with advanced pathologic status and decreased physiologic reserve. Such patients usually are considered to be fragile and beset with multiple system problems that contribute to their presumed increased surgical risk. Yet the risks of surgical therapy generally have decreased progressively because of improved techniques of medical, anesthetic, and surgical management. In cardiac surgical patients, improved monitoring during anesthesia (7, 8) and proved myocardial preservation (9) have been the most significant advances. Notwithstanding, there continues to be a delay in referral of aged cardiac patients for catherterization and angiographic evaluation until they have progressed to an advanced clinical status.

Since the goal of geriatric medicine is to retain the aged in their own community comfortably and as independent and productive citizens, quality of life, in contrast to younger patients, is often a more important consideration than absolute longevity. Therefore, one must take into consideration many factors in determining the physiologic status of an elderly person, such as the activity of the patient before operation, the presence of associated diseases, his or her nutritional status, the patient's mental orientation to the environment and, importantly, his or her level of motivation, including the desire to return to an active, independent life. In this light an additional contraindication to surgery might become limited life expectancy due to senility or the lack of will to live.

PREOPERATIVE EVALUATION

Since anesthetic and surgical risks increase with age, these must be weighed against the relative benefits to the patient (risk:benefit ratio). Preoperative evaluation and preparation and perioperative management play a major role in reducing risk to a minimum, especially in the elderly. The most frequently overlooked aspect of preoperative evaluation in the elderly is the existence of significant noncardiac conditions which are often overshadowed by the urgency of the cardiac disease. The preoperative evaluation must include a thorough history, with particular emphasis on current and recent past medical problems and medications being taken. Of particular importance is information that gauges tolerance to exertion or stress, such as the simple ability to walk up stairs or around the block.

Central Nervous System

One of the most common and devastating postoperative complications in the elderly is cerebral vascular insufficiency, which may vary from limited mental confusion to a hemispheric infarction. Patients who demonstrate evidence of central nervous system disease have increased needs for maintenance of physiologic perfusion pressures during cardiopulmonary bypass and require particular attention to ventilatory and circulatory support in the early postoperative period. A very careful history may indicate that the patient has had symptoms to suggest a transient ischemic attack. Certainly, a remote stroke, with or without residual, has to be carefully evaluated in arriving at a decision about cardiac surgery. It is essential to listen for carotid bruits; should one be present, a cerebral vascular workup that includes duplex scanning or digital subtraction carotid angiography is in order to determine its significance.

Cardiovascular System and Hemodynamic Status

The patient's peroperative hemodynamic status frequently becomes the major consideration in the postoperative management of fluid balance, pulmonary function, the use of vasoactive agents, and the need for circulatory support. The history and timing of a prior myocardial infarction have a significant role in predicting operative risk and hence are important in the decision-making of whether and when to operate, as well as the strategy of operation. While proximity of cardiac surgery to an acute infarction is always a significant risk factor, it is especially a problem for the elderly, and everything should be done to bring elderly patients to a stable state, if possible, before surgery. Evidence of acute ischemia or rhythm and conduction problems must be carefully evaluated by electrocardiogram or thallium-201 perfusion scan or positron emission tomographic (PET) scan.

Two-dimensional echocardiogram or technetium wall motion study can generate an estimate of heart size, regional wall motion, and ejection fraction in the patient with congestive heart failure, or when ventriculography has been omitted because of concern about the radiographic dye. Also, two-dimensional color Doppler flow mapping is rapidly proving to be an excellent noninvasive tool to evaluate stenotic or regurgitant valvular lesions as well as intracardiac shunt, which can be an unexpected and difficult problem to evaluate.

The hypertensive elderly patient requires cardiopulmonary bypass at higher perfusion pressures than usual because his or her major organ systems are so conditioned. Therefore, these patients are much more susceptible to major organ ischemia during brief periods of relative hypotension. A period of preoperative treatment or even hospitalization may be required to control the hypertension and to reduce the patient's mean perfusion pressure to levels that can be more easily maintained during cardiopulmonary bypass and in the postoperative period.

Antihypertensive agents such as reserpine and quanethedine which deplete stores of epinephrine and norepinephrine result in an increased operative risk and in the likelihood of hypotension in the postoperative period. The agents could be discontinued before surgery and an adequate period of time permitted for reversal of their effects. β-Blocking agents are associated with a significant decrease in cardiac function. Clinical experiences indicate that effects from long-acting agents may last at least a week or longer in the elderly. The combination of antiarrhythmic agents and β-blockers is a particularly common preoperative pharmacologic hazard in seriously ill patients and can result in hypotension during cardiopulmonary bypass. The same problem can occur when monamine oxidase inhibitors have been used. Calcium channel blockers should probably be continued up to the time of surgery, because their sudden withdrawal at surgery may adversely affect coronary vascular resistance, resulting in ischemia.

In the postoperative period, elderly hypertensive patients often manifest unpredictable fluctuations in blood pressure, thereby exposing them to a multitude of problems ranging from increased postoperative bleeding to renal dysfunction and cerebral vascular insufficiency.

Pulmonary System

Pulmonary compromise is the most frequent noncardiac complication seen after cardiopulmonary bypass, regardless of previous congestive heart failure or associated valvular disease. Therefore, preoperative pulmonary function is an important consideration because of limitations in pulmonary reserve and the difficulty the elderly have in mobilizing secretions postoperatively.

Again, the history is all-important, and in addition to chest x-ray, pulmonary function tests may be indicated both as a document of the current status of the patient and as a guideline to postoperative ventilatory therapy. Since chronic obstructive lung disease and emphysema are often problems in the aged, one must be sure of adequate function. If pulmonary function is depressed enough to produce hypoxia while breathing room air, operation should be delayed, if possible, until treatment with bronchodilation and respiratory training can improve function to a safer level. Along with hypoxia, wheezing, hypercarbia, or serious depression of pulmonary mechanics all herald significant lung problems. The potential for a problem can be reduced by preoperative chest physiotherapy, especially in heavy-smoking patients. If there is a history of recurrent pulmonary infections or a productive cough, appropriate cultures and antibiotic therapy may even be indicated preoperatively.

During surgery, in addition to avoiding overdistension of the left ventricle and pulmonary venous hypertension, particular attention should be directed to limiting the volume of crystalloid infused. Elderly patients are particularly suscep-

tible to fluid retention, and pulmonary congestion can be the most severe manifestation of excess fluid use. Since prolonged ventilatory support may be necessary, and because nutritional status and wound healing may be compromised, particular attention should be directed to sternal closure, using continuous, braided, vertical wires on either side of the sternum to buttress the usual wire stay sutures.

Use of nasogastric drainage is also an important consideration in regard to pulmonary status. Aspiration of gastric contents can be a very insidious occurrence in aged patients, and the consequences can be devastating. At the least, a nasogastric tube should be in place as long as the patient is on a ventilator or is in a state of altered consciousness. However, the presence of a nasogastric tube in the posterior pharynx, especially when the patient is awake and extubated, can be very annoying and actually contribute to retained pulmonary secretions by interfering with the cough mechanism. Therefore, consideration should be given to the intermittent use of nasogastric suction, as specifically indicated, after intubation.

If the patient's cardiac status is so unstable as not to permit such preparation, the indications for surgery should be reconsidered.

Gastrointestinal Tract and Hemorrhagic Diathesis

Postoperative stress ulceration and gastrointestinal hemorrhage occur in a significant number of patients. Any preoperative history of gastric or duodenal ulcer must be considered as a potential threat and vigorously treated prophylactically in the preoperative and postoperative periods. Control of the gastric pH with antacids may decrease the incidence of postoperative gastrointestinal hemorrhage and is indicated in virtually all cardiovascular surgical patients. Cimetidine (Tagamet) or ranitidine (Zantac) may also be indicated because of their histamine 2 blocking effect and should be given prophylactically in any patients with previous history of peptic ulcer disease. The acid neutralizing effect of feeding is also important, as well as for its nutritional value. Unfortunately, the elderly seem especially prone to anorexia and even nausea, so that one has to be aware of the potential for gastric distension, ileus, and even vomiting. Judicious use of a nasogastric tube is therefore a very important consideration.

Congestive failure may produce derangements in liver function and increase the potential for bleeding at surgery as well as the postoperative susceptibility to anticoagulants. Elderly patients undergoing extracorporal circulation need special attention paid to their coagulation profiles. Platelet count, template bleeding time, prothrombin time, and partial thromboplastin time should be screened routinely for clotting problems. However, if the patient has a *history* of bleeding from minor trauma or from a previous operation, additional studies should be performed, including specific coagulation factor assay and platelet aggregometry. Patients who are taking aspirin regularly should optimally discontinue the drug 2 weeks before operation. Other antiplatelet agents such as dipyridamole and nonsteriodal anti-inflammatory agents should be discontinued at least 72 hr before surgery. If this is not practical, fresh platelets may be necessary at the time of operation, but their use in large quantities may contribute to pulmonary problems. In patients taking warfarin, active reversal with vitamin K_1 may result in "rebound" thrombosis; consequently, natural reversal is favored. However, the urgency for surgery will dictate the decision. Reversal of warfarin effects may require up to 2 weeks if factors X and II are to be completely restored to normal levels (10). The process of reversal can be accelerated by the judicial use of fresh frozen plasma. In more urgent situations vitamin K can be used; and if there is real concern about thrombotic complications, this changeover can be effected with the protective effect of heparin. In short, every step should be taken to normalize clotting mechanisms since bleeding is such a devastating postoperative complication for the elderly.

Nutritional status is often compromised in the elderly, especially in those with long-standing cardiac problems. The importance of nutritional status is highlighted by a recent report that postoperative morbidity and mortality in the elderly are correlated with serum albumin levels on admission (11). As indicated, use of the alimentary tract may be limited for some time after surgery because of ileus and gastric distension. Furthermore, even when tube feedings are started, severe diarrhea can result. Therefore, intravenous hyperalimantation is often a consideration. When indicated, intravenous nutrition should be undertaken but with meticulous attention to details to avoid the potential risks of volume overload and infections.

Renal System

Renal function decreases with aging, as indicated by a progressive decline in the glomerular filtration rate (12). Adequate hydration is of particular importance in preventing perioperative renal dysfunction. Many elderly patients chronically take diuretics for one reason or another, whether to control blood pressure or to treat presumed heart failure; hence, sodium, potassium, and chloride levels may be abnormal. Furthermore, when surgery is undertaken in proximity to cardiac catheterization and angiography, radiographic dye can have a significant deleterious effect on renal function.

Adequate renal function is absolutely necessary for the successful management of cardiopulmonary bypass. The preoperative BUN, creatinine, and creatinine clearance should be obtained on all patients undergoing open-heart surgery. In patients with creatinine clearances of less than 50% of normal for age, the surgeon should be prepared for the likelihood of a period of dialysis or ultrafiltration in the postoperative period. During cardiopulmonary bypass, particular attention should be directed to urine output and appropriate management of perfusion pressures, serum osmolatity, and diuresis. Relatively small amounts of mannitol and lasix can be used to maintain excellent urine output while on cardiopulmonary bypass. The ease of pursuing preventive measures before and during surgery far outweighs the problems of having to resort to dialysis after surgery.

Diabetes Mellitus

In addition to those with established diagnoses, many elderly patients have undiagnosed latent or chemical diabetes. Derangements of carbohydrate metabolism are common during periods of stress, and glucose metabolism is further disturbed during nonpulsatile cardiopulmonary bypass (13). For these reasons, it is necessary to be aware of the patient's status with regard to glucose metbolism. Aside from the nutritional and fluid volume problems that can arise in diabetics, poor resistance to infection is characteristic of the diabetic patient. Aged patients commonly have severe peripheral vascular disease in addition to diabetes mellitus; these coexisting problems can have adverse consequences for wound healing. Finally, the altered pain perception often seen in diabetes can complicate assessment of postoperative convalescence and wound healing.

Screening for Cancer

Undetected neoplastic lesions are not unusual in the elderly. Any aged patient with unexplained fatigue, weight loss, anemia, hemoptysis, or rectal bleeding, as well as painless lymphadenopathy should be worked up for a possible cancer. Those with treated lymphoma or leukemia that are in remission are still candidates for cardiac surgery, but the risk: benefit ratio and anticipated quality of life should be weighed carefully in patients with neoplasms before cardiac surgery.

Summary

There is little specific concern in the evaluation and care of the aged cardiac surgical patient compared to younger patients undergoing cardiac surgery. However, it is necessary to stress attention to detail and the least change in status. This is best illustrated by infection in the elderly, in whom temperature and white blood count elevations may not occur to herald a significant problem. Their margin of tolerance and functional reserve are very limited, often taxing one's clinical judgment. Conversely, an overbearing approach with an elderly cardiac patient who is otherwise relatively heathly can be very destructive to his or her care.

CLINICAL OUTCOMES AFTER SURGERY IN THE ELDERLY

At present, 50% of the cardiac surgical patients at the authors' institution are aged 65 or over. The average age for coronary bypass is 65 years and is steadily increasing.

Coronary Artery Bypass Surgery

Advancing age is a factor in the outcome of coronary artery bypass surgery; but as experience is being accumulated, its significance is lessening. As in other situations, this has occurred as a result of learning from the sharing experiences with the elderly.

The status of complicating medical problems, such as diabetes mellitus and chronic renal disease, as well as an estimate of the mental state and attitude of the patient which would make surgery hazardous have been placed in focus. However, it is necessary to emphasize that the elderly more than younger patients place emphasis on postoperative quality of life than that of an operative mortality. Also, more of them are confronted by the need to correct a concomitant heart valve problem at the time of operation.

The technique of performing coronary artery bypass surgery in the elderly is not different from younger patients. However, a few technical points should be noted. In placing the elderly patient on extracorporeal circulation, one must be especially careful about cannulation. For venous return, the fragile right atrial appendage should probably be avoided, and Teflon felt pledgets may be incorporated into the purse-string suture on the side of the atrium to minimize the possibility of tissue disruption. The ascending sorta is the usual site for arterial return, and one must be cognizant of calcific plaques and soft atheromatous disease involving the intima, which frequently are seen in the aged. Dislodgment of atheromatous emboli and aortic dissection can occur with traumatic cannulations. This is equally true of placement of aortic, combined infusion, ventricular catheters and cross-clamping of the aorta. Also, avulsion of the epicardium can easily occur in the elderly patient if undue tension is employed with retraction of the heart. Because of the high incidence of diffuse calcification of the coronary arteries, the surgeon needs to select the least involved coronary area for the site of anastomosis. In performing the anastomosis, special attention is needed to prevent dissection of the atheromatous intima and media from the adventitia. Likewise, in performing the aortic anastomoses, care needs to be taken to avoid dislodging atheromatous debris into the lumen of the aorta. Although a side-gripping vascular clamp can be used to perform these anastomoses after removing the cross clamp, special care has to be taken to avoid damaging the integrity of the aorta at the margins of the clamp's jaws. In a similar way, vein conduits in the elderly frequently demonstrate loss of elasticity and separation of the intima from the media and adventitia; therefore, sutures have to be carefully placed to correct this when it happens.

In a recent 63-month period of time, isolated coronary artery bypass was performed in 629 patients over age 70 and in 64 patients over age 80. The overall early mortality was 6.2%; 6.5% for septuagenarians and 3.1% for octogenarians. Late mortality during an average 38.2 months of follow-up was 5% for all; 4.6% for septuagenarians and 8.1% for octogenarians. The 3-year probability of survival was 89%. This experience is not significantly different than the 2 to 14% mortality that has been reported from other institutions for patients who are 70 years and over (Table 3.1) (14–18). Our experience supports the contention that when an adequate intensive medical trial in the elderly with angina fails, coronary artery bypass provides an attractive alternative, although such patients do have higher complication rates.

Complications following coronary artery bypass surgery in the aged are extremely important (19). A significant percentage of patients operated on in this age groups have major postoperative complications during the early postoperative period. In our series of 693 operative survivals over age 70, 192 patients (28%) developed major postoperative complications, including postoperative bleeding (5%), sternal dehiscence (3%), renal failure (5%), stroke (3%), sepsis (2%), and postoperative myocardial infarction (10%). One hundred seventy-eight patients (26%) developed minor complications, which included postoperative mental aberrations, pericarditis, small subendocardial myocardial infarctions, and minor wound infections.

TABLE 3.1

OPERATIVE MORTALITY IN PATIENTS AGED OVER 70 YEARS UNDERGOING ISOLATED CORONARY ARTERY BYPASS SURGERY

Reference	Dates of Surgery	No. of Patients	Operative Mortality
Knapp et al (18)	1974–1979	121	1.6
Hochberg et al (24)	1971–1979	75	12.0
Berry et al (17)	1975–1979	65	3.1
Grann et al (16)	1969–1975	30	6.7
Tucker et al (32)	1969–1975	67	4.7
McArthur et al (14)	1970–1975	158	13.9
	1976–1981	1117	4.7
Tsai et al (33)	1980–1986	693	6.2

As a result, lengths of stay were significantly increased over those of younger patients.

The most significant aspect of this experience was that these patients often had well-established histories of coronary atherosclerosis; but their therapy could be described as "expectant" until they became so acute that they frequently could not be discharged from the hospital. Severity of angina was, New York Heart Association (NYHA) class III in 60% and class IV in 25%. This factor, as much as the patients ages, contributed to increased morbidity and mortality.

Valve Replacement Surgery

One of the major problems in performing valvular replacement in the elderly is difficulty in weaning from extracorporeal circulation. Even in patients with normal valvular function, aging results in decreased left ventricular compliance and a decreased ability to respond to stress with an increase in cardiac output. This ability is clearly worse in those with valvular dysfunction. It has been demonstrated that afterload reduction is beneficial in discontinuing cardiopulmonary bypass following valvular replacement or repair. If care is taken to protect the heart with hypothermia and cardioplegia during operation, then medical afterload reduction is often sufficient. If not, inotropic agents, vasopressors, or intraaortic balloon pumping may be needed.

In elderly patients, it is our policy to use a porcine xenograft valve when possible. The hazards of anticoagulation therapy are particularly severe in the elderly. Also, since longevity of the elderly is normally less than 15 years, the concern about valve substitute durability may be less than for the risks of permanent warfarin therapy, However, if these patients have severe compromise of left ventricular function, especially with concomitant coronary atherosclerosis, or if they have a small annulus size, especially with aortic or mitral stenosis, a mechanical valve is indicated. The incidence of thromboembolism with a prothrombin time of 1½ times normal is acceptable, and the incidence of hemorrhagic complications is significantly reduced from that experienced with warfarin to achieve twice control levels of activity.

Aortic Valve Replacement

Aortic valve disease is the most frequent valvular problem in patients over the age of 60. The etiology of aortic stenosis in the elderly patient is uncertain, and as such has no implication for the surgical therapy. Simple wear and tear with secondary fibrocalcific degeneration is probably the most common etiologic factor. More important than aging in determining the value of a surgical approach are such factors as the degree of mental alertness, the presence and seriousness of complicating medical problems, and the attitude of the patient and his or her family toward an operation that carries a sizable risk.

Chest pain suggesting atypical angina is a common presenting symptom followed by chronic congestive heart failure.

Aortic valve surgery should be aggressively recommended to older persons with symptomatic aortic valve disease. Operative mortality has been reported from 4 to 20% (20, 21). At the authors' institution, 30 patients over age 70 were operated during a 45-month period with two operative mortalities (7%). There is a higher incidence of associated coronary artery disease in the aged, and mortality will be increased significantly if aortic valve replacement is combined with coronary artery bypass surgery (22). In 58 such patients, there was a 20% mortality in our series. More advanced cardiac status and prolonged cardiopulmonary bypass time explain much of the difference in the mortalities between these two groups (23).

Mitral Valve Repair or Replacement

Evidence of rheumatic fever occurs in about 4% of necropsies of aged persons. In general, mitral insufficiency is the predominant rheumatic lesion in the elderly. Recently, myoxomatous degeneration and ischemic regurgitation have been recognized as important pathologic processes that cause mitral insufficiency in the elderly. The potential morbidity and mortality of mitral valve replacement or repair in the elderly person are much greater than that in patients with uncomplicated mitral disease, and unless complications precipitate urgent surgery these patients may best be considered for medical management.

Recent reports quote a 10 to 15% operative mortality with mitral valve replacement alone in elderly patients (24, 25). In our 45-month reference period, we operated on 17 patients over age 70 with isolated mitral valve disease. There were five early deaths, for an operative mortality of 29%. A significant cause of mortality was rupture of the posterior atrioventricular groove in patients with a calcified mitral annulus. In 49 patients over age 70, the operative mortality for mitral valve replacement combined with coronary artery bypass surgery was 50% (19 deaths/38 patients). In contrast, the operative mortality for mitral valve repair combined with coronary artery bypass surgery was only 18%. In younger patients, it is generally accepted that preservation of the mitral valve is preferable to replacement; it may turn out that this concept is even more important in the elderly.

Multiple Valve Replacement

Operative mortality for patients undergoing combined aortic and mitral valve replacement has decreased significantly over the past 10 years because of improvements in myocardial protection, the availability of better valve substitutes, and other advances in perioperative care. However, operative mortality in elderly patients is still high (26). Coronary artery bypass surgery combined with aortic and mitral valve replacement can be performed with an acdpetable early mortality rate (12%); but with an appreciable late mortality rate of 28% in a mean follow-up of 40.7 months (27). For most patients, late mortality and morbidity continue to be cardiac in nature or related to complications with anticoagulation therapy.

Pacemaker Therapy

Pacemaker therapy has been widely used for the elderly patient with excellent therapeutic results. Postoperative overdrive pacing using temporary wires has a definite place in the control of arrhythmias and for maximizing cardiac output. Often this technique can preclude the use of antiarrhythmic drugs with their side effects (28).

Aside from postoperative open-heart patients, early use of permanent pacing is the treatment of choice in the elderly because prolonged temporary pacing requires confinement to bed, monitoring, and restriction of movement; and in the aged patient, pneumonia, thrombophlebitis, fecal impaction, psychological decompensation, and other complications are greatly enhanced by prolonged bed rest (29). We feel that the transvenous method is most applicable in elderly patients. At the present time, it is our policy to implant these pacemakers under local anesthesia in an operating room under fluoroscopic control (30).

The indications for permanent pacemaker implantation in the elderly should be extended beyond the treatment of complete AV block to include persistent and symptomatic bradycardia, the sick sinus syndrome, cerebrovascular insufficiency on the basis of low cardiac output, tachyarrhythmias, and certain cases of acute myocardial infarction. An aggressive, definitive approach is indicated in the elderly to help restore effective circulatory function. By increasing the patient's cardiac output, he or she will be able to combat other organ dysfunctions more effectively.

CONCLUSION

When an adequate trial of medical therapy or angioplasty for isolated coronary artery disease in the elderly fails, coronary artery bypass surgery should be pursued for indications that are the same as those for younger patients at a comparable stage in their disease process.

Valve replacement, in the absence of coronary artery disease, can be carried out with acceptable operative mortality and a satisfactory long-term prognosis in the elderly.

In elderly patients requiring combined valve and bypass procedures, early and late mortality is high (23, 31–33). It is generally accepted that the preservation of the mitral valve is preferable to replacement.

The incidence of postoperative complications and related mortality has been significant in the elderly. Prolonged pump time and aortic cross-clamp time are associated with significantly increased mortality. These prolonged times occur predominantly in patients requiring combined procedures.

Therefore, consideration for surgical intervention in the elderly should not be made on the basis of age per se; but rather, case selection should be based on life expectancy in the individual patient in terms of other disease factors. While chronolgic age itself is not a vital factor in prognosis, advanced cardiac status resulting from delay, in deference to advanced age, is a particularly ominous matter.

As we continue to analyze our most recent experience in regard to the timing of operation, it is apparent that the lessons of our earlier experience are resulting in better case selection, more judicious evaluation and surgery, and less morbidity and mortality. As a result, we believe we are better fulfilling the anticipation of the elderly for an independent and improved quality of life when heart disease becomes the limiting factor in their lives.

References

1. Pomerance A. Pathology of the heart with and without cardiac failure in the aged. *Br Heart J* 27:697, 1965.
2. Bjork G: The biology of myocardial infarction. *Circulation* 37:1071, 1968.
3. *Statistical Abstract of the United States.* Washington, DC, U.S. Department of Commerce, 1979, p 17.
4. U.S. Bureau of the Census: Projections of the population of the United States by age and sex, 1964 to 1985. In *Current Population Reports*, Series P23, No. 314. Washington, DC, Government Printing Office, 1965.

5. Cosgrove DM: CABG risk factors change cardiac surgery in 1984. *Cardio* June 1984, p 28.

6. Hamby RI, Wisoff BG, Kolker P, et al: Intractable angina pectoris in the 65 to 79 year age group: a surgical approach. *Chest* 64:46, 1973.

7. Ellison N: Problems in geriatric anesthesia. *Surg Clin North Am* 55:929, 1975.

8. Lorhan PH: Surgery and anesthesia in the octogenarian. *Am J Surg* 114:665, 1967.

9. Elada M, Hall RJ, Gray AG, et al: Coronary revascularization in the elderly patient. *J Am Coll Cardiol* 3:1398, 1984.

10. Koch-Wesser T, Sellers EM: Drug interactions with Coumadin anticoagulants. *N Engl J Med* 285:487, 1971.

11. Rich MW, Keller AJ, Schectman KB, et al: Increased complications and prolonged hospital stay in elderly cardiac surgical patients with low serum albumin. *J Am Coll Cardiol* 2:161A, 1988.

12. Goldman R: Decline in organ functioning with aging. In Rossman I (ed): *Clinical Geriatrics*, ed 2. Philadelphia, JB Lippincott, 1979, pp 23–59.

13. Mills NL, Beandet R, Isom W, et al: Elevated blood sugar levels during cardiopulmonary bypass (Abstr 395). *Circulation* 44 (Suppl II):109 1971.

14. MacArthur A, Elada MA, Hall RJ, et al: Coronary revascularization in the elderly patient. *J Am Coll Cardiol* 3:1398, 1984.

15. Meyer J, Wukasch DC, Seybold-Epting W, et al: Coronary artery bypass in patients over 70 years of age: indications and results. *Am J Cariol* 36:342, 1975.

16. Gann D, Collin C, Hildner FJ, et al: Coronary artery bypass surgery in patients seventy years of age and older. *J Thorac Cardiovasc Surg* 73:237, 1977.

17. Berry BE, Acree PW, Davis PJ, et al: Coronary artery bypass operation in septuagenarians. *Ann Thorac Surg* 31:310, 1981.

18. Knapp WS, Douglas JS, Craver JM, et al: Efficacy of coronary artery bypass grafting in elderly patients with coronary artery disease. *Am J Cardiol* 47:923, 1981.

19. Kuan P, Bernstein SB, Ellestad MH, et al: Coronary artery bypass surgery morbidity. *J Am Coll Cardiol* 3:1391, 1984.

20. Jamieson WR, Dooner J, Munro AI, et al: Cardiac valve replacement in the elderly: a review of 320 consecutive cases. *Circulation* 64(Suppl II):177, 1981.

21. Matloff JM, Czer LSC: Cardiac valve replacement in the presence of coronary atherosclerosis. In Matloff JM (ed): *Cardiac Valve Replacement— Current Status*. Hingham MA, Martinus Nijhoff, 1985, pp 111–122.

22. Nunley DL, Grunkemeier GL, Starr A: Aortic valve replacement with coronary bypass grafting. *J Thorac Cardiovasc Surg* 85:705, 1983.

23. Tsai TP, Matloff JM, Chaux A, et al: Combined valve procedure and coronary artery bypass surgery in septuagenarians and octogenarians—Result in 120 patients. *Ann Thorac Surg* 42:681, 1986.

24. Hochberg MS, Derkac WM, Epstein SE, et al: Mitral valve replacement in elderly patients. Encouraging postoperative clinical and hemodynamic results. *J Thorac Cardiovasc Surg* 77:422, 1979.

25. Teply JF, Grunkemeier GL, Starr A: Cardiac valve replacement in patients over 75 years of age. *J Thorac Cardiovasc Surg* 29:47, 1981.

26. Stephenson LW, Edie RN, Harken AH, et al: Combined aortic and mitral valve replacement: changes in practice and prognosis. *Circulation* 69:640, 1984.

27. Akins CW, Beckley MJ, Daggett WM, et al: Myocardial revascularization with combined aortic and mitral valve replacements. *J Thorac Cardiovasc Surg* 90:272, 1985.

28. Waldo AL, MacLean WA: *Diagnosis and Treatment of Cardiac Arrhythmias Following Open Heart Surgery; Emphasis on the Use of Atrial and Ventricular Epicardial Wire Electrodes*. Mount Kisco, NY, Futura, 1980.

29. Tyers GF: Cardiac pacemakers and cardiac conduction system abnormalities. In *Gibbon's Surgery of the Chest*, ed 4. Philadelphia, WB Saunders, 1983, p 1306.

30. Beller BM, Frates RWM, Wulfsohm N: Cardiac pacemaking in the management of postoperative arrhythmias. *Ann Thorac Surg* 6:68, 1968.

31. Tsai TP, Matloff JM, Gray RJ, et al: Cardiac surgery in the octogenarian. *J Thorac Cardiovasc Surg* 91: 924, 1986.

32. Tucker BL, Lindesmith GG, Stiles QR: Myocardial revascularization in patients 70 years of age and older. *West J Med* 126:179, 1977.

33. Tsai TP, Chaux A, Kass RM, et al: Aortocoronary bypass surgery in septuagenarians and octogenarians. *Chest* 88:47S, 1985.

Section 2
PREOPERATIVE WORKUP

Chapter 4
THE RISK OF SURGERY IN PATIENTS WITH HEART DISEASE

DHUN H. SETHNA, M.D.
RICHARD J. GRAY, M.D.

Operative mortality for cardiac and noncardiac surgery in patients with heart disease has declined progressively over the past decade. The low risk, the gratifying relief of symptoms, and, in the case of open-heart surgery, improved exercise capacity have allowed expansion of the indications for surgery to more patients, including the elderly. Expectations of success are as great in the elderly patient with extensive disease and left ventricular scar as in the younger patient with new onset anginal distress. However, patients, and often their physicians, are unaware of clinical subsets in which operative mortality and morbidity are high. The purpose of this review is to identify high-risk patients so that the physician can make the best therapeutic decision for the cardiac patient scheduled for noncardiac or cardiac operations.

NONCARDIAC SURGERY

Evaluation of patients with heart disease for noncardiac surgery is a common and necessary occurrence. As early as 1929, Howard Sprague made the observations that in these patients, a history of effort tolerance was frequently a better guide than the physical examination, and that congestive heart failure greatly increased complications and mortality from operation (1). Medical treatment of the failing heart could, however, convert a poor risk into a good one. He concluded that, in general, patients who could walk 1 block without dyspnea or chest discomfort, whose diastolic blood pressures were below 120 mm Hg, and who had not had a myocardial infarction within the previous 6 months were reasonable candidates for a necessary surgical procedure.

Goldman and associates, in a recent, large, retrospective study, developed a scoring system for evaluating cardiac risk factors in patients undergoing general noncardiac operations (2). The overall mortality in this group was 5.9% with a cardiac death rate of 1.9%. Points were assigned to each of nine independent correlates of serious cardiac complications (Table 4.1). Factors that did not show independent correlation were controlled diabetes mellitus, presence of a fourth heart sound, controlled hypertension, hyperlipidemia, peripheral vascular disease, and chronic stable class I or class II angina. Patients were divided into four groups (Table 4.2) depending on the number of points; morbidity and mortality were correlated. An

TABLE 4.1

GOLDMAN INDEX RISK FACTORS[a]

Factor	Score
Signs of congestive heart failure	11
Myocardial infarction in the past 6 months	10
Premature ventricular beats (>5/min)	7
Other than sinus rhythm	7
70 or more years old	5
Emergency surgery	4
Vascular, intrathoracic, or upper abdominal surgery	3
Aortic stenosis	3
Poor general condition	3
Total	53

[a]From Goldman L, Caldera DL, Nussbaum SR, et al: Multifactorial index of cardiac risk in noncardiac surgical procedures. *N Engl J Med* 297:845–850, 1977.

excellent prediction of death using this multifactorial risk index was demonstrated in a prospective component of the study. The advantage of this classification was that it gave reproducible, clinical criteria for the identification of the high-risk surgical candidate. It was proposed that if risk factors could be corrected, occurrences of perioperative cardiac complications could be reduced. The usefulness of this index was confirmed by two large studies in which observed risk was comparable to that predicted by the index (3, 4); in one study, patients in the high-risk class IV subset showed a lower than predicted incidence of cardiac events, which was attributed to superior pre- and postoperative care in those already identified to be at higher risk (3).

Geriatric patients are at a higher risk (11%) of major perioperative cardiac complications following abdominal or noncardiac thoracic surgery. In a study of patients aged 65 or older,

TABLE 4.2

GOLDMAN CARDIAC RISK INDEX[a]

Class	Point Total	No or Only Minor Complications	Life-Threatening Complications[b]	Cardiac Death
		%	%	%
I	0–5	99	0.7	0.2
II	6–12	93	5	2
III	13–25	86	11	2
IV	26	22	22	56

[a]From Goldman L, Caldera DL, Nussbaum SR, et al: Multifactorial index of cardiac risk in noncardiac surgical procedures. *N Engl J Med* 297:845, 1977.

inability to do 2 min of bicycle exercise in the supine position to a heart rate greater than 99 beats/min was a strong predictor of perioperative complications (5). When this parameter was tested prospectively, no other clinical or laboratory data, including rest and exercise radionuclide ventriculography or the presence of one or more Goldman indicators, gave any further predictive information. The low sensitivity (31%) of the Goldman index in this study appeared to result from applying an index derived from a general population to a selective geriatric one.

Risks of noncardiac surgery in patients with coronary artery disease depend on symptoms and type and duration of operation. Stable angina with a normal ECG is associated with a 5% death rate after general surgery (6). Data from the Coronary Artery Surgery Study (CASS) show that perioperative mortality is higher (2.4%) in patients who undergo noncardiac surgery without preceding coronary surgery than those who undergo noncardiac surgery after coronary artery bypass grafting (0.9%) (7). However, hospital mortality for bypass surgery averaged 1.4%, so that the combination of the coronary surgery followed by noncardiac surgery appeared no less risky than noncardiac surgery in the medically managed coronary patient. Unstable angina represents a higher perioperative risk and, in these patients, noncardiac surgery should be delayed if possible, and coronary arteriography with myocardial revascularization should be performed if indicated (8). Patients who have undergone previous bypass grafting are less likely to develop myocardial infarction during anesthesia for noncardiac operations than those with angiographic evidence of coronary disease (9). In all patients, antianginal medication should be continued in effective doses during the perioperative period, and this may require institution of topical or parenteral drugs until the resumption of oral medications.

In the absence of a previous myocardial infarction, postoperative infarction occurs in only 0.13% of patients after noncardiac surgery (10). However, in those with a history of recent previous infarction, the postoperative infarction rate can be as high as 66% with a 54% mortality. Proposed mechanisms contributing to this high occurrence of infarction and death include intraoperative tachycardia, hypotension, hypoxia, hemorrhage, or decreased cardiac output. Perioperative myocardial infarction usually occurs within 3 days of operation, and occasionally between the 3rd and 5th postoperative day. In the majority of cases there is no chest pain. Perioperative reinfarction is considerably influenced by the time elapsed between operation and the preceding myocardial infarction (11, 12). Patients operated on within 3 months of a myocardial infarction show a 27 to 37% perioperative reinfarction rate. This decreases to 11 to 14% in the 4th to 6th month after infarction, and stabilizes at 4 to 5% when the myocardial infarction has occurred more than 6 months previously. It has been proposed that continuous, invasive monitoring with aggressive, specific treatment for hemodynamic and arrhythmic abnormalities can further reduce the perioperative reinfarction rate to 5.7% and 2.3% in those who are 0 to 3 and 4 to 6 months following myocardial infarction, respectively (12). Reinfarction is higher in those who have intraoperative hypertension and tachycardia, or hypotension. However, up to one-half of the occurrences of intraoperative ischemia as documented by metabolic, electrocardiographic, or radionuclide criteria may not be associated with changes in heart rate or arterial pressure (13). These events of "silent" ischemia occur despite optimal hemodynamic indices of myocardial oxygen supply and demand, and may well be a manifestation of the coronary artery disease itself, with reductions in regional coronary perfusion occurring unrelated to anesthesia or operation. The above observations indicate that purely elective surgery should normally be delayed until 6 months after a myocardial infarction. Emergency surgery should be performed when necessary, using the best available hemodynamic monitoring. In higher-risk patients who require semielective surgery, cardiac catheterization and coronary bypass surgery may have to be considered before the noncardiac operation.

Patients with congestive heart failure also present increased surgical risk which may be improved by aggressive preoperative management. Patients with preoperative clinical or radiographic heart failure have a higher incidence (16%) of developing pulmonary edema during or after operation, in contrast to those with a prior history but no clinical evidence of heart failure (6%). Patients in New York Heart Association (NYHA) class IV are at a higher risk of pulmonary edema or worsening of heart failure during or after operation (25%) than those who are asymptomatic (3%) (14). In the majority of cases, postoperative pulmonary edema develops within the first 30 to 60 min of termination of anesthesia. Proposed mechanisms are intraoperative fluid overload, cessation of positive pressure ventilation, anesthesia-induced myocardial depression, and postoperative hypertension. Patients with chronic congestive heart failure who are well maintained on medical therapy should have their drugs continued in the perioperative period. Noninvasive studies such as echocardiography and radioisotope angiograms may be necessary in the routine evaluation of these patients. Prophylactic use of digitalis in the absence of definite indications is not recommended (15); digitalization should be done when there is definite congestive heart failure or when the patient has definite cardiac enlargement even without heart failure.

Significant aortic stenosis has been associated with a mortality rate of up to 13% after noncardiac surgery and appears to be an independent cardiac risk factor (14). Doppler and two-dimensional echocardiography should be used to determine the severity of stenosis and myocardial infarction. These patients are very dependent on the atrial contribution to ventricular filling; if atrial fibrillation develops, aggressive attempts to control ventricular rate and restore sinus rhythm should be instituted. In patients with valvular regurgitation, operative risk is related more to the status of left ventricular dysfunction than to the severity of regurgitation (16, 17). The risk of general anesthesia for major noncardiac operations is also low in patients with hypertrophic obstructive cardiomyopathy (18). It should be remembered that specific antibiotic prophylaxis for infectious endocarditis is recommended for patients with prosthetic cardiac valves, rheumatic or other acquired valvular disease, hypertrophic obstructive cardiomyopathy, prior history of bacterial endocarditis, and mitral valve prolapse with insufficiency. Consideration should also be given to the use of anticoagulants in patients with valvular heart disease; in previous reports, anticoagulants have been safely discontinued 3 days before operation, and resumed an average of 2.7 days after surgery without thromboembolic complications (8, 19).

Patients with hypertension who are receiving antihypertensive medication should continue their therapy in the perioperative period. When blood pressure is stable and the diastolic pressure is less than 110 mm Hg, no benefit is derived from postponing elective surgery to achieve better blood pressure control (20). Despite the degree of preoperative control, perioperative alterations in blood pressure will occur in about 25% of hypertensive patients (8). Increases in arterial pressure can be expected during laryngoscopy and intubation, and within the first few hours after anesthesia. Severe hypertension may be treated by intravenous sodium nitroprusside, esmolol, an ultra-short-acting β-blocker, or sublingual nifedipine; the latter has an onset of action within 15 min, with a duration of up to 4 hr (8).

Cardiac arrhythmias occur in the majority of patients who undergo anesthesia and surgery, but only 5% of these are clinically significant (8). Chances of developing new supraventricular arrhythmias after noncardiac surgery are higher when age exceeds 70 years, when preoperative rales are present, and with intraabdominal, intrathoracic, or major vascular surgery (21). Surprisingly, a history of chronic obstructive pulmonary disease or the presence of preoperative atrial premature contractions do not correlate independently with occurrences of postoperative supraventricular arrhythmias.

The clinical importance of ventricular premature contractions is related to the presence or absence of underlying heart disease (8, 22). In the healthy patient without evidence of structural heart disease, complex ventricular ectopy is not associated with perioperative cardiac morbidity or mortality. On the other hand, complex ventricular arrhythmias in patients after myocardial infarction, or in those with severe left ventricular dysfunction due to ischemic heart disease or cardiomyopathy, do increase

the risk of perioperative cardiac complications. Prophylactic perioperative antiarrhythmic therapy is reserved only for patients who have serious arrhythmias, that is, a history of symptomatic ventricular ectopy or sudden death. Hemodynamically significant ventricular arrhythmias may be treated with intravenous antiarrhythmic medications while searching for a possible reversible cause such as hypoxia, electrolyte imbalance, or an acid-base disorder. Even when therapeutic drug levels are maintained, increases in ventricular ectopy due to proarrhythmic drug effects have been observed.

Patients with preoperative sinus bradycardia or chronic bifascicular heart block rarely develop perioperative advanced heart block. In several studies involving patients with chronic bifascicular block, there have been no instances of perioperative heart block (8, 14, 23). Hence, insertion of temporary transvenous pacemakers is not indicated in patients with chronic bifascicular block unless symptoms suggestive of complete heart block are present or the patient has developed a new bifascicular block in the setting of an acute myocardial infarction. Temporary cardiac pacemakers should be inserted preoperatively in patients who fit the criteria for insertion of a permanent pacemaker but in whom the device has not yet been implanted. Patients with permanent cardiac pacemakers should have their pacemakers evaluated for normal pacing and sensing functions prior to operation; in addition, pacemaker type and model number, response to electrical interference, and reprogramming method should be known prior to operation (8).

CARDIAC SURGERY

The clinical profile of patients undergoing coronary artery bypass surgery has altered considerably in the last decade (24). Patients are older and more ill at time of surgery, with increasing severity of congestive heart failure, left ventricular dysfunction, and coronary artery disease, and a higher incidence of emergency operations (24). More patients have associated medical diseases such as diabetes, chronic lung disease, and vascular diseases. Overall operative mortality has increased over the decade, and perioperative morbidity, such as low output syndrome and respiratory and neurologic complications, is more common.

Complications and death after open-heart surgery usually depend on the severity of the patient's illness and on the skill and experience of the anesthesiologist and surgeon. The collaborative study CASS indicated that advanced age, female sex, symptoms of heart failure, left main coronary stenosis, left ventricular dysfunction, and nonelective surgery were associated with higher mortality (25); 40% of patients with left main coronary disease who were operated for "emergency" revascularization died before discharge from hospital. Similar associations have been confirmed between severity of illness and death after operation, identifying as major risk factors advanced age (greater than 65 years), severe obesity (body mass index greater than 30), congestive heart failure, unstable or recent onset angina, left ventricular dysfunction, and reoperation or emergency operation (26). Whereas 12.5% of patients who had two or more risk factors died after surgery, mortality was only 0.4% in those who had none (26).

The importance of anesthetic management has been demonstrated in a recent prospective examination, which showed that postoperative myocardial infarction after coronary bypass surgery occurred when more frequent intraoperative tachycardia and ischemia were permitted (27). Perioperative new S-T segment depression, prolonged global myocardial ischemia from aortic cross-clamp, and the quality of revascularization were important determinants of perioperative infarction. Up to half of the occurrences of intraoperative ischemia as documented by metabolic, electrocardiographic, or radionuclide criteria, however, may not be associated with changes in heart rate or arterial pressure (28).

Advanced age increases the risk of coronary bypass surgery, and the risk is most evident in the oldest patients. In the latter group, surgery is recommended in those who have angina that is unstable or refractory to repeated trials of medical management, and in those with significant left main coronary disease in whom the poor prognosis of these lesions may terminate a long life prematurely. Increased mortality and

morbidity from a variety of complications have been ascribed to surgery performed at extremely advanced ages. In general, hospital mortality for coronary bypass surgery averages 7 to 13% in patients older than 70 years, in contrast to 0 to 3% in those who are 65 years and younger. In the CASS perioperative mortality in patients older than 65 years was 5.2%, which was significantly more than the mortality of 1.9% in patients younger than 65 years (25). There was a trend toward a higher mortality rate at all levels of advancing age; it was 4.6% in patients aged 65 to 69 years, 6.6% in those 70 to 74 years, and 9.5% in those 75 years or older. Duration of hospital stay after operation was also significantly longer for patients 65 years or older than for those younger than 65. Octogenarians undergoing bypass surgery are especially at risk for having major complications in the perioperative period, resulting in increased hospital stay. In one study, the most common problems were atrial arrhythmias and congestive heart failure, each occurring in 48% of patients (29). Bleeding complications necessitating reexploration were also common (36%); other major complications included wound dehiscence or infection, and renal dysfunction. Addition of aortic valve replacement to myocardial revascularization may not increase operative mortality over that for aortic valve replacement alone in those younger than 70 years (30). On the other hand, in those older than 70 years, mortality was higher when it was necessary to add aortic valve replacement to bypass grafting (30). When mitral valve replacement was combined with revascularization there was a higher operative mortality in all age groups over that for bypass surgery alone, and the risk increased with advancing age (30). In the author's experience, the highest risk occurs in elderly females undergoing revascularization combined with mitral valve replacement for ischemic mitral regurgitation.

At any age, operative mortality is higher in females. In the Cleveland Clinic experience, women younger than 60 years who underwent isolated bypass grafting had a higher operative mortality rate than men (2.9 versus 1.3%), despite less severe coronary disease and better left ventricular function (31). When matched for age, severity of angina, and extent of coronary artherosclerosis, women still had twice the operative mortality of men. After 60 years of age, mortality increased in men and differences in this study become insignificant. In the CASS Registry, operative mortality decreased as body height and vessel diameter increased. In a recent analysis at the authors' institution, mortality of isolated coronary bypass in women was twice that of men, a difference that vanished when corrected for preoperative NYHA classification and age. This difference persisted despite correction for body size and technical factors thought previously to be important and strongly suggests that the traditional differences observed reflect a referral bias as regards women.

In older patients, as in younger patients, the prime determinant of survival is left ventricular function. Conventional wisdom and clinical experience suggest that degree of myocardial injury and amount of chronic left ventricular scarring adversely affect perioperative survival. In the CASS Registry, hemodynamic variables that reflected left ventricular dysfunction were associated with more perioperative deaths; these included a cardiothoracic ratio of 0.50 or higher, a left ventricular end-diastolic pressure of 20 mm Hg or greater, and an ejection fraction of less than 50% (25). There was no statistically significant relationship between the left ventricular wall motion score and perioperative risk. The presence of symptoms of congestive heart failure is, for the elderly, a poor prognostic sign. In one study, octogenarians requiring intraaortic balloon counterpulsation for left ventricular dysfunction showed a very high (67%) in-hospital mortality after coronary bypass surgery (29). Nevertheless, with appropriate attention to indications, left ventricular function, and distal coronary artery suitable for bypass grafting, symptomatic relief and quality of life can justify bypass surgery for elderly patients.

Perioperative mortality has also been related to extent and severity of coronary artery disease and extent of involvement of the left main coronary artery. Left main coronary artery stenosis of 50% of more, but less than 70%, is not associated with a higher risk (25). Mortality increases strikingly in those with left main coronary artery stenosis of 70% or more, and with a left

dominant circulation. Fortunately, this condition is uncommon (1.7%). In the CASS Registry, perioperative mortality was 5.7% in patients with single-vessel disease and 3.8% and 5.9% in patients with two-vessel and three-vessel disease, respectively (25). Perioperative mortality was not significantly higher in patients with three-vessel disease than in those who had fewer vessels involved (5.9% versus 4.3%).

Urgency of surgery, not expectedly, has been associated with an increased perioperative risk. In the CASS Registry, mortality was 3.9% in patients who underwent elective surgery, 6.7% in those who had urgent surgery, and 13.7% in patients who had emergency surgery (25). Perioperative deaths have been reported to be as high as 75% in octogenarians undergoing emergency revascularization (29). Stability of preoperative angina pectoris may also influence perioperative deaths associated with coronary bypass grafting. Experience at Toronto General Hospital showed that operative mortality for stable angina was lower than in comparable patients in whom the symptom was unstable (2.9% versus 5.4%) (32). Risk factor analysis revealed that the unstable group had four predictors for operative mortality (age, sex, left ventricular function, and left main coronary stenosis greater than 50%) compared to the stable cohort that had only three predictors (age, sex, and left ventricular function).

The use of platelet inhibitory agents to prevent the progression of coronary artery disease can result in abnormalities of hemostasis after cardiopulmonary bypass. Mediastinal blood loss is significantly greater in patients taking aspirin than in comparable patients who are not on platelet inhibitory agents (33). The degree of mediastinal blood loss does not correlate with patient age, total operative time, bypass time, number of vessels diseased, or number of grafts placed. In addition, routine coagulation studies such as prothrombin time, partial thromboplastin time, platelet count, and template bleeding time are often normal in these patients. There is no difference in bleeding among those who stop using aspirin 5 to 7 days before operation compared to those who discontinue drug use 1 to 4 days preoperatively. It is recommended that aspirin use be discontinued at least 10 days prior to elective open-heart surgery. For emergency operations, platelet transfusions should be available in the operating room at the end of cardiopulmonary bypass. In addition, desmopressin should be considered to assist hemostasis. Mediastinal infections after open-heart surgery are more common in patients who have been in a hospital environment for more than 5 days preceding the operation (34). Other risk factors that predispose to mediastinal infection include obesity, diabetes, reduced serum albumin, female sex, advanced age, and chronic lung disease requiring prolonged ventilation. The use of Dacron or wires to close the sternum, reoperation, external cardiopulmonary massage, and the experience of the surgeon do not appear to relate to sternal wound infections.

References

1. Sprague HB: The heart in surgery. *Surg Gynecol Obstet* 49:54, 1929.
2. Goldman L, Caldera DL, Nussbaum SR, et al: Multifactorial index of cardiac risk in noncardiac surgical procedures. *N Engl J Med* 297:845–850, 1977.
3. Zeldin RA: Assessing cardiac risk in patients who undergo noncardiac surgical procedures. *Can J Surg* 27:402–404, 1984.
4. Detsky AS, Abrams HB, McLaughtlin JR, et al: Predicting cardiac complications in patients undergoing non-cardiac surgery. *J Gen Intern Med* 1:211–219, 1986.
5. Gerson M, Hurst J, Hertzberg V, et al: Cardiac prognosis in noncardiac geriatric surgery. *Ann Intern Med* 103:832–837, 1985.
6. Sapala JA, Ponka JL, Duvernoy WFC: Operative and nonoperative risks in the cardiac patient. *J Am Geriatr Soc* 23:529–534, 1975.
7. Foster ED, Davis K, Carpenter J, et al: Risk of noncardiac operation in patients with defined coronary disease: the Coronary Artery Surgery Study (CASS) Registry experience. *Ann Thorac Surg* 41:42–50, 1986.
8. Weitz HH, Goldman L: Noncardiac surgery in the patient with heart disease. *Med Clin North Am* 71:413–432, 1987.
9. Mahar L, Steen P, Tinker J, et al: Perioperative myocardial infarction in patients with coronary artery disease with and without aortocoronary artery bypass grafts. *J Thorac Cardiovasc Surg* 76:533–537, 1978.
10. Tarhan S, Moffitt E, Taylor W, et al: Myocardial infarction after general anesthesia. *JAMA* 220:1451–1454, 1972.
11. Steen P, Tinker J, Tarhan S: Myocardial reinfarction after anesthesia and surgery. *JAMA* 239:2566–2570, 1978.
12. Rao T, Jacobs K, El-Etr A: Reinfarction following anesthesia in patients with myocardial infarction. *Anesthesiology* 59:499–505, 1983.
13. Slogoff S, Keats AS: Further observations on perioperative myocardial ischemia. *Anesthesiology* 65:539–542, 1986.
14. Goldman L, Caldera D, Southwick F, et al: Cardiac risk factors and complications in non-cardiac surgery. *Medicine* 57:357–370, 1978.
15. Selzer A, Kelly JJ Jr, Gerbode F, et al: Case against routine use of digitalis in patients undergoing cardiac surgery. *JAMA* 195:549–553, 1966.
16. Hirshfield J Jr: Surgery in the patient with valvular heart disease. In Goldman D (ed): *Medical Care of the Surgical Patient.* Philadelphia, JB Lippincott, 1982.
17. Borow KM: Surgical outcome in chronic aortic regurgitation: a physiologic framework for assessing preoperative predictors. *J Am Coll Cardiol* 10:1165–1170, 1987.
18. Thompson R, Liberthson R, Lowenstein E: Perioperative anesthetic risk on noncardiac surgery in hypertrophic obstructive cardiomyopathy. *JAMA* 254:2419–2421, 1985.
19. Tinker JH, Tarhan S: Discontinuing anticoagulant therapy in surgical patients with cardiac valve prostheses. *JAMA* 239:738–739, 1978.
20. Goldman L, Caldera D: Risks of general anesthesia and elective operation in the hypertensive patient. *Anesthesiology* 50:285–292, 1979.
21. Goldman L: Supraventricular tachyarrhythmias in hospitalized adults after surgery. *Chest* 73:450–454, 1978.
22. Goldman L: Cardiac risks and complications of non-cardiac surgery. *Ann Intern Med* 98:504–513, 1983.
23. Pastore J, Yurchiak P, Janis K, et al: The risk of advanced heart block in surgical patients with right bundle branch block and left axis deviation. *Circulation* 57:677–680, 1978.
24. Naunheim KS, Fiore AC, Wadley JJ, et al: The changing profile of the patient undergoing coronary artery bypass surgery. *J Am Coll Cardiol* 11:494–498, 1988.
25. Gersh BJ, Kronman RA, Frye RL, et al: Coro-

nary arteriography and coronary artery bypass surgery: morbidity and mortality in patients age 65 years and older. *Circulation* 67:483–491, 1983.

26. Kennedy JW, Kaiser GC, Fisher LD, et al: Clinical and angiographic predictors of operative mortality from the collaborative study in coronary artery surgery (CASS). *Circulation* 63:793–802, 1981.

27. Paiement B, Pelletier C, Dyrda I, et al: A simple classification of the risk in cardiac surgery. *Can Anaesth Soc J* 30:61–68, 1983.

28. Slogoff S, Keats AS: Does perioperative myocardial ischemia lead to post-operative myocardial infarction? *Anesthesiology* 62:107–114, 1985.

29. Naunheim KS, Kern MJ, McBride LR, et al: Coronary artery bypass surgery in patients aged 80 years and older. *Am J Cardiol* 59:804–807, 1987.

30. Jolly WW, Isch JH, Schumacker HB: Cardiac surgery in the elderly in geriatric cardiology. In Brest A (ed): *Cardiovascular Clinics.* Philadelphia, FA Davis, 1981, pp 195–210.

31. Loop FD, Golding LR, MacMillan JP, et al: Coronary artery surgery in women compared with men: analysis of risks and long term results. *J Am Coll Cardiol* 1:383–390, 1983.

32. Goldman BS, Katz A, Christakis G, et al: Determinants of risk for coronary artery bypass grafting in stable and unstable angina pectoris. *Can J Surg* 28:505–508, 1985.

33. Forraris V, Ferraris SP, Lough FC, et al: Preoperative aspirin ingestion increases operative blood loss after coronary artery bypass grafting. *Ann Thorac Surg* 45:71–74, 1988.

34. Nagachinta F, Stephen M, Reitz B, et al: Risk factors for surgical wound infections following cardiac surgery. *J Infect Dis* 156:967–973, 1987.

Chapter 5
PREPARATION OF THE PATIENT AND FAMILY

DOMENICA L. ROCEY, R.N.

Patients entering the hospital for any reason are subject to unfamiliar, frightening, and stressful experiences. The preoperative period is commonly a stressful, anxiety-ridden time in a patient's life. For a patient facing heart surgery, this experience may be seen as a devastating blow to the patient and his or her family (1); and the initial responses can be disbelief, fear, anxiety, anger, shock, denial, and depression. According to Pitorak, "The psychological responses of any patient who experiences cardiac surgery tends to be more intense [since] everyone associates the heart with life and death and the gamut of emotions" (2).

These responses can be minimized by encouraging the patient to verbalize his or her feelings. Cassady and Altrocchi found that important concerns, in order of their frequency, were physical discomfort, socioeconomic problems, a feeling of helplessness, and fear of disability (3). Other identified sources of anxiety are the uncertainty of the outcome, separation from family, and the possibility of death. Given such a situation, an authoritative, direct, and informed response to each of these concerns, whether stated or not, can be the first step to recovery.

Family reaction to the diagnosis of heart disease and the need for cardiac surgery can be a traumatic life event that presents a threat not only to the patient but also to the integrity of the family system. It is important to remember that response to stressful situations and the coping patterns that emerge will vary with families; the behavior patterns exhibited often reflect the ways in which a family has sought to protect and preserve its integrity in the past. Previous experience with illness and surgery, in particular, will influence current responses and the ability of both the patient and family to cope. According to Lazarus and coworkers, coping is a dynamic process that continually reshapes how people choose to deal with events, the concerns they express, and their emotional responses over time (4–6). Among the coping strategies of cardiac surgical patients and their families, information seeking is used most often in the preoperative period. It has been suggested that information seeking is most important when uncertainty is the greatest (7). Knowledge of what is about to happen and how it will be felt can replace the insecurity that accompanies uncertainty, resulting in a more positive experience. It is for this reason that people are interested in obtaining information before surgery. Preoperative education programs, including the personal contacts involved, can meet these needs and be used as a means to reduce anxiety (8). The importance of developing an accepting and warm relationship in this process must be emphasized.

Unfortunately, such education programs may

not always achieve the same level of success, because teaching is a highly individualistic and creative matter, and flexibility is essential to capture the enthusiasm of the learner. While the important person in the teacher-learner situation is the learner, the teacher must have sufficient skills and experience to "read" the learner. Therefore, a cardiac surgical teaching program must consider what the patients and families want to know, as well as what the health care staff think they need to know. It must be appreciated that not all patients truly desire a great deal of information during the preoperative period, and thus the patient's readiness to learn is important. For example, the acutely ill patient requiring emergency surgery is rarely ready to learn. Finally, it must be recognized that some families are not capable of understanding or accepting the information that needs to be transmitted. This situation constitutes an extremely difficult environment, with the potential for misunderstanding, anguish, and even conflict.

Regardless, because of their importance as part of the health care team, the family should be included whenever possible in all teaching components. The teacher must be aware of the importance of family support to patients. Supportive relationships help to diminish anxiety by reducing the feeling of alienation upon coming to the hospital.

SUPPORT SYSTEMS

By the time a decision to have cardiac surgery is reached, *existing* support systems, which involve a spouse, other family members, friends, neighbors, family physicians, and clergymen have usually been activated. On admission to the hospital, *additional* support systems come into focus. These obviously include the surgeon, cardiologist, and anesthesiologist. However, these systems must be considered incomplete unless they also involve cardiac care nurses, dieticians, social services, liaison psychologists, other cardiac care specialists, hospital support groups, and the cardiac surgery liaison nurse. All of these specialists will care for both the physical and emotional needs of the patient and his or her family, but the liaison nurse becomes the focal point for the hospital support. The cardiac surgery liaison nurse fulfills a unique position. While he or she has a primary role in patient and family education, there are also many collateral responsibilities that make this an indispensable position. As the primary educator for patients and families, the liaison nurse is responsible for developing and implementing all education programs for patients and their families, including those prior to coming to the hospital, during the hospital stay, and after discharge. Liaison nurses are usually responsible for emphasizing the dos and don'ts of preadmission protocols, of coordinating surgical schedules, of making admission appointments, and of coordinating the many elements of the health care team at the time of admission. Thus, they serve as advocates for patients and families in times of uncertainty or difficulty, especially including assistance to the family during the grieving and loss process, if the patient should die. They provide access to other hospital and community services and provide liaison with family physicians or others designated by the patient or his or her family. Finally, they provide continuity of care by coordinating follow-up telephone calls and postsurgical follow-up visits. Through these interactions they have the opportunity to become best acquainted with the patient and family.

While some anxiety is normal in such circumstances, the patient or family with excessive fears may significantly increase the risk of surgical morbidity or mortality, possibly by some direct effect of psychic stimuli on the cardiovascular system (9, 10). Thus, an extreme fear of surgery is a potentially dangerous problem that must be taken seriously. When such fears are exhibited, their importance must be recognized and referral to liaison psychiatry or the department's psychologist is indicated.

At the author's center, Heart Families is a unique program of specially trained volunteers who have experienced heart surgery either personally or in their families. Through this personal experience and extensive training they are able to provide the families of patients with support and information, thereby helping to reduce the anxiety associated with cardiac surgery. They also help family members make better use of available hospital services and acquaint them with practical methods to simplify home convalescent care.

The Department of Medical Social Service should be able to provide many additional services where indicated. These include counseling for financial problems, coordinating with available community services, medical transportation, transfers to other health facilities, and personal counseling.

TEACHING AND COORDINATION PRIOR TO HOSPITALIZATION

The liaison nurse's involvement begins when the decision for surgery is made and a tentative date is chosen. The liaison nurse does the initial scheduling and sees the patient, and preferably the family as well, to prepare for admission. In the initial interview with patient and family, the liaison nurse establishes an accepting and reassuring relationship, gathers information about the patient and his or her support systems, his or her past experience with illness and hospitalization, and any unique financial problems. At this time, the patient's knowledge and understanding of the cardiac diagnosis and impending surgery, as well as his or her fears and concerns, are assessed. Wherever possible, misconceptions are clarified and appropriate information is given. Existing medication schedules are reviewed and specifics of these are repeated. Where there are potential problems, as with aspirin or other antiplatelet agents or anticoagulants, these are identified and appropriate steps taken to make everyone aware of potential problems. The need for smoking cessation, dental clearance for valve replacement patients, and the tests performed in the hospital before the patient is actually admitted are discussed.

Based on the initial contact, the liaison nurse then formulates an individualized teaching plan that will best meet the needs of the patient and family and makes referrals as appropriate. These may include such diverse matters as referral for financial counseling or making appointments in the blood bank. During the initial patient contact, the liaison nurse reviews the sequence of events that will occur from preadmission to discharge and rehabilitation, giving explanations

and the rationale for each step. To the extent that it can be done prior to the scheduled surgery, the patient and family are introduced to the staff who will be involved in that patient's care, are shown an educational movie on cardiac surgery and recovery, and tour the cardiac surgical unit and step-down area. Finally, each patient is sent a letter confirming the surgical date, stating when to come to the hospital, where to report, and what items to bring.

BLOOD TRANSFUSION THERAPY

One of the more significant preparations for cardiac surgery involves a discussion of blood transfusion therapy, including the possible need for components (red cells, fresh frozen plasma, and platelets), and acquisition of blood. Several factors make it difficult to conduct such surgery without the use of blood. Increasingly, cardiac surgery is being carried out in emergency situations involving a more elderly population with more complex problems, often following inpatient therapy. All of these circumstances can result in decreased blood volumes and anemia, with altered clotting mechanisms from the use of antiplatelet agents, anticoagulants, and thrombolytic agents.

In an emergency there is usually no option but to use hospital bank blood. Although all donors are screened for history of tranfusion-mediated disease and HTLV-III antibody, under ideal circumstances it is still preferred to use either autologous or directed donor blood.

ON ARRIVAL AT THE HOSPITAL

The patient and family are familiarized with some of the equipment they will see in use later in the cardiac surgical intensive care unit. If the patient or family is unable to tour the area, a description of what to expect should be provided. The patient should be told that when he or she awakes following surgery, an endotracheal tube may be in place and attached to a respirator to assist in breathing. The patient should be made aware that in this instance he or she will not be able to talk until the tube is removed and he or she must communicate by writing notes. The patient and family should be made aware of all additional devices that may be used; these include a nasogastric tube, chest tubes, Foley catheter, intravenous lines, an arterial line, a Swan-Ganz catheter, and temporary pacing wires. The purpose for each should also be explained as indicated.

The family should be aware that body temperature may be reduced during surgery, necessitating a heating blanket postoperatively; that there may be a need for soft hand restraints; that most of the (uncomfortable) devices will be removed in a day or two; that while there may be some pain it is generally well controlled by medication and comfort measures; and that the duration of a typical stay in the intensive care unit is 2 days.

It should be explained that while in the intensive care unit the patient is awakened frequently for important nursing care, such as taking of vital signs, turning, coughing, and deep breathing. Immediately after surgery, diet is limited to fluids, but as soon as feasible it will be changed to a regular diet, albeit low in sodium and cholesterol.

The use of incentive spirometry is demonstrated preoperatively; and the vital importance of its use to promote deep breathing and coughing, and that of respiratory therapy to minimize postoperative lung complications such as atelectasis, infection, and pneumonia is emphasized.

OTHER TEACHING TOPICS

For patients scheduled for valve surgery, the differences between valvular repair and replacement are introduced. Models of the prosthesis to be used should be demonstrated and their characteristics defined. Patients receiving a defibrillator or pacemaker implant should be allowed to see actual units similar to the ones they will receive.

Other matters to be discussed include possible confusion or disorientation, which resolves prior to discharge; extreme weakness and fatigability experienced by all patients, with resolution a few weeks after discharge, coinciding with resumption of normal hemoglobin levels; decreased appetite (family should be encouraged to bring favorite foods from home); and depres-

sion and mild visual disturbances, which usually resolve shortly after discharge. Activities that can be expected after leaving intensive care include sitting in a chair for all meals, progressing to self-care in the bathroom, perhaps sitting in a chair initially; walking 5 times per day before discharge; and showering before discharge.

At the completion of the preoperative interviews and teaching sessions the liaison nurse may wish to prepare a teaching checklist. This checklist is used to communicate to other members of the health care team what has been taught and what areas need additional reinforcement. A copy of the checklist used at the authors' institution is shown in Figure 5.1.

DURING SURGERY

During surgery the patient's family and friends are requested to wait in a lobby where they can be periodically informed as to the progress of surgery. The liaison nurse should report to the family as frequently as indicated, even on an hourly basis.

Shortly after surgery is completed, the liaison nurse should escort the family members to meet with the surgeon to discuss the operation, and then on to visit briefly with the patient (usually no more than two family members at a time). The telephone number of the intensive care unit should be provided to family members. Visiting restrictions should be substantially relaxed following transfer from the intensive care unit to the patient's regular room.

AFTER SURGERY

Throughout the hospital stay, patient and family should be followed by the liaison nurse on a daily basis. Daily classes are provided on nutrition, stress management, discharge instructions, coping after heart surgery, and topics of special interest (for a full discussion, see Chapter 27). As part of the postoperative teaching, each patient receives a copy of the "Heart to Heart" booklet, which discusses in detail the postoperative recovery period.

Even after the patient is discharged, continuation of telephone contact and making of referrals for such support as community-based

FIGURE 5.1

	PATIENT I.D.
PATIENT EDUCATION RECORD **PREOPERATIVE INTERVIEW**	

PURPOSE:

1.) To orient the patient and family to the routine preoperative and postoperative procedues and the CSICU environment thus promoting active participation and cooperation during hospitalization.

2.) To provide the opportunity for the patient and family to verbalize feelings and concerns in an attempt to lessen preoperative anxiety.

CONTENT REVIEWED:

PREOPERATIVE EXPECTATIONS	YES	NO	POSTOPERATIVE EXPECTATIONS	YES	NO
Preparation (skin & bowel)	☐	☐	Waking up - Can't talk	☐	☐
NPO/No Smoking	☐	☐	Coughing/Triflo	☐	☐
CSICU Environment/Tour	☐	☐	Discomfort/Splinting	☐	☐
Visiting Hours	☐	☐	Pain Medication	☐	☐
Expected Length of Stay	☐	☐	Sutures/Staples/Dressings	☐	☐
Family Waiting Area	☐	☐	Pacing wires	☐	☐
Sedation	☐	☐	IV's/Drainage Tubes/Catheters	☐	☐
IV's; Oxygen	☐	☐	Respiratory Treatments	☐	☐
Belongings	☐	☐	Progressive Ambulation	☐	☐

PATIENT/FAMILY OBJECTIVES:

COMPLETED	YES	NO
1.) Able to describe routine preoperative preparation and procedures in general terms;	☐	☐
2.) Able to describe postoperative expectations in general terms;	☐	☐
3.) Verbalize feelings and concerns regarding hospitalization and surgery;	☐	☐
4.) Verbalize understanding of surgical procedure in general terms.	☐	☐

REFERRALS:

Blood Donation: _____

Social Service: _____

Heart Families: _____

Nutritionist: _____

Outpatient Cardiac Program: _____

SUPPORT SYSTEM:

_____

_____

ADDITIONAL COMMENTS:

_____

_____

Date: _____ Signature of Cardiac Liaison Nurse _____ R.N.

Patient education record, preoperative interview.

nursing care and rehabilitation programs can be of great assistance. The need for a coordinated pre- and postoperative education program to help with the stress of this time period has been reconfirmed in a recent publication (11).

SUMMARY

The main goal of the preoperative program is to ensure that patients and their family members are fully and accurately informed about what to expect to achieve peace of mind and to make a good psychological adjustment to surgery. There is sufficient evidence, both from the literature and the authors' personal experience, to believe that whenever the program is fully implemented its aims can be attained.

A major limitation is in cases in which, because of an emergency, the program cannot be fully implemented. This is increasingly common and presents our greatest challenge. Ironically, when the surgery is performed on an emergency basis, the fear of death may be much greater than otherwise, and both patient and family are often in a state of disbelief or denial as they come face to face with the seriousness of the illness that necessitates cardiac surgery. It is in these cases that extra efforts must be made to provide a state of hopefulness, encouragement, and crisis support. Through continuing efforts, the educational program must be updated to remain current with new trends in medical and surgical practice.

References

1. Rognoz B: Nursing care of the cardiac surgery patient. *Nurs Clin North Am* 4:631, 1969.
2. Pitorak E: Open-ended care for open-heart patient. In Lewis EP (ed): *Nursing in Cardiovascular Disease.* New York, AJN, 1971.
3. Cassaday J, Altrocchi J: Patient concerns about surgery. *Nurs Res* 9:220, 1960.
4. Lazarus RS: *Psychological Stress and the Coping Process.* New York, McGraw Hill, 1966.
5. Lazarus RS, Averill JR, Opton EM Jr: The psychology of coping, issues of research and assessment. In Godho GV, Hamburg DA, Adorus JE (eds): *Coping and Adaptation.* New York, Basic Books, 1974, p 249.
6. Lazarus RS, Folkman S: *Stress, Appraisal and Coping.* New York, Springer Verlag, 1984.
7. King KB: Measurement of coping strategies, concerns and emotional response in patients undergoing coronary artery bypass grafting. *Heart Lung* 14:579, 1985.
8. Fuerst EV, Wolff LV, Weitzel MH: The nurse or a health teacher. In *Fundamentals of Nursing.* Philadelphia, JB Lippincott, 1974, p 148.
9. Kornfeld DS: The influence of emotions on the outcome of cardiac surgery. (Discussion of paper by Dr. Janet A. Kennedy and Hyman Bakst.) *Bull NY Acad Med* 42:846, 1966.
10. Kimball CP: Psychological responses to the experience of open heart surgery. I. *Am J Psychiatry* 126:348, 1969.
11. Gilliss CL, Sparacino PSA, Gortiner SR, et al: Events leading to the treatment of coronary artery disease: implications for nursing care. *Heart Lung* 14:250, 1985.

Section 3
MEDICAL AND SURGICAL MANAGEMENT DURING ANESTHESIA

Chapter 6
TECHNICAL ASPECTS OF CARDIOPULMONARY BYPASS

CARLOS BLANCHE, M.D.
JACK M. MATLOFF, M.D.
DANIEL A. MacKAY

Cardiopulmonary bypass is the technique by which systemic venous blood is diverted extracorporeally through a system of tubes and devices that remove carbon dioxide from the blood and replenish its oxygen content and then return it to the body. These devices are generically known as pump oxygenators. By substituting for the gas exchange function of the lungs, the oxygenator accounts for the lung portion of the heart-lung machines. Blood is returned from the extracorporeal apparatus through the action of a mechanical pump that simulates cardiac function by virtue of circulating blood through the arterial circulation, through the capillaries, and to the venous circulation.

The concept of extracorporeal circulation was envisioned by Dr. John Gibbon of Philadelphia in the late 1930s. Using the technique of total extracorporeal cardiopulmonary bypass that he had developed in the laboratory, his pioneering experimental work culminated in the first successful repair of an intracardiac lesion, a large atrial septal defect in an 18-year-old woman in 1953. Thus, Gibbon, with this unprecedented achievement, opened a new therapeutic era that eventually resulted in the development of modern cardiac surgery.

Along the way, many scientific investigations have defined the body's physiologic response to extracorporeal circulation and has led to the development of a variety of other devices such as heat exchangers, oxygenators, and improved in-line monitors that have allowed the uses of the technique to be extended. Refinements of anesthetic and surgical techniques and improved understanding of the use of blood have made cardiopulmonary bypass the safe and predictable technique known and practiced today throughout the world. Standard cardiopulmonary bypass is essential for most intracardiac operations today; when properly conducted, it is tolerated by virtually all patients with minimal risks and complications.

This chapter will review the various components of the extracorporeal circulatory system (Fig. 6.1) and will describe the conduct of cardiopulmonary bypass with attention to different techniques of myocardial preservation.

COMPONENTS AND METHODOLOGY OF EXTRACORPOREAL CIRCULATION

With the exception of the pumps, most of the apparatus is now made of disposable plastics

FIGURE 6.1

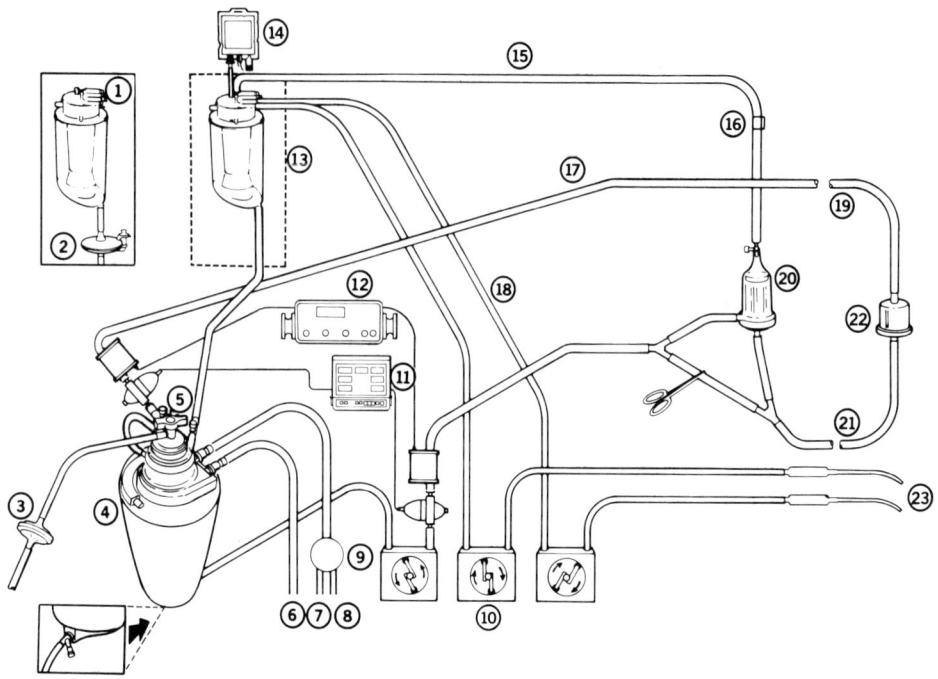

The recommended extracorporeal circuit. **1**, BCR-3000 cardiotomy reservoir; **2**, PF-427 bypass blood filter; **3**, GF-10 biologic gas line filter; **4**, Bentley 10 PLUS adult blood oxygenator; **5**, pO_2 controller; **6**, Water out; **7**, Water in—hot; **8**, Water in—cold; **9**, Temperature regulator (pressure limited to 75 psi); **10**, Pump heads; **11**, Gas STAT—for blood gas analysis; **12**, OxySAT monitor; **13**, BCR-3500 cardiotomy reservoir with filter; **14**, Blood and/or priming solution; **15**, Arterial filter purge line; **16**, 20-4672 Cutter one-way check valve; **17**, To venous cannulae; **18**, Suction lines; **19**, Connect for recirculation process; **20**, AF-1025, AF-1040 arterial blood filter; **21**, To arterial cannula; **22**, RF-10 recirculation filter; **23**, BDS-100 disposable suckers. (From the *Bentley 10 PLUS Adult Blood Oxygenator Instruction Booklet*. Irvine, CA, Baxter Healthcare Corporation, p 31.)

for one-time use. In the past, oxygenators were made of glass and metal and were designed for multiple uses. One of the most significant advances in the development of extracorporeal circulation has been the discarding of these disk oxygenators in favor of disposable plastic units.

Tubing for Extracorporeal Circulation

All pump tubing in the cardiopulmonary bypass circuit is single-use polyvinyl chloride that will not change stiffness at low temperature. The venous line is ½ inch by ³⁄₃₂ inch, the arterial line is ³⁄₈ inch by ³⁄₃₂ inch, and the cardiotomy suction and left ventricular lines are of ¼ inch by ¹⁄₁₆ inch tubing.

Venous Cannulation

Venous blood returning to the right atrium is usually diverted from the right atrium and the

venae cavae individually to the heart-lung machine. This is accomplished either with a single cannula placed in the right atrium or with two venous cannulae placed through the right atrium into the superior vena cava and into the inferior vena cava. Single cannulae are sometimes constructed with two separate openings, one in the right atrium and one into the inferior vena cava. More recently, single cannulae are avialable in which there are two extensions that can be placed directly into the superior and inferior venae cavae. Right atrial cannulae are usually introduced through purse-string sutures in the lateral wall of the right atrium to preserve the right atrial appendage. This can be prudent if a dual-chamber, atrioventricular pacemaker is subsequently needed. The tip of the right atrial appendage is an excellent site for placement of the atrial lead. This consideration has been modified to a degree with the availability of screw-in atrial leads. In patients undergoing coronary artery bypass or aortic or mitral valve surgery, a single right atrial venous cannulation technique is adequate. In cases in which a right atriotomy or ventriculotomy is anticipated, double venous cannulation to the inferior and superior venae cavae is always necessary. By placing ensnaring tapes externally around the venae cavae, total cardiopulmonary bypass can be achieved. This method is also used when retroperfusion of the coronary sinus is anticipated for delivery of cardioplegia. An alternative approach for intitiating cardiopulmonary bypass early in the conduct of surgery may employ cannulation through one or both femoral veins. When the venous cannula is advanced, this drains the inferior vena cava extremely well.

For most bypass and valve operations the single venous cannulation techniques is adequate. A large-bore, two-stage catheter is introduced through a stab wound within a circular purse-string suture placed in the anterolateral aspect of the right atrium. The tip of the cannula is advanced 1 to 2 cm into the inferior vena cava so that the built-in cage lies in the middle of the right atrium ensuring maximum decompression of the right atrium and the superior vena cava. Improper positioning could impair hepatic venous return, with serious consequences. Furthermore, adequate venous return is needed to prevent retrograde flow through the coronary sinus to the left side of the heart. In addition to making visualization of the coronary arteriotomy difficult, retrograde blood flow can also wash out cardioplegia, with deleterious effects. For this reason, some surgeons prefer to use total cardiopulmonary bypass during the performance of bypass surgery. Although the use of the single right atrial cannula does not technically constitute total cardiopulmonary bypass since blood can enter the lungs and left side of the heart via the tricuspid valve and the coronary sinus, the proper use of a two-stage single cannula of size 51 French is virtually equivalent to total cardiopulmonary bypass. To compensate for any blood that may bypass the venous cannula, some form of left-heart venting is advised.

When two venous cannulae are used separately, they are placed near the caval-atrial junction and are advanced 2 to 3 cm into the respective vena cava. As indicated, tapes placed around the venae cavae can be tightened with snares so that all the blood is diverted from the venae cavae to the heart-lung machine. This gives the driest operative field and also allows for procedures on the right side of the heart. Furthermore, using total cardiopulmonary bypass of this nature avoids the possibility of introducing air to the right atrium, which can interfere with the vacuum effect on venous return.

As noted, in special circumstances venous return may be obtained by cannulating the femoral vein and passing the tip of the catheter into the inferior vena cava. This approach is especially useful in emergent situations in which extracorporeal circulation is needed prior to the sternotomy incision, as occasionally occurs in complicated situations involving the ascending aorta or in reoperations. The femoral vessels are readily accessible with a cutdown, ensuring rapid cannulation. The distal end of the femoral vein can be clamped safely, and a snare passed around the vein proximally ensures the vacuum effect that gives gravity drainage. The size of the cannula to be used in these circumstances will depend on the size of the patient and the catheter internal diameter necessary to achieve satisfactory flow.

In situations in which a persistent left superior vena cava is present, it can be cannulated either directly along its course or through the right atrium, by advancing the catheter through the coronary sinus and into the left superior vena cava.

Venous Reservoirs

All venous blood directed from the right atrium enters the venous side of the oxygenating system. When a bubble oxygenator is used, the venous blood enters directly into the oxygenating port and therefore a venous reservoir is not needed. With membrane oxygenators, a venous reservoir is needed to collect the blood before it is pumped through the membrane itself. There are two types of venous reservoirs. One is a soft and sometimes heparin-coated bag. The other is a rigid plactic shell; this shell in some cases is an integral part of the whole oxygenator. The capacity of these venous reservoirs varies from approximately 400 ml to a maximum of 3000 ml. The reservoir is positioned below the level of the right atrium to allow blood to drain by gravity. When a bubble oxygenator is used, blood exits from the defoamer and the heat exchanger into an arterial reservoir. The blood is pulled from the arterial reservoir by an arterial pump that advances it through an arterial filter and into the arterial cannula. In the membrane oxygenator, the venous reservoir is used after blood goes through the defoamer and heat exchanger. The blood then goes through a pump that drives the blood through a hollow fiber membrane oxygenator. From this oxygenator blood again goes through the arterial filter and returns to the arterial cannula.

Oxygenators

The two most commonly used types of oxygenators for cardiopulmonary bypass are the generic bubble and membrane oxygenators. A brief description of their mechanism of action is appropriate. In **bubble oxygenators**, venous blood enters the oxygenator by gravity, and thus the bubble oxygenator acts simultaneously as a venous reservoir. Blood is oxygenated by direct contact with oxygen. Unoxygenated blood mixes with fine oxygen-containing bubbles, resulting in oxygen diffusion out of the bubbles into the blood; carbon dioxide diffuses in the opposite direction.

After the bubbles and blood are thoroughly mixed in the oxygenator chamber, the bubbles are removed by the trapping action of mesh filters treated with an antifoam compound. These substances alter the surface tension of the bubbles, allowing them to break up. The oxygenated blood is then passed through a heat exchanger, allowing gas and heat exchange to occur simultaneously. When this process is complete the blood enters an arterial reservoir before being pumped through the arterial filter back to the patient.

In **membrane oxygenators** there is no direct contact between the gas and blood; oxygen is separated from the blood by a semipermeable capillary membrane. The oxygen diffuses through the microporous membrane from the oxygenation module into the blood compartment, while carbon dioxide diffuses in the opposite direction. Blood is spread over a large surface area for this process to occur efficiently. The transfer of gases across the membrane is primarily determined by the nature, surface area, thickness, and pressure differential across this microporous barrier; this is particularly true with carbon dioxide. Oxygen transfer is determined mainly by the thickness of the blood flow path (1). Some membrane oxygenators have a heat exchanger as an integral component.

Trauma and destruction of platelets and other blood elements during cardiopulmonary bypass can lead to serious postoperative coagulation problems and organ dysfunction. Although still controversial, bubble oxygenators do not appear to cause more trauma to red cells, leukocytes, and platelets than do membrane oxygenators when perfusion time is less than 3 hr (2). Intense blood-air contact during cardiotomy suction is considered to be a major destructive force for blood elements (3). Since the extent of platelet and erythrocyte damage depends on the total volume of cardiotomy suction, it may be that the apparent hematologic superiority of membrane oxygenators is explained by the greater volume of intracardiac suction known to occur during longer perfusion times (4).

At the authors' institution, the Bentley 10 bubble oxygenator is used in low-risk patients with a predicatable short cardiopulmonary bypass time. This device has the advantages of being simple to use and assemble, relatively inexpensive, and efficient; in addition, it can be rapidly primed. In high-risk patients, such as in the elderly, in reoperations, and with complex surgical procedures, we favor the use of membrane oxygenators. The device used is the Bentley BOS-CM 50, which provides an exchange surface area of approximately 5.3 m^2 and a blood flow of 2.7 liters min.

With advancing technology, it is apparent that hybrid oxygenators will encompass the best features of bubble and membrane formats, avoiding any presumed advantage of one over the other. These devices should result in significant financial savings in regard to manufacturing costs and personnel time for setup. In the present atmosphere of cost containment, these may become increasingly important considerations in deciding which device will be used.

Heat Exchangers

Heat exchangers are used to control blood temperatures during extracorporeal circulation. Since most intracardiac operations are now done with hypothermia to reduce systemic metabolic requirements, thereby increasing margins to safety, cooling and rewarming are necessary and can be easily and precisely adjusted with efficient heat exchangers. These are now available as separate, disposable or reusable units. Whichever is used, the heat exchanger is an integral component of most bubble and membrane oxygenator systems. Nasopharyngeal temperature can be decreased to the range of 20 to 25°C at the rate of 0.7 to 1.5°C min. This is usually accomplished in about 10 min, allowing arterial blood temperature to drop as low as 17 to 20°C.

Rewarming is done at a slower rate, usually 1°C over each 3 to 5 min. The heat exchanger is not allowed to go over 42°C and, as a consequence, rewarming is a slower process than cooling. The water bath temperature to nasopharyngeal temperature gradient is kept under 6 to 8°C, and blood temperature is never raised above 4°C because blood proteins may denature at 44°C (5). The ways in which temperature is monitored will be discussed separately.

Arterial Pumps

The arterial roller pumps that are most commonly used today are not different than those originally introduced by Dr. Michael DeBakey in 1934 (6). These pumps deliver continuous, nonpulsatile flow. The advantages of such pumps are their simplicity to operate, their accurate perfusion rates, and their proven reliability. Perfusion flow rate can be accurately controlled by altering the speed of rotation of the pump head and by adjusting the degree of compression that the pump exerts on the arterial tubing that traverses the pump.

The concept of pulsatile perfusion during cardiopulmonary bypass has gained increasing clinical interest, expecially with the desire for prolonged pump support. The latter is particularly true in the situation in which the need for a bridge to a cardiac transplant is entertained. Further studies are needed to establish the importance and the precise role of this technique.

Centrifugal Pumps

In contrast to the roller pump, blood in a centrifugal pump is moved by an impeller or a vortexing motion. These pumps are used extensively for long-term cardiac assist because they appear to be less traumatic to blood than roller pumps. Centrifugal pumps are gaining popularity for routine cardiac cases; however, the additional costs of these plastic disposable units may not be warranted.

Arterial Filters

The most common arterial filters have a pore size of 25 to 40 μm. They are placed in the extracorporeal circulation system to remove particulate matter. They also act as a bubble trap if air accidentally enters the circuit.

Arterial Cannulation

The arterial cannula is usually placed in the ascending aorta proximal to the take-off of the innominate artery. Enough room has to be left so that the aorta can be cross-clamped proximal to this site, an aortic infusion-suction vent can be inserted, and proximal coronary artery bypass anastomosis or work on the aortic valve can be done.

The aortic cannula is usually secured in place with two Teflon pledgeted purse-string sutures that encircle and are secured to the cannula and to the edge of the sternotomy incision. Careful insertion of the tip of the cannula is important to avoid trauma to the intima which could initiate an aortic dissection. Care also has to be taken not to dislodge intimal plaques which may embolize and cause cerebral vascular accidents. For the same reasons, inadvertent placement of the tip into the brachiocephalic vessels, against the inner wall of the aorta, or with the cannula directed proximally must be avoided. When the aortic cannula tip lies freely in the aortic lumen and is directed toward the aortic arch, the downstream blood flow is unobstructed. Pressure in the arterial cannula has to be extremely carefully monitored, especially at the onset of cardiopulmonary bypass.

For most patients, a tapered, angled no. 24 French catheter with a 9.5 mm internal diameter gives satisfactory flow with minimal resistance. If needed, a wide variety of aortic cannula sizes are available. Occasionally, the femoral artery needs to be used for arterial cannulation. Cases in which such a technique is valuable include those in which there is a severely calcified ascending aorta, or when operations on the aortic arch and brachiocephalic vessels are anticipated such as for resection of an aneurysm of the ascending aorta. This technique is also useful when some control may be needed before dividing the sternum. Rarely, the axillary artery can be used when no other appropriate site for cannulation is available.

Left Ventricular, Left Atrial, and Aortic Venting

Additional venting of blood from within the heart or the ascending aorta is commonly employed in cardiac interventions. There are several practical and physiologic advantages associated with the use of venting: (a) Such venting can facilitate exposure, especially for aortic valve replacement or when an absolutely blood-free, dry operative field is desired for coronary anastomoses; (b) it reduces the rate of myocardial rewarming during aortic cross-clamping by effectively draining blood return to the left ventricle; (c) it prevents blood from washing out cardioplegia solution if the blood enters the aorta and traverses the coronary arteries; and (d) it prevents left ventricular distension, particularly significant in the presence of aortic insufficiency. Occasionally, left atrial venting will accomplish the same goal. There is conclusive evidence in the literature that left ventricular distension reduces subendocardial perfusion, causing persistent ischemia that may result in impaired left ventricular performance (7).

However, venting is not without risk, and complications may arise, particularly due to the introduction of air into the left ventricle or

aorta with subsequent air embolization to the systemic circulation. In addition, the venting site may create a potential source of bleeding, may produce myocardial or aortic damage, may dislodge endocardial thrombus, and may be associated with arrhythmias or pulmonary venous obstruction. Despite these potential risks, venting is advisable, if not essential, in most operations requiring cardiopulmonary bypass.

Venting of the left ventricle can be accomplished with a catheter introduced into the right superior pulmonary vein, across the mitral valve, and into the cavity of the left ventricle, or by placing an aortic root vent through a purse-string suture. Blood from the ventricular chamber is vented by gravity or by mild negative suction into the pump oxygenator. Routinely, during coronary revascularization and valvular cases venting is carried out with a dual-purpose aortic root cannula that permits the infusion of cardioplegia solution as well as venting. Venting of the aorta is extremely helpful when air may have been introduced into the heart. When the aortic clamp is removed and the circulation reestablished, any air that is in the heart or pulmonary veins has the potential to be removed by placing suction on the aortic vent. The left ventricular vent is also useful for removing air, as well as for decompressing the left ventricle, particularly after aortic or mitral valve surgery.

Priming Solutions

Pump oxygenators require a priming volume, which is most often a crystalloid solution. The resulting hemodilution that occurs has beneficial effects. These include a reduction in the amount of blood needed to prime the circuit and a reduction in viscosity of the perfusate. While reducing exposure to whole blood and the probability of transfusion-related reactions (8), the use of crystalloid priming solution also reduces the potential for coagulation abnormalities and the possibility of bleeding. Hemodilution increases renal clearance of sodium, potassium, creatinine, and free water, and also increases urinary output. It also reduces the incidence of acute tubular necrosis (5). Furthermore, hemodilution tends to balance certain adverse effects of hypothermia, primarily increased blood viscosity, the shifting of the oxy-hemoglobin dissociation curve to the left, dimunition of blood flow to the brain, and direct tissue trauma. It also counteracts adverse effects of the pump oxygenerator, such as microemboli, consumption of coagulation components, hemolysis of red cells, and denaturation of serum proteins (9). Part of these benefits result from improved microcirculation due to a reduction in blood viscosity (10).

The disadvantages of hemodilution include the reduction of plasma colloid-osmotic pressure with subsequent increased visceral water content that is greatest in gastrointestinal organs, myocardium, and lung. It also reduces oxygen-carrying capacity, but the advantages outweigh these problems (9).

The bubble oxygenator is primed with 1800 ml of Plasmalyte-A solution, a balanced electrolyte solution similar to plasma with a pH of 7.40, and 44.6 mEq of sodium bicarbonate. Mannitol, 12.5 gm, is added to the initial prime. Depending on the situation of urine output and the length and complexity of the surgery, additional Mannitol is given just prior to release of the aortic cross-clamp. Membrane oxygenators are primed with the same components, except that a priming volume of 2200 ml of Plasmalyte-A solution is required. In addition, antibiotics are added to the prime, usually 1 gm of Ancef, or 500 mg of vancomycin in patients allergic to penicillin.

The overall need for whole blood has been much reduced by the use of nonblood priming solutions, as noted; but an essential contribution to this reduced use has been a result of increased preoperative hematologic evaluation, improved intraoperative technique, greater attention to hemostasis, more appropriate use of heparin and protamine, improved understanding of platelet function and how to enhance it, and the use of a variety of methods to conserve shed blood for reinfusion. Except in unusual cases in which patients begin surgery with anemia, when surgery is complex and lengthy, or when done in juxtaposition with catheterization or the use of thrombolytic agents, almost no transfusions are needed during surgery or in the operating room. Beyond this, the potential for adverse reactions has been further diminished by the use of autotransfusion and directed donor programs to obtain blood for surgery (11). Autotransfused blood, where feasible, is clearly the ideal substitute. Directed donor blood, from donors who are well known to the recipient, is also recommended. However, the safety of the blood supply should be greater now than at any time in the past; all donors are closely evaluated, including screening for human immunodeficiency virus (HIV) antibodies.

Intrapericardial (Coronary) Suction

In most cardiac procedures, blood is shed into thee pericardium or may be found in a chamber which is open. This blood is conserved to maintain the patient's own blood volume. Traditionally, devices to accomplish this are termed coronary suction catheters. Any blood that is recovered from the pericardium or the chambers of the heart must be filtered to remove particulate foreign material that might become the source of an embolus once it is returned to the systemic circulation. Although essential to any cardiac surgical procedure, these suction devices are recognized as one of the most traumatic elements of the extracorporeal circulatory system. The intense blood-air interface induces turbulence and high shear stresses, particularly at the suction catheter tip (4), and this can be quite destructive to the formed blood elements.

Autotransfusion and Blood Conservation Systems

These have already been mentioned. Although not part of the extracorporeal circuit, an autotransfusion system is an important component of cardiopulmonary bypass. It is worth reemphasizing that blood preservation is achieved by harvesting blood from the operative field, processing it by centrifugation, and returning it to the patient as packed red blood cells. The standard cell-saver device is able to process 250 ml of blood and have it available for transfusion in 8 to 10 min. A more efficient system with a 3- to 4-min processing time is available for trauma cases, or when a higher amount of blood loss is anticipated.

CONDUCT OF CARDIOPULMONARY BYPASS

Heparin and Protamine

Heparin is given by the anesthesiologist soon after the chest is opened. After a control activated clotting time (ACT) is obtained, a loading dose of 3 mg/kg of heparin is given through a central venous line. The ACT is checked prior to going on bypass, and if levels are less than 480 seconds, additional heparin is given according to a heparin dose-response curve.

Activating clotting time is checked at 30-min intervals while on cardiopulmonary bypass; it is kept at the level of 480 seconds or greater. Once bypass is terminated, and after removal of the venous cannula, protamine is given to reverse heparin, usually during a 5- to 10-min period. The reversing dose approximates 1.3 mg of protamine for 1 mg of heparin. A more accurate technique for controlling and reversing heparin effects involves a heparin dose response and protamine reversal titration, such as with the Hepcon device. At present, this technique has not received widespread use due to higher cost.

The ACT is checked twice before the operation is concluded, and if the ACT has not returned to control level after the initial dose of protamine, additional protamine is given. The arterial cannula should be removed only after the protamine dose is given because of possible hypotension or anaphylaxis, particularly in the insulin-dependent diabetic. The history of diabetes mellitus and protamine zinc insulin usage, or allergies to fish, should arouse concern. Furthermore, with increasing likelihood of prior exposure to heparin, whether from repeat catheterization, angioplasties, reoperations, or as primary therapy for coronary atherosclerotic disease, the potential for reactions to protamine is increasing. Should hypotension occur it usually responds to infusions of volume, vasoactive agents, steroids, and antihistamines. When reaction is anticipated, pretreatment is recommended. With the potential of a severe reaction based on a prior experience, consideration should be given to using the original agent for reversal of heparin, that is, Polybrene.

Monitoring Parameters during Cardiopulmonary Bypass

Safe cardiopulmonary bypass depends, in great part, on continuous and accurate monitoring of several physiologic and biochemical parameters. Thus, continuous communication among the members of the cardiac and surgical team, including the surgeon, anesthesiologist, perfusionist, and nurses, about the patient's physiologic requirements and response to cardiopulmonary bypass is essential for a successful outcome. Monitoring during surgery and hemodynamic manipulation are discussed in detail in Chapter 7 and 8, respectively.

General Considerations. The electrocardiogram is monitored continuously during the operative procedure, not only for rate and rhythm, but also for QRS and S-T segment morphology. Arterial blood pressure is monitored with a radial or femoral line, and both mean pressures and systolic-diastolic variations are noted. Central venous pressure and pulmonary artery and wedge pressure are monitored with a balloon flotation pulmonary arterial catheter via the jugular or subclavian vein. Urinary output is measured with a Foley catheter that simultaneously monitors bladder (core) temperature. Nasopharyngeal temperature is monitored with an esophageal probe.

When hemodynamic monitoring is performed, cardiac output and derived indices such as cardiac index, stroke volume, left ventricular stroke work index, systemic vascular resistance, and pulmonary vascular resistance should be obtained. After baseline values are obtained, they are repeated prior to intubation, before and after cardiopulmonary bypass, and at the end of the case when the chest is closed. Of course, measurements are obtained, as indicated, at any time during the course of surgery. Continuous monitoring of the arterial pressure in the extracorporeal circulation circuit is essential to detect sudden or gradual changes in the peripheral vasculature or the arterial cannula, especially at the site of insertion. Because of the tapered construction of the arterial cannula, a gradient between the proximal portion attached to the extracorporeal pump and the distal aortic lumen is expected. For this reason, arterial circuit line pressures of 100 to 250 mm Hg are acceptable. Higher pressures may indicate obstruction to the arterial flow and must be corrected.

Perfusion Flow Rate.   Perfusion flow rates during cardiopulmonary bypass vary from 1.8 to 2.5 liters/min/m^2. Increased lactic acid production, low oxygen consumption, and acidosis will develop with flow rates of less than 1.6 liters/min/m^2 at normothermia (12). A flow rate of approximately 2.0 liters/min/m^2 is recommended, although lower flows can be used as body temperature decreases, such as at 23 to 25°C.

Perfusion Pressures.   During cardiopulmonary bypass a mean arterial pressure of 50 to 75 mm Hg is preferred. However, in special circumstances such as significant carotid occlusive disease, the mean arterial pressure should be kept at 75 to 80 mm Hg.

Pharmacologic manipulation of the arterial blood pressure may be needed, as changes in the systemic vascular resistance occur during extracorporeal circulation. Soon after initiation of cardiopulmonary bypass, the systemic vascular resistance falls abruptly, followed by a gradual increase toward normal or even exceeding normal levels. Although considerable variation exists, patients with coronary artery disease tend to develop a higher level of systemic vascular resistance during cardiopulmonary bypass (10).

The central venous pressure during cardiopulmonary bypass is kept as low as possible, preferably less than 10 mm Hg. This is done to minimize cerebral edema and decrease accumulation of extracellular fluid in the most dependent parts of the body. For the same physiologic reasons, left atrial pressure is kept as close to zero as possible, to avoid the accumulation of interstitial water in the lung parenchyma.

Hypothermia reduces systemic metabolic requirements during extracorporeal circulation; for every decrease of 10°C in body temperature, oxygen requirements decrease approximately 50% (5). This immproves tolerance to low systemic flow, which decreases noncoronary collateral flow and bronchial flow, and thereby facilitates exposure in the operative field.

Temperature.   During cooling or rewarming, the body temperature does not change uniformly. Changes in organ temperature will depend on organ blood flow per unit of mass. Highly perfused organs such as the brain, heart, and kidneys will then change temperature more rapidly than less-perfused organs like skin and skeletal muscle (5). Nasopharyngeal temperature closely reflects the brain temperature, whereas urinary bladder temperature usually reflects the temperature in the lesser perfused organs. Patients are routinely cooled to 25°C with cardiopulmonary bypass. This is accomplished in approximately 10 min, allowing blood temperature to drop to 17 to 20°C. Rewarming is done in a much slower fashion. The differential temperature between the blood and the water bath in the heat exchanger can by easily controlled and is not allowed to exceed 6 to 8°C to prevent gaseous emboli and direct tissue trauma.

Urinary Output.   The urinary output is a good indicator of peripheral perfusion. Hemodilution is known to increase renal clearance of sodium, potassium, creatinine, and free water by producing an increase in urinary output (5). In addition, Mannitol is used in the oxygenator prime solution, and it is therefore not unusual to observe large amounts of urinary output during extracorporeal circulation.

Prolonged cardiopulmonary bypass is associated with increased destruction of blood elements, resulting in increased hemolysis and hemoglobinemia. Free plasma hemoglobin can precipitate in the renal tubules, particularly when the urine output is decreased. Microemboli and microdebris may selectively embolize the outer renal cortex, thereby contributing to postoperative renal dysfunction (5). Aside from some preoperative variables, the incidence of postoperative acute renal failure predictably correlates with the duration of cardiopulmonary bypass (13) and with sustained profound depression of cardiac function and subsequent low output in the postoperative period (14). Furosemide or Mannitol is routinely added to maintain urinary output during cardiopulmonary bypass, providing it has not increased with changes in perfusion flow rate or pressure. Occasionally, preexisting anuria or oliguria in a patient with chronic renal failure on chronic dialysis will necessitate relentless dialysis or ultrafiltration during cardiopulmonary bypass.

Hematocrit.   During cardiopulmonary bypass, the perfusate is diluted to a hematocrit of about 20%. Ordinarily, hematocrit is checked every hour while on cardiopulmonary bypass. Hematocrit can be assessed continuously during bypass using a photometric device such as that manufactured by American Bentley (Oxy-Sat II). Blood is added to a circuit if the hematocrit falls below 20%, especially in patients over the age of 65. After bypass, any blood remaining in the circuit is centrifuged in the cell saver and transfused as washed packed red cells.

Glucose, Potassium, and Ionized Calcium. Monitoring of glucose and potassium and, perhaps more importantly, of ionized calcium has been made much easier by the availability of a variety of newer devices that enable a quick determination to be performed in the operating room.

The glucose concentration is kept at 100 to 200 mg/dl during bypass. No glucose solution is added to the prime in diabetics, and insulin is given if blood glucose levels exceed 200 mg/dl. Potassium is kept in the normal physiologic range and frequently has to be added to the perfusate because of increased urinary losses that occur during cardiopulmonary bypass. Glucose and potassium are monitored hourly during extracorporeal circulation, and special attention is given to diabetic patients and those with preexisting renal dysfunction.

Arterial Blood Gases. Continuous in-line monitoring of the arterial blood gases and mixed venous saturation is done during cardiopulmonary bypass. With efficient oxygenators the PaO_2 and the $PaCO_2$ can be adjusted to desired levels. A PaO_2 lower than 85 mm Hg results in a rapid decline in arterial oxygen content and mixed venous desaturation (10). The PaO_2 should be kept at about 150 to 250 mm Hg on bypass, ensuring an optimal margin of safety. Higher oxygen concentration is unnecessary and may be toxic. The $PaCO_2$ is kept at a normal physiologic level of 35 to 40 mm Hg during cardiopulmonary bypass.

TECHNIQUES OF MYOCARDIAL AND PERIPHERAL TISSUE PRESERVATION

The primary goal of specific myocardial protection is to avoid or minimize myocardial necrosis and thereby to preserve myocardial function, by maintaining metabolic substrate and ultrastructure during an extended period of induced myocardial ischemia. Myocardial preservation during cardiopulmonary bypass is achieved by systemic and topical hypothermia and infusion of cold cardioplegic solution into the coronary arteries.

Hypothermia

The protective effects of hypothermia are secondary to an induced reduction in basal cellular metabolism. Current techniques to produce myocardial hypothermia include total body hypothermia with extracorporeal circulation, direct myocardial cooling with intermittent or continuous bathing of the heart with cold saline solution or the use of a cooling pad, direct intracavitary irrigation, and infusion of cold cardioplegic solution through the coronary ostia.

The optimal temperature for myocardial preservation is not known, but clinical and experimental studies suggest that myocardial temperatures between 15 and 20°C during global ischemic arrest are satisfactory for preservation of ventricular function (15). Myocardial temperatures of 20°C or more do not reduce cardiac metabolism sufficiently to achieve maximum protection during ischemic arrest. Temperatures lower than 10°C do not result in better preservation of glycogen stores (16) and may cause detrimental changes in left ventricular compliance (15).

Unfortunately, systemic and topical hypothermia cool the heart unevenly because of the presence of noncoronary collateral flow, ventricular hypertrophy, and critical coronary stenoses at unpredictable locations. Thus, a temperature gradient within the myocardium can be produced, particularly in the subendocardial layers and areas distal to severe coronary stenoses (15, 16).

To obtain more uniform and even cooling, a combination of different methods to produce cardiac hypothermia is preferable to using one technique alone. One recommended approach consists of lowering body temperature to 25°C during cardiopulmonary bypass. Approximately 1000 ml of 4°C crystalloid cardioplegia is infused through the aortic root initially, and supplemented with intermittent infusions of 100 to 150 ml every 20 to 30 min, given through the vein grafts, and occasionally through the aortic root. Also, the heart is bathed intermittently with cold saline solution, and cold-soaked packs are placed surrounding the heart during the course of positioning for exposure to the various structures being operated upon.

In aortic valve surgery, particularly for aortic insufficiency, cold cardioplegic solution is infused directly into the coronary ostia soon after cross-clamping. Polystan catheters, with pressure-dependent occluding balloons just proximal to the catheter tips, are particularly effective.

An alternative approach, although its role is still not clearly defined in clinical practice, is retrograde perfusion through the coronary sinus. This technique appears to have some advantages, such as more uniform delivery of the cardioplegic solution and superior myocardial protection in the presence of critical coronary stenoses. However, the right ventricle may be inadequately protected because of the venous drainage communications that bypass the coronary sinus, and potential injury to the coronary sinus can occur with subsequent conduction abnormalities (10).

Profound Hypothermia and Circulatory Arrest

In special circumstances, such as during repair of aortic arch aneurysm, profound hypothermia and circulatory arrest has proved to be a safe and reliable technique. This technique may involve initial surface cooling with ice packs surrounding the head and body. Core cooling is then accomplished on cardiopulmonary bypass until the nasopharyngeal temperature reaches 15 to 18°C. Perfusion is then stopped, and repair is accomplished usually within 60 min of circulatory arrest. Upon its completion, bypass is restarted and rewarming is begun. This technique greatly facilitates exposure and provides myocardial protection with no clinical or structural cerebral dysfunction when properly conducted (17).

Cardioplegic Solutions

The clear need for myocardial preservation during global cardiac ischemia was recognized in the early days of coronary revascularization surgery. This was clinically evident by the significant incidence of electrocardiographic or enzymatic evidence of perioperative myocardial necrosis. Myocardial edema, in greater or lesser degrees, is uniformly present after aortic cross-clamping. Severe myocardial edema reduces ventricular compliance with subsequent reduction in stroke volume and cardiac output (18). Induce global ischemia produces complex changes in myocardial cell metabolism and ultrastructure. Its most important sequela is myocardial necrosis and its incidence and extent depend in great part on the duration of the ischemic arrest (18).

Metabolically, ischemia produces an increase in anaerobic metabolism with depletion of high energy stores, intracellular acidosis, and inhibition of essential metabolic enzymes (16). The accumulation of lactate and acidosis interferes with normal aerobic metabolism and energy production, further compounding the metabolic problem. These biochemical and ultrastructural changes are more evident clinically during reperfusion when myocardial function is depressed and cannot accommodate increased metabolic demand.

The concept of specific cardioplegia to minimize or avoid these deleterious anatomic, metabolic, and physiologic sequelae was introduced by Melrose in 1955. He described a hyperosmolar, hyperkalemic solution that subsequent clinical experience proved to be harmful because of excessive concentration of potassium *citrate* (16). Bretschneider and Kirsh in Europe introduced improved cardioplegic solutions in the 1960s based on intracellular formulas, with improved clinical results. In 1973, Gay and Ebert (19) reintroduced potassium cardioplegia in the United States, using a solution containing potassium *chloride*. Subsequent clinical results have been excellent, and the technique quickly gained widespread exceptance. The combination of myocardial hypothermia and rapid potassium diastolic arrest has become the most widely employed method of myocardial protection during cardiopulmonary bypass.

Several modifications have been made throughout the years with uniformly good clinical results. Multiple crystalloid cardioplegic solutions are now available for clinical practice, differing in their composition and concentration of various elements; most of them use buffered extracellular formulas for hyperkalemic diastolic arrest, differing primarily in the osmolarity and pH of the solution. They contain different elements such as potassium, sodium, magnesium, calcium, and bicarbonate, as well as lactate, glucose, procaine, lidocaine, steroids, and calcium channel blockers.

Buckberg and colleagues in 1978 (20) introduced cold blood cardioplegia with similarly good clinical results. Its use is based on the potential advantages of using blood as a vehicle for cardioplegic arrest and for making oxygen available to the heart during this process. The heart is arrested in an oxygen-rich environment, so that no ATP is depleted prior to asystole. Autologous blood, being the most physiologic of all solutions, supposedly provides a medium rich in oxygen for replenishment of cellular energy levels to maintain aerobic metabolism during ischemic arrest. Although hypothermia shifts the oxyhemoglobin dissociation curve to the left, there is probably enough oxygen dissolved in the blood to maintain metabolism. Blood provides a physiologic metabolic substrate with normal osmolarity and excellent buffering capability. Disadvantages include sludging at low temperature and rouleau formation, but these have proved to be relatively insignificant problems. Rosenkrantz and Buckberg and colleagues (21) also introduced the concept of normothermic glutamate-enriched blood cardioplegia. They base their hypothesis on the observation that warm cardioplegia improves tolerance of known infarcted muscle to subsequent ischemia during aortic cross-clamping in patients with cardiogenic shock who undergo coronary revascularization.

The "safe" duration of cardioplegic arrest is not known, and most likely is variable from patient to patient. It is clear, though, that intermittent infusion of cardioplegic solution approximately every 20 to 30 min after the initial dose for diastolic arrest is necessary for maintenance of myocardial hypothermia and cardioplegic arrest (16).

Clinical experience with cardioplegic solutions in conjunction with other methods of myocardial protection has given excellent clinical results, and further refinements in technique will probably improve myocardial protection, particularly in patients with preexisting depressed cardiac function. Controversy still exists over the advantages of one type of cardioplegia or the other, and further studies are needed to determine whether there is even a superiority of blood versus crystalloid cardioplegic, let alone the merits of one specific type or another. To emphasize the uncertainty of this issue, it should be noted that excellent results are still obtained at major medical centers using systemic and topical hypothermia, intermittent cross-clamping, and ischemic ventricular fibrillation.

A popular agent is St. Thomas asanguinous cardioplegic solution, given with a pressurized bag, as previously described. It contains 20 mEq/liter of potassium chloride, 147 mEq/liter of sodium chloride, 32 mEq/liter of magnesium chloride, 4 mEq/liter of calcium chloride, and 0.03 mg/dl of procaine with a pH of 7.4 and an osmolality of 300 mosmol.

DISCONTINUATION OF CARDIOPULMONARY BYPASS

One of the most important aspects of cardiopulmonary bypass is the process by which it is discontinued. It is a time that is not fully appreciated for its critical importance to the surgery; and very little has ever been reported concerning this aspect of heart surgery.

After completion of the surgical procedure and while the patient is being rewarmed on cardiopulmonary bypass, air is evacuated from the aorta, the venous coronary bypasses, and the cardiac chambers. Air is vented from the venous bypasses using a no. 25 needle in multiple areas. Air is removed from the left ventricle by direct aspiration of the apex with a large-bore needle or through a left ventricular vent prior to discontinuing bypass. Simultaneously, the anesthesiologist ventilates the lungs with positive pressure to allow air contained in the pulmonary veins to escape. Air can also be vented from the stab wound in the right superior pulmonary vein into which the left ventricular vent was placed or from the left atriotomy, if there is one. Furthermore, the left atrial appendix should be compressed several times for the same purpose. In cases in which there is a very large left atrium, it may be appropriate to vent the left atrium superiorly, between the aorta and superior vena cava. Moving the table into a variety of positions, beginning in the Trendelenburg position and moving to the reversed Trendelenburg position, with the left side down, may be helpful while the aortic vent is on full suction. The aortic vent is always removed last. The presence of intracardiac air can be ascertained by the use of a transesophageal or epicardial Doppler probe. Changes in the ECG, especially in the inferior leads, corresponding to right coronary air embolism, may be heralded by acute ischemic changes in the S-T segments or T waves.

After all air is evacuated and the vent lines removed, and upon reaching normothermia by bladder and nasopharyngeal temperature monitoring for a minimum of 5 min cardiopulmonary bypass may be gradually discontinued by progressively occluding the venous outflow line and allowing the heart to "override" the pump. Approximately 12 to 15 min after the aortic clamp has been removed, any residual effect of the cardioplegia can be neutralized by systemic administration of from ½ to 2 gm of calcium chloride.

Successful weaning from cardiopulmonary bypass requires complete washout of cardioplegic solution, adequate rewarming, a stable cardiac rhythm, and strong and forceful right and left ventricular function. Atrial, ventricular or atrioventricular sequential pacing may be required, and temporary pacing wires (two atrial and one or two ventricular) are routinely placed (22). Where heart block of varying degress may be present, the calcium chloride often reverses this affect.

After placing the patient on partial cardiopulmonary bypass as noted by partially occluding the venous cannula and allowing some of the venous return to go through the heart, visual inspection of cardiac size and activity is of paramount importance. It will determine, along with the standard hemodynamic parameters, the feasibility of further discontinuing cardiopulmonary bypass. Bypass is terminated at a relatively low arterial systemic pressure (80 to 100 mm Hg) with appropriate right and left atrial pressures. Optimal filling pressures will depend on ventricular compliance and func-

tion; thus, considerable variation will exist from patient to patient. In general, right atrial and left atrial pressures are adjusted between 10 and 14 mm Hg with volume infusion and by pharmacologically manipulating preload and afterload. Large doses of nitroglycerin may allow greater fluid administration and the ability to empty all of the blood and priming solution into the vasculature. Moderate doses of mephenteramine (Wyamine) may be particularly useful in stabilizing the patient's blood pressure at this point.

If cardiac performance is inadequate, a longer period may be in order to allow the heart to recover further on cardiopulmonary bypass, provided the surgical repair is satisfactory. This "ride" should be pursued before beginning any more advanced pharmacologic therapy. Severe depression of ventricular performance is initially managed pharmacologically, as discussed in Chapter 8; but if inotropic support does not significantly improve cardiac function, mechanical assistance will then be required.

Introaortic balloon pumping (IABP) is based on the principle of diastolic counterpulsation, to achieve improved coronary blood flow and increased systemic perfusion. IABP augments diastolic coronary perfusion pressure, reduces systolic afterload, and thereby improves myocardial metabolism, augmenting cardiac output. There are no metabolic "costs" of IABP. For these reasons, the intraaortic balloon pump is a valuable clinical tool for patients with severely impaired cardiac function preoperatively and with patients with poor ventricular performance who cannot be weaned off cardiopulmonary bypass, as discussed in Chapter 14.

SUMMARY

In the 35 years from its inception in 1953, cardiopulmonary bypass has progressively evolved to be the safe, common, indispensible surgical adjunct that it is today. Changes have occurred in our understanding of the metbolic and physiologic consequences of artificial circulation, in conception and fabrication of the equipment, in experience and, perhaps most important, in respect for the technique. When appropriately and carefully used, it has contributed more to improving quality of life and sustaining longevity of life than any other biomedical device. When used inappropriately, it can result in unequaled morbidity and mortality. What it achieves is not intrinsic to the device itself, but to how it is used.

References

1. Davis C: Extracorporeal circulation. In Sabiston DC Jr (ed): *Textbook of Surgery*, ed 10.
2. Clark RE, Beauchamp RA, McGrath RA, et al: Comparison of bubble and membrane oxygenators in short and long perfusions. *J Thorac Cardiovasc Surg* 78:655–666, 1979.
3. DeJong JC, Ten-Ovis HJ, Smit Sibinga CT, et al: Hematologic aspects of cardiotomy suction in cardiac operations. *J Thorac Cardiovasc Surg* 79:227–236, 1980.
4. Boonstra PW, Vermenlen FEE, Levsink JA, et al: Hematological advantage of a membrane oxygenator over a bubble oxygenator in long perfusions. *Ann Thorac Surg* 41:297–300, 1986.
5. Glenn WWC, Baue AE, Geha AS, et al: *Thoracic and Cardiovascular Surgery*, ed 4. East Norwalk, CT, Appleton-Century-Crofts, 1983, pp 1091–1106.
6. DeBakey M: A single continuous flow blood transfusion instrument. *New Orleans Med Surg J* 87:386, 1934.
7. Lucas SK, Schaff HV, Flaherty JT, et al: The harmful effects of ventricular distention during post ischemic reperfusion. *Ann Thorac Surg* 32:486–493, 1981.
8. Verska JJ, Luchington LG, Brewer LA III: A comparative study of cardiopulmonary bypass with nonblood and blood prime. *Ann Thorac Surg* 18:72–80, 1974.
9. Utley JR, Wachtel C, Cain RB, et al: Effects of hypothermia, hemodilution and pump oxygenation on organ water content, blood flow and oxygen delivery and renal function. *Ann Thorac Surg* 31:121–133, 1981.
10. Kirklin JW, Barrat-Boyes BG: *Cardiac Surgery*, ed 1. New York, John Wiley & Sons, 1986, pp 29–82.
11. Cove H, Matloff JM, Sacks HJ, et al: Autologous transfusion in coronary artery bypass surgery. *Transfusion* 16(3):245–248, 1976.
12. Sabiston DC Jr, Spencer FC: *Gibbon's Surgery of the Chest*, ed 4. Philadelphia, WB Saunders, 1983, pp 909–925.
13. Abel RM, Buckley MJ, Austen WG, et al: Etiology, incidence and prognosis of renal failure following cardiac operations. *J Thorac Cardiovasc Surg* 71:323–333, 1976.
14. Hilberman M, Derby GC, Spencer RJ, et al: Sequential pathophysiological changes characterizing the progression from renal dysfunction to acute renal failure following cardiac operation. *J Thorac Cardiovasc Surg* 79:838–844, 1980.
15. Balderman SC, Binette JP, Chan AWK, et al: The optimal temperature for preservation of the myocardium during global ischemia. *Ann Thorac Surg* 35:605–614, 1983.
16. Lazar HL, Roberts AJ: Recent advances in cardiopulmonary bypass and the clinical application of myocardial protection. *Surg Clin North Am* 65:455–470, 1985.
17. Ergin MA, O'Connor J, Guinto R, et al: Experience with profound hypothermia and circulatory arrest in the treatment of aneurysm of the aortic arch. *J Thorac Cardiovasc Surg* 84:649–655, 1982.
18. Kirklin JW, Barrat-Boyes BG: *Cardiac Surgery* ed 1. New York, John Wiley & Sons, 1986, pp 83–108.
19. Gay WA, Ebert PA: Functional, metabolic and morphologic effects of potassium-induced cardioplegia. *Surgery* 74:284–290, 1973.
20. Follettee DM, Mulder DG, Maloney JV, et al: Advantages of blood cardioplegia over continuous coronary perfusion or intermittent ischemia. Experimental and clinical study. *J Thorac Cardiovasc Surg* 76:609–619, 1978.
21. Rosenkranz ER, Buckberg GD, Laks H, et al: Warm induction of cardioplegia with glutamate-enriched blood in patients with cardiogenic shock who are dependent on inotropic drugs and intraaortic balloon support. *J Thorac Cardiovasc Surg* 86:507–518, 1983.
22. Fields J, Berkovits BV, Matloff JM: Surgical experience with temporary and permanent AV sequential demand pacing. *J Thorac Cardiovasc Surg* 66:865, 1973.

Chapter 7
HEMODYNAMIC MONITORING DURING AND AFTER CARDIAC SURGERY

ARNOLD FRIEDMAN, M.D.
HERMAN BERNSTEIN, M.D.

In patients undergoing cardiac surgery, hemodynamic monitoring is necessary to obtain continuous information that can be used to prevent and dictate treatment of hemodynamic abnormalities before they proceed to catastrophic cardiac events. Methods currently available to monitor the cardiovascular system range from those that are noninvasive—such as the electrocardiogram (ECG), cuff blood pressure, transesophageal echocardiography, and radionuclear ventriculography—to those that are invasive, such as arterial cannulation and central venous and pulmonary arterial catheterization. This chapter will concentrate on invasive monitoring during and after cardiac surgery.

ARTERIAL BLOOD PRESSURE

Direct measurement of arterial blood pressure is essential in cardiac surgery in which beat-to-beat pressure must be continuously monitored to detect and treat rapid changes that may occur. Arterial cannulation also allows ready access to blood sampling for blood gas analysis, electrolyte and glucose determinations, and assessment of anticoagulation and coagulopathies. In addition, detailed visual analysis of the arterial waveform can provide information about cardiovascular function. The upstroke of the pulse pressure wave is related to aortic blood flow acceleration and reflects the rate of rise of left ventricular pressure. The peak of the waveform corresponds to the ejection of blood from the left ventricle and volume displacement within the aorta. The downslope of the pulse pressure is interrupted by the dicrotic notch and a decline in the amplitude of the pulse pressure to the end of diastole. This segment of the pressure wave correlates with diastolic runoff determined, in part, by systemic vascular resistance. Besides these components of the arterial waveform, marked beat-to-beat changes are associated with cardiac dysfunction or, if seen during ventilation, can indicate hypovolemia, cardiac tamponade, or increased intrathoracic pressure (1).

ARTERIAL CANNULATION

The radial artery is the most common site for arterial blood pressure monitoring during cardiac surgery because it is readily accessible, is large enough to produce accurate pressures (2), and is associated with few significant complications because of adequate collateral flow. Adequacy of collateral circulation to the hand may be determined by the Allen or modified Allen test using Doppler plethysmography (3, 4), finger pulse transducer (5), or pulse oximetry (6) and should be demonstrated prior to cannulation. Factors that might deter selection of a radial artery include lack of collateral circulation through the ulnar artery (abnormal Allen test), Raynaud's phenomenon of the hand or fingers, vasculitis of the extremity, brachial artery cutdown for coronary angiography, stenosis of the subclavian or axillary artery, recent cannulation of the same radial artery, or infection near the cannulation site.

Complications

Major complications of arterial cannulation are ischemia or necrosis secondary to thrombosis (7, 8), embolism, or compartment syndrome from extravasation of intravenous fluids or blood; hemorrhage; hematoma; infection; retrograde air embolism into the central circulation (9); aneurysm; arteriovenous fistula; foreign body from sheared-off end of catheter; and vasovagal syncope. The incidence of radial artery thrombosis, the most frequent complication, has been reduced when 20-gauge, nontapered Teflon catheters are used and left in place for less than 40 hr (10, 11). Another study has demonstrated that the Allen test is not predictive of ischemic damage to the hand and that the size, shape, and material of the catheter do not influence the development of ischemia (12). Other factors that may be associated with abnormal flow are hematoma formation, extracorporeal circulation, female sex, vascular disease of the same extremity, low flow states requiring vasopressors, and surgical trauma to the artery by cutdown or ligation (13). Whenever ischemia occurs, the catheter should be removed immediately. In an attempt to remove intraarterial thrombus, vigorous aspiration is applied during decannulation (14).

Technique of Cannulation

Selection of an appropriate site and good technique are necessary to obtain a high degree of success and low risk of complications in arterial cannulation. The preferred side for cannulation of the radial artery is the nondominant hand unless contraindications or site of surgery (i.e., descending thoracic aortic aneurysm or patent ductus arteriosus) dictate a specific extremity. The patient's hand is extended over a roll of gauze and dorsiflexed at the wrist approximately 60° with both the hand and lower forearm immobilized on a short arm board. The hand is then checked to make sure arterial flow or pulsations are not compromised and the radial artery is located just proximal to the head of the radius. The area is cleansed with providone iodine solution and draped with sterile towels. Under sterile technique, the skin over the artery is infiltrated with 1% lidocaine and nicked with an 18-gauge needle. A short, 20-gauge, nontapered Teflon catheter and needle stylet is inserted at a 15 to 30° angle to the surface of the skin until blood appears in the hub of the needle. The angle between the needle and skin is reduced to 10° and, while the needle is held in a fixed position, the outer catheter is advanced over the needle into the artery. If blood should stop dripping, the needle may have penetrated the back wall and should be removed. The catheter is then pulled back until a brisk spurt of blood occurs and then is advanced slowly up the artery. If there is no return of blood, the needle is advanced farther (through-and-through technique); the catheter can then be successfully advanced when blood return occurs during withdrawal. If the catheter cannot be advanced when pulsatile blood flow is obtained, a 0.021 inch × 35 cm soft-tip guide wire is advanced into the artery. The catheter is then advanced over the guide wire and attached to nondistensible 4-inch extension tubing with a Luer-Lok connection. The wrist is fixed in a neutral position to avoid median nerve damage, and povidone iodine ointment and a sterile dressing are applied at the insertion site.

Alternate Sites

If neither radial artery can be cannulated, alternative sites include the ulnar, brachial, axillary, femoral, dorsalis pedis, and superficial temporal arteries.

Femoral artery cannulation is used as the most frequent alternative to radial artery cannulation (15). Moreover, the femoral artery can be a useful monitoring site during descending thoracic aorta aneurysm to assess distal perfusion. This artery is identified approximately 2 cm below the inguinal ligament and prepared around the insertion site as described for radial artery cannulation. Under sterile technique, the overlying skin is infiltrated with 1% lidocaine. Since the Seldinger technique is used, skin and artery are entered with an 18-gauge needle at about a 45° angle. As soon as blood spurts from the end of the needle, a J-wire is inserted through the needle into the femoral artery and the needle is removed. The wire must pass without any resistance into the lumen of the artery because insertion of the wire against resistance may lead to intramural dissection. After nicking the skin and subcutaneous tissue with a no. 11 blade, a 6- or 8-inch 18-gauge catheter is advanced up the artery. Rarely, arteriosclerosis, tortuosity of the artery, or hematoma can prevent a successful cannulation. The catheter is sutured in place with 3-0 silk and covered with providone iodine ointment and a sterile dressing. Complications of femoral arterial cannulation include thrombosis, embolism, hematoma, hemorrhage, dissection, arteriovenous fistula, aneurysm, pseudoaneurysm, and sepsis.

The technique, contraindications, and complications for ulnar artery cannulation are similar to those for the radial artery. It may be the preferred cannulation site when the palmar arch is supplied primarily by the radial artery. Although the brachial artery is a larger-diameter vessel and can be successfully used for monitoring in cardiac surgery (16, 17) additional risk occurs because of lack of collateral flow to the hand and thromboemboli resulting in radial or ulnar artery occlusion. The axillary artery can be cannulated using the Seldinger technique, as a 6- or 8-inch 18-gauge Teflon catheter is inserted into the aortic arch via the axillary artery (18, 19). Complications include embolism, direct injury to the brachial plexus, and axillary sheath hematoma with brachial plexus compression. Because of anticoagulation and bleeding diathesis during and after cardiac surgery, the axillary artery is avoided as a site for intraarterial monitoring. Although cannulation of the dorsalis pedis artery is another alternative to radial artery cannulation (20), this site is not

preferred because of discrepancies of systolic and diastolic pressure with aortic pressure and the high incidence of thrombotic occlusion (21).

Sources of Error

Direct measurement of BP requires a catheter, stopcock, fluid-filled extension tubing, continuous flush device, pressure transducer, and pressure monitor with display. The major problems of accurate BP measurement with this system are (a) improper baseline zero and baseline drift, (b) improper transducer or monitor calibration (c) inadequate dynamic response, and (d) improepr determination of derived data from the available pressure signals (22, 23). The disparity between direct and indirect pressure measurements can be minimized by observing the following: (a) allow the transducer and amplifier to warm up at least 10 min before establishing baseline zero and calibration; (b) mechanically zero the transducer; (c) electrically zero and calibrate the recording system with a mercury manometer; (d) frequently recheck the mechanical and electrical zero position and recalibrate during surgery; (e) use stiff, noncompliant extension tubing of shortest possible length (24); (f) avoid the use of more than one stopcock between the catheter and transducer; (g) keep the tubing stopcocks, and domes completely free of bubbles; (h) avoid aspirating blood samples the full length of tubing; (i) flush the catheter so that clotting does not occur; (j) use the transducer with the highest frequency response; and (k) ensure that the recorded waveforms and derived parameters are adequate by using a fast-flush test (25).

CENTRAL VENOUS PRESSURE MONITORING

Normal Venous Waveform

The central venous pressure (CVP) is an indicator of right ventricular preload in a supine patient and reflects the balance between blood volume, venous capacitance, and cardiac function. If the right ventricular function, pulmonary vascular resistance, and mitral valve are normal, the CVP also provides an estimate of left ventricular preload (26). Besides pressure measurements, CVP monitoring allows observation of venous waveform and respiratory fluctuation, venous access for rapid infusion of fluids, administration of vasoactive drugs and pharmaceutical agents with undesirable effects in high concentration, removal of autologous blood, and aspiration of air emboli.

The normal CVP tracing consists of three positive waves (a, c, and v) and two negative descents (x and y). The a wave is produced by retrograde transmission of the pulse pressure resulting from right atrial contraction. With atrial relaxation, the venous pulse descends from the summit of the a wave and is interrupted by a second positive venous pulse, the c wave. This wave is most likely produced by right ventricular systole and bulging of the tricuspid valve into the right atrium. Following the summit of the c wave, the venous pulse contour descends and forms the x descent, which is produced by downward displacement of the base of the ventricle and tricuspid valve during ventricular systole and continued atrial relaxation. The v wave is formed by the increasing pressure as blood continues to fill the caval veins and right atrium while the tricuspid valve is closed. After the peak of the v wave is reached, the pressure in the right atrium begins to fall initially as the result of decreased bulging of the tricuspid valve into the right atrium. Shortly afterward, the y descent occurs when the tricuspid valve opens and blood flows into the right ventricle.

Observation and recording of these venous pressure waves can be very useful in cardiac surgery. Large a waves, which are the result of the right atrium contracting against increased resistance, are present with tricuspid or pulmonary stenosis, pulmonary hypertension, and acute pulmonary embolism, whereas absence of the a wave is observed with atrial fibrillation. Cannon a waves occur when the right atrium contracts against a closed tricuspid valve and can be regular or irregular. Regular cannon waves are seen in nodal rhythm and 2:1 atrioventricular block with or without tachycardia. Irregular cannon waves are associated with complete heart block, ventricular tachycardia, and ventricular pacemaker. In cardiac tamponade and constrictive pericarditis, the right atrial, right ventricular end diastolic, pulmonary artery diastolic,

and pulmonary wedge pressures are elevated and nearly equal except, for example, when blood clots produce localized tamponade. In constrictive pericarditis, x and y descents are exaggerated and very rapid, while the prominent y descent is absent in cardiac tamponade. When large v waves are seen, the diagnosis of tricuspid regurgitation should be considered.

For CVP monitoring, the central venous catheter is connected with extension tubing to a properly calibrated transducer placed at the level of the right atrium or midaxillary line and is displayed on a recorder. Normal mean central venous pressure measured at end expiration is 3 mm Hg with a range of 1 to 7 mm Hg. However, measurements can be interpreted only within the context of overall cardiovascular function and with a thorough understanding of the limitations and possible errors in measurement.

Technique of Cannulation

Numerous routes for central venous catheterization include the internal and external jugular, median basilic, subclavian, and femoral veins. The internal jugular vein is the usual choice for central venous cannulation during cardiac surgery because of accessibility to the anesthesiologist, high success rate, low incidence of complications, and suitability for longterm catheterization. The right side is preferred because it is a relatively straight line to the superior vena cava and right atrium, the dome of the right lung and pleura is lower than on the left side, and the thoracic duct is on the left.

The three main routes for cannulating the right internal jugular vein are the posterior, central, and anterior. Each approach is effective in experienced hands, and the route selected depends on the experience and preference of the operator. The internal jugular vein (Fig. 7.1) runs medial to the sternocleidomastoid muscle in its upper part and under the medial portion of the clavicular head of the sternocleidomastoid muscle in its lower part. The carotid artery is consistently deep and medial to the internal jugular vein as both are contained within the cartoid sheath.

The patient is first attached to an ECG for

FIGURE 7.1

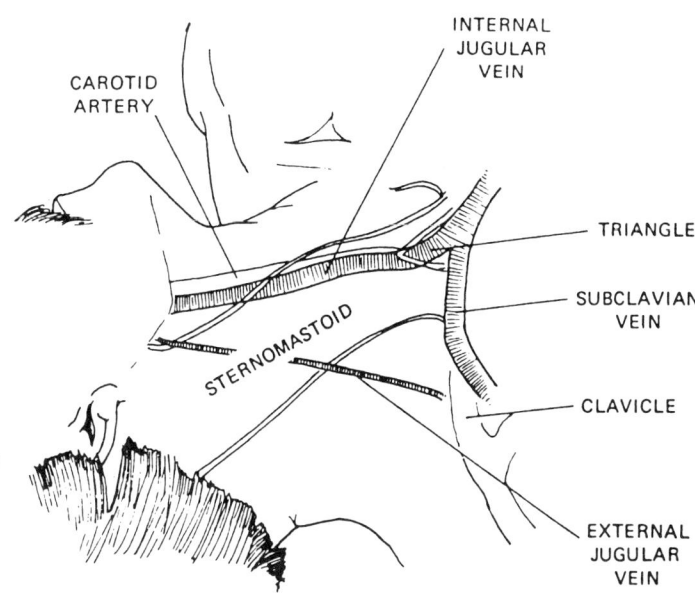

Anatomy of neck and upper thorax demonstrating relationships to internal jugular vein.

continuous monitoring throughout the procedure. The patient is then placed in a 15° Trendelenburg position with the neck extended and turned toward the left. Because of a high incidence of hypoxemia during insertion of monitoring lines after morphine and scopolamine premedication, arterial oxygen saturation should be continuously monitored with a pulse oximeter, and supplemental oxygen should be administered to maintain SaO_2 at 95% or higher (27). Sufficient premedication and local anesthesia by experienced personnel should minimize increases in blood pressure and heart rate during the insertion of lines (28). After the area has been prepared with antiseptic solution, the surrounding area is covered with sterile drapes and sterile technique is maintained throughout the procedure. Regardless of approach, the skin and subcutaneous tissue are then infiltrated with 1% lidocaine.

In the posterior approach (Fig. 7.2), a 25-gauge, 1½-inch exploring needle is introduced under the lateral border of the sternocleidomastoid muscle about 5 cm above the clavicle or just above the point where the external jugular vein crosses the sternocleidomastoid muscle. The needle is advanced caudally and

ventrally toward the suprasternal notch at an angle of 45° to the sagittal and horizontal planes and 15° forward angulation in the frontal plane. This should allow entry of the vein within 5 to 7 cm (29, 30).

With the central approach (Fig. 7.3), the needle is inserted at the apex of the triangle formed by the two heads of the sternocleidomastoid muscle and the clavicle and directed caudally and laterally toward the ipsilateral nipple at a 45° angle with the frontal plane. If the carotid artery pulse is located within the triangle, the artery should be retracted medially so that inadvertent puncture is avoided. If the vein is not entered after a few centimeters, the needle should be reinserted and advanced 5 to 10° more in the lateral direction (31–33).

With the anterior approach (Fig. 7.4), the left index and middle fingers are placed on the carotid artery, which is retracted medially from the medial border of the sternocleidomastoid muscle at the level of the superior border of the thyroid cartilage. The needle is advanced inferiorly and laterally under the posterior aspect of the muscle and enters the internal jugular vein at its widest diameter (34, 35).

After identifying the vein with the exploring

FIGURE 7.2

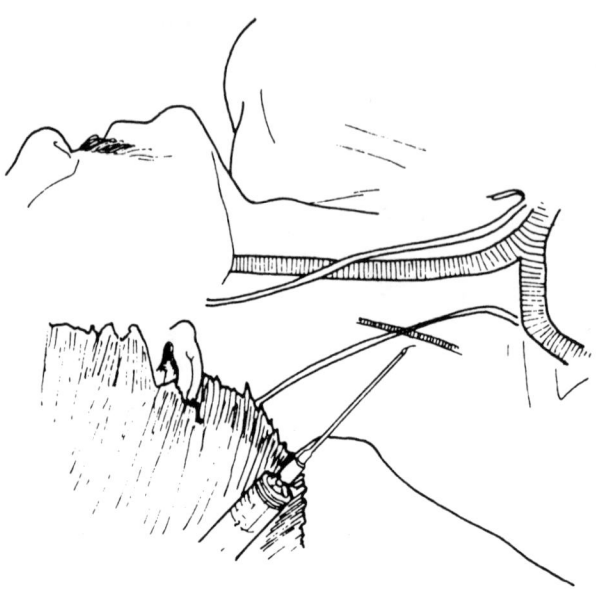

Posterior approach for internal jugular venipuncture.

needle, an 18-gauge, 2½-inch, thin-wall needle is advanced while maintaining a slight negative pressure on the syringe as a pop through the carotid sheath and vein wall is usually felt. If blood has not been aspirated after advancement of the needle, the needle should be slowly withdrawn while maintaining negative pressure, as the needle may have penetrated the back wall

FIGURE 7.3

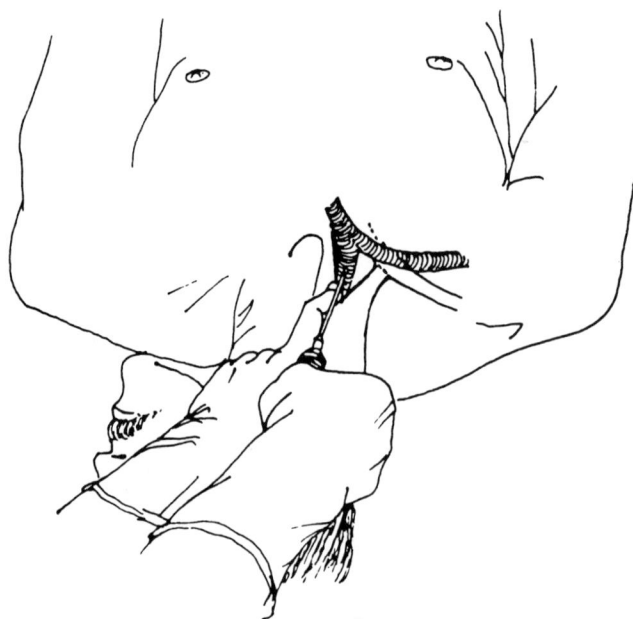

Central approach for internal jugular venipuncture.

FIGURE 7.4

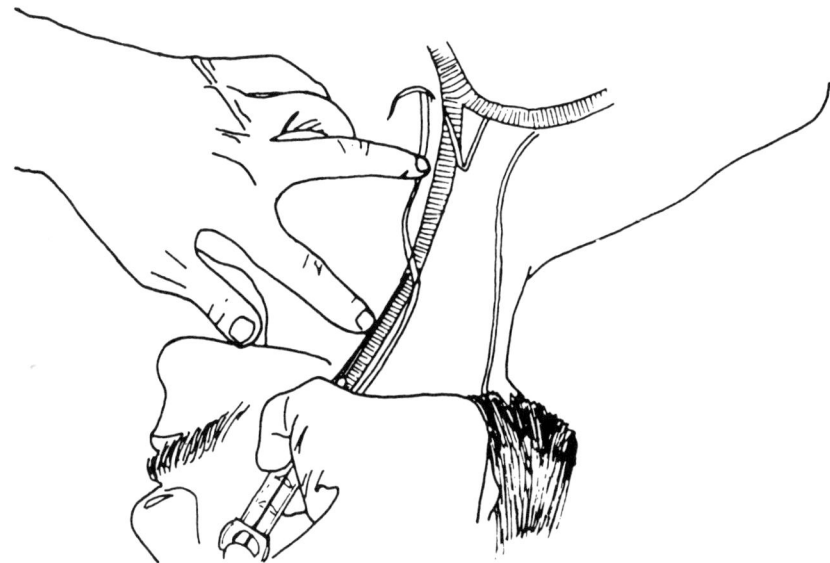

Anterior approach for internal jugular venipuncture.

of the vein. Occasionally a steeper Trendelenburg position or a Valsalva maneuver by the patient will distend the vein. When blood is aspirated, heparin flush solution (5000 units of heparin in 500 ml of normal saline) remaining in the syringe will make the entering blood initially appear bright red, but venous-colored blood will be evident as additional blood is withdrawn. Occasionally the color of the aspirated blood can be deceptive as the PVO_2 will be elevated because the patient is breathing supplemental oxygen or has a high cardiac output or, conversely, the arterial blood may be desaturated. If there is any question of the venous location of the needle in the absence of pulsatile flow, the pressure waveform can be checked by connecting the needle to a transducer or the PO_2 of the blood from the needle can be compared to the PaO_2 from the arterial line. If numerous attempts at identifying the right internal jugular vein fail, ultrasonic localization of the vein can facilitate central venous cannulation (36, 37).

After entering the vein, a 0.035-inch × 45-cm J-wire or 0.035-inch × 40-cm straight guide wire is passed through the needle into the vein approximately 20 cm (Seldinger technique). The needle is removed over the guide wire and a 2- to 3-mm puncture of the skin around the guide wire is made with a no. 11 scalpel blade. A 14-gauge, 12-cm polyurethane catheter is threaded over the guide wire and advanced with a rotary motion to aid passage through tissue into the vein. The guide wire is removed and extension tubing with a stopcock and syringe are attached to the hub of the catheter. Blood is then aspirated to verify free flow from the catheter and a dilute heparin flush solution is used to clear the tubing of aspirated blood. An intravenous infusion or extension tube with transducer is then attached to the CVP line. A 4-0 silk suture secures the hub of the catheter to prevent accidental removal, and the insertion site is cleaned of blood and allowed to dry. A small amount of povidone iodine ointment and a water-vapor-permeable, transparent, adhesive membrane is applied over the skin and catheter.

Success of internal jugular venous cannulation in adults is 90 to 98% and the complication rate is 2 to 3%. Principal complications include carotid artery puncture, pneumothorax, local or systemic infection, air embolism, catheter shearing, brachial plexus injury, Horner's syndrome, hydrothorax, hemothorax, cardiac tamponade, tracheal laceration, hematoma causing respiratory distress or vocal cord paralysis, arteriovenous fistula, thrombosis of the internal jugular vein, and ventricular or supraventricular arrhythmias (38).

Alternate Sites

The external jugular vein is the main alternate site for central venous cannulation. Although external jugular vein cannulation is satisfactory, the success rates are lower than for internal jugular vein cannulation and it presents a less reliable conduit for pulmonary artery catheterization.

The external jugular vein begins at the angle of the mandible and runs obliquely across the body of the sternocleidomastoid muscle toward the middle of the clavicle where it penetrates the deep fascia of the subclavian triangle and enters the subclavian vein. After preparation of the patient as discussed previously, the vein is fixed and distended with the left index finger, and an 18-gauge, 1¼-inch needle is inserted into the vein. Difficulty in cannulation can occur because the vessel is thin-walled and movable in the subcutaneous tissue. When free flow of blood is aspirated, a 0.035-inch × 45-cm flexible J-tipped wire is advanced through the needle into the external jugular and subclavian veins. Because of venous valves and acute angulation where the external jugular vein joins the subclavian vein, rotating the J-wire while simultaneously moving the wire in and out or internally rotating the ipsilateral shoulder with upward pressure on the scapula can facilitate passage of the guide wire. The CVP catheter is attached to tubing with a stopcock and syringe, secured with sutures, and dressed with sterile technique as previously described. Success rates of 70 to 95% are reported in adults using the J-wire (39, 40). Complications include local hematoma, thrombosis of the vein, perforation of the vessel wall, sepsis, and vein wall entrapment between the guide wire and needle wall (41).

When a neck vein on either side is not available, other choices for central venous cannulation include the subclavian, basilic, and femoral veins. With the infraclavicular subclavian approach, the patient is prepared under sterile conditions and placed in Trendelenburg position with the head turned away from the venipuncture site. The needle is inserted 1 cm below the junction of the middle and medial third of the clavicle and advanced medially and slightly cephalad behind the clavicle toward the posterior-superior aspect of the sternal end of the clavicle in the frontal plane. Once the vein has been entered and blood aspirated, the bevel of the needle should be rotated caudally so the guide wire can be inserted into the brachiocephalic vein. Although the success rate is 80 to 95%, specific complications of this approach include pneumothorax, hemothorax from subclavian artery puncture, subclavian arteriovenous fistula, subclavian vein thrombosis, mediastinal hemorrhage, and air entrainment through the puncture site around the catheter (42–44).

Basilic vein cannulation has the advantages of simplicity, low complication rate, easily visible landmarks, and cannulation in the sitting position. Disadvantages of this approach include low success rate (60 to 75%), inaccessibility to the anesthesiologist, and the specific complications of thrombophlebitis and hematoma at the puncture site.

The advantages of femoral vein cannulation include simplicity, high success rate, and low immediate complication rate. However, this is rarely used because of inaccessibility to the anesthesiologist and the extremely high incidence of later complications, which include deep vein thrombosis or thrombophlebitis, pulmonary embolism, and sepsis.

PULMONARY ARTERY CATHETERIZATION

The introduction of the balloon-tipped thermodilution pulmonary artery (Swan-Ganz) catheter has been one of the major advances in the perioperative care of the cardiac surgical patient. By measuring the right atrial pressure, pulmonary arterial pressure, pulmonary capillary wedge pressure, and cardiac output, the dynamic variables of systemic and pulmonary vascular resistances, stroke volume index, and stroke work index can be calculated and altered by pharmacologic interventions to achieve a more physiologic state. Commercially available systems incorporating a hand-held programmable calculator can derive these variables and permit digital and graphic display of ventricular function curves and indices of cardiovascular performance (45). Moreover, samples of mixed venous blood for measurements of PVO_2, intrapulmonary shunt, and cardiac output by the Fick principle can be obtained and drugs can be administered directly into the pulmonary artery. Waveform analysis can aid in the diagnosis of tricuspid and mitral regurgitation, and oxygen stepup from the right atrium to the right ventricle can be diagnostic of a ventricular septal defect.

Modifications in the catheter allow on-line mixed venous oxygen saturation (46), atrial and ventricular pacing (47), measurement of right ventricular ejection fraction (48), monitoring of the intracardiac electrogram (49), performance of angiography (50, 51), calculation of lung water (52), and detection and aspiration of venous air emboli (53, 54).

Indications for preoperative insertion of the pulmonary artery (PA) catheter in cardiac surgery differ among anesthesiologists, cardiologists, and cardiac surgeons. Indications used at the author's center for pulmonary artery catheterization are listed in Table 7.1. Preinduction insertion allows the cardiovascular team to follow hemodynamic measurements in the awake supine position, during anesthetic induction, during endotracheal intubation, during the prebypass and postbypass periods, and in the intensive care unit.

Technique of Cannulation

The patient is first attached to an ECG for continuous monitoring throughout the procedure. Defibrillation and synchronized cardioversion equipment should be available for immediate use. Sites for insertion of the PA catheter are identical to those described for central venous cannulation. Because of the high success rate and accessibility to the anesthesiologist, the right internal jugular vein is preferred. After the initial steps of locating and inserting an 18-gauge, 2½-inch, thin-wall needle into the vein (as described previously in cannulation techniques for CVP monitoring),

TABLE 7.1

INDICATIONS FOR PULMONARY ARTERY CATHETERIZATION DURING CARDIAC SURGERY

1. Coronary artery revascularization with
   a. Poor left ventricular function (left ventricular ejection fraction <0.4, left ventricular end-diastolic pressure >16 mm Hg, cardiac index <2 liters/min/m², stroke volume index <35 ml/beat, left ventricular end-diastolic pressure increases more than 10 mm Hg during the ventriculogram)
   b. Left main coronary lesion
   c. Recent myocardial infarction (<6 months)
   d. Complications of myocardial infarction (ventricular septal defect, mitral regurgitation, ventricular aneurysm or pseudoaneurysm, rupture of the free wall of the ventricle, Dressler's syndrome with moderate to severe pericardial effusion, cardiogenic shock, right ventricular infarction)
   e. Ischemic papillary muscle dysfunction
   f. Diffuse coronary artery atherosclerosis in the distal vessels where inadequate myocardial preservation with cold cardioplegic solution or incomplete revascularization is expected
2. Significant aortic or mitral disease
3. Tricuspid insufficiency
4. Pulmonary hypertension
5. Intraaortic balloon counterpulsation
6. Hemodynamic instability
7. Hypertrophic obstructive cardiomyopathy
8. Cardiac tamponade
9. Pericardiectomy in patients with chronic constrictive pericarditis or cardiac tamponade
10. Patients undergoing arrhythmia surgery (intraoperative electrophysiologic mapping with ventricular resection or implantation of automatic implantable defibrillator or both), especially with poor left ventricular function
11. Thoracic aortic aneurysm

a 0.035-inch × 40-cm, straight, flexible guide wire is inserted through the needle and advanced approximately 20 cm into the vein. After removing the needle, a no. 11 scalpel blade is used to widen the puncture site around the guide wire. If the blade has not been inserted directly against the wire or the slit around the guide wire is too small, a skin tag or subcutaneous tissue will prevent easy passage of the dilator and sheath. A size 8.5 French sheath and dilator are placed over the guide wire; the external tip of the guide wire must extend above the dilator where it can be held and eventually withdrawn. The dilator-sheath assembly is inserted through the skin and advanced with a twisting motion through the subcutaneous tissue to facilitate entry into the vein. After the assembly is in the vein, the sheath is advanced while grasping the dilator and guide wire. This prevents catheter embolism and ensures that the flexible catheter, rather than the stiffer dilator, will come in contact with and not rupture the thin vein wall (this is especially important when inserting the assembly in the left internal jugular vein). When the sheath is inserted to 10 cm, its placement is verified by aspirating venous blood through the side port.

The PA catheter is tested before insertion by (*a*) inflating the balloon to the recommended inflation volume to check for air leaks, (*b*) connecting the catheter connector cable from the cardiac output computer to the thermistor attachment of the pulmonary artery catheter to check electrical integrity, and (*c*) flushing the CVP (proximal) and PA (distal) lumens with heparinized saline, which removes air bubbles. With the pressure transducer open to the fluid-filled PA lumen, a pressure tracing that reflects motion of the catheter tip is seen on the oscilloscope screen.

The curved tip of the catheter should be inserted into the introducer sheath at a 10 o'clock position, which is the orientation of the right ventricle to the right atrium. Once the catheter is past 20 cm, the balloon should be inflated with 1.5 ml of air. Blood should be aspirated from the PA lumen to ensure there are no air bubbles. Location of the catheter tip in a central vein can be verified by pressure changes related to respiration or coughing. When the right atrium is entered, venous waveforms can be visualized. As the catheter is advanced into the right ventricle and pulmonary artery, characteristic phasic pressures are visualized. The catheter is then slowly advanced until it wedges in a branch of the pulmonary artery. Approximate distances from various insertion sites are listed in Table 7.2. If the catheter wedges at 43 cm or less, inaccurate thermodilution cardiac output measurements can occur since the right atrial port is inside the introducer sheath and located near the venous infusion port or side arm of the introducer sheath (55). Proper placement in the wedge position is documented by (*a*) the char-

TABLE 7.2

DISTANCE TO RIGHT ATRIUM, RIGHT VENTRICLE, AND PULMONARY ARTERY

Vein	Right Atrium	Right Ventricle	Pulmonary Artery
	cm	*cm*	*cm*
Internal jugular			
Right	20	30	45
Left	25	35	50
Antecubital			
Right	40	50	65
Left	45	55	70
Femoral	30	40	50
Subclavian	15	25	40

acteristic atrial pressure pattern transmitted retrograde from the left atrium, (*b*) the withdrawal of arterialized blood from the PA lumen, and (*c*) a mean pressure lower than the mean pulmonary arterial pressure. Deflation of the balloon identifies a typical phasic pulmonary arterial tracing. Once the catheter is satisfactorily positioned, a sterile sleeve is secured over the PA catheter to allow for sterile repositioning. The sheath is then secured to the skin with a suture to avoid dislodgment, and the puncture site is covered with a sterile dressing.

Right heart catheterization is usually accomplished in less than 2 min. However, difficult passage of the PA catheter can occur in low cardiac output states, tricuspid regurgitation, pulmonary hypertension, or congenital cardiac defects. Advancement of the catheter can be facilitated by (*a*) passing the catheter during deep inspiration which increases blood flow through the right heart, (*b*) using a different orientation of the catheter tip, (*c*) changing the patient to a 5° head-up and right lateral tilt position, (*d*) rotating the catheter during its passage, (*e*) flushing the catheter with cold solution to stiffen it, and (*f*) using the maximum recommended inflation volume in the balloon. When the catheter becomes more compliant at body temperature or the right ventricular end-diastolic volume is decreased, the catheter can advance into a continuous or intermittent wedge position (especially during positive pressure ventilation) and must be withdrawn to prevent pulmonary infarction.

Continuous analysis of the pulmonary artery

waveform and pressure is important to detect inadvertent wedging and errors in measurement. Technical difficulties leading to inaccurate measurement include improperly calibrated transducer, air bubbles in the transducer or tubing, inaccurate zero reference point, distant location of the PA catheter tip relative to the left atrial level, overwedging, changes in intramural pressure with respiration, and clotting within or at the tip of the catheter.

Complications

The most frequent complications of PA monitoring (excluding those mentioned with central venous cannulation) include air embolism, arrhythmias, conduction disturbances, intracardiac knotting, pulmonary artery perforation, thromboembolism, pulmonary infarction, infection, balloon rupture, and failure to advance the catheter in the pulmonary artery.

Although documented cases of air emboli during insertion are rare (56, 57), this complication can be minimized by (a) placing the insertion site below the level of the right atrium to increase venous pressure (Trendelenburg position for internal jugular or subclavian vein cannulation), (b) removing the guide wire or dilator or both during a Valsalva maneuver in a spontaneously breathing patient or during a positive-pressure breath in a patient on controlled mechanical ventilation, (c) reducing the time the hub of a needle or cannula in a vein is open to the atmosphere by keeping the hub occluded by a syringe or gloved finger, and (d) using a self-sealing valve in the sheath. Rupture of the balloon with introduction of small volumes of air into the venous system can lead to coronary or cerebral ischemia in patients with right-to-left intracardiac shunts. Predisposing factors leading to balloon rupture include excessive storage temperatures and exceeding the maximum inflation volume of the balloon (58). Failure to wedge, absence of inflation resistance, lack of spontaneous air return into the inflating syringe, or blood appearing at the inflation port indicates balloon rupture. When this complication occurs, the stopcock is turned off to the patient and the catheter is removed as early as possible. If the PA catheter is needed in a patient with an intracardiac right-to-left shunt, carbon dioxide can be used for balloon inflation to protect against systemic air embolism.

Transient atrial and ventricular premature contractions are common during catheter insertion. Nonsustained ventricular tachycardia is not uncommon, but atrial or ventricular fibrillation is rare (59, 60). Prophylactic lidocaine has been shown to be ineffective in preventing arrhythmias during preoperative insertion (61). Balloon inflation prevents the tip of the catheter from contacting the ventricular endocardium and should reduce the incidence of arrhythmias; however, the balloon or free portion of the catheter, especially if coiled, will stimulate arrhythmias. To minimize supraventricular arrhythmias, the balloon should be inflated at 20 cm and passed quickly through the right atrium and ventricle under continuous ECG monitoring. When ventricular tachycardia occurs, the balloon should be deflated and the catheter withdrawn into the superior vena cava. Persistent ventricular tachycardia should be treated with intravenous lidocaine (1 mg/kg) or electrical cardioversion.

During passage through the right ventricle, approximately 5% of patients will sustain a transient right bundle-branch block due to contact with the septum. In patients with preexisting left bundle-branch block, there is a relatively high incidence of developing complete heart block (5 to 20%) (62). In this subset of patients, a multipurpose (pacing) Swan-Ganz catheter or pacing electrode can be used prophylactically. Left fascicular or left bundle-branch block can also occur with PA catheter insertion, as trauma to the bundle of His has been implicated (63).

Coils and knots of the catheter can cause arrhythmias and conduction disturbances and prevent transmission of pressure tracings or proper placement of the catheter tip (64). Coiling of the catheter should be suspected when an unusually long length of catheter is needed (10 cm greater than the normal distance expected from the insertion site to right atrium, right ventricle, pulmonary artery, and wedge position) or when recurrent ventricular arrhythmias occur with pressure tracing indicating the tip of the catheter in the right atrium. To avoid knotting, the catheter should be withdrawn and stiffened with cold flush solution. Success is enhanced when the catheter is reoriented and the patient is repositioned. Occasionally, knots may incorporate papillary muscle, chordae tendineae, or cardiac pacemaker leads or rupture a tricuspid leaflet (65). Knots are verified from postinsertion x-rays and resistance during catheter withdrawal. Although the knot may be tightened into the sheath and withdrawn, most are removed with fluoroscopic techniques or operative intervention (66, 67).

Pulmonary artery perforation is a rare but well-known serious complication. Hemoptysis related to balloon inflation, catheter manipulation, or flushing the catheter in a wedge position is a common manifestation. Risk factors include advanced age, pulmonary hypertension, hypothermia, and female sex. Additional technical factors include numerous and prolonged inflation times, inflation of a wedged catheter, eccentric balloon inflation, initial balloon inflation with a small volume of air associated with subsequent migration of the PA catheter into a smaller vessel, high balloon pressure during inflation, distal catheter tip migration during balloon deflation, and larger pressure gradients across the inflated balloon in pulmonary hypertensive patients (68–70).

To minimize the occurrence of this complication, several precautions should be taken. When the PA catheter is initially inserted, 1.5 ml of air is used to inflate the balloon so the catheter does not pass into a smaller, more distal vessel. When a wedge pressure is required, the catheter can be advanced if necessary to the wedge position through a sterile external sheath that protects the catheter. Because of catheter tip migration, the minimum balloon volume needed to obtain a wedge pressure should be used with each measurement rather than some fixed predetermined volume. To minimize the number of subsequent balloon inflations, routine wedge pressures prior to cardiopulmonary bypass are not recommended if the initial pulmonary artery diastolic pressure agrees with the pulmonary capillary wedge pressure in the absence of increased pulmonary vascular resistance. Since distal catheter migration occurs during bypass and upward retraction of the heart, the PA catheter should be withdrawn 5 cm prior

to bypass (71). After bypass, the catheter should be carefully repositioned since there is frequently an increased pulmonary artery diastolic–wedge pressure difference due to changes in pulmonary vascular resistance (72). Unless a phasic pulmonary artery pressure is visible, the balloon should not be inflated because a and v waves from a wedge tracing may incorrectly give the appearance of a pulmonary artery pressure tracing. Overwedging from a distal location of the catheter tip results from impingement of the tip against the vessel wall or herniation of the balloon over the catheter tip and warrants immediate withdrawal of the catheter until a normal wedge tracing is seen.

If massive intrabronchial bleeding occurs, treatment includes insertion of a double-lumen endotracheal tube with isolation of the bleeding lung or advancement of a single-lumen endotracheal tube advanced into the main-stem bronchus of the noninvolved lung, reversal of heparin anticoagulation, blood and fluid replacement, positive end-expiratory pressure applied to the involved lung to compress the bleeding sites, and surgical intervention (68).

As with any foreign object in the vascular system, the catheter serves as a nidus for clot propagation. Several studies have documented that PA catheters are thrombogenic and may be the source of pulmonary embolism (73, 74). The incidence of thrombus formation is a function of the time the catheter remains within the patient, the presence of a coagulopathy (i.e., disseminated intravascular coagulation) or hypercoagulable state, low cardiac output, congestive heart failure, catheter material, and intimal damage. The thrombi can be the cause of damped pressure tracings, degraded thermistor performance with inability to detect temperature changes during cardiac output measurements, and inability to aspirate blood for venous sampling. Although the morbidity from these clots is unknown, internal jugular (29, 75) or subclavian (76) vein thrombosis is seen at the insertion site and may result in the development of upper extremity edema, neck pain, or venous distension. Prophylactic measures to decrease thromboembolic complilcations include heparin impregnation of the catheter (77), heparin flush solutions, systemic heparinization, and removal of the catheter after 24 to 48 hr. In addition to clot formation, thrombocytopenia has been related to PA catheterization in humans (78). Although its clinical relevance is unknown, it may be one of the many factors leading to thrombocytopenia and postoperative bleeding in cardiac surgical patients.

Pulmonary infarction may result from catheter occlusion of a branch of the pulmonary artery, migration of catheter-induced thrombus during removal, emboli from in situ catheter or venous thrombi, guide wire embolism, latex embolism from a deteriorating balloon, thrombotic endocardial vegetations, and right-sided endocarditis (79, 80). To diminish this complication, balloon inflation periods should be as short as possible; the number of balloon inflations should be minimized; the PA catheter should be withdrawn when spontaneous catheter wedging occurs; heparin-bonded PA catheters should be used; and the use of the balloon lumen valve should be avoided.

Infectious complications include bacterial colonization, contamination, cellulitis, thrombophlebitis, bacteremia, septic shock, and endocarditis (81–83). Infections can be minimized by inserting the catheter and performing thermodilution cardiac output with aseptic technique; by changing dressings, infusion sets, transducers, and calibration equipment daily; and by removing the catheter within 72 hr. If sepsis develops in spite of appropriate antibiotics or without any obvious source of infection, the central lines should be removed. If the PA catheter is necessary for monitoring, the replacement should be inserted at a later time through a new site.

Uncommon complications associated with PA catheters include Horner's syndrome, nerve injury, catheter fracture, bradycardia secondary to cardiac output measurement, arteriovenous fistula, suturing the catheter to a vessel or the heart, freezing a segment of the catheter to the heart during cryoblation, intraoperative transection of the catheter, starch thrombosis, and decreases in arterial oxygen partial pressure or end tidal concentration of carbon dioxide during balloon inflation (84–88).

Since the benefit of monitoring must be weighed against the many potential complications and added cost factor to the patient, future methods for assessing ventricular function and ischemic regional wall motion abnormalities should be noninvasive, portable, inexpensive, risk-free, rapid, and applicable to the perioperative cardiac surgical patient. Techniques currently being investigated include two-dimensional transesophageal echocardiography, cardiokymography, and radionuclide scintigraphy. In spite of these numerous technological advances, the bedside clinician still remains the mainstay for diagnosis and decision making in cardiac surgery.

References

1. Brunner JMR: *Handbook of Blood Pressure Monitoring.* Littleton, MA, PSG Publishing, 1978, p 174.
2. Ryan JF, Raines J, Dalton BC, et al: Arterial dynamics of radial artery cannulation. *Anesth Analg* 52:1017–1025, 1973.
3. Mozersky DJ, Buckley CJ, Hagood CO Jr, et al: Ultrasonic evaluation of the palmar circulation. A useful adjunct to radial artery cannulation. *Am J Surg* 126:810–812, 1973.
4. Kamienski RW, Barnes RW: Critique of the Allen test for continuity of the palmar arch assessed by Doppler ultrasound. *Surg Gynecol Obstet* 142:861–864, 1976.
5. Brodsky JB: A simple method to determine patency of the ulnar artery intraoperatively prior to radial artery cannulation. *Anesthesiology* 42:626–627, 1975.
6. Nowak GS, Moorthy SS, McNiece WL: Use of pulse oximetry for assessment of collateral arterial flow. *Anesthesiology* 64:527, 1986.
7. Bedford RF, Wollman H: Complications of radial artery cannulation. *Anesthesiology* 38:228–236, 1973.
8. Downs JB, Rackstein AD, Klein EF, et al: Hazards of radial artery catheterization. *Anesthesiology* 38:283–286, 1973.
9. Lowenstein E, Little JW, Lo HH: Prevention of cerebral embolization from flushing radial artery cannulas. *N Engl J Med* 285:1414–1415, 1971.
10. Bedford RF: Radial arterial function following percutaneous cannulation with 18- and 20-gauge catheters. *Anesthesiology* 47:37–39, 1977.
11. Bedford RF: Percutaneous radial artery cannulation. Increased safety using Teflon catheters. *Anesthesiology* 42:219–222, 1975.
12. Slogoff S, Keats AS, Arlund C: On the safety

of radial artery cannulation. *Anesthesiology* 59:42–47, 1983.

13. Kim JM, Arakawa K, Bliss J: Arterial cannulation: factors in the development of occlusion. *Anesth Analg* 54:836–841, 1975.

14. Bedford RF: Removal of radial artery thrombi following percutaneous cannulation for monitoring. *Anesthesiology* 46:430–432, 1977.

15. Colvin MP, Curran JP, Jarvis D, et al: Femoral artery pressure monitoring. Use of the Seldinger technique. *Anaesthesia* 32:451–455, 1977.

16. Barnes RW, Foster EJ, Janssen GA, et al: Safety of brachial artery catheters as monitors in the intensive care unit—prospective evaluation with the Doppler ultrasonic velocity detector. *Anesthesiology* 44:260–264, 1976.

17. Comstock MK, Ellis T, Carter JG, et al: Safety of brachial vs. radial arterial catheters. *Anesthesiology* 51:S158, 1979.

18. Adler DC, Bryan-Brown CW: Use of the axillary artery for intravascular monitoring. *Crit Care Med* 1:148–150, 1973.

19. DeAngelis J: Axillary arterial monitoring. *Crit Care Med* 4:205–206, 1976.

20. Husum B, Palm T, Ericksen J: Percutaneous cannulation of the dorsalis pedis artery. *Br J Anaesth* 51:1055–1058, 1979.

21. Youngberg JA, Miller ED: Evaluation of percutaneous cannulations of the dorsalis pedis artery. *Anesthesiology* 44:80–83, 1976.

22. Gardner RM, Hollingsworth KW: Optimizing the electrocardiogram and pressure monitoring. *Crit Care Med* 14:651–658, 1986.

23. Toll MO: Direct blood-pressure measurements: Risks, technological evolution and some current problems. *Med Biol Eng Comput* 22:2–5, 1984.

24. Boutros A, Albert S: Effect of the dynamic response of transducer tubing system on accuracy of direct blood pressure measurement in patients. *Crit Care Med* 11:124–127, 1983.

25. Gardner RM: Direct blood pressure measurement—dynamic response requirements. *Anesthesiology* 54:227–236, 1981.

26. Otto CW: Central venous pressure monitoring. In Blitt CD (ed): *Monitoring in Anesthesia and Critical Care Medicine*, New York, Churchill Livingstone, 1985, p 121.

27. Hensley FA Jr, Dodson DL, Martin DE, et al: Oxygen saturation during preinduction placement of monitoring catheters in the cardiac surgical patient. *Anesthesiology* 66:834–836, 1987.

28. Waller JL, Zaidan JR, Kaplan JA, et al: Hemodynamic responses to preoperative vascular cannulation in patients with coronary artery disease. *Anesthesiology* 56:219–221, 1982.

29. Jernigan WR, Gardner WC, Mahr MM, et al: Use of the internal jugular vein for placement of central venous catheter. *Surg Gynecol Obstet* 130:520–524, 1970.

30. Brinkman AJ, Costley DO: Internal jugular venipuncture. *JAMA* 223:182–183, 1973.

31. Daily PO, Griepp RB, Shumway NE: Percutaneous internal jugular vein cannulation. *Arch Surg* 101:534–536, 1970.

32. English ICW, Frew RM, Pigott JF, et al: Percutaneous catheterization of the internal jugular vein. *Anaesthesia* 24:521–531, 1969.

33. Prince SR, Sullivan RL, Hackel A: Percutaneous catheterization of the internal jugular vein in infants and children. *Anesthesiology* 44:170–174, 1976.

34. Mostert JW, Kenny GM, Murphy GP: Safe placement of central venous catheter into internal jugular veins. *Arch Surg* 101:431–432, 1970.

35. Boulanger M, Delva E, Maille JG, et al: Une nouvelle voie d'abord de la veine jugulaire interne. *Can Anaesth Soc J* 23:609–615, 1976.

36. Bazaral M, Harlan S: Ultrasonographic anatomy of the internal jugular vein relevant to percutaneous cannulation. *Crit Care Med* 9:307–310, 1981.

37. Legler D, Nugent M: Doppler localization of the internal jugular vein facilitates central venous cannulation. *Anesthesiology* 60:481–482, 1984.

38. Hug CC Jr: Monitoring. In Miller RD (ed): *Anesthesia*, 3d 2. New York, Churchill Livingstone, 1986, p 411.

39. Giesy J: External jugular vein access to central venous system. *JAMA* 219:1216–1217, 1972.

40. Blitt CD, Wright WA, Petty WC, et al: Central venous catheterization via the external jugular vein: a technique employing the J-wire. *JAMA* 229:817–818, 1974.

41. Hey NT, Mahood JHS, Pictak SP: A complication of external jugular cannulation. *Anesthesiology* 64:836–837, 1986.

42. Moosman DA: The anatomy of infraclavicular subclavian vein catheterization and its complications. *Surg Gynecol Obstet* 136:71–74, 1973.

43. Borja AR, Hinshaw JR: A safe way to perform infraclavicular subclavian vein catheterization. *Surg Gynecol Obstet* 130:673–676, 1970.

44. Kloosterboer TB, Springman SR, Coursin DB: Subclavian vein catheter as a source of air emboli in the sitting position. *Anesthesiology* 64:411, 1986.

45. Barash PG, Chen Y, Kitahata LM, et al: The hemodynamic tracking system: a method of data management and guide for cardiovascular therapy. *Anesth Analg* 59:169–174, 1980.

46. Krauss XH, Verdouw PD, Hugenholtz PG, et al: On-line monitoring of mixed venous oxygen saturation after cardiothoracic surgery. *Thorax* 30:636–643, 1975.

47. Zaidan JR: Experience with the pacing pulmonary artery catheter. *Anesthesiology* 53:S118, 1980.

48. Kay H, Afshari M, Barash P, et al: Measurement of ejection fraction by thermal dilution techniques. *J Surg Res* 34:337–346, 1983.

49. Chatterjee K, Swan HJC, Ganz W, et al: Use of a balloon-tipped flotation electrode catheter for cardiac monitoring. *Am J Cardiol* 36:56–61, 1975.

50. Berry AJ: Pulmonary embolism during spinal anesthesia: angiographic diagnosis via a flow-directed pulmonary artery catheter. *Anesthesiology* 57:57–59, 1982.

51. Orta DA Jr, Eisen S, Yergin BM, et al: Segmental pulmonary angiography in the critically-ill patient using a flow-directed catheter. *Chest* 76:269–273, 1979.

52. Lewis F, Elings VB, Sturm JA: Bedside measurement of lung water. *J Surg Res* 27:250–261, 1979.

53. Bedford RF, Marshall WK, Butler A, et al: Cardiac catheters for diagnosis and treatment of venous air embolism. *J Neurosurg* 55:610–614, 1981.

54. Munson ES, Paul WL, Perry JC, et al: Early detection of venous air embolism using a Swan-Ganz catheter. *Anesthesiology* 42:223–226, 1975.

55. Curley J, Harte F, Sheikle F: Erroneous cardiac output determination due to pulmonary artery catheter proximal port dysfunction. *Anesthesiology* 64:662, 1986.

56. Doblar DD, Hinkle JC, Fay ML, et al: Air embolism associated with pulmonary artery introducer kit. *Anesthesiology* 56:307–309, 1982.

57. Peters JL, Armstrong R: Air embolism occurring as a complication of central venous catheterization. *Ann Surg* 187:375–378, 1978.

58. Latex balloons on wedge-pressure catheters. *Health Devices* 6:123–124, 1977.

59. Sprung CL, Pozen RG, Rozanski JJ, et al: Advanced ventricular arrhythmias during bedside pulmonary artery catheterization. *Am J Med* 72:203–208, 1982.

60. Katz JD, Cronau LH, Barash PG, et al: Pulmonary artery flow-guided catheters in the perioperative period. *JAMA* 237:2832–2834, 1977.

61. Salmenpera M, Peltola K, Rosenberg P: Does prophylactic lidocaine control cardiac arrhythmias associated with pulmonary artery catheterization? *Anesthesiology* 56:210–212, 1982.

62. Thomson IR, Dalton BC, Lappas DG, et al: Right bundle-branch block and complete heart block caused by the Swan-Ganz catheter. *Anesthesiology* 51:359–362, 1979.

63. Castellanos A, Ramirez AV, Mayorga-Cortes A, et al: Left fascicular blocks during right-heart catheterization using the Swan-Ganz catheter. *Circulation* 64:1271–1276, 1981.

64. Iberti TJ, Jayagopal SG: Knotting of a Swan-Ganz catheter in the pulmonary artery. *Chest* 83:711, 1983.

65. Schwartz KV, Garcia FG: Entanglement of Swan-Ganz catheter around an intracardiac structure. *JAMA* 237:1198–1199, 1977.

66. Dach JL, Galbut DL, Lepage JR: The knotted Swan-Ganz catheter: new solution to a vexing problem. *AJR* 137:1274–1275, 1981.

67. Mond HG, Clark DW, Nesbitt SJ, et al: A technique for unknotting an intracardiac flow-directed balloon catheter. *Chest* 67:731–732, 1975.

68. Barash PG, Nardi D, Hammond G, et al: Catheter-induced pulmonary artery perforation. Mechanisms, management, and modifications. *J Thorac Cardiovasc Surg* 82:5–12, 1981.

69. McDonald DH, Zaidan JR: Pressure-volume relationships of the pulmonary artery catheter balloon. *Anesthesiology* 59:240–243, 1983.

70. Johnston WE, Royster RL, Vinten-Johansen J, et al: Influence of balloon inflation and deflation on location of pulmonary artery catheter tip. *Anesthesiology* 67:110–115, 1987.

71. Johnston WE, Royster RL, Choplin RH, et al: Pulmonary artery catheter migration during cardiac surgery. *Anesthesiology* 64:258–262, 1986.

72. Heinon J, Salmenpera M, Takkunen O: Increased pulmonary artery diastolic–pulmonary wedge pressure gradient after cardiopulmonary bypass. *Can Anaesth Soc J* 32:165–170, 1985.

73. Hoar PF, Stone JG, Wicks AE, et al: Thrombogenesis associated with Swan-Ganz catheters. *Anesthesiology* 48:445–447, 1978.

74. Park GR, Scott DHT: Complication of the reuse of flow-directed pulmonary artery catheters. *Br Med J* 284:258–259, 1982.

75. Chastre J, Cornud F, Bouchama A, et al: Thrombosis as a complication of pulmonary-artery catheterization via the internal jugular vein. *N Engl J Med* 306:278–281, 1982.

76. Dye LE, Segall PH, Russell RO Jr, et al: Deep venous thrombosis of the upper extremity associated with use of the Swan-Ganz catheter. *Chest* 73:673–675, 1978.

77. Hoar PF, Wilson RM, Mangano DT, et al: Heparin bonding reduces thrombogenicity of pulmonary artery catheters. *N Engl J Med* 305:993–995, 1981.

78. Kim YL, Richman KA, Marshall BE: Thrombocytopenia associated with Swan-Ganz catheterization in patients. *Anesthesiology* 53:261–262, 1980.

79. Foote GA, Schabel SI, Hodges M: Pulmonary complications of the flow-directed balloon-tipped catheter. *N Engl J Med* 290:927–931, 1974.

80. McCloud TC, Putman CE: Radiology of the Swan-Ganz catheter and associated pulmonary complications. *Radiology* 116:19–22, 1975.

81. Pinilla JC, Ross DF, Martin T, et al: Study of the incidence of intravascular catheter infection and associated septicemia in critically ill patients. *Crit Care Med* 11:21–25, 1983.

82. Singh S, Nelson N, Acosta I, et al: Catheter colonization and bacteremia with pulmonary and arterial catheters. *Crit Care Med* 10:736–739, 1982.

83. Greene JF Jr, Fitzwater JE, Clemmer TP: Septic endocarditis and indwelling pulmonary artery catheters. *JAMA* 233:891–892, 1975.

84. Keefer JR, Barash PG: Pulmonary artery catheterization. In Blitt CD (ed): *Monitoring in Anesthesia and Critical Care Medicine.* New York, Churchill Livingstone, 1985, p 177.

85. Pace NL: A critique of flow-directed pulmonary arterial catheterization. *Anesthesiology* 47:455–465, 1977.

86. Zahl K, Murray T, Jobes DR: Frozen pulmonary artery catheter: a complication associated with cryoablation of the ventricle. *Anesthesiology* 64:662–663, 1986.

87. Kainuma M, Shimada Y: Decreased partial pressure of oxygen in arterial blood secondary to inflation of a pulmonary artery flow-directed catheter balloon. *Anesthesiology* 66:214–216, 1987.

88. Dobi S, Ishizawa Y, Saito S: Changes in pulmonary oxygenation and hemodynamic responses during pulmonary arterial occlusion pressure measurements. *Anesthesiology* 66:216–220, 1987.

Chapter 8
HEMODYNAMIC MANIPULATION OF THE PATIENT DURING ANESTHESIA

ARNOLD S. FRIEDMAN, M.D.
DHUN H. SETHNA, M.D.

Anesthesia for heart disease is complex and has undergone significant evolution with greater understanding of hemodynamic principles, the introduction of new anesthetic agents, and an improved ability to monitor and pharmacologically manipulate the cardiovascular system. To provide circulatory stability the anesthesiologist must (a) understand the pathophysiology of coronary artery and valvular heart disease; (b) know what anesthetic agents, drugs, and surgical interventions alter cardiovascular function; and (c) provide the patient with adequate sedation, analgesia, amnesia, and protection of vital organs. The purpose of this chapter is to provide an appreciation of the approach used in anesthetizing patients with the commonly encountered acquired cardiac diseases undergoing cardiac surgery.

GENERAL CONSIDERATIONS

Anesthesia of the patient scheduled for cardiac surgery is predicated on the history and physical examination, electrocardiogram, chest x-ray, laboratory studies, noninvasive cardiac tests, cardiac catheterization, type of operation, surgeon, and pharmacologic agents used before, during, and after surgery.

Management of Preoperative Drugs

β-Blocker drugs should be maintained up to the morning of surgery because propranolol withdrawal has been associated with intermediate coronary syndrome, myocardial infarction, ventricular arrhythmia, and sudden death (1). These drugs may be further beneficial in reducing perioperative double product (heart rate times systolic blood pressure), arrhythmias, and myocardial ischemia (2). However, they may cause less inotropic response to β-agonist drugs, greater vasoconstriction to α-agonist drugs, and bronchospasm.

Calcium entry blocking drugs are also continued to surgery because abrupt withdrawal has been associated with myocardial ischemia (3), which may be precipitated by α_2-adrenoceptor affinity for agonist and platelet hyperactivity (4). Since smoking-induced coronary vasoconstriction can be prevented by calcium antagonist drugs, their continuation may improve myocardial oxygen supply in cigarette smokers (5). Interaction with anesthetic drugs can occur

(6–8), but therapeutic effects outweigh their potential risks.

Antihypertensive drugs are continued to surgery unless systolic arterial pressure is less than 110 mm Hg because rebound hypertension, myocardial ischemia, and arrhythmias can occur with abrupt withdrawal (9, 10). These medications can also reduce the perioperative hemodynamic instability and dosage of anesthetic drugs (11–15). Diuretics are discontinued the night prior to surgery unless patients have congestive heart failure. This approach avoids loss of potassium and magnesium (especially relevant in digitalized patients) and marked hypovolemia.

Antiarrhythmic drugs should also be prescribed to the time of surgery, with the exception of patients scheduled for intraoperative electrophysiologic studies. It is not clearly known whether volume of distribution or clearance of these drugs requires changes in dosage or dosing schedules in the perioperative period. Effects of antiarrhythmic drugs which could influence anesthetic management during cardiac surgery include augmentation of nondepolarizing neuromuscular blockade (16, 17), enhancement of cardiovascular and electrophysiologic effects of anesthetic agents (18); proarrhythmia induction (19); induced supraventricular arrhythmias in digitalized patients given pancuronium (20); and hypotension associated with bretylium (21).

Patients with atrial fibrillation may be given dioxin the morning of surgery to control ventricular rate. Since digitalis preparations have a low therapeutic to toxic ratio, they are usually discontinued the night prior to surgery in stable patients with chronic congestive heart failure because rhythms related to digitalis toxicity are difficult to diagnose in the perioperative period and are aggravated by intravenous calcium salts or diuretic-induced hypokalemia and hypomagnesemia (22, 23). These arrhythmias include sinus bradycardia, sinoatrial exit block, AV nodal block, atrial or ventricular ectopic beats, junctional tachycardia, paroxysmal atrial tachycardia with AV block, ventricular tachycardia, and ventricular fibrillation (24).

Although nitrate preparations are usually continued until the morning of surgery, it is difficult to recommend a definitive dose or dosage schedule because of nitrate-induced vascular hyporesponsiveness related to sustained plasma and tissue concentrations of nitrate and relative depletion of thiol groups within vascular smooth muscle cells (25). Adverse reactions to nitrates include hypotension, bradycardia, methemoglobinemia (26, 27), prolonged template bleeding time (28), increased intracranial pressure (29), acute ethanol intoxication from the diluent (30), and rash from their topical application.

Intravenous heparin is often continued until surgery in patients with unstable angina. When surgery is anticipated, heparin is substituted for warfarin in patients whose anticoagulation therapy should not be interrupted. Partial thromboplastin times (PTT) are maintained at approximately twice control values in these high-risk patients. In addition to bleeding, complications of heparin include increased oxygen consumption secondary to release of lipoprotein lipase (31), thrombocytopenia due to increased platelet levels of IgG and C_3 (32, 33) and synthesis of thromboxane A_2 by platelets, and neutralization of the antiaggregating effects of PGI_2 (34, 35), which may lead to arterial or venous thrombosis (36).

Premedication

Preoperative medication is given to produce amnesia and reduce anxiety and discomfort associated with invasive monitoring. Choice and dose of drugs are dependent on the patient, type of operation, myocardial function, and coexisting lung or neurologic disease. Patients with normal or moderately depressed left ventricular function and no pulmonary disease should be given heavy premedication with morphine, scopolamine, and a benzodiazepine. When left ventricular or respiratory function is depressed, minimal premedication and reassurance during the preoperative visit can allay anxiety and minimize myocardial oxygen demand. Disadvantages of these drugs include respiratory depression, dysphoria, prolonged postoperative confusion, and an intense antisialagogue action. Supplemental oxygen should be administered because of potential hypoxemia associated with premedication (37).

Monitoring

Intraoperative electrocardiography (ECG) is used for detection of myocardial ischemia, arrhythmias, conduction abnormalities, electrolyte changes, or pacemaker dysfunction and intraaortic balloon triggering. Multiple-lead ECG systems used in the operating room consist of five electrodes allowing seven different ECG leads (I, II, III, aVR, aVL, aVF, and V_5) to be monitored.

Studies in patients undergoing exercise stress testing show that lead V_5 is more sensitive in detecting ST segment abnormalities and reflects disease of the left anterior descending or circumflex coronary arteries (38, 39). Factors influencing the sensitivity and specificity of the ECG for diagnosing myocardial ischemia include depth of horizontal or down-sloping ST segment depression measured 0.08 second after the J point, amplitude of ST segment elevation, integration of all ST amplitude and slope changes during exercise and recovery, and decreased heart rate response to stress (40–43). Evaluation of ST segments may be obscured by drugs and electrolyte abnormalities, conduction disturbances, ventricular hypertrophy, preexcitation syndromes, distortion of the ST segment by low-frequency filters of the ECG circuitry, and size of the QRS tracing on the oscilloscope. Artifacts that may prevent reliable interpretation of myocardial ischemia or stimulate arrhythmias include muscle tremors, movement of the diaphragm, respiratory-induced alterations in electrical axis, loose electrodes or broken leads, faults in ECG monitors, roller pumps of cardiopulmonary bypass machines, electrocautery, or 60 Hz alternating current associated with improper grounding (44–46).

Accurate assessment of ST segment changes requires that the ECG monitor be properly calibrated so that a signal of 1 mV will produce a deflection of 10 mm. The seven leads should be recorded prior to operation for baseline reference. Cardiac surgical patients may arrive in the operating room with greater ST segment depression than was present in their preoperative ECG (47). Two leads (modified V_5, II) should be monitored simultaneously during surgery to enhance detection of ischemia of the anterolateral and inferior myocardial wall (48).

In some patients true posterior and right ventricular ischemia and arrhyrthmias can be diagnosed with an esophageal ECG (49, 50). Recognition and quantitation of ischemia may be facilitated by modified microcomputer-based ECGs with ST segment trend monitoring which allow early ischemia detection and consequent pharmacologic intervention (51, 52). Since perioperative myocardial ischemia as diagnosed by ECG can be associated with higher myocardial infarction rates in patients undergoing myocardial revascularization (47), it is important for anesthesiologists to have a simple, artifact-free, instantaneous ECG to detect early myocardial ischemia. Unfortunately, diagnosing myocardial ischemia by ECG is less sensitive than detection of regional wall motion abnormalities by transesophageal echocardiography (53) or cardiokymography (54).

Intraoperative arrhythmias are frequently seen during anesthesia and occur most commonly with insertion of pulmonary artery catheters, endotracheal intubation and extubation, surgical manipulation of the heart, reperfusion after release of aortic cross-clamp, and episodes of myocardial ischemia. ECG lead II is usually selected for arrhythmia detection since P wave morphology is better visualized and junctional or ventricular rhythms can be more easily identified. Invasive electrocardiographic monitoring, such as esophageal ECG or intracardiac electrograms with a multipurpose pulmonary artery catheter, can enhance diagnosis of complex arrhythmias and heart block (55). Automatic arrhythmia detection systems may enhance the accuracy of arrhythmia detection (56).

Invasive arterial cannulation (see Chapter 7) is necessary for continuous blood pressure monitoring and frequent arterial blood gas measurements. Pulmonary artery catheters (indications during cardiac surgery are listed in Table 7.1) are useful in cardiac surgery because hemodynamic variables can be calculated and altered by pharmacologic interventions to achieve a more physiologic state (57), left ventricular filling pressures can be optimized, and hemodynamic abnormalities can be more readily detected (58). Cost-benefit analysis of hemodynamic invasive monitoring is difficult to ascertain but benefits must be balanced by the potential complications discussed in the previous chapter. These catheters should be placed by experienced personnel using adequate local anesthesia after patients have been effectively premedicated (59). Additional monitoring used during cardiac surgery includes urine output; esophageal, bladder, or rectal temperature; serum electrolyte (potassium, calcium, and sodium) and glucose determinations; tests of coagulation; electroencephalogram (which may detect potential cerebral insult, determine adequate dose of barbiturates for cerebral protection, or monitor anesthetic depth) (60, 61); and measurement of lower esophageal contractility as a reflection of anesthetic depth.

ANESTHETIC INDUCTION AND MAINTENANCE

Patients should be preoxygenated prior to induction of anesthesia, because hypoexmia and hypercarbia from premedications or intravenous sedation can lead to hypertension and tachycardia. Thiopental (1 to 4 mg/kg), diazepam (0.5 mg/kg), midazolam (0.2 mg/kg), and etomidate (0.3 mg/kg) have been used effectively as induction agents in premedicated patients. Supplemental intravenous narcotics (fentanyl, sufentanil, alfentanil) or inhalational anesthetics provide greater anesthetic depth to attenuate reflex response to laryngoscopy and endotracheal intubation, surgical incision, and sternotomy. Doses can be titrated by continuous monitoring of heart rate, arterial and pulmonary capillary wedge pressures, ST segments on ECG, and level of consciousness with consequent changes in sympathetic and parasympathetic tone, and alterations in intravenous volume may lead to hemodynamic instability. Young patients, hypertensives, patients with good left ventricular function, and those not receiving β-blockers or calcium antagonists require greater anesthetic depth to attenuate reflex responses to stimuli. Elderly patients, patients with depressed left ventricular function, and those with diminished coronary vascular reserve usually need smaller doses of anesthetic drugs.

Laryngoscopy and tracheal intubation can cause reflex sympathetic or parasympathetic stimulation with resultant tachycardia, brady-

cardia, hypertension, arrhythmias, myocardial ischemia, and ventricular failure (62, 63). Attenuation or treatment of hypertension is achieved by short-duration laryngoscopy (less than 15 seconds), intravenous lidocaine (2 mg/kg) or laryngotracheal lidocaine spray (2 mg/kg) prior to laryngoscopy (64, 65), intravenous nitroglycerin or nitroprusside prior to or after laryngoscopy (66), greater depth of anesthetic agents prior to or after intubation, and intravenous esmolol prior to intubation (67). Increases in heart rate can be attenuated with lidocaine spray, short-duration laryngoscopy (less than 15 seconds), and appropriate combination of narcotics (fentanyl, sufentanil, and alfentanil) and neuromuscular relaxants. Tachycardia can be treated with increasing depths of anesthesia with a volatile agent or intravenous esmolol (67). When severe bradycardia and hypotension occur, heart rate can be increased with atropine (0.5 mg intravenous doses), gallamine (10 to 20 mg in patients not receiving β-blockers), or pacing. If ventricular arrhythmias occur, lidocaine (1 mg/kg) can be given while treating predisposing factors.

No technique employing single or multiple anesthetic drugs has been shown to be clearly superior (68). Advantages of fentanyl, sufentanil, or alfentanil alone for cardiac surgery are minimal myocardial depression, hemodynamic stability, good control of heart rate, and reduction of endocrine and metabolic response to surgery; disadvantages include awareness, muscle rigidity, increased volume requirements, hypertension during or after sternotomy, and postoperative respiratory depression (69). Advantages of inhalational anesthetics include reduction of myocardial oxygen consumption, unconsciousness, muscle relaxation, easy titration, suppression of reflex responses to noxious stimulation, rapid recovery of respiratory function, and easy airway management; disadvantages are arrhythmias, myocardial depression, and lack of sustained analgesia during the postoperative phase (70).

Cannulation of the heart for cardiopulmonary bypass frequently results in supraventricular arrhythmias. Synchronized cardioversion or rapid initiation of cardiopulmonary bypass should be instituted if hypotension occurs. When patients with supraventricular tachycardia remain normotensive and have rapid ventricular rates, verapamil, propranolol, or esmolol may be given cautiously to slow ventricular response.

Initiation of Cardiopulmonary Bypass

After a control activated clotting time (ACT) is determined, and prior to insertion of venous and arterial cannulae, a loading dose of heparin (300 units/kg or 3 mg/kg) is given through a central venous line. Variation in heparin dose-response curves (71), heparin potency of each lot (72), biologic half-lives of heparin, antithrombin III levels (73, 74), and volumes of distribution have encouraged the use of the Hemochron system to measure ACT and determine the effectiveness of anticoagulation. Procoagulant activity during cardiopulmonary bypass is prevented by maintaining an ACT greater than 480 seconds. Patients refractory to heparinization may have low antithrombin III levels (73, 74), sepsis (75, 76), prior heparin treatment (77), or concomitant intravenous nitroglycerin therapy (78), and may require higher doses of heparin or fresh frozen plasma or both. Just prior to instituting cardiopulmonary bypass, the accuracy of all the monitors are checked, the need for additional muscle relaxants is determined, inhalational anesthetics are stopped, and prebypass fluid administration and urine output are recorded. Upon initiation of cardiopulmonary bypass (CPB), transient hypotension is common and may be due to decreased blood viscosity from the blood-free prime or release of vasoactive substances secondary to the reaction of serum proteins, blood cells, or platelets with the foreign surface of the heart-lung machine. Further management during CPB is discussed in Chapter 6.

Weaning from Cardiopulmonary Bypass

Prior to separation from bypass, one should recalibrate the monitoring system; rewarm the patient to a body temperature above 35°C; check the ventilator, endotracheal tube, and oxygen source; ensure an adequate blood volume in the pump reservoir; turn off the vaporizer on the pump during rewarming; record the ECG in multiple leads; and check arterial blood gas, hematocrit, and potassium. If the heart does not spontaneously defibrillate or revert to sinus rhythm with lidocaine (2.5 mg/kg intravenously) (79), it is electrically defibrillated with 5 to 10 J applied internally across the ventricles. Supraventricular arrhythmias can be controlled with atrial, ventricular, or AV sequential pacemaker, esmolol, verapamil, or edrophonium. Recurrent ventricular ectopy may require lidocaine, procainamide, or bretylium, or treatment of myocardial ischemia. Electrocardiographic ST segment elevation after CPB indicates air or particulate emoblization of the coronary circulation, coronary artery spasm, mechanical obstruction of the graft, inadequate myocardial protection during aortic cross-clamp, or inhomogeneous reperfusion. Prevention of myocardial ischemia begins with adequate myocardial preservation as treatment includes intravenous or intracoronary nitroglycerin, calcium entry blockers, intracoronary papaverine, higher perfusion pressure after aortic cross-clamp on CPB, or even surgical correction.

Systolic pressure differences between the central aorta and radial artery can be significant (greater than 12 mm Hg) and are temporally associated with rewarming at the end of CPB and alterations of forearm vascular resistance (80). Although central aortic and radial artery pressures usually equilibrate after 10 to 60 min following CPB, occasionally a patient will require a direct aortic pressure line or insertion of a femoral artery catheter for accurate systemic pressure measurement.

Upon separation from CPB an assessment of cardiac function is performed. If a pulmonary artery catheter has been inserted, ventricular filling pressures, systemic arterial blood pressure, cardiac index, and systemic vascular resistance should be measured and optimized. Alternatively, central venous and arterial pressures may be optimized by directly inspecting the heart. Transfusion through aortic or atrial cannulae can optimize preload, but excessive volume may cause ventricular distension with increasing myocardial oxygen demand and decreasing stroke volume. Intravenous calcium chloride (5 to 7 mg/kg) can improve myocardial performance but is not needed routinely (8). Additional calcium chloride requirements are determined by serum ionized calcium level.

Hemodynamic calculations can determine subsets of hypotension and dictate appropriate pharmacologic intervention. If patients have low cardiac output, high systemic vascular resistance, and optimal preload, vasodilator therapy and inotropic support may improve cardiac performance. If patients have low cardiac output and systemic vascular resistance with an optimal preload, inotropic support and vasopressor therapy may be used to maintain hemodynamic stability. Persistent low cardiac output after cardiopulmonary bypass may require other treatment. Potentially correctable medical causes of low cardiac output after CPB include hypoxemia, arrhythmias, acid-base abnormalities, hypocalcemia, hyperkalemia, sepsis, inhalation anesthetics, drug-induced myocardial depression, anaphylaxis, or anaphylactoid reactions. Surgically correctable lesions of low cardiac output include previously undiagnosed valvular lesions (mitral regurgitation, aortic regurgitation and stenosis, or tricuspid regurgitation), hypertrophic obstructive subaortic stenosis, atrial or ventricular septal defect, and kinked or clotted grafts. Other myocardial factors associated with low cardiac output include preoperative ventricular dysfunction, perioperative myocardial infarction, the duration of ischemic aortic cross-clamping, adequacy of cardioplegia during aortic cross-clamping, inadequate myocardial revascularization, coronary air or particulate embolism, and coronary artery spasm. If medical treatment or surgical intervention is ineffective in restoring blood pressure and cardiac output, mechanical support with intraaortic balloon counterpulsation or left or right ventricular assist should be considered (see Chapters 13, 14, and 18).

Afterload reduction can significantly improve cardiac performance as immediate postoperative hypertension can be treated with anesthetic drugs, intravenous nitroglycerin or nitroprusside, and β or calcium entry blockers. Nitroglycerin is preferred in nonhypertensive coronary artery bypass grafting (CABG) patients because it dilates epicardial coronary arteries, reduces preload and myocardial wall tension, redistributes coronary blood flow to the subendocardium, has less effect on intrapulmonary shunting, and has minimal toxicity (82).

Nitroprusside is a more effective arteriolar vasodilator and decreases afterload in hypertensives or, in combination with inotropes, improves cardiac performance in patients with low cardiac output and high systemic vascular resistance. Adverse effects of nitroprusside include cyanide and thiocyanate toxicity, inhibition of hypoxic pulmonary vasoconstriction, and baroreflex-induced sinus tachycardia (see Chapters 13 and 15).

Rarely, a hyperdynamic left ventricle syndrome—characterized by excessive contractility, high systemic vascular resistance, and normal stroke volume—is seen in patients with left ventricular hypertrophy. If nitroprusside is used to maintain mean arterial pressure between 90 and 110 mm Hg, there will be progressive increases in stroke volume, pulse pressure, and heart rate, and a fixed mean arterial pressure. This can result in myocardial ischemia since myocardial oxygen demand increases secondary to increasing systolic pressure and heat rate and coronary artery oxygen supply is reduced by decreasing diastolic blood pressure and filling time. Treatment includes β-blockade with incremental doses of intravenous esmolol or propranolol and/or infusion of the ganglionic blocker trimethaphan (250 mg in 250 ml D_5W) to reduce mean arterial pressure and pulse pressure (83).

Before reversal of anticoagulation, an ACT allows one to calculate residual heparin according to a heparin dose-response curve (84). For heparin neutralization, 1.3 mg of protamine is given for each 1 mg of residual heparin after removal of cannulae. Because ACT determined by standard Hemochron may be in substantial error due to hemodilution, hypothermia (85), and hypofibrinogenemia (86) and does not measure plasma heparin levels, calculated doses of protamine for heparin reversal may be inaccurate. An alternative method for calculating protamine needed to reverse circulating heparin and determining adequacy of heparin neutralization is a test of automated heparin-protamine titration as measured by the Hepcon (87).

Intravenous protamine reactions can be classified as systemic hypotention from rapid intravenous administration, anaphylactic or anaphylactoid reaction, catastrophic pulmonary vasoconstriction, or noncardiogenic pulmonary edema. Hypotension can be avoided by slow infusion of protamine over 15 to 30 min, intraaortic or left atrial infusion of protamine, and dilution of protamine during infusion. Although anaphylactic or anaphylactoid reactions occur more frequently in patients with fish allergy, vasectomy, prior intravenous exposure to protamine (cardiac cathertization, previous cardiac or vascular surgery), and diabetics given NPH (3 to 6 μg protamine per unit insulin) or protamine zinc insulin (PZI) (10 to 15 μg protamine per unit insulin), there are no prospective studies in large patient populations allowing estimation of risk or recommendation of prophylactic measures such as antihistamine or steroid administration in these patient subsets. Treatment includes oxygen, volume infusion, epinephrine, steroids, antihistamines, aminophylline (for severe or sustained bronchospasm), and norepinephrine (if needed to maintain coronary perfusion pressure) (88, 89). Catastrophic pulmonary vasoconstriction has been described in patients with pulmonary hypertension and mitral valve disease without documented prior exposure to the drug. This response is characterized by right ventricular dilation, pulmonary arterial hypertension, decreased left ventricular filling pressure, and systemic hypotension as diagnosis is aided by the pulmonary artery catheter. Treatment includes isoproterenol, epinephrine, and calcium chloride (90).

Additional coagulation tests that can be useful in the perioperative evaluation of the whole blood hemostatic process are thromboelastography and Sonoclot. The thromboelastogram, which measures viscoelastic clot strength, can assess initial procoagulant activation through fibrin cross-linking and clot lysis and detect abnormalities of coagulation factors, platelets, fibrinogen, and fibrinolysis (91, 92). The Sonoclot, which also measures changes in the viscoelastic properties of plasma as it is recalcified, measures recalcification time, fibrin polymerization, incorporation of platelets in the clot, and retraction of the clot, and corresponds to quantitative and qualitative abnormalities of platelets (93).

ANESTHETIC MANAGEMENT OF THE PATIENT WITH CORONARY ARTERY DISEASE

Elective Coronary Artery Revascularization

Pathophysiology.   Maintenance of myocardial oxygen balance is essential to avoid myocardial ischemia. Major determinants of myocardial oxygen consumption include heart rate, afterload, preload, and contractility (94), while myocardial oxygen supply is dependent on coronary blood flow and oxygen content of arterial blood. Since the myocardium at rest extracts most of the oxygen from the coronary arterial blood, increases in myocardial work and oxygen demand are balanced by autoregulation and increases in coronary blood flow. With coronary artery disease and reduced coronary blood flow reserve, myocardial oxygen demand may exceed oxygen supply and produce ischemia (95).

Intraoperative—Prebypass.   Unpremedicated or poorly premedicated patients are prone to higher heart rates and arterial pressure with increases in myocardial oxygen demand that can provoke ischemia. Premedications for CABG patients with good to moderately depressed left ventricular function include oral diazepam (0.1 to 0.15 mg/kg), morphine (0.1 to 0.15 mg/kg intramuscularly) and scopolamine (0.2 to 0.4 mg intramuscularly). If patients have severely depressed left ventricular function or general debility, light premedication and reassurance during the preoperative visit can minimize anxiety. Patients should arrive in the operating room with supplemental oxygen, be monitored with a pulse oximeter to maintain an SaO_2 level of at least 95% (37), and have an arterial blood gas determination after insertion of the arterial catheter.

Upon arrival in the operating room, an ECG lead should be immediately displayed on the oscilloscope because patients undergoing coronary artery bypass surgery have frequent preoperative episodes of myocardial ischemia, most of which are silent (96). Since electrocardiographic evidence for perioperative myocardial ischemia on arrival in the operating room can occur in 18% of patients during CABG, knowledge of preoperative ECG allows one to diagnose myocardial ischemia, which can be associated with a threefold increase in perioperative myocardial infarction (47).

Arterial cannulae will most frequently be inserted in the radial artery. With dissection of the internal thoracic artery, the Favalaro retractor can produce stress on the sternum and subclavian artery, which may reduce flow and loss of arterial pressure waveform (97). To avoid this problem, the radial artery opposite the side of dissection should be used for pressure monitoring or the Chaux retractor should be substituted for the Favalaro retractor (98). In addition to inaccuracies of transducer position, calibration, and dynamic response of the recording system, which may create significant measurement errors, radial artery pressures may not accurately reflect intraaortic pressure since the radial artery catheter is peripherally located from the central circulation. Moreover, some patients may have diminished radial arterial pulses due to previous arterial cannulation or repeated cardiac catheterizations (Sones technique). If both internal thoracic arteries are used for grafting, the arterial catheter can be placed in a femoral artery (see Chapter 7).

There are no prospective studies that demonstrate reduction in morbidity or mortality in patients who routinely have a pulmonary artery catheter (PAC) inserted for CABG. Nevertheless, common criteria for PAC insertion include poor left ventricular function, left main coronary artery lesion, recent myocardial infarction, complications of myocardial infarction, concomitant valvular lesions, reoperation, unstable angina, and pulmonary hypertension (see Table 7.1). Additional advantages of PAC insertion during CABG include early detection of myocardial ischemia as diagnosed by prominent a and v waves seen on the pulmonary capillary wedge pressure (PCWP) tracing (99), measurement of elevated PCWP or depressed cardiac output (58), calculation of hemodynamic indices which can be used for therapeutic interventions (57), and assessment of ventricular distension from noncoronary collateral flow during CPB.

Since CABG patients have compromised coronary flow reserve, induction of anesthesia and endotracheal intubation should be accomplished with minimal cardiovascular instability. Often an increase in sympathetic tone with resultant vasoconstriction and hypovolemia can be anticipated before induction. Since abolition of high central sympathetic tone and changes in baroreceptor function occur with loss of consciousness and with administration of anesthetics, cardiac filling pressures and peripheral resistance should be normalized before induction.

Hypertension and tachycardia in CABG patients can be associated with profound decreases in left ventricular performance during endotracheal intubation (100). Forty-five percent of CABG patients evaluated by thallium-201 perfusion imaging showed regional myocardial hypoperfusion immediately after intubation despite stable hemodynamics (101). When patients with coronary artery disease having laryngoscopy and intubation for vascular surgery were studied with ECG, cardiokymography, and myocardial lactate metabolism, those who became ischemic demonstrated immediate decreases in coronary sinus blood flow during laryngoscopy. When the laryngoscope was removed, coronary sinus blood flow returned to baseline levels in ischemic patients despite progressive increases in mean arterial pressures, PCWP, and heart rate (102).

Increased myocardial oxygen demand can be minimized by keeping heart rate low and controlling systolic blood pressure to within 20% of preinduction levels. This is achieved by reducing preinduction anxiety, ensuring an adequate level of anesthesia, and continuing preoperative β-blocker, antihypertensive, nitrate, and calcium channel blocker drugs until the time of surgery. Myocardial oxygen supply can be maximized by keeping diastolic arterial pressure normal or slightly high and heart rate low, using nitroglycerin to reduce preload and redistribute coronary blood flow to the subendocardium, and ensuring adequate oxygen content with 100% FiO_2, satisfactory hemoglobin (more than 10 to 12 mg/100 ml), and cessation of smoking at least 18 hr prior to anesthesia.

There were no signs of myocardial ischemia or anaerobic metabolism during sternotomy in CABG patients receiving halothane–nitrous oxide–oxygen anesthesia (103) or enflurane-oxygen anesthesia (104). However, in a study comparing high-dose morphine–nitrous oxide–oxygen anesthesia with halothane–nitrous oxide–oxygen anesthesia (105), greater elevations in myocardial oxygen extraction occurred in the halothane group during sternotomy despite comparable increases in coronary blood flow. Myocardial oxygenation was inadequate, resulting in ECG changes or lactate production in 10 of 14 patients anesthetized with halothane–nitrous oxide and 8 of 12 patients with morphine–nitrous oxide anesthesia. Thus, myocardial ischemia can occur during laryngoscopy, intubation, and surgical stimulation regardless of anesthetic technique and may not be associated with any systemic hemodynamic changes. Moreover, varying skills between anesthesiologists in managing patients may be as important as choice of anesthetic agents (47).

Since no anesthetic technique has been shown clearly to affect outcome during CABG, selection of technique should be made on the nature and severity of coronary artery anatomy and pathophysiology; left and right ventricular function; concomitant valvular lesions; loading conditions of the myocardium; patient's age, body mass, and debility; other medical problems or drugs; and pharmacokinetics and pharmacodynamics of anesthetic drugs (see Chapter 10). Stable induction can be achieved with fentanyl, sufentanil, or alftentanil. After the induction dose of opiates, deepening of the anesthetic state and reducing baseline systolic blood pressure by 20% with enflurane or halothane can minimize reflex hypertension and tachycardia associated with intubation. Further opiates or inhaled anesthetic agents or both may be given to prevent autonomic response and decrease cardiac work and myocardial oxygen consumption. The combined opiate–inhalation agent techniques can maintain a hypodynamic circulation and reduce myocardial oxygen consumption while preserving myocardial oxygen supply in CABG patients. The combined technique allows good titration of agents and cessation of inhaled agents to lighten the anesthetic level when hemodynamics become depressed. Patients with good ventricular function require and tolerate higher doses of anesthesia than those with poor ventricular function. Since isoflurane has been shown to dilate normal segments of the coronary vascular bed in patients with coronary artery disease with subsequent redistribution of myocardial blood flow and possible regional myocardial ischemia (·106, 107), it is not recommended as the sole anesthetic agent in patients with coronary artery disease. Nevertheless, there are no prospective studies with isoflurane demonstrating a higher risk of myocardial ischemia or infarction or an adverse outcome in CABG patients.

Neuromuscular blocking drugs can produce adverse cardiovascular effects in patients with coronary artery disease (108). Metocurine-pancuronium mixtures (109), vecuronium (110), and atracurium allow hemodynamic stability and should be used to avoid tachycardia and hypotension. Some patients using β-adrenergic and calcium entry blockers who have sinus bradycardia may require pancuronium to avoid further slowing of heart rate and concomitant hypotension.

Arterial pressure should be maintained within 20% of baseline value and heart rate between 50 and 70 beats/min to reliably preserve myocardial oxygen demand and supply. If excessive sympathetic stimulation occurs, increasing depth of inhaled anesthetics or vasodilators can control hypertension. Nitroglycerin is preferred because it decreases myocardial oxygen consumption, is more effective in treating myocardial ischemia, is less likely to produce coronary steal, and has less toxicity (82, 111).

In a canine model with fixed coronary artery stenosis, myocardial ischemia occurred when the mean arterial pressure:heart rate ratio was below 1 (112). When tachycardia allows the mean arterial pressure:heart rate ratio to be less than 1, propranolol (0.5 to 1 mg intravenous doses) or esmolol can be used to control heart rate, while increasing depth of inhaled anesthetics can be used if hypertension accompanies the change in heart rate. If hypotension and an elevated preload occur with tachycardia, phenylephrine may be used to augment coronary perfusion along with nigroglycerin to decrease preload and enhance coronary blood flow to the subendocardium (113).

Hypotension with a low preload associated with opiates and benzodiazepines can be treated with fluids, Trendelenburg position, ephedrine

(5 to 10 mg intravenously), mephenteramine (3 to 6 mg intravenously) or phenylephrine (25 to 50 μg intravenously). If inhaled agents produce hypotension, they should be reduced or withdrawn until arterial pressure returns to acceptable levels. When bradycardia is associated with hypotension, heart rate should be increased to maintain an adequate arterial pressure using atropine (0.5 mg intravenously), gallamine (10 to 20 mg intravenously in patients without β-blockers) (108), atrial or ventricular pacing, or cessation of vagally mediated maneuver.

Clinical studies demonstrate that the majority of perioperative ECG abnormalities occur without acute hemodynamic changes prior to the onset of ischemia (47, 96). When ischemia occurs, hemodynamic instability should be corrected, if present. If ischemia persists or occurs without hemodynamic abnormalities, nitroglycerin and calcium entry blockers can be used to reverse imbalances of regional coronary blood flow and myocardial oxygen demand because these drugs ameliorate coronary artery spasm or silent ischemia and attenuate ischemic manifestations induced by pacing or exercise in patients with fixed coronary artery stenosis (114, 115). They may also be useful in decreasing the risk of intraoperative myocardial ischemia during CABG even though this has only been demonstrated in noncardiac surgery (116, 117).

Weaning from Bypass. A modification of the hemodynamic tracking profile obtained by plotting left ventricular stroke work index (LVSWI), cardiac index, or stroke volume index against PCWP can be used to determine cardiovascular therapy and effectiveness of intervention during weaning from CPB (57, 118). Depending on ventricular function (groups 1 through 3), suggested treatment is based on location within the quadrant as shown in Figure 8.1: **A**, adequate depth of anesthesia or no treatment; **B**, vasodilators or diuretics; **C**, volume administration or pacing; and **D**, inotropes with or without vasodilators, IABP, or ventricular assist devices. By monitoring the trend of intervention, a patient in quadrant C with normal ventricular function (group 1) and low LVSWI and PCWP will be given fluid and move to quadrant A or B, where vasodilator or increased depth

of anesthesia may be required for further cardiovascular therapy. In contrast, a patient in quadrant C with poor ventricular function (group 3) and low LVSWI and PCWP will move to quadrant D when given fluid and will require inotropes with or without vasodilators, intraaortic balloon pumping, or ventricular assist devices.

In a study evaluating cardiovascular performance immediately after CPB, CABG patients with good preoperative ventricular function (left ventricular ejection fraction [LVEF] greater than 0.55 and no significant dyssynergy) have left and right ventricular function curves that are 75% and 60% of preoperative control, respectively. In comparison, patients with preoperative left ventricular dysfunction (LVEF less than 45% or dyssynergy) have left and right ventricular function curves reduced to 40% and 30% of preoperative control immediately after CPB (119). Moreover, ventricular dysfunction is transient in those patients with good ventricles, and recovery to 90% of control occurs within 4 hr of revascularization. In comparison, ventricular dysfunction, (in the group with severely depressed ventricular function) persists for 24 hr after revascularization with only 60% recovery of preoperative ventricular function (119). Thus, CABG patients with good and those with depressed preoperative left ventricular function will have hemodynamic profiles best described by groups 2 and 3, respectively. Further, patients after CBP in quadrant C will respond differently to volume infusion than normal patients. In a study evaluating ventricular function curves immediately after CPB, volume infusion increases end-diastolic and systolic volume index, PCWP, and stroke volume index as LVEF decreases despite reductions in systemic vascular resistance. Thus, augmentation of stroke volume achieved by increasing preload may be accompanied by a decrease in LVEF, and the Frank-Starling mechanism with augmentation of stroke volume and LVEF may occur at different preloads when comparing volume infusion in the intensive care unit with that done immediately after CPB (120).

Since CABG patients are dependent on the relationship of both global and regional myocardial oxygen supply and demand, pharma-

FIGURE 8.1

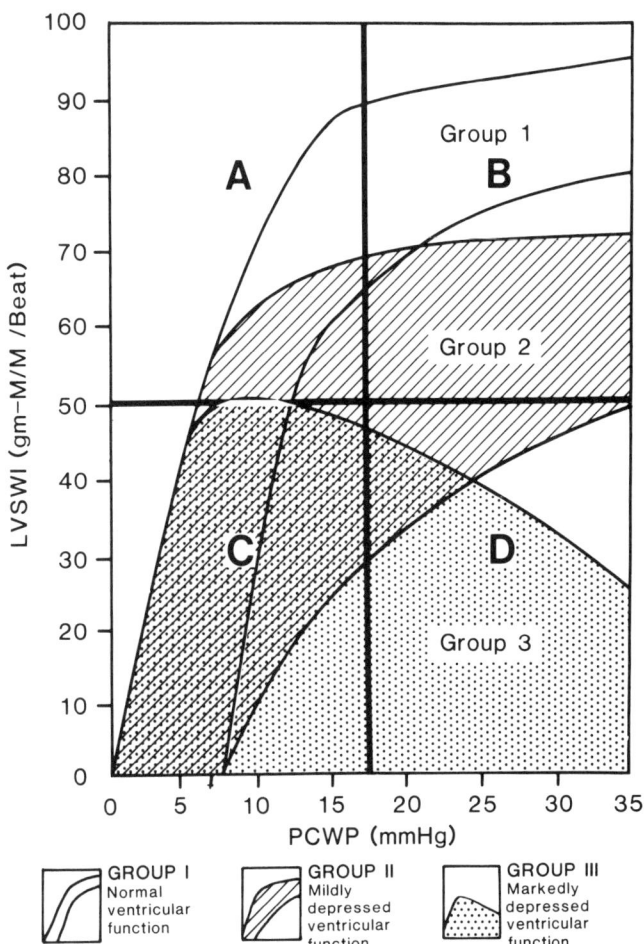

Modification of hemodynamic tracking profile for weaning patients from cardiopulmonary bypass. Depending on ventricular function (groups 1 through 3) and provisions to maintain coronary perfusion pressure, suggested treatment is based on location within quadrants as follows: (**A**) adequate depth of anesthesia or no treatment; (**B**) vasodilators or diuretics; (**C**) volume administration or pacing; and (**D**) inotropes with or without vasodilators, IASP, or ventricular assist devices. (From Barash PG, Chen Y, Kitahata LM, et al: The hemodynamic tracking system: a method of data management and guide for cardiovascular therapy. *Anesth Analg* 59:169–174, 1980, with permission; and O'Conner JP, Wynands JE: Anesthesia for myocardial revascularization. In Kaplan JA (ed): *Cardiac Anesthesia*. Orlando, FL, Grune & Stratton, 1987, p 577, with permission.)

cologic efficacy of inotropes is dependent on such factors as coronary perfusion pressure, drug effect on vessel conductance, coronary and regional perfusion, myocardial contractility and oxygen consumption, and dose-response curve. Saphenous vein graft (SVG) and internal thoracic artery (ITA) flow immediately after myocardial revascularization has received scant attention after CPB. In a canine model that maintained constant systemic hemodynamics, norepinephrine increased ITA and SVG flow,

as phenylephrine decreased flow in both grafts. However, norepinephrine increased rate of rise of ventricular pressure (dp/dt) and myocardial oxygen consumption, which might worsen perioperative ischemia. In contrast, epinephrine increased ITA flow but decreased SVG flow. Because dp/dt did not increase, epinephrine would have theoretical advantages in the treatment of postoperative hypotension, especially if large areas of myocardium are revascularized with an ITA (121). However, studies of epinephrine demonstrate increased contractility and myocardial oxygen consumption, which might provoke ischemia in a larger revascularized area with SVG (122). In another canine model, dopamine, dobutamine, and isoproterenol produced maldistribution of coronary blood flow (CBF) distal to fixed coronary artery stenosis by increasing the resistance to flow through a stenotic coronary artery. This redistribution was dependent on dose of drug, reductions of the distal diastolic coronary pressure-time index, and decreases in the ratio of distal diastolic coronary pressure-time index to tension-time index (123). Effects of inotropes may thus be important in patients with incomplete revascularization or with collateral-dependent areas of native circulation and poor distal runoff of new grafts.

In patients after CABG surgery, dobutamine increased CBF, consistent with its augmentation of myocardial oxygen consumption (MVO_2). In comparison, increases in CBF were attenuated with dopamine despite increases in MVO_2, thus suggesting direct vasoconstrictor effects on the coronary vasculature (124). Effects on the coronary vasculature may be dose dependent, as low doses (1 to 3 μg/kg/min) of dopamine stimulate specific postjunctional dopaminergic receptors (DA_1-receptors) and inhibit prejunctional receptors (DA_2-receptors) of norepinephrine release in coronary arterial beds which can both produce vasodilation. At higher doses, dopamine stimulates α-adrenergic receptors, which override DA_2-receptor effects and produce vasoconstriction.

In another animal model of reperfused myocardium after acute coronary occlusion, dobutamine enhanced cardiovascular performance, similar to the clinical situation of ischemia and stunned myocardium after aortic cross-clamp, as the contractile response to reperfusion and inotropic stimulation was greatly affected by the method of reperfusion (125).

When myocardial injury occurs, it is essential to ensure the supply of nutrients to the myocardium for protein synthesis. Glucose-insulin-potassium (GIK) infusions may benefit ischemic myocardium by increasing availability of glucose and storage of glycogen, decreasing availability of free fatty acids, stabilizing cell membrane, and favorably influencing prosta-

glandin synthesis (126–128). Because carnitine is a carrier for mitochondrial transmembrane movement of free fatty acids, administration of L-carnitine in the ischemic myocardium may result in increased fatty acid oxidation and lower intracellular concentrations of free fatty acids, decreased myocardial lactate concentration, and enhanced myocardial utilization of available oxygen (129).

Coronary artery spasm immediately after myocardial revascularization has been associated with profound hypotension, atrioventricular block, ventricular tachycardia, and inferior ST segment elevation on ECG and may be provoked by α-agonist drugs or intravenous calcium (130–132). Treatment includes intravenous or intracoronary nitroglycerin, intracoronary papaverine, and calcium entry blockers.

Air emboli during CABG surgery may be introduced through the left ventricular vent site, air trapped in a coronary bypass graft at the time of anastomosis, temperature-related and solubility changes of gases coming out of solution to form microbubbles, the oxygenator during extracorporeal circulation, or venous air which can enter the systemic circulation through interatrial or interventricular septal defects. Recommendations for reducing microemboli with extracorporeal circulation include using lower gas to blood flow ratios, maintaining high reservoir volumes, judicious cooling and rewarming to prevent large gradients between cold blood and warm tissues, priming the circuit and evacuating air in the prebypass period, and using membrane oxygenators and arterial line filtration (133). By using two-dimensional transesophageal echocardiography to detect trapped air in the left heart (134), surgical maneuvers to prevent coronary artery air emboli include filling, venting, and compressing the chambers of the heart prior to weaning from cardiopulmonary bypass; slowly releasing the aortic cross-clamp after several beats of the heart while gently pinching the proximal right coronary artery and using an aortic root vent; and using a 25-gauge needle inserted into the graft to dissipate any residual air (135). The anesthesiologist should increase airway pressure during the venting procedure to force flood with residual air bubbles from the pulmonary veins into the left ventricle and avoid nitrous oxide which would significantly enlarge any residual air. If suspected coronary air embolus occurs, the patient should be placed in Trendelenburg position with evacuation of air from the left ventricle and/or graft, have CPB flow increased to two times normal, and be given intracoronary or intravenous nitroglycerin or calcium channel blockers. Regardless of the cause of the observed ECG changes, creatine phosphate (MB fraction) levels will be significantly higher postoperatively in patients with ST segment elevation than in patients who do not have ST segment elevation after coronary artery bypass (136).

When weaning from CPB is completed and heparin reversed with protamine as monitored by ACT and Hepcon, the patient can be evaluated for additional anesthesia by electroencephalogram (EEG) or esophageal depth of anesthesia monitor. Since all patients have some ventricular dysfunction after CPB, additional inhaled anesthetics, β-blockers, and calcium entry blockers should be given with caution.

Reoperation for Coronary Artery Bypass Grafting

During the early 1970s, incomplete revascularization during primary CABG and early graft closure were the major indications for repeat CABG. In more recent years, CABG is most often performed for progressive coronary atherosclerosis and/or graft atherosclerosis and thrombosis (137). Although there have been decreases in mortality and morbidity in primary revascularization over the past 15 years, significant increases in perioperative myocardial infarction, postoperative respiratory insufficiency, perioperative hemorrhage, post-CPB requirement for IABP and/or inotropes, and mortality have been noted in reoperation when compared to those undergoing primary revascularization (137–139).

Preoperative Assessment. Since reoperation entails certain unique risks, evaluation must be focused accordingly. The indications for reoperation, analysis of recent cardiac catheterization report and diagnostic noninvasive cardiac tests, chest x-ray, and review of the operative note and anesthetic record relating to previous cardiac surgery are especially important. The cardiac catheterization report should indicate patency or occlusion of native vessels and grafts, collateral circulation of native vessels, and assessment of right and left ventricular systolic and diastolic function.

Occult constrictive pericarditis is a rare but important complication of previous CABG (140, 141). This diagnosis is suggested during right heart catheterization by right atrial pressure usually above 15 mm Hg, pulmonary artery systolic pressure less than 50 mm Hg, PCWP minus the right ventricular end-diastolic pressure less than 6 mm Hg, normal to low cardiac output, and a dip and plateau pattern in the right ventricular pressure tracing. Frequently, the only clue to occult constrictive pericarditis may be equally high right and left ventricular end-diastolic pressures during acute volume loading. Patients with right atrial and ventricular enlargement, such as those with tricuspid regurgitation and pulmonary hypertension, ascending aortic aneurysms or dilated aortas, multiple cardiac surgical procedures, anatomic abnormality of the chest wall, or previous mediastinal irradiation appear to be at greater risk for catastrophic hemorrhage during sternotomy.

Operative reports of previous surgeries can give information regarding ventricular function, technical difficulties during operation, distal runoff of the coronary arteries, quality of the aorta, graft conduits, difficult weaning from CPB, or other postoperative complications. Surgical closure of the pericardium allows less sternal adhesions and noncoronary collateral blood flow within the mediastinum, which makes sternal reentry and dissection technically easier. It is important to know if the ITA was used as a bypass conduit because (*a*) a patient ITA graft during sternotomy or mediastinal dissection may be damaged, leading to myocardial ischemia that requires rapid institution of CPB via the femoral route; (*b*) the initiation of cardioplegic cardiac arrest may require greater amounts of cold potassium cardioplegic solution in a heart being perfused with a patent ITA pedicle; or (*c*) more need for IABP support has been attributed to suboptimal myocardial preservation in the presence of a patent ITA graft (142).

Monitoring. Two 14-gauge venous catheters are placed for volume expansion, one catheter should preferentially be placed in the right upper extremity because left innominate vein tears may occur during sternotomy. Intravenous fluid bags connected to these catheters should be placed in blood pump bags. Due to the high incidence of perioperative ischemia in patients for CABG reoperation, two ECG leads (V_5, II) are recommended to measure ST segment changes and trends, and a pulmonary artery catheter is placed in all patients. If evidence of heart block, left bundle-branch block, or symptomatic bifascicular block is present prior to surgery, a five-lead multipurpose pulmonary artery catheter, which allows atrial, ventricular, or AV sequential pacing, should be selected for hemodynamic monitoring (143). Because epicardial atrial and ventricular pacing leads after CPB are often difficult to secure successfully in the fibrosed epicardium and myocardium during repeat CABG, it may be necessary to continue endocardial pacing into the postoperative period after reoperations.

Transthoracic external defibrillation pads (R_2 Corporation, Morton Grove, IL) placed in a V_5 apex-posterior configuration can be used for rapid defibrillation once the operation is under way but before the heart has been dissected free enough to allow placement of internal paddles. Additional monitoring with two-dimensional transesophageal echocardiography can allow visualization of global left ventricular function, detection of regional wall motion abnormalities from myocardial ischemia, evaluation of mitral insufficiency and repair, detection of residual air emboli before weaning from cardiopulmonary bypass, or diagnosis of aortic dissection at the aortic cannulation site (144).

Anesthetic Technique. The lungs should be kept deflated during sternotomy, and the heparin dose should be calculated and ready to administer immediately in the event that catastrophic hemorrhage would require urgent CPB. Heparin should be administered through the distal port of the pulmonary artery catheter if surgical repair without cardiopulmonary bypass is not possible. The groin can be exposed and the arterial perfusion cannula placed in the femoral artery. A right ventriculotomy may be used as venous return for cardiopulmonary bypass and additional heparin can be added to the prime by the perfusionist. After heparinization, shed blood may be scavenged to the pump.

High-dose narcotic anesthetic techniques may be preferred to inhalational techniques to provide more stable hemodynamics and to facilitate pulmonary ventilation through the evening of surgery. Because of higher incidence of postoperative respiratory insufficiency, blood requirements, and reexploration for postoperative bleeding, these patients are less suitable candidates for early extubation.

Since myocardial blood supply may be primarily dependent on previous vein grafting, repeat CABG patients are at greater risk for acute myocardial ischemia from graft laceration (145) or distal embolization of friable atheromata that may occur with manipulation of the heart or grafts prior to CPB (146). These episodes of acute transmural ischemia may be diagnosed by ST segment elevation on the ECG, a finding in distinct contrast to the more typical subendocardial ischemia with ST segment depression observed during primary CABG. Although treatment with phenylephrine, nitroglycerin, or nifedipine can normalize ST segment elevation, perioperative myocardial infarction can still occur because of a possible vasospastic component associated with apparent coronary artery embolization during mediastinal dissection (147).

Repeat CABG patients are at greater risk for perioperative bleeding than patients undergoing primary revascularization. Those with previous ITA implant, those receiving antiplatelet drugs or other medications with adverse effects on clotting mechanisms, and patients who have their reoperation shortly after the first procedure can bleed excessively. Preoperative coagulation tests are performed to detect bleeding tendencies and prepare blood components prior to surgery. Nonessential drugs that interfere with the clotting mechanism should be discontinued prior to surgery.

Intraoperative autotransfusion can be performed following induction of anesthesia (148). One or two units of blood can be withdrawn from the patient and replaced with 1½ times the volume using crystalloid or colloid solutions to maintain normovolemia. Blood is stored at room temperature to preserve clotting factors and platelets. After separation from CPB and reversal of heparinization, this fresh autologous blood is reinfused. Patients with good ventricular function usually increase their cardiac output and maintain arterial pressure during normovolemic hemodilution and allow adequate oxygen delivery despite reductions in oxygen content. Optimal hematocrit in humans is approximately 30% to maintain adequate oxygen delivery (149). With poor ventricular function, hemodilution to a hematocrit of 30% allows increase in cardiac output and maintenance of arterial pressure. At a hematocrits of 20%, significant decreases in arterial pressure and systemic vascular resistance occur with normovolemic hemodilution which cannot be compensated by increasing cardiac output (150). Thus, responses to intraoperative hemodilution are determined by ventricular function and preoperative hematocrit. Although intraoperative autotransfusion can reduce homologous blood transfusion and improve postoperative hemostasis, meticulous surgical hemostasis to minimize intraoperative blood loss is just as important.

Systems have also been developed for retransfusion of shed mediastinal blood as it is lost in the intensive care unit (151, 152). When postoperative chest tube drainage exceeds 500 ml/hr or is 200 ml/hr for over 3 hr with no evidence of a coagulopathy, the patient should have an exploratory mediastinotomy for surgical control of bleeding. Since postoperative hypertension increases the amount of bleeding, adequate control of blood pressure is imperative for reducing blood loss following reoperations (see Chapter 15).

Emergency Coronary Artery Revascularization

Acute myocardial infarction is the principal cause of death in the United States. Efforts to decrease mortality have focused on reducing the extent of myocardial injury by decreasing myocardial oxygen demand and improving myocardial oxygen supply. Recent therapeutic interventions, such as thrombolytic agents, percutaneous transluminal coronary angioplasty (PTCA), and emergency surgical revascularization, are being used more frequently for evolving acute myocardial infarction. The scientific premise for these interventions is the belief that

infarction is an evolving process and that infarct size and pump dysfunction can be limited if the acute occlusion can be reopened or bypassed before the onset of irreversible myocardial cellular damage. Whatever intervention is used to reestablish coronary blood flow, patients with acute myocardial injury are being seen more frequently for emergency revascularization.

Emergency CABG during the evolving myocardial infarction is thus performed in one of the following settings: (a) immediately after cardiac catheterization as the primary means of reestablishing coronary perfusion; (b) following successful thrombolytic therapy in patients at risk for reocclusion; (c) following unsuccessful thrombolytic therapy because of continued myocardial ischemia or hemodynamic instability; (d) because of a failed PTCA or complications of the PTCA associated with continued myocardial ischemia or hemodynamic instability; or (e) after a complication of cardiac cathertization associated with myocardial ischemia or hemodynamic instability.

Anesthesia in Emergency CABG. Once the decision is made to operate on the patient with acute myocardial infarction, the anesthesiologist should be involved with further resuscitation and hemodynamic management in an attempt to shorten the time between the initial ischemic event and surgery. Although these patients frequently have femoral artery and vein sheaths, additional intravenous and monitoring catheters can be inserted in the catheterization laboratory while the operating room is prepared for surgery. Vascular sheaths from the catheterization site are not removed because these patients may have recent thrombolytic or heparin therapy and rapid access to the aorta may be needed for insertion of an intraaortic balloon. These patients may also require surgical repair of the femoral artery and vein which can best be managed after emergency CABG surgery. Occasionally endotracheal intubation is indicated in the catheterization laboratory. Problems during anesthesia in these patients arise from evolving myocardial infarction with hemodynamic instability and arrhythmias, full stomach with the risk of pulmonary aspiration, hemorrhage due to thrombolytic agents or heparin, no preoperative preparation or control of medication, no immediate availability of blood products, and lack of time for appropriate monitoring. Transfer of patients from the cardiac catheterization laboratory to the operating room should be done with monitoring of heart rate, rhythm, and intraarterial blood pressure, and supplemental oxygen. In patients with hemodynamic instability, therapy should include inotropes or vasodilators or both and the use of an intraaortic balloon. Since hemorrhage and coagulation disturbances may occur, blood products should be ordered at this time. Patients with a full stomach should be given 30 ml of 0.3 M sodium citrate orally and 10 to 20 mg metoclopramide intravenously to increase gastric pH and reduce gastric volume by increasing motility and emptying. In patients receiving dopamine, metoclopramide is contraindicated because it is a dopamine antagonist. Histamine$_2$ inhibitors and anticholinergics have a slow onset of action and may not be effective under these conditions.

Monitoring.   Monitoring of the ECG should consist of leads II and V_5 unless maximal ST elevation is seen in another lead. Although pulmonary artery catheterization can be performed with minimal risks in patients having coagulopathies, anesthesia should be rapidly induced with an arterial and a central venous pressure catheter to minimize time to cardiopulmonary bypass. Two-dimensional transesophageal echocardiography can be used later during the perioperative period because ECG changes can normalize despite continued wall motion abnormalities (53, 145). If further hemodynamic monitoring is required, a left atrial catheter to assess left ventricular volume and a pulmonary artery thermistor to measure cardiac output can be placed during separation from cardiopulmonary bypass.

Induction and Maintenance.   In a patient with a full stomach and an evolving myocardial infarction, the main objective is to maintain coronary perfusion pressure and hemodynamic stability while preventing aspiration by rapid control of the airway. A rapid-sequence induction can be performed with 2 mg/kg thiopental and 5 μg/kg fentanyl (153) or 2 mg/kg thiamylal and 2 μ/kg sufentanil (154) combined with cricoid pressure (Sellick's maneuver). However,

these techniques have been investigated only in patients with American Society of Anesthesiologists (ASA) 1 and 2 classifications. Another rapid-sequence induction technique uses etomidate (0.3 mg/kg) and succinylcholine combined with a Sellick's maneuver (155). In patients scheduled for elective CABG, rapid infusion of fentanyl (50 μg/kg) can result in satisfactory induction of anesthesia, although occasionally patients may develop a transient, moderate drop in blood pressure due to loss of sympathetic tone (156). Another acceptable induction to maintain hemodynamic stability is adequate preoxygenation followed by rapid infusion of fentanyl (10 to 25 μg/kg) over 2 to 3 min, neuromuscular relaxants, and Sellick's maneuver. Since these patients have higher heart rates than patients coming to the operating room for elective CABG, rapid neuromuscular paralysis can be achieved with succinylcholine or a priming dose of vecuronium or atracurium (157).

Hemodynamic stability and adequate coronary perfusion pressure can be achieved with a combination of opiate narcotic and inhalational anesthetics. Halothane has been extensively studied in canine models of acute coronary insufficiency and has been found to (*a*) decrease heart rate, systolic arterial blood pressure, and rate-pressure product index; (*b*) reduce summation of ST segment elevation; and (*c*) reduce myocardial infarction size when compared to awake control animals (158–160). Although halothane can beneficially reduce myocardial oxygen consumption, excessive anesthetic-induced myocardial depression and vasodilation may compromise coronary perfusion and oxygen balance. In another canine model of myocardial ischemia, increasing halothane concentration was associated with severe ventricular dysfunction in the ischemic myocardial region when blood pressure and left ventricular contraction were reduced and left ventricular preload was increased (161, 162). Thus, opiates during the induction and intubation and additional opiates alone or with inhalation anesthetics for maintenance of anesthesia can achieve adequate hemodynamic stability and coronary perfusion pressure prior to cardiopulmonary bypass in patients with acute myocardial infarction.

Weaning from Cardiopulmonary Bypass. Patients undergoing emergency myocardial revascularization require inotropes and intraaortic balloon pulsation more frequently than elective CABG patients (163). Occasionally, left or right ventricular assist devices can be effective in selected patients with poor cardiac function.

Patients with prior thrombolytic therapy have more postoperative hemorrhage, greater activated clotting times, and higher blood requirements (163, 164). Since streptokinase indirectly activates the endogenous fibrinolytic system, patients having thrombolytic therapy may require extensive therapy with fresh frozen plasma, platelets, cryoprecipitate, and epsilon-aminocarproic acid to reverse their postbypass coagulopathy. A rational approach to therapy is based on prothrombin time, partial thromboplastin time, platelet count, template bleeding time, fibrinogen, thrombin time, fibrin split products, and D-dimers. Occasionally, patients undergoing emergency CABG within 24 hr of intracoronary thrombolysis can be managed with no increase in bleeding or blood product use (165). Variations in postoperative transfusion practices and institutional biases toward frequent transfusions can contribute to differences in reported transfusion requirements.

AORTIC STENOSIS

Progressive obstruction to left ventricular ejection with increased pressure overload stimulates concentric left ventricular hypertrophy. Because diastolic compliance is decreased in hypertrophy, adequate blood volume and an effective, well-timed left atrial contraction are necessary for the left ventricle to maintain preload and stroke volume. Normal cardiac performance is achieved at a greater expenditure of energy and lesser efficiency as ventricular wall tension and area under the pressure-volume loop increase. Eventually, ejection fraction decreases as compensatory left ventricular dilation and elevated end-diastolic volume are necessary to maintain stroke volume. In end-stage aortic stenosis, stroke volume decreases (166).

Coronary vascular reserve is diminished in aortic stenosis because left ventricular pressures can be much higher than coronary perfusion pressures, prolongation of systole occurs at the expense of diastole, the growth of the coronary circulation in the hypertrophied left ventricle does not match the increase in left ventricular mass, and the Venturi phenomenon may impair flow into the coronary orifices (167, 168). Moreover, a 30 to 50% incidence of coexistent coronary artery disease enhances vulnerability to myocardial ischemia (167).

If preoperative myocardial ischemia is present, sufficient premedication should be given to prevent increasing myocardial oxygen demand from anxiety-induced hypertension and tachycardia. Patients with critical outflow obstruction, low blood pressure, and congestive heart failure are dependent on sympathetic tone and should be given light preoperative sedation with intravenous supplementation on arrival in the operating room.

Intraoperative monitoring should include a continuous ECG display of modified V_5 and aVF. Since these patients usually exhibit a pattern of left ventricular hypertrophy with secondary ST segment changes, intraoperative ischemia can be difficult to diagnose. In such cases, pseudonormalization of repolarization abnormalities, changes of QRS vector, or elevations of ST segment could indicate myocardial ischemia.

Direct arterial pressure monitoring is necessary because these patients are vulnerable to hypotension, leading to decreased coronary perfusion pressure, myocardial ischemia, decreased stroke volume, and further hypotension. Ventricular filling pressure should also be monitored because central venous pressure underestimates left ventricular filling pressure in patients with a hypertrophied, noncompliant left ventricle. Management of intravascular volume, cardiac output, and derived hemodynamic parameters during induction and surgery is facilitated by a pulmonary artery catheter (PAC) inserted preoperatively. Ventricular arrhythmias during the insertion of PACs, though rare, could precipitate hypotension and myocardial ischemia. An alternative to insertion of PAC is placement by the surgeon of a left atrial catheter for postbypass monitoring.

Sinus rhythm is essential since preload and

stroke volume decrease without coordinated atrial systole. Factors that predispose to arrhythmias (i.e., alkalosis, endogenous or exogenous catecholamines, hypoxemia, digitalis toxicity, and halothane) should be avoided. Supraventricular or ventricular tachycardia that produces hypotension or ischemic ST segment changes should be converted using synchronized DC cardioversion. If patients are normotensive without electrocardiographic evidence of ischemia, ventricular arrhythmias can be treated with intravenous lidocaine (1 mg/kg) or procainamide (10 mg/kg at a rate of 50 mg/min), and supraventricular arrhythmias can be treated with intravenous digoxin (0.25 mg), verapamil (2.5 mg), or small doses of propranolol-esmolol, or procainamide.

Sinus tachycardia is not well tolerated because it causes more-frequent energy-consuming contractions with compensatory increases in pressure gradients to maintain stroke volume and may result in ischemic induced anaerobic metabolism (169). Myocardial oxygen supply decreases with tachycardia because coronary blood flow is reduced by shorter diastolic filling time and more frequently compression of coronary vessels within the ventricular wall. Stroke volume also decreases as heart rate increases if there is inadequate time for the compensatory pressure gradient across the valve to increase in systole and for passive filling of the left ventricle in diastole. Sinus tachycardia and hypertension associated with surgical stimulation and intubation must be avoided.

Patients with good ventricular function can be induced with fentanyl to prevent further impairment of left ventricular emptying and marked decreases in systemic vascular resistance which may lead to coronary hypoperfusion. Although the role of inhalational anesthetics may be added to blunt autonomic reflexes which may exacerbate myocardial ischemia and the transvalvular pressure gradient. Patients with critical aortic stenosis or left ventricular dysfunction benefit from the hemodynamic stability and lack of myocardial depression that are characteristic of a pure narcotic technique. Those with or without associated aortic regurgitation have been induced with 0.5 to 1 mg/kg of intravenous morphine, which increases cardiac index and

stroke volume index and reduces systemic vascular resistance (170). Morphine has also been used as an adjunct to diazepam–nitrous oxide during induction in patients with aortic stenosis, resulting in an increased cardiac index and heart rate, decreased systemic vascular resistance, left ventricular stroke work index, and systolic blood pressure, and an unchanged pulmonary capillary wedge pressure. Surgical stimulation was associated with an increased systolic blood pressure, left ventricular stroke work index, and systemic vascular resistance; and an adverse relationship between myocardial oxygen supply and demand was reflected by an increase in the rate pressure product and a decrease in the endocardial viability ratio indices (171). Since a 10% incidence of morphine-induced hypotension (systolic blood pressure less than 70 mm Hg) can occur in patients undergoing valvular surgery (172), high-dose fentanyl (50 μg/kg), which is associated with minimal changes in cardiovascular dynamics, is preferred. Addition of intravenous diazepam (10 mg), which by itself has minimal cardiovascular effects, can cause significant depression of arterial blood pressure, stroke volume, and cardiac output when added to high-dose fentanyl (173). Although halothane and enflurane have been used in patients with valvular heart disease, adverse changes in hemodynamics can occur (174, 175). Nitrous oxide should be avoided because it can increase systemic vascular resistance when added to narcotics (176).

In a randomized study of neuromusclear blocking agents in patients with aortic stenosis induced with fentanyl (50 μ/kg) (177), vecuronium (0.12 mg/kg), which does not release histamine or demonstrate autonomic effects, produced the most stable hemodynamics. Atracurium (0.4 mg/kg) also demonstrated clinical stability except for one patient who developed hypotension. Pancuronium and pancuronium-metocurine caused significant increases in heart rate, which can predispose to myocardial ischemia. Metocurine produced mild vasodilation with minimal increases in heart rate in patients given morphine and diazepam. When increases in heart rate occur, they can be treated with intravenous esmolol or small increments of edrophonium (1 mg). Excessive β blockade can be detrimental in patients with congestive heart failure dependent on endogenous catecholamine stimulation to maintain stroke volume.

Because stroke volume is relatively fixed in aortic stenosis, cardiac output is rate dependent and severe bradycardia can lead to hypotension or electrocardiographic evidence of myocardial ischemia. Patients can develop bradycardia and asystole from vagotonia associated with sternotomy or rapid administration of sufentanil and vecuronium during induction (178).

Patients with mild to moderate aortic stenosis can be given hydralazine or prazosin to decrease systemic vascular resistance and improve cardiac performance. Since cardiac index and stroke volume increase and systemic vascular resistance and mean arterial pressure decrease predictably, it is concluded that these patients may respond favorably to reductions in systemic vascular resistance and that resistance to ventricular emptying is determined predominantly by systemic vascular resistance rather than by aortic valve area (179). In patients with critical aortic stenosis, judicious titration of nitroprusside reduced mean arterial pressure, left ventricular systolic pressure, systemic vascular resistance, left ventricular end-diastolic pressure, left ventricular stroke work index, and left ventricular oxygen consumption; cardiac index and heart rate were unaltered, and subendocardial perfusion index (diastolic pressure time index/systolic pressure time index) was decreased. Compared to lesser degrees of obstruction, afterload on the left ventricle in severe aortic stenosis appears to be affected predominantly by the impedance at the aortic valve rather than the arterial system (180). Since cardiac performance may be limited by a left ventricle that has maximally used its Frank-Starling preload reserve, there are often minimal changes in left ventricular end-diastolic volume or stroke volume. Since the hypertrophied left ventricle requires an adequate diastolic blood pressure for coronary perfusion, intraoperative vasodilators should be avoided because they can produce hypotension, myocardial ischemia, ventricular dysfunction, and ventricular fibrillation. Intraoperative hypotension should be treated rapidly with phenylephrine, an α-adrenergic agonist,

to maintain coronary perfusion pressure. After restoring hemodynamic stability, the precipitating cause can be treated by using rapid volume infusion or Trendelenburg position for low preload or by using synchronized cardioversion or antiarrhythmic drug for arrhythmia.

Nitroglycerin for treating subendocardial ischemia is controversial in patients with aortic stenosis (181, 182). If significant increments in heart rate or reduction in aortic diastolic pressure do not occur, nitroglycerin may reduce myocardial oxygen demand and favorably influence myocardial oxygen balance. Since compliance of the hypertrophied left ventricle is diminished, significant hypotension can occur if left ventricular end-diastolic volume and pressure are too low.

A mild decrease in left ventricular contractility will be seen immediately after aortic valve replacement, possibly due to myocardial ischemia or edema during cardiopulmonary bypass, which may persist for several days. Because of left ventricular hypertrophy and diminished compliance, these patients are still susceptible to hypotension due to arrhythmias and loss of atrial systole. Since impedance to the hypertrophied left ventricle is significantly reduced, the same stroke volume can be ejected with a much small left ventricular systolic pressure, and cardiac index eventually increases. Postoperative hypertension can be seen and may require vasodilators to reduce afterload, which is now predominantly determined by the impedance of the arterial system.

Combined Aortic Stenosis and Aortic Regurgitation

Significant regurgitant flow adds to the forward flow across the stenotic aortic valve. For a given aortic valve area, the left ventricle must generate higher systolic pressure than would be necessary in pure stenosis of equal severity. Because of the regurgitant flow, left ventricular end-diastolic volume increases and left ventricular diastolic and systolic tension are significantly augmented. This causes pulmonary congestion and myocardial ischemia to occur at a larger aortic valve area than in pure aortic stenosis.

Combined Aortic Stenosis and Mitral Stenosis

With combined aortic and mitral stenosis, limitation of flow through the mitral valve diminishes flow across the aortic valve. This results in a smaller pressure gradient across the aortic valve for a given degree of aortic stenosis and significantly less compensatory left ventricular hypertrophy.

Combined Aortic Stenosis and Mitral Regurgitation

If mitral regurgitation is present with aortic stenosis, the high peak left ventricular systolic pressure augments regurgitant volume across the mitral valve during systole. Mitral regurgitation is diminished after replacement of the aortic valve, but improvement is less predictable when patients have moderate to severe mitral regurgitation associated with acquired mitral valve disease.

Aortic Regurgitation

Chronic aortic regurgitation results in left ventricular volume overload with an increase in ventricular wall tension and myocardial fiber length and a decrease in effective stroke volume. When diastolic regurgitant flow increases, total ventricular stroke volume and afterload are increased and stimulate left ventricular hypertrophy, which attempts to normalize systolic wall tension. Compensatory increases in diastolic compliance cause significant elevations in left ventricular end-diastolic volumes with minimal changes in end-diastolic pressures. Since myocardial fiber shortening is relatively energy inexpensive in this setting, cardiac output can be maintained with small increases in myocardial oxygen consumption. With further worsening of diastolic filling, ventricular volume becomes more dependent on atrial systole to maintain an adequate stroke volume. As end-systolic volume increases and contractility diminishes, left atrial pressure increases and cardiac output and stroke volume are reduced (166).

In acute aortic regurgitation, left ventricular end-diastolic pressure rises precipitously since the diastolic volume overload is imposed on a noncompliant, normal-sized left ventricle. Because of limitations imposed by the Frank-Starling mechanism, the left ventricle cannot support an effective stroke volume, and systolic arterial pressure and cardiac output are maintained by reflex increases in systemic vascular resistance and heart rate. Although initial, premature closure of the mitral valve may prevent the elevated left ventricular end-diastolic pressure from being transmitted to the pulmonary capillaries, left ventricular filling from the left atrium is also impaired, which can limit forward flow across the valve. Since the left ventricle compensates acutely by increasing end-diastolic volume with a relatively unchanged ejection fraction, left ventricular distension can lead to mitral annular enlargement, functional mitral regurgitation, fulminant pulmonary edema, and eventual increased right ventricular afterload (183).

Light preoperative sedation is preferred to minimize myocardial depression and avoid hypoxemia. However, high sympathetic tone and elevated systemic vascular resistance will enhance regurgitation across the aortic valve.

Precordial ECG lead V_5 is monitored intraoperatively for signs of subendocardial ischemia, which can occur because of an increase in basal myocardial oxygen requirements and a reduction in coronary vascular reserve. Arterial and pulmonary artery catheters are useful to assess preload and maximize cardiac output. In acute aortic regurgitation, the pulmonary capillary wedge pressure may significantly underestimate left ventricular end-diastolic pressure because of early closure of the mitral valve.

The determinants of regurgitant volume include duration of diastole, the mean diastolic pressure gradient from aorta to left ventricle, and the regurgitant valve area. Beneficial effects of increasing heart rate in chronic atrial fibrillation are uncertain. Although pacing-induced tachycardia can decrease left ventricular end-diastolic pressure and volume, total stroke volume, and the ratio of regurgitant volume to total stroke volume with increases in forward cardiac output, the regurgitant volume/min is unchanged. Improvements in forward cardiac output are maximal in patients with sinus bradycardia who are atrially paced to rates of 75 to 85 beats/min; moderate increases occur with rates between 85 and 110 beats/min; and no change or decreases occur when rates exceed 110 beats/min (184). In patients with preexisting left bundle-branch blocks (185); combined aortic regurgitation, coronary artery disease, and AV block (186); previous cardiac surgical procedures and a history of AV block; or hemodynamically significant sinus bradycardia, insertion of thermodilution pulmonary artery pacing catheters may allow more precise control of heart rate and antrioventricular synchrony, especially when parasympathomimetic drugs are used. If pacing is not readily available when hemodynamically significant severe bradycardia occurs, atropine, β-chronotropic agonists, or parasympatholytic muscle relaxants, such as pancuronium or gallamine, can be efficacious. However, pharmacologic control is less predictable and may lead to myocardial ischemia, accelerated junctional arrhythmias, or myocardial dysfunction. Although supraventricular arrhythmias are better tolerated in patients with aortic regurgitation than in those with aortic stenosis, maintenance of atrial systole is important since forward filling is impeded by regurgitant flow.

Since the diastolic pressure gradient across the aortic valve is a significant determinant of regurgitant volume, changes in systemic vascular resistance play an important role in these patients. In the awake state, patients with chronic aortic regurgitation and congestion heart failure have high systemic vascular resistances secondary to elevated circulating catecholamines and enhanced activity of the renin-angiotensin system, preoperative anxiety, and shivering from exposure to a cold environment. Since these patients may have been on vigorous diuretic therapy, their initially large circulating blood volume can become lower than normal. Arterial vasodilators, such as nitroprusside, phentolamine, and hydralazine, can improve forward cardiac output and stroke volume and reduce systemic vascular resistance, left ventricular end-diastolic volume, and regurgitant volume. These effects are even more significant in patients with elevated left ventricular end-diastolic pressures and depressed ejection fractions. In a study evaluating afterload reduction during aortic valve replacement, nitroprusside prevented systemic vascular resistance from exceeding preoperative

control levels, but stroke volume fell and heart rate increased (187). With concurrent preload augmentation and afterload reduction, systemic vascular resistance was controlled within the normal physiologic range without inducing hypotension or tachycardia, as cardiac index and stroke volume index significantly increased during anesthesia and surgery (188). Since the left ventricle is very compliant in chronic aortic regurgitation, large amounts of intravenous fluids may be required to augment preload and produce an increase in pulmonary capillary wedge pressure. It is necessary to maintain arterial diastolic and mean pressures during afterload reduction and preload augmentation because the hemodynamic situation can deteriorate rapidly if coronary hypoperfusion occurs.

Induction with narcotics (e.g., fentanyl or morphine) supplemented with judicious use of vasodilators and preload augmentation can control the response to intubation and surgical stimulation effectively and reduce systemic vascular resistance and regurgitant fraction while enhancing forward flow. Halothane and enflurane may be hazardous in patients with severe aortic regurgitation because of their negative inotropic action. Although isoflurane may reduce systemic vascular resistance and augment forward flow, it could also alter coronary autoregulation and further compromise the reduced coronary vascular reserve to produce myocardial ischemia. Nitrous oxide should be avoided because it increases systemic vascular resistance and depresses contricality (176).

In a randomized study comparing the hemodynamic effects of neuromuscular relaxants on patients with aortic regurgitation, vecuronium (0.12 mg/kg) and pancuronium-metocurine combination (0.04 mg/kg pancuronium–0.16 mg/kg metocurine) produced minimal chronotropic changes during high-dose fentanyl induction and intubation. Assessment of the pancuronium group was obscured since baseline control measurements demonstrate higher heart rates and decreased stroke volumes when compared to the other groups. For unexplained reasons, atracurium caused an elevated mean arterial pressure that could potentially augment regurgitant volume and increase left ventricular end-diastolic pressure (177).

Severely symptomatic patients tolerate narcotic anesthetics better than volatile anesthetic agents which can depress myocardium, decrease total stroke volume, and augment regurgitant volume. Induction doses of narcotics (e.g., sufentanil) and neuromuscular agents (e.g., vecuronium) could induce vagotonia and provoke bradycardia (178) and thus exacerbate left ventricular end-diastolic pressure, diastolic wall tension, and myocardial oxygen demand while reducing diastolic coronary perfusion pressure gradient. Thus, neuromuscular relaxants which can alter chronotropic responses to vagal stresses may be very useful in this subset of patients. Inotropic drugs may be needed to improve systolic blood pressure and forward cardiac output. Intraaortic balloon counterpulsation is contraindicated in aortic regurgitation because it augments regurgitation and causes left ventricular distension.

After aortic valve replacement, inotropic support is often necessary. Occasionally, vasodilators with or without inotropes may be used because of the increased impedance to left ventricular ejection and relative safety of the higher aortic diastolic pressure. Patients with chronic aortic regurgitation and reduced contractility may require higher filling pressures after CPB. In contrast, patients with acute aortic regurgitation will have relatively normal left ventricular contractility and diastolic properties and can usually be maintained at a normal left ventricular end-diastolic pressure.

Mitral Stenosis

Progressive obstruction of the mitral valve impairs left atrial emptying and left ventricular filling, resulting in low stroke volumes. Increases in left atrial and pulmonary artery pressures lead to redistribution of blood flow to the upper lobes and perivascular edema with decreased pulmonary compliance and increased work of breathing. Elevations in pulmonary artery pressure and resistance with impedance to the right ventricle also result in right ventricular dilation and hypertrophy, right ventricular failure, and functional tricuspid regurgitation (166). Since ventricular filling is rate dependent, increases in heart rate cause obligatory increases in left atrial and pulmonary artery pressures with

reductions in left ventricular stroke volume and arterial pressure. Rapid ventricular rates and atrial fibrillation are thus poorly tolerated in these patients (189).

Light premedication (e.g., benzodiazepine) with a preoperative visit to allay anxiety is preferred because excessive premedication can result in hypoxemia, hypercarbia, increased pulmonary vascular resistance, and decreased right ventricular performance. Patients should have supplemental oxygen after premedication and be kept in a reverse Trendelenburg position to reduce hypoxemia and the work of breathing.

Inferior or esophageal ECG leads should be monitored for arrhythmias or ischemic ST segment changes. Arterial monitoring is necessary because patients are hemodynamically labile and at risk for oxygen desaturation. Although pulmonary capillary wedge pressures do not reflect left ventricular end-diastolic pressure when a pressure gradient exists across the mitral valve, insertion of pulmonary artery catheters prior to induction permit measurements of right ventricular preload and afterload, evaluation of tricuspid regurgitation, and trends of cardiac output. This allows precise management with vasodilator and inotropic agents, mechanical ventilation, and the reverse Trendelenburg position. Patients with high left ventricular end-diastolic pressure at cardiac catheterization usually have coexisting mitral regurgitation, aortic valve disease, or primary myocardial disease. Occasionally, the pulmonary artery catheter may be difficult to pass into the right ventricle or pulmonary artery because these patients often have pulmonary hypertension, low cardiac output, tricuspid regurgitation, atrial fibrillation, and right ventricular dilation. Since these patients are at increased risk for pulmonary artery perforation, the catheter should be withdrawn into the proximal pulmonary artery before cardiopulmonary bypass and wedged only when necessary after weaning from bypass.

Because sinus tachycardia is poorly tolerated by patients with mitral stenosis, esmolol or propranolol in small doses may be useful to decrease heart rate, pulmonary artery and capillary wedge pressures, and mitral valve gradient without changing left ventricular end-diastolic pressure or stroke volume (190). Patients with severe mitral stenosis often have chronic atrial fibrillation. Since rapid ventricular rates cause greater decompensation than loss of atrial systole, verapamil, digitalis, or esmolol can be beneficial in reducing left atrial pressures and improving stroke volumes that vary directly with the length of the preceding diastolic filling period (166, 191). Digitalized patients who arrive in the operating room with rapid atrial fibrillation may need supplemental intravenous digoxin (0.125 mg), esmolol, or verapamil. Repletion of total body potassium and magnesium in patients with chronic diuresis and atrial fibrillation is important to avoid digitalis-induced arrhythmias. In patients who deteriorate from normal sinus rhythm to atrial fibrillation with hemodynamic instability prior to cardiopulmonary bypass, synchronized DC cardioversion is indicated.

Selection of neuromuscular relaxants and anesthetic agents should be limited to those least likely to produce tachycardia. Vecuronium and atracurium would appear to be ideal since they have no effect on chronotropy (108). When combined with fentanyl analgesia, they tend to maintain or slightly decrease the ventricular response to atrial fibrillation. Conversely, when severe reductions in heart rate are associated with hypotension, thermodilution pulmonary artery pacing catheters can be used to increase ventricular rate and maintain cardiac output.

Because existing elevation in pulmonary vascular resistance may impair right ventricular performance, high-dose narcotics are preferred to inhalation agents which can depress the myocardium. Occasionally, low concentrations of inhalation agents are necessary in patients with good ventricular function to supplement narcotic analgesia to prevent sympathetic stimulation. Nitrous oxide should be avoided in pulmonary hypertension because associated increments of pulmonary vascular resistance in patients receiving narcotic analgesia may cause right ventricular failure (176). Since endogenous release of catecholamines with surgical stimulation increases systemic and pulmonary vascular resistance and depress the myocardium (192). Reduction of systemic vascular resistance by nitroprusside in patients with isolated mitral stenosis can decrease pulmonary artery and capillary wedge pressures and increase heart rate with no

effect on cardiac output, whereas cardiac index may increase when severe pulmonary hypertension or some mitral regurgitation coexists with mitral stenosis (193). Moreover, nitroprusside can be efficacious in reducing pulmonary vascular resistance and impedance to right ventricular ejection. Nitroglycerin is associated with decreases in pulmonary arterial, left atrial, and left ventricular end-diastolic pressures and mitral valve gradients without changes in heart rate and cardiac index. These effects can improve right ventricular performance and occasionally improve symptoms of congestive heart failure. However, side effects of vasodilators may cause tachycardia or reductions in left ventricular preload or left atrial pressure, resulting in severe hypotension. Patients who benefit most from afterload reduction include those with combined mitral stenosis and insufficiency and those with pure mitral stenosis, severe pulmonary hypertension, and adequate arterial pressure. Since systemic pressures are essential for perfusion of the right ventricle, vasodilator therapy should be started gradually in patients with good cardiovascular reserve. Inotropic support may be necessary if both cardiac index and blood pressure remain low despite manipulation of preload and afterload. During the perioperative period, hypoxemia, hypercarbia, acidosis, hypothermia, and release of endogenous α-adrenergic catecholamines, which can increase pulmonary vascular resistance and precipitate right ventricular failure, should be avoided. Vasoconstrictors must be used cautiously to treat hypotension because they could markedly elevate pulmonary vascular resistance and induce right ventricular failure.

After cardiopulmonary bypass, there is usually an immediate decrease in left atrial pressure followed by a more gradual decline in pulmonary vascular resistance. However, if pulmonary capillary wedge pressure and pulmonary vascular resistance remain elevated and lead to clinical deterioration, the use of dobutamine, isoproterenol, and amrinone, which are inotropes and pulmonary vasodilators, can improve hemodynamics. In right ventricular failure, pulmonary arterial vasodilators (i.e., isoproterenol, dobutamine, nitroglycerin, phentolamine, amrinone, or prostaglandin E_1) can be infused into a right atrial line. Simultaneously, inotropic drugs (i.e., epinephrine, norepinephrine) for left ventricular and systemic support can be given directly through a separate left atrial line. In one study of patients developing refractory right heart failure and pulmonary hypertension after mitral valve replacement, prostaglandin E_1 (30 to 150 ng/kg/min), a potent pulmonary vasodilator, was infused into a central venous line and norepinephrine (up to 1 μg/kg/min) was given through a left atrial line. All patients had rapid pulmonary vasodilator responses with marked improvement in right ventricular performance (194). If pulmonary vascular resistance remains elevated and is associated with normal or elevated pulmonary capillary wedge pressure and blood pressure, the use of pulmonary vasodilators, such as nitroprusside and phentolamine, along with preload augmentation can increase stroke volume and cardiac output. However, these drugs improve pulmonary blood flow, blunt hypoxic pulmonary vasoconstriction, and increase intrapulmonary shunting, which decrease arterial oxygen saturation.

There will be a residual gradient across the mitral valve after surgery because of incomplete mitral commissurotomy or intrinsic obstruction of the mitral prosthesis. Therefore, wedge pressure will continue to overestimate left ventricular end-diastolic pressure, especially in patients with atrial fibrillation. Because of this persistent gradient, patients will elevate left atrial pressure when the diastolic flow period is reduced during tachycardia. Hence, tachycardia should be avoided even after mitral valve replacement.

Preoperative decreases in vital capacity and lung compliance and increases in shunting and work of breathing, typical of mitral valve disease, are accentuated in the postoperative period. Since residual narcotics and benzodiazepines depress the CO_2 response curve postoperatively, patients usually require longer periods of mechanical ventilation postoperatively.

Mitral Regurgitation

Chronic mitral regurgitation results in left ventricular volume overload and dilation. Since filling of the left atrium begins immediately with ventricular systole, there is no isovolumic con-

traction, and 50% of regurgitant flow occurs before aortic valve opening. This dissipates myocardial wall tension and minimizes energy expenditure of the left ventricle. Regurgitant flows depend on flow ventricular volume, mitral valve orifice size, pressure gradient across the mitral valve, left atrial and pulmonary compliance, changes in pulmonary blood volume, and impedance to ejection into the aorta. Left ventricular ejection fraction is often in the normal range, but low normal left ventricular ejection fractions (less than 0.55) indicate significant deterioration of myocardial contractility (166).

Acute mitral regurgitation—usually secondary to myocardial ischemia, acute myocardial infarction, chordal rupture in mitral valve prolapse, or bacterial endocarditis—results in acute volume overload with decreases in forward stroke volume. There is compensatory tachycardia, increased contractility, and left ventricular dilation. Because regurgitation occurs into a small, noncompliant left atrium, left ventricular end-diastolic, left atrial, and pulmonary venous pressures are high. This results in pulmonary congestion and edema, pulmonary artery hypertension, acute right ventricular failure, and low cardiac output (195).

Heavy premedication is given to patients with chronic mitral regurgitation and good left ventrical function or angina, and patients with mitral valve prolapse. Minimal or no premedication should be given to patients with acute mitral regurgitation or chronic mitral regurgitation and poor left ventricular function.

A modified V_5 and inferior ECG lead is monitored to detect myocardial ischemia, P wave morphology, and arrhythmias. Direct arterial pressure monitoring is essential because these patients require hemodynamic and arterial blood gas determinations. Preoperative insertion of a pulmonary artery catheter is also essential because it allows optimal preload augmentation, assessment of systemic vascular resistance and regurgitant v waves, and accurate titration of vasodilators and inotropic agents. Intraoperative changes in the height of the v wave or the mean pulmonary capillary wedge pressure should be noted because they may reflect increased intravascular volume, altered loading conditions of the left ventricle, dynamic change in the mitral valve orifice size, or diminished compliance of the left atrium and ventricle.

Intraoperatively, patients with nonischemic mitral regurgitation should have their heart rate maintained between 70 and 90 beats/min. When coronary artery disease is associated with mitral regurgitation, heart rates between 50 and 70 may result in a more favorable myocardial oxygen balance. Vercuronium, pancuronium-metocurine combination, and atracurium are preferred neuromuscular blockers because of their cardiovascular stability and minimal effect on myocardial oxygen consumption.

Since patients with acute or chronic mitral regurgitation and depressed ventricular function are dependent on sympathetic tone to maintain function, anesthetic techniques that avoid myocardial depression and decrease afterload are preferred. Narcotic analgesics (e.g., fentanyl, sufentanil), arterial vasodilators (e.g., nitroprusside), and preload augmentation (187, 188) can be used to decrease impedance to left ventricular ejection, improve forward stroke volume and cardiac output, and decrease mitral orifice size. Nitrous oxide should be avoided because it increases systemic and pulmonary vascular resistance and depresses myocardial contractility when added to narcotic analgesia in patients with pulmonary hypertension (176, 192). In patients with mitral regurgitation and myocardial ischemia or infarction, left ventricular function may be severely impaired. Although vasodilators are useful in maintaining forward stroke volume, systemic hypotension may ensue and inotropic drugs or intraaortic balloon may be required to prevent coronary hypoperfusion and further clinical deterioration.

In patients with mitral valve prolapse, ventricular volume determines the extent of the prolapse. Increases in left ventricular volume associated with slower heart rate and adequate preload diminish prolapse of the redundant mitral leaflets into the left atrium (196). Tachycardia, hypovolemia, decreased venous return, vasodilation, excessive airway pressure, and reverse Trendelenburg position should be avoided because they decrease ventricular volume and increase mitral regurgitation and prolapse of the mitral valve leaflets. Vecuronium, pancuronium-metocurine, and atracurium for neuromuscular relaxation are preferred since they have no detrimental cardiovascular effects. By decreasing catecholamine excess from surgical stimulation and depressing contractility, enflurane, which has the least effect on systemic vascular resistance of the inhalation anesthetics, may augment ventricular volume and theoretically reduce prolapse of the mitral valve leaflets. If arrhythmias develop, the usual causes (i.e., light anesthesia, hypoxemia, hypercarbia, sympathetic stimulation) should be corrected. If the arrhythmias persist, intravenous esmolol or propranolol is the drug of choice. If unsuccessful, ventricular arrhythmias may require lidocaine; supraventricular arrhythmias, depending on the type, may be treated with intravenous verapamil, digoxin, or pronestyl.

After cardiopulmonary bypass and mitral valve replacement, left ventricular afterload can no longer be dissipated through regurgitation into the low-pressure left atrium. Since the left ventricle is hypocontractile and the entire stroke volume is now ejected against aortic resistance, inotropic drugs with or without vasodilators are often required to increase contractility and reduce afterload. If systemic hypotension and coronary hypoperfusion persist (seem primarily in ischemic mitral regurgitation), additional intraortic balloon support or left or right ventricular assist may be necessary. Occasionally, elevated pulmonary vascular resistance and right ventricular failure may be the cause of the low cardiac output syndrome, and inotropes with pulmonary vasodilating properties may be beneficial. After cardiopulmonary bypass, patients with chronic mitral regurgitation and impaired cardiac function usually need a high preload, while patients with acute mitral regurgitation and good left ventricular function require normal filling pressures.

References

1. Miller RR, Olson HG, Amsterdam EA, et al: Propranolol-withdrawal rebound phenomenon. *N Engl J Med* 293:416–418, 1975.
2. Slogoff S, Keats AS, Ott E: Preoperative propranolol therapy and aortocoronary bypass operations. *JAMA* 240:1487–1490, 1978.
3. Subramanian VB, Bowles MJ, Khurmi NS, et al:

Calcium antagonist withdrawal syndrome: objective demonstration with frequency-modulated ambulatory ST-segment monitoring. *Br Med J* 286:520–521, 1983.

4. Mehta J, Lopez LM: Calcium-blocker withdrawal phenomenon: increase in affinity of alpha$_2$ adrenoceptors for agonist as a potential mechanism. *Am J Cardiol* 58:242–246, 1986.

5. Winniford MD, Jansen DE, Reynolds GA, et al: Cigarette smoking-induced coronary vasoconstriction in atherosclerotic coronary artery disease and prevention by calcium antagonists and nitroglycerin. *Am J Cardiol* 59:203–207, 1987.

6. Kapur PA, Bloor BC, Flacke WE, et al: Comparison of cardiovascular responses to verapamil during enflurane, isoflurane, or halothane anesthesia in the dog. *Anesthesiology* 61:156–160, 1984.

7. Kapur PA, Campos JH, Tippit SE: Influence of diltiazem on cardiovascular function and coronary hemodynamics during isoflurane anesthesia in the dog: correlation with plasma diltiazem levels. *Anesth Analg* 65:81–87, 1986.

8. Merin RG: Calcium channel blocking drugs and anesthetics: is the drug interaction beneficial or detrimental? *Anesthesiology* 66:111–113, 1987.

9. O'Connor DE: Accelerated acute clonidine withdrawal during coronary artery bypass surgery. *Br J Anaesth* 53:431–433, 1981.

10. Katz JD, Croneau LH, Barash PG: Postoperative hypertension: a hazard of abrupt cessation of antihypertensive medication in the preoperative period. *Am Heart J* 92:79–80, 1976.

11. Ghignone M, Quintin L, Duke PC, et al: Effects of clonidine on narcotic requirements and hemodynamic response during induction of fentanyl anesthesia and endotracheal intubation. *Anesthesiology* 64:36–42, 1986.

12. Prys-Roberts C, Meloche R, Foex P: Studies of anaesthesia in relation to hypertension. 1. Cardiovascular responses of treated and untreated patients. *Br J Anaesth* 43:122–137, 1971.

13. Goldman L, Caldera DL: Risks of general anesthesia and elective operation in the hypertensive patient. *Anesthesiology* 50:285–292, 1979.

14. Flacke JW, Bloor BC, Flacke WE, et al: Reduced narcotic requirement by clonidine with improved hemodynamic and adrenergic stability in patients undergoing coronary bypass surgery. *Anesthesiology* 67:11–19, 1987.

15. Ghignone M, Cavillo O, Quinton L: Anesthesia and hypertension: the effect of clonidine

on perioperative hemodynamics and isoflurane requirements. *Anesthesiology* 67:3–10, 1987.

16. Harrah MD, Way WL, Katzung BG: The interaction of d-tubocurarine with antiarrhythmic drugs. *Anesthesiology* 33:406–410, 1970.

17. Miller RD, Way WL, Katzung BG: The potentiation of neuromuscular blocking agents by quinidine. *Anesthesiology* 28:1036–1041, 1967.

18. Pratila MG, Pratilas V: Anesthetic agents and cardiac electromechanical activity. *Anesthesiology* 49:338–360, 1978.

19. Horowitz LN, Zipes DP (eds): A symposium: perspectives on proarrhythmia. *Am J Cardiol* 59:1E–56E, 1987.

20. Bartolone RS, Rao TLK: Dysrhythmias following muscle relaxant administration in patients receiving digitalis. *Anesthesiology* 58:567–569, 1983.

21. Alfery DD, Denlinger JK: Profound hypotension following a "test dose" of bretylium tosylate. *Anesth Analg* 58:516–518, 1979.

22. Shapiro W: Correlative studies of serum digitalis levels and the arrhythmias of digitalis intoxication. *Am J Cardiol* 41:852–859, 1978.

23. Iseri LT, Freed J, Bures AR: Magnesium deficiency and cardiac disorders. *Am J Med* 58:837–846, 1975.

24. Beller GA, Smith TW, Abelmann WH, et al: Digitalis intoxication. *N Engl J Med* 284:989–997, 1971.

25. Abrams J: Tolerance to organic nitrates. *Circulation* 74:1181–1185, 1986.

26. Fibuch EE, Cecil WT, Reed WA: Methemoglobinemia associated with organic nitrate therapy. *Anesth Analg* 58:521–523, 1979.

27. Zurick AM, Wagner RH, Starr NJ, et al: Intravenous nigroglycerin, methemoglobinemia, and respiratory distress in a postoperative cardiac surgical patient. *Anesthesiology* 61:464–466, 1984.

28. Lichtenthal PR, Rossi EC, Louis G, et al: Dose-related prolongation of the bleeding time by intravenous nitroglycerin. *Anesth Analg* 64:30–33, 1985.

29. Ghani GA, Sung YF, Weinstein MS, et al: Effects of intravenous nitroglycerin on the intracranial pressure and volume pressure response. *J Neurosurg* 58:562–565, 1983.

30. Shook TL, Kirshenbaum JM, Hundley RF, et al: Ethanol intoxication complicating intravenous nitroglycerin therapy. *Ann Intern Med* 101:498–499, 1984.

31. Jung RT, Shetty PS, James WPT: Heparin, free fatty acids and an increased metabolic demand for oxygen. *Postgrad Med J* 56:330–332, 1980.

32. Cines DP, Kaywin P, Bina M, et al: Heparin-associated thrombocytopenia. *N Engl J Med* 303:788–795, 1980.

33. Trowbridge AA, Caraveo J, Green JB, et al: Heparin-related immune thrombocytopenia. *Am J Med* 65:277–283, 1978.

34. Anderson WH, Mohammad SF, Chuang HYK, et al: Heparin potentiates synthesis of thromboxane A_2 in human platelets. *Adv Prostaglandin Thromboxane Res* 6:287–291, 1980.

35. Saba HI, Saba SR, Blackburn CA, et al: Heparin neutralization of PGI_2: Effects upon platelets. *Science* 205:499–501, 1979.

36. Makhoul RG, McCann RL, Austin EH, et al: Management of patients with heparin-associated thrombocytopenia and thrombosis requiring cardiac surgery. *Ann Thorac Surg* 43:617–621, 1987.

37. Hensley FA Jr, Dodson DL, Martin DE, et al: Oxygen saturation during preinduction placement of monitoring catheters in the cardiac surgical patient. *Anesthesiology* 66:834–836, 1987.

38. Robertson D, Kostuk WJ, Ahuja SP: The localization of coronary artery stenosis by 12 lead ECG response to graded exercise test: support for intercoronary steal. *Am Heart J* 91:437–444, 1976.

39. Kaplan JA, King SB: The precordial electrocardiographic lead (V_5) in patients who have coronary artery disease. *Anesthesiology* 45:570–574, 1976.

40. Kattus AA: Exercise electrocardiography: recognition of the ischemic response, false positive and negative patterns. *Am J Cardiol* 33:721–731, 1974.

41. Hollenberg M, Budge WR, Wisneski JA, et al: Treadmill score quantifies electrocardiographic response to exercise and improves test accuracy and reproducibility. *Circulation* 61:276–285, 1980.

42. Hollenberg M, Zoltick JM, Go M, et al: Comparison of a quantitative treadmill exercise score with standard electrocardiographic criteria in screening asymptomatic young men for coronary artery disease. *N Engl J Med* 313:600–606, 1985.

43. Cohn K, Kamm B, Feteih N, et al: Use of treadmill score to quantify ischemic response

and predict extent of coronary disease. *Circulation* 59:286–296, 1979.

44. Borrello G: ECG artifacts simulating atrial flutter. *JAMA* 223:439, 1973.

45. Shapiro LA, Jedeikin R, Hoffman S: Misdiagnosis due to ECG failure. *Anesthesiology* 60:166, 1984.

46. Doss JD, McCabe CW, Weiss GK: Noise-free data during electrosurgical procedures. *Anesth Analg* 52:156–160, 1973.

47. Slogoff S, Keats AS: Does perioperative myocardial ischemia lead to postoperative myocardial infarction? *Anesthesiology* 62:107–114, 1985.

48. London MJ, Hollenberg M, Wong MG, et al: Intraoperative myocardial ischemia: localization by continuous 12-lead electrocardiography. *Anesthesiology* 69:232–241, 1988.

49. Kates RA, Zaidan JR, Kaplan JA: Esophageal lead for intraoperative electrocardiographic monitoring. *Anesth Analg* 61:781–785, 1982.

50. Trager MA, Feinberg BI, Kaplan JA: Right ventricular ischemia diagnosed by an esophageal electrocardiogram and right atrial pressure tracing. *J Cardiothorac Anesth* 1:123–125, 1987.

51. Kotrly KJ, Kotter GS, Mortara D, et al: Intraoperative detection of myocardial ischemia with an ST segment trend monitoring system. *Anesth Analg* 63:343–345, 1984.

52. Kotter GS, Kotrly KJ, Kalbfleisch JH, et al: Myocardial ischemia during cardiovascular surgery as detected by an ST segment trend monitoring system. *J Cardiothorac Anesth* 1:190–199, 1987.

53. Smith JS, Cahalan MK, Benefiel DJ, et al: Intraoperative detection of myocardial ischemia in high-risk patients: electrocardiography versus two-dimensional transesophageal echocardiography. *Circulation* 72:1015–1021, 1985.

54. Bellows WH, Bode RH Jr, Levy JH, et al: Noninvasive detection of periinduction ischemic ventricular dysfunction by cardiokymography in humans: preliminary experience. *Anesthesiology* 60:155–158, 1984.

55. Mantle JA, Massing GK, James TN, et al: A multipurpose catheter for electrophysiologic and hemodynamic monitoring plus atrial pacing. *Chest* 72:285–290, 1977.

56. Yanowitz F, Kinias P, Rawling D, et al: Accuracy of a continuous real-time ECG dysrhythmia monitoring system. *Circulation* 50:65–72, 1974.

57. Barash PG, Chen Y, Kitahata LM, et al: The hemodynamic tracking system: A method of

data management and guide for cardiovascular therapy. *Anesth Analg* 59:169–174, 1980.

58. Waller JL, Johnson SP, Kaplan JA: Usefulness of pulmonary artery catheters during aortocoronary bypass surgery. *Anesth Analg* 61:221–222, 1982.

59. Waller JL, Zaidan JR, Kaplan JA, et al: Hemodynamic responses to preoperative vascular cannulation in patients with coronary artery disease. *Anesthesiology* 56:219–221, 1982.

60. Nussmeier NA, Arlund C, Slogoff S: Neuropsychiatric complications after cardiopulmonary bypass: cerebral protection by a barbiturate. *Anesthesiology* 64:165–170, 1986.

61. Rampil IJ, Matteo RS: Changes in EEG spectral edge frequency correlate with the hemodynamic response to laryngoscopy and intubation. *Anesthesiology* 67:139–142, 1987.

62. Bassel GM, Lin YT, Oka Y, et al: Circulatory response to tracheal intubation in patients with coronary artery disease and valvular disease. *Bull NY Acad Med* 54:842–848, 1978.

63. Fox EJ, Sklar GS, Hill CH, et al: Complications related to the pressor response to endotracheal intubation. *Anesthesiology* 47:524–525, 1977.

64. Denlinger JK, Ellison N, Ominsky AJ: Effects of intratracheal lidocaine on circulatory responses to tracheal intubation. *Anesthesiology* 41:409–412, 1974.

65. Stoelting RK: Circulatory changes during direct laryngoscopy and tracheal intubation: influence of duration of laryngoscopy with or without prior lidocaine. *Anesthesiology* 47:381–383, 1977.

66. Stoelting RK: Attenuation of blood pressure response to laryngoscopy and tracheal intubation with sodium nitroprusside. *Anesth Analg* 58:116–119, 1979.

67. Menkhaus PG, Reves JG, Kissin I, et al: Cardiovascular effects of esmolol in anesthetized humans. *Anesth Analg* 64:327–334, 1985.

68. Roizen MF: Does choice of anesthetic significantly affect cardiovascular outcome after cardiovascular surgery. In Estafanous FG (ed): *Opioids in Anesthesia*. Boston, Butterworth, 1984, pp 180–189.

69. Bovill JG, Seber PS, Stanley TH: Opioid analgesics in anesthesia: with special reference to their use in cardiovascular anesthesia. *Anesthesiology* 61:731–755, 1984.

70. Hug CC Jr: Pharmacology—anesthetic drugs. In Kaplan JA (ed): *Cardiac Anesthesia*. New York, Grune & Stratton, 1979, pp 3–37.

71. Bull BS, Korpman RA, Huse WM, et al: Heparin therapy during extracorporeal circulation. I. Problems inherent in existing heparin protocols. *J Thorac Cardiovasc Surg* 69:674–684, 1975.

72. Brozovic M, Baugham DR: Standards for heparin. In Bradshaw RA, Wessler S (eds): *Heparin—Structure, Function and Clinical Implications*. New York, Plenum, 1975, p 163.

73. Mabry CD, Read RC, Thompson BW, et al: Identification of heparin resistance during cardiac and vascular surgery. *Arch Surg* 114:129–134, 1979.

74. Anderson EF: Heparin resistance prior to cardiopulmonary bypass. *Anesthesiology* 64:504–507, 1986.

75. Blauhut B, Necek S, Kramar H, et al: Activity of antithrombin III and effect of heparin on coagulation in shock. *Thromb Res* 19:775–782, 1980.

76. Chung F, David T, Watt J: Excessive requirement for heparin during cardiac surgery. *Can Anaesth Soc J* 28:280–282, 1981.

77. Esposito RA, Culliford AT, Colvin SB, et al: Heparin resistance during cardiopulmonary bypass. *J Thorac Cardiovasc Surg* 85:346–353, 1983.

78. Habbab MA, Haft JI: Heparin resistance induced by intravenous nitroglycerin: a word of caution when both drugs are used concomitantly. *Arch Intern Med* 147:857–860, 1987.

79. Morrell DF, Harrison GG: Lignocaine kinetics during cardiopulmonary bypass. *Br J Anaesth* 55:1173–1177, 1983.

80. Stern DH, Gerson JI, Allen FB, et al: Can we trust the direct radial artery pressure immediately following cardiopulmonary bypass? *Anesthesiology* 62:557–561, 1985.

81. Drop LJ: Ionized calcium, the heart, and hemodynamic function. *Anesth Analg* 64:432–451, 1985.

82. Flaherty JT, Magee PA, Gardner TL, et al: Comparison of intravenous nitroglycerin and sodium nitroprusside for treatment of acute hypertension developing after coronary artery bypass surgery. *Circulation* 65:1072–1077, 1982.

83. Sladen RN: Management of the adult cardiac patient in the intensive care unit. In Ream AK, Fogdall RP (eds): *Acute Cardiovascular Management*. Philadelphia, JP Lippincott, 1982, pp 510–512.

84. Bull BS, Huse WM, Brauer FS, et al: Heparin therapy during extracorporeal circulation. II. The use of a dose-response curve to individualize heparin and protamine dosage. *J Thorac Cardiovasc Surg* 69:685–689, 1975.

85. Culliford AT, Gitel SN, Starr N, et al: Lack of correlation between activated clotting time and plasma heparin during cardiopulmonary bypass. *Ann Surg* 193:105–111, 1981.
86. Glass DD: Management of blood and coagulation. In Kaplan JA (ed): *Cardiac Anesthesia—Cardiovascular Pharmacology*. New York, Grune & Stratton, 1983, p 456.
87. Jobes DR, Schwartz AJ, Ellison N, et al: Monitoring heparin anticoagulation and its neutralization. *Ann Thorac Surg* 31:161–166, 1981.
88. Horrow JC: Protamine: a review of its toxicity. *Anesth Analg* 64:348–361, 1985.
89. Horrow JC: Protamine allergy. *J Cardiothorac Anesth* 2:225–242, 1988.
90. Lowenstein E, Johnston WE, Lappas DG, et al: Catastrophic pulmonary vasoconstriction associated with protamine reversal of heparin. *Anesthesiology* 59:470–473, 1983.
91. Spiess BD, Tuman KJ, McCarthy RJ, et al: Thromboelastography as an indication of post-cardiopulmonary bypass coagulopathies. *J Clin Monit* 3:25–30, 1987.
92. Tuman KJ, Spiess BD, McCarthy RJ, et al: Effects of progressive blood loss on coagulation as measured by thromboelastography. *Anesth Analg* 66:856–863, 1987.
93. Saleem A, Blifeld C, Saleh S, et al: Visoelastic measurement of clot formation: a new test of platelet function. *Ann Clin Lab Sci* 13:115–124, 1983.
94. Braunwald E: Control of myocardial oxygen consumption. *Am J Cardiol* 27:416–432, 1971.
95. Hoffman JIE: Maximal coronary flow and the concept of coronary vascular reserve. *Circulation* 70:153–159, 1984.
96. Knight AA, Hollenberg M, London MJ, et al: Perioperative myocardial ischemia: importance of the preoperative ischemic pattern.
97. Kinzer JB, Lichtenthal PR, Wade LD: Loss of radial artery pressure trace during internal mammary artery dissection for coronary artery bypass graft surgery. *Anesth Analg* 64:1134–1136, 1985.
98. Chaux A, Blanche C: A new concept in sternal retraction: applications for internal mammary artery dissection and valve replacement surgery. *Ann Thorac Surg* 42:473–474, 1986.
99. Kaplan JA, Wells PH: Early diagnosis of myocardial ischemia using the pulmonary artery catheter. *Anesth Analg* 60:789–793, 1981.
100. Giles RW, Berger HJ, Barash PG, et al: Continuous monitoring of left ventricular performance with the computerized nuclear probe during larygnoscopy and intubation before coronary artery bypass surgery. *Am J Cardiol* 50:735–741, 1982.
101. Kleinman B, Henkin RE, Glisson SN, et al: Qualitative evaluation of coronary flow during anesthetic induction using thallium-201 perfusion scans. *Anesthesiology* 64:157–164, 1986.
102. Reiz S, Rydvall A, Haggmark S: Coronary haemodynamic effects of surgery during enflurane-nitrous oxide anaesthesia in patients with ischaemic heart disease. *Acta Anaesthesiol Scand* 29:106–112, 1985.
103. Hilfiker O, Larsen R, Sonntag H: Myocardial blood flow and oxygen consumption during halothane-nitrous oxide anaesthesia for coronary revascularization. *Br J Anaesth* 55:927–932, 1983.
104. Moffitt EA, Imrie DD, Scovil JE, et al: Myocardial metabolism and haemodynamic responses with enflurane anaesthesia for coronary artery surgery. *Can Anaesth Soc J* 31:604–610, 1984.
105. Wilkinson PL, Hamilton WK, Moyers JR, et al: Halothane and morphine–nitrous oxide anesthesia in patients undergoing coronary artery bypass operation: patterns of intraoperative ischemia. *J Thorac Cardiovasc Surg* 82:372–382, 1981.
106. Reiz S, Balfors E, Sorensen MB, et al: Isoflurane—a powerful coronary vasodilator in patients with coronary artery disease. *Anesthesiology* 59:91–97, 1983.
107. Moffitt EA, Barker RA, Glenn JJ, et al: Myocardial metabolism and hemodynamic responses with isoflurane anesthesia for coronary arterial surgery. *Anesth Analg* 65:53–61, 1986.
108. Savarese JJ, Lowenstein E: The name of the game: no anesthesia by cookbook. *Anesthesiology* 62:703–705, 1985.
109. Thomson IR, Putnins CL: Adverse effects of pancuronium during high-dose fentanyl anesthesia for coronary artery bypass grafting. *Anesthesiology* 62:708–713, 1985.
110. Morris RB, Cahalan MK, Miller RD, et al: The cardiovascular effects of vecuronium and pancuronium in patients undergoing coronary artery bypass grafting. *Anesthesiology* 58:438–440, 1983.
111. Chiariello M, Gold HK, Leinbach RC, et al: Comparison between the effects of nitroprusside and nitroglycerin on ischemic injury during acute myocardial infarction. *Circulation* 54:766–773, 1976.

112. Buffington CW: Hemodynamic determinants of ischemic myocardial dysfunction in the presence of coronary stenosis on dogs. _Anesthesiology_ 63:651–662, 1985.

113. Borer JS, Redwood DR, Levitt B, et al: Reduction in myocardial ischemia with nitroglycerin or nitroglycerin plus phenylephrine administered during acute myocardial infarction. _N Engl J Med_ 293:1008–1012, 1975.

114. Rosenthal SJ, Ginsburg R, Lamb IH, et al: Efficacy of diltiazem for control of symptoms of coronary artery spasm. _Am J Cardiol_ 46:1027–1032, 1980.

115. Petru MA, Crawford MH, Sorenson SG, et al: Short- and long-term efficacy of high-dose oral diltiazem for angina due to coronary artery disease: a placebo-controlled, randomized, double-blind cross-over study. _Circulation_ 68:139–147, 1983.

116. Coriat P, Daloz M, Bousseau D, et al: Prevention of intraoperative myocardial ischemia during noncardiac surgery with intravenous nitroglycerin. _Anesthesiology_ 61:193–196, 1984.

117. Godet G, Coriat P, Baron JF, et al: Prevention of intraoperative myocardial ischemia during noncardiac surgery with intravenous diltiazem: a randomized trial versus placebo. _Anesthesiology_ 66:241–245, 1987.

118. O'Connor JP, Wynands JE: Anesthesia for myocardial revascularization. In Kaplan JA (ed): _Cardiac Anesthesia._ Orlando, FL, Grune & Stratton, 1987, pp 551–588.

119. Mangano DT: Biventricular function after myocardial revascularization in humans: deterioration and recovery patterns during the first 24 hours. _Anesthesiology_ 62:571–577, 1985.

120. Mangano DT, Van Dyke DC, Ellis RJ: The effect of increasing preload on ventricular output and ejection in man. Limitations of the Frank-Starling mechanism. _Circulation_ 62:535–541, 1980.

121. Jett GK, Arcidi JM Jr, Dorsey LMA, et al: Vasoactive drug effects on blood flow in internal mammary artery and saphenous vein grafts. _J Thorac Cardiovasc Surg_ 94:2–11, 1987.

122. Vasu, MA, O'Keefe DD, Kapellakis GZ, et al: Myocardial oxygen consumption: effects of epinephrine, isoproterenol, dopamine, norepinephrine, and dobutamine. _Am J Physiol_ 235:H237–H241, 1978.

123. Warltier DC, Zyvoloski M, Gross GJ, et al: Redistribution of myocardial blood flow distal to a dynamic coronary arterial stenosis by sym-

pathomimetic amines. _Am J Cardiol_ 48:269–279, 1981.

124. Fowler MB, Alderman EL, Oesterle SN, et al: Dobutamine and dopamine after cardiac surgery: greater augmentation of mycardial blood flow with dopamine. _Circulation_ 70(Suppl I):I103–I111, 1984.

125. Bertizbeitia LD, Piccione W, Austin JC, et al: Inotropic response of the salvaged myocardium after acute coronary occlusion. _Ann Thorac Surg_ 41:58–64, 1986.

126. Rogers WJ, Russell RO Jr, McDaniel HG, et al: Acute effects of glucose-insulin-potassium infusion on myocardial substrates, coronary blood flow and oxygen consumption in man. _Am J Cardiol_ 40:421–428, 1977.

127. Prather JW, Russell RO Jr, Mantle JA, et al: Metabolic consequences of glucose-insulin-potassium infusion in treatment of acute myocardial infarction. _Am J Cardiol_ 38:95–99, 1976.

128. Haider W, Eckersberger F, Wolner E: Preventive insulin administration for myocardial protection in cardiac surgery. _Anesthesiology_ 60:422–429, 1984.

129. Thomsen JH, Shug AL, Yap VU, et al: Improved pacing tolerance of the ischemic human myocardium after administration of carnitine. _Am J Cardiol_ 43:300–306, 1979.

130. Buxton AE, Goldberg S, Harken A, et al: Coronary artery spasm immediately after myocardial revascularization. _N Engl J Med_ 304:1249–1253, 1981.

131. Skarvan K, Graedel E, Hasse J, et al: Coronary artery spasms after coronary artery bypass surgery. _Anesthesiology_ 61:323–327, 1984.

132. Boulanger M, Maille JG, Pelletier GB, et al: Vasospastic angina after calcium injection. _Anesth Analg_ 63:1124–1126, 1984.

133. Kurusz M: Gaseous microemboli: Sources, causes, and clinical considerations. _Med. Instrum_ 19:73–76, 1985.

134. Oka Y, Moriwaki KM, Hong Y, et al: Detection of air emboli in the left heart by M-mode transesophageal echocardiography following cardiopulmonary bypass. _Anesthesiology_ 63:109–113, 1985.

135. Lawrence GH, McKay HA, Sherensky RT: Effective measures in the prevention of intraoperative aeroembolus. _J Thorac Cardiovasc Surg_ 62:731–735, 1971.

136. Thomson IR, Rosenbloom M, Cannon JE, et al: Electrocardiographic ST-segment elevation after myocardial reperfusion during coronary ar-

tery surgery. *Anesth Analg* 66:1183–1186, 1987.

137. Lytle BW, Loop FD, Cosgrove DM, et al: Fifteen hundred coronary reoperations: results and determinants of early and late survival. *J Thorac Cardiovasc Surg* 93:847–859, 1987.

138. Estafanous FG: Anesthesia and heart reoperations. *Cleve Clin Q* 48:93–96, 1981.

139. Brummett C, Reves JG, Lell WA, et al: Patient care problems in patients undergoing reoperation for coronary artery grafting surgery. *Can Anaesth Soc J* 31:213–220, 1984.

140. Kutcher MA, King SB III, Alimurung BN, et al: Constrictive pericarditis as a complication of cardiac surgery: recognition of an entity. *Am J Cardiol* 50:742–748, 1982.

141. Ng AS, Dorosti K, Sheldon WC: Constrictive pericarditis following cardiac surgery—Cleveland Clinic experience: report of 12 cases and review. *Cleve Clin Q* 51:39–45, 1984.

142. Baillot RG, Loop FD, Cosgrove DM, et al: Reoperation after previous grafting with the internal mammary artery: technique and early results. *Ann Thorac Surg* 40:271–273, 1985.

143. Zaidan JR: Experience with the pacing pulmonary artery catheter. *Anesthesiology* 53:S118, 1980.

144. Visser CA, Koolen JJ, Van Wezel HB, et al: Transesophageal echocardiography: technique and clinical applications. *J Cardiothorac Anesth* 2:74–91, 1988.

145. Dobell ARC, Jain AK: Catastrophic hemorrhage during redo sternotomy. *Ann Thorac Surg* 37:273–278, 1984.

146. Keon WJ, Heggtveit HA, Leduc J: Perioperative myocardial infarction caused by atheroembolism. *J Thorac Cardiovasc Surg* 84:849–855, 1982.

147. Camann WR, Wojtowicz SR, Mark JB: Reoperation for coronary artery bypass grafting: anesthetic challenge. *J Cardiothorac Anesth* 1:458–467, 1987.

148. Kaplan JA, Cannarella C, Jones EL, et al: Autologous blood transfusion during cardiac surgery: a reevaluation of three methods. *J Thorac Cardiovasc Surg* 74:4–10, 1977.

149. LeVeen HH: Normovolemic hemodilution and autotransfusion in surgery. In Hauer JM (ed): *Autotransfusion.* New York, Elsevier/North Holland, 1981, p 71.

150. Estafanous FG, Selim W, Tarazi RC: Effects of cardiac depression on hemodynamic responses to hemodilution. *Anesthesiology* 63:A38, 1985.

151. Hauer JM, Schaff HV, Bell WR, et al: Reinfusion of shed mediastinal tube blood following open heart surgery: a prospective study. *Circulation* 56(Suppl III):250, 1977.

152. Carter RF, McArdle B, Morritt GM: Autologous transfusion of mediastinal drainage blood: a report of its use following open-heart surgery. *Anaesthesia* 36:54–59, 1981.

153. Cork RC, Weiss JL, Hameroff SR, et al: Fentanyl preloading for rapid-sequence induction of anesthesia. *Anesth Analg* 63:60–64, 1984.

154. Kleinman J, Marlar K, Silva DA, et al: Sufentanil attenuation of the stress response during rapid sequence induction. *Anesthesiology* 63:A379, 1985.

155. Gooding JM, Weng JT, Smith RA, et al: Cardiovascular and pulmonary responses following etomidate induction anesthesia in patients with demonstrated cardiac disease. *Anesth Analg* 58:40–41, 1979.

156. Murkin JM, Moldenhauer CC, Hug CC Jr: High-dose fentanyl for rapid induction of anesthesia in patients with coronary artery disease. *Can Anaesth Soc J* 32:320–325, 1985.

157. Schwarz S, Ilias W, Lackner F, et al: Rapid tracheal intubation with vecuronium: the priming principle. *Anesthesiology* 62:388–391, 1985.

158. Bland JHL, Lowenstein E: Halothane-induced decrease in experimental myocardial ischemia in the non-failing canine heart. *Anesthesiology* 45:287–293, 1976.

159. Davis RF, DeBoer LWV, Rude RE, et al: The effect of halothane anesthesia on myocardial necrosis, hemodynamic performance, and regional myocardial blood flow in dogs following coronary artery occlusion. *Anesthesiology* 59:402–411, 1983.

160. MacLeod BA, Augereau P, Walker MJA: Effects of halothane anesthesia compared with fentanyl anesthesia and no anesthesia during coronary ligation in rats. *Anesthesiology* 58:44–52, 1983.

161. Lowenstein E, Foex P, Francis CM, et al: Regional ischemic ventricular dysfunction in myocardium supplied by a narrowed coronary artery with increasing halothane concentration in the dog. *Anesthesiology* 55:349–359, 1981.

162. Francis CM, Foex P, Lowenstein E, et al: Interaction between regional myocardial ischaemia and left ventricular performance under halothane anaesthesia. *Br J Anaesth* 54:965–980, 1982.

163. Hill RF, Kates RA, Davis D, et al: Anesthetic

implications for the management of patients with acute myocardial infarction: a matched cohort study of patients undergoing emergency myocardial revascularization. *J Cardiothorac Anesth* 2:23–29, 1988.

164. Skinner JR, Phillips SJ, Zeff RH, et al: Immediate coronary bypass following failed streptokinase infusion in evolving myocardial infarction. *J Thorac Cardiovasc Surg* 87:567–570, 1984.

165. Mantia AM, Lolley DM, Stullken EH Jr, et al: Coronary artery bypass grafting within 24 hours after intracoronary streptokinase thrombolysis. *J Cardiothorac Anesth* 1:392–400, 1987.

166. Schlant RC, Nutter DO: Heart failure in valvular heart disease. *Medicine* 50:421–451, 1971.

167. Lombard JT, Seltzer A: Valvular aortic stenosis: a clinical and hemodynamic profile of patients. *Ann Intern Med* 106:292–298, 1987.

168. Marcus ML, Doty DB, Hiratzka LF, et al: Decreased coronary reserve: a mechanism for angina pectoris in patients with aortic stenosis and normal coronary arteries. *N Engl J Med* 307:1362–1366, 1982.

169. Trenouth RS, Phelps NC, Neill WA: Determinants of left ventricular hypertrophy and oxygen supply in chronic aortic valve disease. *Circulation* 53:644–650, 1976.

170. Lowenstein E, Hallowell P, Levine FH, et al: Cardiovascular response to large doses of intravenous morphine in man. *N Engl J Med* 281:1389–1393, 1969.

171. Knight PR, Kroll DA, Nahrwald ML, et al: Comparison of cardiovascular responses to anesthesia and operation when intravenous lidocaine or morphine sulfate is used as adjunct to diazepam–nitrous oxide for cardiac surgery. *Anesth Analg* 59:130–139, 1980.

172. Conahan TJ, Ominsky AJ, Wollman H, et al: A prospective random comparison of halothane and morphine for open-heart anesthesia: one year's experience. *Anesthesiology* 38:528–535, 1973.

173. Stanley TH, Webster LR: Anesthetic requirements and cardiovascular effects of fentanyl-oxygen and fentanyl-diazepam-oxygen anesthesia in man. *Anesth Analg* 57:411–416, 1978.

174. Stoelting RK, Reiss RR, Longnecker DE: Hemodynamic responses to nitrous oxide–halothane and halothane in patients with valvular heart disease. *Anesthesiology* 37:430–435, 1972.

175. Christensen V, Sorenson MB, Klauber PV, et al: Haemodynamic effects of enflurane in patients with valvular heart disease. *Acta Anaesth Scand* (Suppl)67:34–37, 1978.

176. Stoelting RK, Gibbs PS: Hemodynamic effects of morphine and morphine-nitrous oxide in valvular heart disease and coronary artery disease. *Anesthesiology* 38:45–52, 1973.

177. Sethna DH, Starr JN, Estafanous FG: Cardiovascular effects of nondepolarizing neuromuscular blockers in patients with aortic valve disease. *Can J Anaesth* 34:582–588, 1987.

178. Starr NJ, Sethna DH, Estafanous FG: Bradycardia and asystole following the rapid administration of sufentanil with vecuronium. *Anesthesiology* 64:521–523, 1986.

179. Greenberg BH, Massie BM: Beneficial effects of afterload reduction therapy in patients with congestive heart failure and moderate aortic stenosis. *Circulation* 61:1212–1216, 1980.

180. Awan NA, DeMaria AN, Miller RR, et al: Beneficial effects of nitroprusside on left ventricular dysfunction and myocardial ischemia in severe aortic stenosis. *Am Heart J* 101:386–394, 1981.

181. Perloff JG, Ronan JA Jr, deLeon AC Jr: The effect of nitroglycerin on left ventricular wall tension in fixed orifice aortic stenosis. *Circulation* 32:204–213, 1965.

182. Grose R, Nivatpumin T, Katz S, et al: Mechanism of nitroglycerin effect in valvular aortic stenosis. *Am J Cardiol* 44:1371–1377, 1979.

183. Morganroth J, Perloff JK, Zeldis SM, et al: Acute severe aortic regurgitation. Pathophysiology, clinical recognition, and management. *Ann Intern Med* 87:223–232, 1977.

184. Judge TP, Kennedy JW, Bennett LJ, et al: Quantitative hemodynamic effects of heart rate in aortic regurgitation. *Circulation* 44:355–367, 1971.

185. Thomson I, Dalton BC, Lappas DG, et al: Right bundle-branch block and complete heart block caused by the Swan-Ganz catheter. *Anesthesiology* 51:359–362, 1979.

186. Latson TW, Lappas DG: Use of a pacing catheter to control heart rate in a patient with aortic insufficiency and coronary artery disease. *Anesthesiology* 63:712–715, 1985.

187. Stone JG, Faltas AN, Hoar PK: Sodium nitroprusside therapy for cardiac failure in anesthetized patients with valvular insufficiency. *Anesthesiology* 49:414–418, 1978.

188. Stone JG, Calabro JR, Hoar PF, et al: Afterload reduction and preload augmentation improve the anesthetic management of patients

with cardiac failure and valvular regurgitation. *Anesth Analg* 59:737–742, 1980.

189. Arani DT, Carleton RA: The deleterious role of tachycardia in mitral stenosis. *Circulation* 36:511–516, 1967.

190. Meister SG, Engel TR, Feitosa GS, et al: Propranolol in mitral stenosis during sinus rhythm. *Am Heart J* 94:685–688, 1977.

191. Beiser GD, Epstein SE, Stampfer M, et al: Studies on digitalis. XVII. Effects of ouabain on the hemodynamic response to exercise in patients with mitral stenosis in normal sinus rhythm. *N Engl J Med* 278:131–137, 1968.

192. Hilgenberg JC, McCammon RL, Stoelting RK: Pulmonary and systemic vascular responses to nitrous oxide in patients with mitral stenosis

and pulmonary hypertension. *Anesth Analg* 59:323–326, 1980.

193. Stone JG, Hoar PF, Faltas AN, et al: Nitroprusside and mitral stenosis. *Anesth Analg* 59:662–665, 1980.

194. D'Ambra MN, LaRaia PJ, Philbin DM, et al: Prostaglandin E_1. A new therapy for refractory right heart failure and pulmonary hypertension after mitral valve replacement. *J Thorac Cardiovasc Surg* 89:567–572, 1985.

195. DePace NL, Nestico PF, Morganroth J: Acute severe mitral regurgitation. Pathophysiology, clinical recognition, and management. *Am J Med* 78:293–306, 1985.

196. Jeresaty RM: *Mitral Valve Prolapse.* New York, Raven Press, 1979, pp 1–251.

Chapter 9
CARDIOVASCULAR AND METABOLIC RESPONSES TO GENERAL ANESTHESIA

DHUN H. SETHNA, M.D.
EMERSON A. MOFFITT, M.D.
JOHN BUSSELL, M.D.

In patients with coronary artery disease, especially those who have had recent myocardial infarctions, postoperative ischemia, including reinfarction, is more likely and mortality is increased (1). Intraoperative cardiovascular instability (tachycardia, hypertension, or hypotension) is associated with a higher occurrence of postoperative myocardial infarction, and invasive hemodynamic monitoring and aggressive cardiovascular therapy during surgery have been shown to reduce postoperative cardiac morbidity (2). Over the past decade, animal experiments and clinical studies have indicated that the anesthetic chosen in patients with coronary disease should allow heart pump function and arterial pressure to be controllably depressed during operation; that is, myocardial oxygen consumption (MVO_2) should not be allowed to rise, since oxygen supply (coronary blood flow) to myocardial ischemic areas may not increase sufficiently (3). This chapter summarizes clinical studies examining the effects of anesthesia and surgical stimulation on cardiac rhythm, systemic and coronary hemodynamics, and myocardial oxygen balance in patients undergoing cardiac surgery; some comments will also be made on coincident hormonal responses.

EFFECTS ON CARDIAC RHYTHM AND CONDUCTION

Clinical Studies

Postinduction arrhythmias are obvious on an oscilloscope in 18% of patients, but the incidence increases to 60% when Holter monitoring is used (4). Slow sinus rhythms, suppression of the primary pacemaker leading to AV nodal escape beats, and ventricular premature beats are common during inhalation anesthesia. Isorhythmic dissociation, a rhythm more often observed than classified, is a frequent accompaniment (5). In this type of AV nodal dissociation, the dissociated and upright P wave approaches the QRS complex, disappears within it for several beats, then reappears and recedes from the QRS. The sequence may be repeated. If the P waves progress beyond the QRS complex, they remain upright. If the moment of dissociation is missed, the oscilloscope pattern is one of QRS complexes without visible P waves and may be misread as an AV nodal rhythm. Long tracings and an awareness of the phenomenon usually increase its recognition. Attenuation of sympathetic tone by anesthesia, and anesthetic depression of SA node may cause or contribute to isorhythmic dissociation. Less commonly seen are true AV nodal rhythms or a wandering pacemaker.

Halothane sensitizes the myocardium to the arrhythmogenic properties of catecholamines to a greater extent than equipotent isoflurane, enflurane, or the equivalent narcotic–nitrous oxide anesthesia (6). The mechanisms remain unclear: norepinephrine reuptake is not affected by halothane, nor are receptor number and binding affinity of β-adrenergic receptors when examined by radioligand binding on membrane preparations from canine myocardium; observations that catecholamine-induced adenylate cyclase activity is reduced have not been substantiated. Since plasma catecholamines are reduced during deep halothane anesthesia, the sensitization mechanism may not depend on increases in neurotransmitter level. Clinically, if subcutaneous epinephrine is required for local hemostasis in the presence of halothane, the dose should not exceed 1 μg/kg over 10 min. Twice this can be used if injected with 0.5% lidocaine. Halothane also sensitizes the myocardium to the arrhythmogenic properties of dopamine, phenylephrine, metaraminol, cocaine, and aminophylline, while bretylium and guanethidine provoke arrhythmias with the agent by releasing catecholamines from adrenergic storage sites. Ten days of imipramine pretreatment renders dogs more susceptible to epinephrine-induced arrhythmias during halothane anesthesia.

Arrhythmias associated with digitalis result from enhancement of phase 4 depolarization in Purkinje fibers and, therefore, enhanced automaticity (4). Halothane, which depresses phase 4 depolarization, has been shown to moderate the cardiotoxic effects of digitalis and may even have a therapeutic value in ouabain-induced ventricular tachycardia. Enflurane and isoflurane also increase tolerance to ouabain toxicity and restore sinus rhythm when administered during ouabain-induced ventricular tachycardia

(4). They do not antagonize the AV nodal depression effect of digitalis.

Electrophysiologic Studies

Inward calcium currents that generate the "slow" action potential in sinoatrial nodal tissue were inhibited by halothane, leading to dose-dependent reductions in the maximum rate of rise (Vmax) of phase 4 and phase 0 of the action potential and to a negative chronotropic action (4, 7). This has been demonstrated in single sinoatrial nodal fibers, and can be partially attenuated by calcium and potentiated by verapamil. Enflurane and isoflurane also depressed sinoatrial nodal discharge rates in isolated guinea pig SA node preparations, without effects on resting membrane or threshold potentials (7). Rabbit atrial fibers, however, appeared to be less sensitive, and resting membrane potential and action potential amplitude showed little change with 2% halothane and even higher doses of enflurane (4).

His bundle electrograms confirmed that halothane caused dose-dependent slowing of cardiac conduction and prolonged A-H and H-V intervals, that persisted after atropine administration, thereby suggesting direct effects on the refractory period rather than a vagotonic action (4, 7). Propranolol further slowed conduction, indicating that sympathetic enhancement of AV conduction was still present even at a 2% halothane concentration. Enflurane increased A-H interval but not H-V interval in some studies (4), and depressed atrial effective refractory period, functional refractory period of the AV node, and AV nodal conductivity. Isoflurane was found to have no effect on AV nodal or His-Purkinje conduction time in spontaneously beating dog hearts (7).

Recent studies in chronically instrumented dogs, however, have shown prolongation of AV nodal, His-Purkinje and ventricular activation times by all three inhalation agents, when compared to the awake state in spontaneously beating hearts (7). These effects were due, in part, to direct depressant actions on AV nodal conduction, but predominantly from removal of sympathetic tone, without effects on the vagal tone.

The effects of halothane on single Purkinje

fibers have been inconsistent (4). Thus, resting membrane potential and rate of phase 4 depolarization were unaltered in canine tissue, whereas increased Vmax and enhanced membrane responsiveness were observed in other studies. In contrast, dose-dependent reductions in the rate of spontaneously beating fibers occurred in sheep Purkinje tissue, with increases in membrane threshold potential and attenuation of the rate of rise of phase 4 depolarization and action potential duration. Enflurane enhanced the rate of phase 4 depolarization of spontaneously beating Purkinje fibers, and reduced the threshold potential. Intraventricular conduction was slowed by halothane, and ventricular automaticity was depressed in isolated ventricular cell preparations and in intact animals (4). Enflurane had little effect on the resting membrane potential of normal guinea pig ventricular muscle, and the amplitude and Vmax of the action potential were virtually unaffected by even a 6% concentration.

HEMODYNAMIC EFFECTS AND MYOCARDIAL OXYGEN BALANCE

Inhalational Anesthesia

Halothane and Enflurane

Clinical observations that halothane causes myocardial depression have been substantiated by echocardiography and radionuclide angiography (8, 9). Proposed mechanisms include inhibition of release of membrane-bound calcium during excitation-contraction coupling, and reduced sensitivity of β-adrenergic receptors to norepinephrine leading to decreased intracellular cyclic AMP. Effects of halothane on baroreceptor mechanism, which are difficult to interpret, include sensitization of the afferent nerve endings and depression of the central reflex.

Decrease in cardiac index and stroke work index with halothane induction are associated with substantial reductions in myocardial oxygen needs (MVO_2) and significant increases in coronary sinus oxygen content without myocardial lactate production (3). Titration of halothane in anticipation of surgical stimulation adequately controls heart rate and arterial pressure and maintains global myocardial oxygen balance (10). In patients with left ventricular failure, reductions in coronary blood flow accompany those in mean arterial pressures, but MVO_2 also decreases without changes in coronary sinus lactate and hypoxanthine levels (11). It has been suggested that an unloading effect on the failing left ventricle by systemic vasodilation with halothane may predominate in some patients over direct cardiodepressant action by the agent.

Equipotent doses of enflurane can depress the mechanics and contractility of cardiac muscle more than halothane (12). Myocardial work and oxygen demands are reduced during enflurane anesthesia, and oxygen needs are fulfilled by proportional reductions in oxygen extraction and myocardial blood flow (3). However, if enflurane reduces arterial pressures substantially, myocardial ischemia can occur (13). Mean arterial pressure and stroke work index have been shown to be below awake values during sternotomy; that is, sympathetic responses to surgical stimulation remain attenuated with this agent (3). Normal myocardial lactate extraction usually continues during and after enflurane anesthesia.

Isoflurane

Like other inhaled agents, isoflurane depresses contractility in isolated papillary heart muscles; in patients, cardiac output is usually sustained with isoflurane because increases in heart rate and reductions in peripheral resistance compensate for decreases in stroke volume (14). Arterial pressure and peripheral vascular resistance are reduced in a dose-related manner, and can reach 50% of awake control values at high inspired concentrations. Blood flow to skeletal muscle is particularly enhanced, despite the drop in perfusion pressure by general vasodilation.

In a study examining myocardial oxygen balance in unpremedicated patients with coronary disease, isoflurane decreased coronary perfusion pressure by a combination of systemic vasodilation and reductions in cardiac performance (3, 15). Coronary blood flow did not change; consequently, coronary vascular resistance was calculated as being reduced. Despite reductions in MVO_2 and myocardial oxygen extraction, patients developed ischemic ECG changes with marked decreases in myocardial lactate extraction. Electrocardiographic changes reverted to baseline when the agent was discontinued, thus implicating isoflurane with myocardial ischemia, presumably due to reduced perfusion pressures or coronary flow redistribution or both. Patients without ECG changes had unchanged myocardial lactate extraction. In a follow-up report in which regional blood flow and metabolites were also measured, isoflurane–nitrous oxide anesthesia caused reductions in regional flow and oxygen extraction, so that calculated MVO_2 decreased in this area of the heart (16). More than half the patients showed ECG (V_5) signs of ischemia with reductions in myocardial lactate extraction, and one heart produced lactate. Other investigators have also observed myocardial lactate production with isoflurane, despite reductions in global MVO_2 (17, 18), in 30% of patients, indicating that isoflurane, under similar clinical conditions as halothane or enflurane, is more frequently associated with regional myocardial ischemia in the presence of coronary artery disease. On the other hand, examination of myocardial function by transesophageal echocardiography in similar patients failed to show new regional wall motion abnormalities with isoflurane-fentanyl anesthesia (19).

Nitrous Oxide

Nitrous oxide depresses myocardial contractility and increases sympathetic activity, resulting in peripheral vascular constriction and elevated serum levels of norepinephrine (9). Addition of nitrous oxide to opioid or enflurane anesthesia causes dose-dependent reductions in cardiac index and arterial pressure. In patients with valvular heart disease anesthetized with halothane, the weak sympathomimetic actions of nitrous oxide appear to improve the myocardial depression caused by halothane alone. In patients with coronary artery disease, however, addition of nitrous oxide to halothane (3) or enflurane (13) results in further myocardial depression and regional myocardial ischemia. Reductions in coronary blood flow caused by nitrous oxide are not accompanied by concom-

itant reductions in MVO_2 as seen with other inhaled agents; hence, myocardial oxygen supply decreases without a reduced oxygen demand, and myocardial lactate production occurs in the absence of ECG signs of ischemia. Patients anesthetized with halothene–nitrous oxide or morphine–nitrous oxide show ECG signs of ischemia or myocardial lactate production frequently during anesthesia or with surgical stimulation, and this may be attributed to the nitrous oxide (20).

Narcotic "Anesthesia"

Morphine

Intravenous morphine reduces arterial pressure due to venodilation, while decreases in heart rate result from stimulation of the medullary vagal nucleus and, partly, from direct actions on the SA node (9, 21). Reduced sympathetic tone to peripheral veins from a selective CNS effect is believed to be the mechanism of venodilation; hypotension may be enhanced by histamine release and bradycardia. Venoconstrictor responses to carbon dioxide and tilt are attenuated by morphine, whereas those associated with deep breathing are preserved.

Slow injections of "anesthetic" doses (1 to 2 mg/kg intravenously) decrease myocardial oxygen demand more than supply (3); however, when used as the sole anesthetic, morphine does not prevent increases in heart rate and systemic vascular resistance or maintain myocardial oxygen balance during surgical stimulation (3, 21). Reductions in arterial pressures at induction often lead to decreases in mean coronary flows (myocardial oxygen supply); however, myocardial oxygen balance is usually maintained because there are greater reductions in MVO_2 and increases in coronary sinus oxygen content. Sternotomy increases heart rate and arterial pressure over awake values, with most patients requiring vasodilator therapy. Myocardial oxygen extraction also increases with stimulation, and myocardial lactate extraction may be greatly reduced with the random production of myocardial lactate. This can occur without ECG (V_5) signs of ischemia, indicating that a normal S-T segment may not be an assurance of adequate myocardial oxygenation (3). Several studies have confirmed that elevations of heart rate and arterial pressure with surgical stimulation during morphine anesthesia may be associated with ischemic S-T segment depression or myocardial lactate production (3, 21). Pretreatment with propranolol appears to permit better control of hemodynamics and myocardial oxygen balance during operation (3).

In contrast to clinical experience, large doses of morphine (2 to 10 mg/kg) reduced coronary blood flow and caused myocardial lactate production even in unstimulated, anesthetized animals (22). In a study involving conscious dogs with presumably normal coronary arteries, morphine injection was associated with decreases in coronary blood flow and increases in coronary vascular resistance (22).

Fentanyl and Sufentanil

Fentanyl, even in large doses, maintains cardiovascular stability during induction (21). Myocardial function is preserved, and systemic vascular resistance is unchanged because the drug has minimal effects on vascular smooth muscle or histamine release. Bradycardia, from stimulation of the central vagal nucleus, is common but usually not severe, and can be readily reversed by anticholinergics, sympathomimetics, or drugs having vagolytic properties (e.g., pancuronium).

Low-dose fentanyl and sufentanil show no differences in systemic and coronary hemodynamic responses (21). Clinical experience with higher doses in patients undergoing cardiac surgery is, however, inconsistent in the nature and degree of cardiovascular stability provided (21). Whereas some reports indicate that sufentanil allows more-stable hemodynamics with less-frequent intraoperative hypertension, others show that the latter is common with either drug and requires treatment with vasodilators or other anesthetics. In a double-blind protocol in which fentanyl and sufentanil dosages were varied, hypertension occurred in all groups, usually with sternotomy or aortic cannulation, and as high as 30 µg/kg of sufentanil failed to prevent hypertension (21, 23). It has been suggested that hypertension associated with mammary artery dissection or aortic manipulation may not be due to inadequate anesthesia, but rather to ac-

tivation of sympathetic reflexes that are not blocked by these drugs. Hypertension with stimulation occurs frequently during fentanyl anesthesia in healthier patients who have good ventricular function or who are not on β-adrenergic blocker therapy. Also, sudden decreases in arterial pressure or bradycardia have been associated with sufentanil in patients with slow heart rates from chronic β-adrenergic blocker therapy (24).

Premedicated patients on β-adrenergic blocker drugs show minimal changes in heart rate on induction or intubation with high-dose fentanyl; in fact, heart rate may even decrease at sternotomy (3). Despite reductions in MVO_2 below awake values from reduced oxygen extraction, random instances of myocardial lactate production may be encountered with electrocardiographic normal S-T segments (3). Other studies have found no significant changes in coronary flow or MVO_2 (25), or reductions in MVO_2 (26), with normal myocardial lactate extraction in patients with coronary disease.

These observations, showing that fentanyl generally maintains myocardial oxygen balance during anesthesia and surgical stimulation, contrast with an earlier report that even large doses produce incomplete anesthesia and fail to protect the myocardium from ischemia in patients with coronary disease (3), the majority of whom produced myocardial lactate on sternotomy. The relative absence of anaerobic glycolysis in the other studies may have been due to heavier premedication, higher drug doses at induction, and more complete β-adrenergic blockade.

Experience with sufentanil infusions in patients with coronary artery disease show that ventricular function is usually preserved and global and regional myocardial perfusion is maintained (27). However, reductions in MVO_2 preclude random occurrences of myocardial lactate production.

Fentanyl-Enflurane and Fentanyl-Halothane Combinations

Fentanyl with either enflurane or halothane produces stable and comparable cardiovascular effects (3). Steady and controlled decreases of cardiac index from awake levels account for lowered arterial pressures. Coronary sinus oxygen content usually increases on induction, but gradually returns to awake levels before cardiopulmonary bypass. Myocardial lactate extraction usually remains unchanged, but rare instances of myocardial lactate production do occur despite stable systemic hemodynamics and a reduced global MVO_2.

NONNARCOTIC INTRAVENOUS ANESTHESIA

Thiopental, an ultra-short-acting barbiturate, and etomidate, a carboxylated imidazole, are usually used for induction of anesthesia (9, 14). Thiopental causes dose-dependent decreases in arterial pressures, partly from a direct myocardial depressant action and from venodilation due to an effect on the medullary sympathetic center. The severity of hypotension depends on the dose and rate of injection, and is more pronounced in those who are hypovolemic, hypertensive, or have myocardial dysfunction. Systemic vascular resistance shows no change or may be minimally increased. Effects on heart rate are inconsistent, with increases being usually observed. Myocardial oxygen consumption and coronary blood flows are increased in healthy patients, and lactate extraction remains unchanged (28).

Lack of cardiovascular effects is claimed to be one of the main features of etomidate (14). More recent observations, however, indicate that hemodynamic complications such as hypotension may be more common with this drug than was previously thought (29). In healthy patients, MVO_2 is usually preserved, and the drug may show weak coronary vasodilator effects.

Diazepam, even in large doses, maintains cardiovascular stability when combined with nitrous oxide in patients with coronary disease (30). Smaller doses have been shown to increase coronary blood flow, reduce myocardial oxygen consumption, and decrease elevated left ventricular end-diastolic pressures (9). Reductions in stroke volume may occur from lower ventricular filling pressures rather than from impaired myocardial contractility: animal studies have shown transient decreases, no change, or augmentation of myocardial contractility after administration of the drug.

ENDOCRINE RESPONSES TO SURGERY AND ANESTHESIA

Surgery and cardiopulmonary bypass are associated with raised serum levels of ADH, ACTH, cortisol, aldosterone, epinephrine, and norepinephrine, which allow increased water retention through decreased water clearance (ADH effect); greater reabsorption of sodium and excretion of potassium and hydrogen ions (aldosterone); and elevations in heart rate, peripheral vascular resistance, and myocardial contractility (catecholamine effect) (31). In addition, energy sources are mobilized from liver, fat, and muscle under the influence of catabolic hormones, and insulin activity is suppressed. These responses, selectively evolved by the body to restore homeostasis in the healthy subject, may not be well tolerated in patients with ischemic or myopathic heart disease: thus, increased sodium and fluid retention may aggravate heart failure, and elevations in circulating catecholamines can increase cardiac work and oxygen consumption and lower the myocardial excitability threshold with arrhythmogenesis. Mechanical hyperventilation, oxidation of citrate from blood transfusion and lactate from intravaneous fluids, removal of gastric juice by nasogastric suction, and diminished ability of the kidneys to excrete alkaline urine (aldosterone effect) often lead to significant perioperative alkalosis which can be associated with arrhythmias, cerebral vasoconstriction, and reduced peripheral oxygenation.

Endocrine effects of anesthetics are generally smaller than those from surgical stimulation, and serum hormone levels are not suppressed by commonly used agents during operation and cardiopulmonary bypass. Differences in the preoperative state of the patient (apprehension, dehydration, starvation), the dose of anesthetic, the type of surgery, and degree of associated stimulation of afferent pathways may all influence the type and magnitude of hormonal responses. Effects of opioids are inconsistent, usually short-lived, and related to narcotic potency (21, 31). Morphine usually suppresses cortisol and, in higher doses, growth hormone secretion during operation; plasma catecholamine, renin, and ADH levels are not influenced. The more potent opioids fentanyl and sufentanil further attenuate rises in plasma cortisol, glucose, growth hormone, norepinephrine, ADH, renin, and aldosterone responses during surgery. In addition, sufentanil but not fentanyl may reduce ADH and growth hormone levels during cardiopulmonary bypass.

Effects of inhaled agents after induction of anesthesia are variable (9, 14, 31). Halothane increases ACTH, cortisol, and ADH secretion but has no effect on growth hormone. During isoflurane anesthesia, in contrast, plasma growth hormone and insulin are elevated with minimal effect on adrenocortical hormones. Enflurane is associated with small changes in ADH, ACTH, and cortisol secretions. Dose-dependent reductions in plasma epinephrine and norepinephrine, compared to the conscious state, occur in unstimulated humans and rats during inhalation anesthesia with halothane, enflurane, and isoflurane. Decreases in catecholamine levels with halothane are also observed in adrenalectomized animals. Proposed mechanisms of this decrease include reduced central sympathetic discharge, lowered production, increased reuptake, or increased destruction of catecholamines at the nerve endings.

SUMMARY

An appreciation of the effects of anesthetics on hemodynamics, cardiac rhythm, and myocardial oxygen balance is an ideal basis for choice of anesthetic in patients with heart disease. However, the existing clinical evidence is derived from unrandomized, noncomparative studies done in small numbers of selected patients, usually not elderly and with good ventricular function, with varying degrees of functional coronary stenoses, collateral flow, and coronary vascular reserve. Differences in preoperative medications, drug doses and protocols, the use of nitrous oxide, and nonuniformity of criteria established to define hemodynamic instability, and the need for interventions, also account for differences in results between studies. Applications to general practice are hence difficult.

It appears that there is no ideal anesthetic agent or technique for cardiac surgery. Halothane and enflurane depress heart pump function and arterial pressure and, with titration, allow control of cardiovascular responses to surgical stimulation. On the other hand, hypertension requiring vasodilator therapy occurs frequently during surgery with narcotic anesthesia, especially in those who have good ventricular function. Myocardial oxygen balance is comparably maintained by these agents, although myocardial ischemia will occur in response to hemodynamic abnormalities. However, in some patients, decreases in regional coronary blood flow probably occur despite adequate systemic hemodynamics, resulting in random instances of myocardial ischemia even in the presence of a reduced global MVO_2. Isoflurane seems to be associated more frequently with regional myocardial ischemia in patients with coronary artery disease, and some studies show that myocardial ischemia without ECG changes can occur when nitrous oxide is added to halothane or enflurane. Agents other than isoflurane or nitrous oxide may hence be preferable in patients with coronary artery disease. Skill and care in administration of anesthesia remains as critical to cardiovascular outcome as choice between agents.

References

1. Tarhan S, Moffitt EA, Taylor WF, Guiliani ER. Myocardial infarction after general anesthesia. JAMA 220:1451–1454, 1972.
2. Pierce EC Jr: Anesthesiology. JAMA 254:2317–2318, 1985.
3. Moffitt EA, Sethna DH: Myocardial metabolism in coronary artery disease: effects of anesthesia. *Anesth Analg* 65:395–410, 1986.
4. Pratila MG, Pratilas V: The effects of the volatile anesthetics on the heart. In Sperelakis N (ed): *Physiology and Pathophysiology of the Heart.* Boston, Martinus Nijhoff, 1984, pp 617–635.
5. Sethna DH, DeBoer G, Millar RA: Observations on junctional rhythms during anesthesia. *Br J Anaesth* 56:924–925, 1984.
6. Maze M, Mason DM Jr: Etiology and treatment of halothane-induced arrhythmias. *Clinics in Anesthesiology* 1:301–322, 1983.
7. Atlee JL III: *Perioperative Cardiac Dysrhythmias:*

Mechanisms, Recognition, Management. Chicago, Year Book, 1985, pp 151–167.

8. Chraemmer-Jorgensen B, Moilund-Carlsen PF, Marving J, Pederson JF: Left ventricular performance monitored by radionuclide cardiography during induction of anesthesia. *Anesthesiology* 62:278–286, 1985.

9. Hug CC Jr: Pharmacology—anesthetic drugs. In Kaplan JA (ed): *Cardiac Anesthesia.* New York, Grune & Stratton, 1979, pp 3–38.

10. Hilfiker O, Larsen R, Sonntag H: Myocardial blood flow and oxygen consumption during halothane–nitrous oxide anesthesia for coronary revascularization. *Br J Anaesth* 55:927–932, 1983.

11. Reiz S, Balfors E, Gustavsson B, et al: Effects of halothane on coronary haemodynamics and myocardial metabolism in patients with ischaemic heart disease and heart failure. *Acta Anaesthesiol Scand* 26:133–138, 1982.

12. Brown BR Jr, Crout RJ: A comparative study of the effects of general anesthetics on myocardial contractility. *Anesthesiology* 34:236, 1971.

13. Rydvall A, Haggmark S, Nyhman H, Reiz S: Effects of enflurane on coronary haemodynamics in patients with ischaemic heart disease. *Acta Anaesthesiol Scand* 28:690–695, 1984.

14. Churchill-Davidson HC: *A Practice of Anesthesia.* Chicago, Year Book, 1984.

15. Reiz S, Balfors E, Sorenson MB, Ariola S, Friedman A, Truedsson H: Isoflurane—a powerful coronary vasodilator in patients with coronary artery disease. *Anesthesiology* 59:91–97, 1983.

16. Reiz S, Ostman M: Regional coronary hemodynamics during isoflurane–nitrous oxide in patients with ischemic heart disease. *Anesth Analg* 64:570–576, 1985.

17. Larsen R, Hilfiker O, Merkel G, Sonntag H, Drobnik L: Myocardial oxygen balance during enflurane and isoflurane anesthesia for coronary artery surgery. *Anesthesiology* 61:A4, 1984.

18. Moffitt EA, Barker RA, Glenn JJ, et al: Myocardial metabolism and hemodynamic responses with isoflurane anesthesia for coronary artery surgery. *Anesth Analg* 65:53–61, 1986.

19. Smith JS, Cahalan MK, Benefid DJ, et al: Fentanyl vs. fentanyl and isoflurane in patients with impaired left ventricular function. *Anesthesiology* 63:A18, 1985.

20. Wilkinson PL, Hamilton WK, Moyers JR, et al: Halothane and morphine–nitrous oxide anesthesia in patients undergoing coronary artery bypass operation. *J Thorac Cardiovasc Surg* 82:372–382, 1981.

21. Bovill JG, Sebel PS, Stanley TH: Opioid analgesics in anesthesia: with special reference to their use in cardiovascular anesthesia. *Anesthesiology* 61:731–755, 1984.

22. Sethna DH, Moffitt EA, Gray RJ, et al: Cardiovascular effects of morphine in patients with coronary arterial disease. *Anesth Analg* 61:109–114, 1982.

23. Rosow CE, Philbin DM, Moss J, et al: Sufentanil vs fentanyl: suppression of hemodynamic responses. *Anesthesiology* 59A:323, 1983.

24. Starr NJ, Sethna DH, Estafanous FG: Bradycardia and asystole following the rapid administration of sufentanil with vecuronium. *Anesthesiology* 64:521–526, 1986.

25. Skourtis CT, Nissen M, McGinish LA, et al: The effect of high-dose fentanyl on cardiac metabolic balance and coronary circulation in patients undergoing coronary artery surgery. *Anesthesiology* 61:A6, 1984.

26. Gilbert M, Christianson O: High dose fentanyl reduces myocardial oxygen consumption and changes myocardial substrate. *Acta Anesth Scand* 27:A161, 1983.

27. Lappas DG, Palacios I, Athanasiadis C, et al: Sufentanil dosage and myocardial blood flow and metabolism in patients with coronary artery disease. *Anesthesiology* 63:A58, 1985.

28. Sonntag H, Hellberg K, Schenk HD, et al: Effects of thiopental on coronary blood flow and myocardial metabolism in man. *Acta Anesthesiol Scand* 19:69–78, 1975.

29. Criado A, Maseda J, Navarro E, et al: Induction of anesthesia with etomidate: hemodynamic study of 36 patients. *Br J Anaesth* 52:803, 1980.

30. McCammon RL, Hilgenberg JC, Stoelting RK: Hemodynamic effects of diazepam and diazepam–nitrous oxide in patients with coronary artery disease. *Anesth Analg* 59:438–441, 1980.

31. Kaufman L: The endocrine response to surgery and anesthesia. In Scurr S, Feldman S (eds): *Scientific Foundations of Anaesthesia.* Chicago, Year Book, 1982, pp 290–308.

Chapter 10
ANESTHETIC TECHNIQUES FOR CARDIAC SURGERY

DHUN H. SETHNA, M.D.
EMERSON A. MOFFITT, M.D.
ERROLL L. HACKNER, M.D.

The aims of anesthesia for cardiac surgery are to provide unconsciousness, amnesia, analgesia, and muscular relaxation while preserving hemodynamic stability and myocardial oxygen balance. In this chapter, the principles of preanesthetic evaluation and preparation of patients with heart disease are described, along with anesthetic techniques best suited to achieve these goals.

PREOPERATIVE PREPARATION

Premedication to decrease anxiety and induce sedation is beneficial in patients scheduled for elective operations. Unpremedicated patients are likely to have higher heart rates, arterial pressures, and MVO_2 on arrival to the operating room than those who are sedated (1). Premedication for cardiac patients has typically been morphine sulfate and scopolamine, perhaps supplemented with diazepam. Alternatively, diazepam or lorazepam may be given orally as the only drug 2 to 3 hr before operation. Doses should be markedly reduced and narcotics avoided in patients with severe valvular dysfunction or cardiac failure. Additional diazepam or morphine should be given intravenously in the operating room if the patient is not relaxed and drowsy. Sublingual nitroglycerin should be available during transport to the operating room; the value of topical nitroglycerin application at the time of premedication remains to be proved.

In general, preoperative medications should be continued up to the day of operation. Antihypertensive, antiarrhythmic, β-adrenergic, and calcium channel blocker therapy should be continued up to the morning of operation without reductions in dose. Acute withdrawal of β-adrenergic blockers often will precipitate severe angina, arrhythmias, or myocardial infarction, and withdrawal of antihypertensive drugs may lead to labile intraoperative arterial pressures. Digitalis is discontinued 24 to 48 hr before operation since a greater sensitivity to digoxin-associated arrhythmias may be seen after cardiopulmonary bypass.

Practices for monitoring patients during cardiac operations may vary. A seven-lead ECG system is usual, with lead V_5 continuously monitored since observations on exercising patients have indicated that 89% of ischemic S-T changes detected by a 12-lead ECG can be seen in this lead. A continuous two-lead ECG display is desirable. A large-bore peripheral intravenous catheter, a percutaneous radial artery cannula on the side opposite a previous brachial arteriotomy, and a multilumen central venous catheter placed before induction of anesthesia are considered by many physicians to be satisfactory for monitoring and intravenous access. Pulmonary artery (Swan-Ganz) catheters are used routinely at some centers, but at others are reserved for reoperations and for patients with severe ventricular dysfunction, recent myocardial infarction, or valvular lesions, and are always inserted before anesthesia is given. In unstable patients in whom it is crucial to proceed to cardiopulmonary bypass quickly, anesthesia can be safely administered without a pulmonary artery catheter, using instead a left atrial catheter and a catheter-thermistor inserted directly into the pulmonary artery after sternotomy.

Phenylephrine or nitroglycerin (100 μg/ml) should be available in labeled syringes for treatment of cardiovascular instability, along with lidocaine, esmolol, calcium chloride, and atropine. Nitroglycerin and nitroprusside for infusion should be prepared before induction, especially with narcotic anesthesia. Preparation of other drugs for infusion should be based on the patient's baseline hemodynamic status as determined in the operating room.

INDUCTION AND INTUBATION

Selection of an anesthetic technique for cardiac patients should be based on the nature and severity of the heart disease and on the type of cardiovascular response most beneficial to the affected heart. Patients with critical coronary artery stenosis or severe ventricular hypertrophy, in whom the capacity for additional coronary vasodilation ("coronary reserve") is forfeited, are dependent on mechanical factors such as duration of diastole and arterial pressure to maintain blood flow to potentially ischemic areas of the myocardium. Tachycardia (which increases MVO_2 and compromises coronary flow by reducing diastolic perfusion time) and hy-

potension (which may further reduce coronary flow) may cause myocardial ischemia and should be avoided during operation.

Patients with aortic stenosis have fixed cardiac outputs which they are often unable to increase in response to surgical stress. Hence they tolerate hypovolemia due to fluid loss poorly, and may suffer cardiovascular collapse in response to vasodilator drugs. In addition, reductions in left ventricular compliance secondary to left ventricular hypertrophy requires careful maintenance of volume status. These patients are very dependent on the atrial contribution to ventricular filling; if atrial fibrillation develops, an aggressive attempt to control ventricular rate and restore sinus rhythm should be instituted. Patients with aortic or mitral regurgitation, on the contrary, should benefit from lowered arterial pressure ("afterload" reduction), which decreases the regurgitant fraction. Shortening of diastole by increasing heart rate usually has little effect on aortic regurgitation since only the last part of diastole, in which the least regurgitant flow occurs, would be eliminated. Operative risk seems to be related more to the status of left ventricular function than to the severity of valvular regurgitation. In patients with mitral stenosis, volume status is also an important factor in the perioperative period. Fluid overload must be avoided because it may further elevate left atrial pressure and result in pulmonary edema. Conversely, inappropriate diuresis or fluid restriction may decrease left ventricular volume with resultant decreases in left ventricular end-diastolic pressure and cardiac output. Tachycardia is poorly tolerated because as heart rate increases diastolic filling time decreases, thereby reducing the time for blood flow across the mitral valve.

Patients with cardiomyopathy require elevated left ventricular end-diastolic pressures to generate an adequate cardiac output; high ventricular filling pressures should therefore be maintained. Management of patients with idiopathic hypertrophic subaortic stenosis entails controlled depression of myocardial contractility by anesthetic drugs, maintenance of ventricular filling pressures with fluid infusions, and use of vasopressors that act selectively on α-adrenergic receptors to elevate systemic vascular resistance. Drugs that increase myocardial contractility may increase the ventricular outflow gradient and should be avoided. Any situation that reduces left ventricular preload (i.e., hypovolemia, venodilation, or loss of sinus rhythm) will decrease left ventricular filling and increase the dynamic pressure gradient.

Anesthetic drugs should be given slowly with continuous monitoring of heart rate, arterial and central venous pressures, and level of consciousness. Younger patients, hypertensives, patients with good ventricular function, and those not on treatment with β-adrenergic blockers require relatively greater anesthetic depth to attenuate reflex response to intubation; whereas agents that can cause myocardial depression should be avoided in those with diminished ventricular reserve. Inhalation agents can be given if used cautiously in patients treated with calcium channel blockers because of the potential for additive vasodilator, negative inotropic, or atrioventricular blocking actions. For unstable patients requiring emergency operation, anesthesia can be induced with diazepam, etomidate, or fentanyl. Volatile agents should be given only in low concentrations if ventricular function is compromised or unknown. If a high-dose narcotic technique such as fentanyl is selected, the opioid alone may be used for induction, given slowly to assess tolerance of the circulation.

Laryngoscopy usually raises arterial pressure and heart rate, from sympathetic stimulation in patients who are not completely β-blocked (2). The risk of such a major response, particularly in patients with coronary disease or hypertension, is a myocardial oxygen deficit—that is, myocardial oxygen supply is exceeded by a greatly increased consumption, causing ischemia. Methods of attenuating this response include deep anesthesia, lidocaine (by topical laryngeal spray or intravenously), neuromuscular blockers, β-adrenergic blocking agents, and vasodilators (2).

TECHNIQUES OF NARCOTIC ANESTHESIA

Intravenous morphine has lost favor for cardiac anesthesia. When used as the sole anesthetic agent, 0.5 to 3.0 mg/kg is given intravenously at a rate of 5 mg/min; even with these doses, amnesia is often incomplete and hypotension or hypertension is frequent during operation (3). Larger doses prevent cardiovascular responses to stimulation, but at the price of marked increases in perioperative blood and fluid requirements and prolonged postoperative respiratory depression (3).

Butorphanol and pentazocine produce cardiovascular effects that may not be suitable for patients with coronary disease (4). Both drugs elevate systemic and pulmonary vascular resistance and produce myocardial depression associated with reduced cardiac index and increased left ventricular end-diastolic pressure. Buprenorphine maintains hemodynamic stability and is well tolerated by patients with severe coronary disease, but lacks sufficient potency to be used as the only anesthetic agent (4). Initial experience with alfentanil by a variable-rate infusion technique for cardiac anesthesia has been encouraging (3). Fentanyl and its analogue sufentanil are the opioids most frequently administered for cardiac operations.

Fentanyl

Fentanyl, a synthetic narcotic 50 to 100 times more potent than morphine, has lipophilic properties facilitating rapid movement across biologic membranes (3, 4). Plasma fentanyl concentrations are proportional to and change in parallel with concentrations in the brain within 10 to 15 min of drug injection, and correlate closely with CNS effects (anesthesia, respiratory depression). Peak uptake occurs in heart, brain, and lung within 90 seconds, and most of the drug is redistributed from plasma within 60 min to inactive sites in skeletal muscle and fat. Fentanyl is predominantly biotransformed in the liver; pharmacokinetics are not altered in renal disease since only small amounts of drug are eliminated unchanged by the kidneys. Liver disease and factors that reduce hepatic flow (heart failure, advanced age, vasoconstrictor therapy, cardiopulmonary bypass) increase duration of drug effect, and drugs that can increase hepatic blood flow (e.g., dopamine, isoproterenol) may reduce fentanyl elimination (4).

There are varying opinions regarding the dose

and technique of administering fentanyl for use as the sole anesthetic. Vasodilators are so frequently required with fentanyl-oxygen anesthesia to treat hypertension that they are an essential component of this technique, especially in patients with good ventricular function or those not on β-adrenergic blocker therapy. Doses up to 150 μg/kg have been used, but prolonged respiratory depression is common at higher doses, while cardiovascular stability and amnesia cannot be ensured. An initial bolus or rapid infusion (30 to 75 μg/kg given over 3 to 20 min) is usually followed by a slower infusion (10 to 30 μg/kg/hr). Unconsciousness can be induced by a dosage range of 11 to 18 μg/kg, the latter being associated with average plasma levels of 34 ng/ml. Plasma concentrations between 20 and 25 ng/ml usually maintain heart rate and arterial pressure within 20% of preanesthetic levels; higher plasma levels seem to provide more cardiovascular stability until a ceiling effect is reached, after which hemodynamic responses to stimulation may not be effectively controlled. Infusions of fentanyl at three different rates, 0.3, 0.4, and 0.5 μg/kg/min after loading doses of 30, 40, and 50 μg/kg respectively, still permitted stimulation-related hypertension in 9 of 10 patients at the lowest dose, in 70% of patients in the intermediate group, and in 50% at the highest dose (5). In another study, patients became hypertensive during surgical stimulation despite mean plasma concentrations of 25 ng/ml, but fewer showed blood pressure elevations when plasma levels exceeded 30 ng/ml (6). Thus, although plasma levels are usually higher than necessary for unconsciousness when greater than 30 μg/kg of fentanyl are given at induction, they may provide needed protection during early periods of operation when strong stimulation such as tracheal intubation or sternotomy occur. However, considerable variation is seen in patient responses, and a stable hemodynamic circulation is not ensured at any dose. Critically ill patients or those with severely impaired cardiovascular function appear to require lower doses of fentanyl for total anesthesia (7).

Fentanyl can be infused at fixed rates to provide predictable mean plasma concentrations (4). Pharmacokinetic data from human volunteers show that stable peak and maintenance plasma fentanyl levels can be expected after a loading dose of 50 μg/kg followed by an infusion of 0.3 μg/kg/min (4). Fentanyl 75 μg/kg followed by a constant-rate infusion at 10 μg/kg/hr allows a stable hemodynamic course when given to premedicated patients on chronic β-adrenergic blocker therapy (8). Maintenance infusions are usually discontinued on rewarming after cardiopulmonary bypass or when a total fentanyl dose of 100 μg/kg has been given. Recently, a three-dose technique has been described in which fentanyl was injected at induction, at sternotomy, and before cardiopulmonary bypass (9). Cardiovascular stability usually extends into the postoperative period; patients can be extubated 12 to 18 hr after operation, at which time serum fentanyl levels are often below 2 ng/ml.

Fentanyl-oxygen anesthesia is often supplemented with volatile agents. Some supplementary drugs are not always beneficial in patients receiving fentanyl (2). The addition of nitrous oxide produces significant myocardial depression with elevation in systemic vascular resistance, leading to decrease in cardiac output and arterial pressure. Diazepam decreases myocardial contractility when combined with fentanyl in isolated heart muscle preparations, and may be associated with severe hypotension in some patients who have received fentanyl. Scopolamine and droperidol are useful and safe adjuncts to opioids.

Sufentanil

Sufentanil, a synthetic fentanyl analogue, has a selective affinity for "mu" opioid receptors that is 5 to 10 times greater than that of fentanyl (3, 4). Peak uptake occurs in heart, brain, lung, and liver within 2 min of injection in rats, and most of the drug is excreted within 24 hr. It is rapidly metabolized to virtually inactive compounds, and only small amounts are excreted unchanged. Although its elimination half-life is shorter than that of fentanyl, patients anesthetized with sufentanil for coronary bypass surgery do not usually show much difference in recovery time from anesthesia or time to extubation compared to fentanyl.

Several doses and techniques have been proposed for sufentanil when used as the sole anesthetic for cardiac operations (3, 4). In premedicated patients, failure to respond to command occurs after 4.2 μg/kg. Doses between 7 and 30 μg/kg given over 4 to 20 min have been used for induction, usually followed by a continuous infusion, or supplemental boluses (50 to 200 μg) given when arterial pressures rise. Premedicated patients with valvular heart disease can be anesthetized with 15 μg/kg and maintained on a constant-rate infusion (0.075 μg/kg/min) until rewarming during cardiopulmonary bypass (10). Similar to fentanyl, a three-dose method has been described in which sufentanil was given at induction (10 to 12 μg/kg), at sternotomy (3 to 5 μg/kg), and before cardiopulmonary bypass (5 to 7 μg/kg); anesthesia is supplemented at the onset of cardiopulmonary bypass by a single dose of diazepam or lorazepam, and vasodilators are used to control intraoperative hypertension (9). Thus, sufentanil is also unable to predictably prevent a hyperdynamic circulation regardless of dose or technique.

When injected rapidly in cardiac patients on preoperative β-adrenergic blocker therapy, sufentanil can cause severe hypotension with short periods of asystole (11). When combined with diazepam at induction, hypotension can also occur, so induction with sufentanil should always be slow with careful monitoring of arterial pressure.

INHALATION ANESTHESIA

Noninflammable, volatile, and stable fluorinated hydrocarbons such as halothane or enflurane are acceptable, and regularly used, inhalation agents for cardiac anesthesia, after an induction with etomidate, thiopental, or a moderate dose of fentanyl (1). Inspired gas concentrations controlled by a vaporizer in the breathing circuit are titrated during induction and operation to maintain a stable, mild depression of hemodyamics. When depth of anesthesia is judged to be adequate after induction, the patient's ability to respond to stimulation may be evaluated by insertion of a urinary catheter. If arterial pressure does not increase, laryngoscopy and intubation are performed; otherwise, depth of anesthesia is increased.

The concentration of inhaled agent can usually be titrated to avoid severe myocardial depression and hypotension, but supplemental intravenous agents can be given. Isoflurane in patients with coronary artery disease seems to be associated more frequently with regional myocardial ischemia, both on induction and later than the other two volatile agents (1). There is evidence that hemodynamic depression and ischemia can occur when nitrous oxide is added to halothane or enflurane (1), so its use and that of isoflurane cannot be recommended in coronary patients. Fentanyl, given at induction and followed by maintenance with halothane or enflurane, allows good control of hemodynamics and myocardial oxygen balance during and after cardiac operations (1).

SELECTION OF NEUROMUSCULAR BLOCKING DRUGS

Intravenous nondepolarizing neuromuscular blocking drugs that provide muscular relaxation can produce adverse cardiovascular effects in patients with heart disease (12). Curare can decrease arterial pressure due to histamine release and blocking effects on sympathetic ganglia. Pancuronium increases heart rate from vagolytic actions on cardiac muscurinic receptors and from effects on sympathetic nerve terminals, where it facilitates norepinephrine release and blocks norepinephrine reuptake. Since increases in heart rate have been associated with ischemic S-T segment depressions on Holter monitor recordings, avoidance of pancuronium in patients with coronary disease has been advocated (13). Other studies have not documented heart rate increases from pancuronium in well β-blocked patients, and the drug remains widely used. Tachycardia is also poorly tolerated by patients with critical aortic stenosis, and neuromuscular blockers other than pancuronium may be preferable in these cases (14). Combinations of neuromuscular blockers allow lower doses with reductions in dose-dependent cardiovascular effects, and pancuronium-metocurine mixtures have been advocated (12). Vecuronium, which does not release histamine or show autonomic effects, usually permits a stable cardiovascular course. Constant-rate infusions of atracurium give a similar effect, although hypotension has been reported after atracurium administration, presumably from histamine release.

There appears to be no consensus regarding equipotency of doses of different neuromuscular blocking drugs (12, 15). However, under narcotic–nitrous oxide anesthesia, vecuronium has been shown to be almost as potent as pancuronium, and the two have been regarded as equipotent (13, 16). Atracurium can be given in doses up to 0.4 mg/kg for endotracheal intubation; higher doses are associated with more instances of histamine release and cardiovascular instability.

BENZODIAZEPINES

Benzodiazepines are used as pre- and postoperative tranquilizers and hypnotics, anesthetic induction agents, and adjuvants to the maintenance of cardiac anesthesia. When given orally in sedative or hypnotic doses they do not produce significant hemodynamic or respiratory changes. The benzodiazepines are also excellent amnesic agents (17, 18).

Diazepam is available in parenteral and oral form. It is not water soluble. The parenteral form is dissolved in a vehicle that has irritating tissue properties, resulting in painful intramuscular and intravenous injections, occasionally leading to phlebitis (19). Oral use results in reliable and predictable effects (20); it is a good amnesic agent and is useful as a supplement to high-dose narcotic anesthesia, with which recall has been reported. The amnesic properties are potentiated by scopolamine (21).

Diazepam, even in small doses (0.125 mg/kg), produced significant decreases in mean arterial pressure and systemic vascular resistance, accompanied by decreases in plasma epinephrine and norepinephrine when administered during fentanyl infusion (22). Intravenous diazepam (0.5 mg/kg) with 50% nitrous oxide has been used as an induction agent in patients undergoing coronary bypass grafting. It produced small but significant decreases in mean arterial pressures, rate pressure product, and left

and right stroke work indices (23). Although moderate systolic hypotension can be beneficial to some patients with coronary artery disease, adequate coronary perfusion should be maintained. Diazepam-induced cardiac depression is more pronounced when left ventricular end-diastolic pressures are elevated (24). It should be used with caution in patients with increased "filling" pressures receiving high-dose fentanyl-oxygen anesthesia.

Lorazepam is available in both oral and parenteral forms. It should not be used with scopolamine as premedication because the combination may result in agitation. When compared with diazepam, it has a delayed onset and more prolonged duration of action (25), and is less associated with phlebitis or painful injection. As an adjunct to high-dose fentanyl anesthesia, it does not produce significant untoward hemodynamic effects (26).

Midazolam is available only in water-soluble parenteral form and does not have the prolonged duration of action of lorazepam or result in painful injections (27). Its short half-life (120 min) is prolonged (to 281 min) by slower metabolism following cardiopulmonary bypass (28). It is three times as potent as diazepam (27) and is suitable as an intravenous agent in patients with ischemic heart disease (29). When compared with diazepam, it produced small but significant increases in heart rate. Both midazolam and diazepam produced small but statistically significant reductions in systemic and pulmonary artery pressures. Cardiac index, however, was maintained with both drugs (30). Effects of midazolam on the coronary circulation are minimal, and the drug can be used safely in patients with coronary artery disease. Midazolam caused decreases in coronary sinus blood flow and myocardial oxygen consumption. Coronary vascular resistance did not change, but coronary sinus oxygen tension increased slightly, suggesting mild alterations in autoregulation. No evidence of myocardial ischemia occurred as judged by the absence of changes in the ECG and in the myocardial lactate extraction and relaxation time constants (31). Radionuclide cineangiography studies have demonstrated that, like diazepam, midazolam does not influence left ventricular ejection fraction and does not induce regional myocardial dysfunction in patients with coronary artery disease (32).

Repeated doses of midazolam after open-heart surgery produced stable concentrations within 4 hr with no tendency to cumulation, and the drug was rapidly cleared following discontinuation. Similar doses of diazepam given at the same frequency produced plasma concentrations that were still increasing at the time of drug discontinuation (33). Midazolam is thus a better choice in the postoperative period when patients may require sedation for short-term ventilatory support.

Midazolam is a safe induction agent for emergency cardiac surgery in which hemodynamic stability is crucial, and the drug can be effectively used in a rapid sequence induction (34). In combination with ketamine as an induction agent, it effectively attenuates the cardiostimulatory responses and unpleasant emergency reactions associated with ketamine (34, 35). A midazolam-ketamine anesthetic regimen has been successfully used in a patient with documented opiate allergy undergoing coronary artery bypass surgery (36).

ANESTHESIA FOR CARDIAC TRANSPLANTATION

Since immunosuppressive therapy with cyclosporin is started before operation, strict asepsis must be maintained during preoperative insertion of the radial artery and multilumen CVP catheters. Pulmonary artery catheters are avoided at some centers because they may increase the incidence of perioperative infection and require removal with the recipient heart. Left atrial catheters and thermistor-catheters inserted directly in the pulmonary artery may be used for perioperative monitoring of cardiovascular function.

Because the actual timing of transplantation cannot be anticipated, recipients of heart transplants are considered to have a full stomach and, after preoxygenation, are made unconscious and intubated rapidly with etomidate and succinylcholine (A Govier, personal communication). Diazepam is then given in incremental doses up to 0.3 mg/kg to maintain anesthesia, perhaps supplemented with fen-

tanyl, or etomidate may be used alone. After transplantation with a healthier heart, fentanyl and isoflurane may be used. Phenylephrine is frequently required to raise arterial pressure after cardiopulmonary bypass. Low doses of dopamine, furosemide, and mannitol are given during operation to reduce postoperative cyclosporin-related renal failure.

References

1. Moffitt EA, Sethna DH: The coronary circulation and myocardial metabolism in coronary artery disease: effects of anesthesia. Anesth Analg 65:395–410, 1986.
2. Moffitt EA, Sethna DH, Bussell J, et al: Effects of intubation on coronary flow and myocardial oxygenation. Can Anaesth Soc J 32:105–111, 1985.
3. Moldenhauer CC: New narcotics in cardiac anesthesia. In Kaplan JA (ed): Cardiovascular Pharmacology. New York, Grune & Stratton, pp 31–78, 1983.
4. Bovill JG, Sebel PS, Stanley TM: Opioid analgesics in anesthesia: with special reference to their use in cardiovascular anesthesia. Anesthesiology 61:731–755, 1984.
5. Sprigge JM, Wynands JE, Whalley DG, et al: Fentanyl infusion anesthesia for aortocoronary bypass surgery: plasma levels and hemodynamic responses. Anesth Analg 61:972–978, 1982.
6. Wynands JE, Townsend GE, Wong P, et al: Blood pressure response and plasma fentanyl concentrations during high- and very high-dose fentanyl anesthesia for coronary artery surgery. Anesth Analg 62:661–665, 1983.
7. Wynands JE, Wong P, Whalley DG, et al: Fentanyl infusion anesthesia for patients with poor ventricular function undergoing aortocoronary bypass surgery. In Abstracts, 4th Annual Meeting, Society of Cardiovascular Anesthesiologists, Washington DC, May 3–5, 1982, pp 85–86.
8. Moffitt EA, Scovil JE, Barker RA, et al: Myocardial metabolism and hemodynamics responses during high dose fentanyl anesthesia for coronary patients. Can Anaesth Soc J 31:611–618, 1984.
9. Howie MB, McSweeney TD, Lingam RP, et al: A comparison of fentanyl-O_2 and sufentanil-O_2 for cardiac anesthesia. Anesth Analg 64:877–887, 1985.
10. Samuelson PN, Reves JG, Kirklin JK, et al: Sufentanil infusion anesthesia in patients undergoing valvular heart surgery. Anesthesiology 63:A74, 1985.

11. Starr NJ, Sethna DH, Estafanous FG: Brady-cardia and asystole following the rapid administration of sufentanil with vecuronium. *Anesthesiology* 64:521–523, 1986.

12. Sethna DH, Estafanous FG, Starr NJ: Cardiovascular effects of nondepolarizing neuromuscular blockers in patients with coronary artery disease. *Can Anaesth Soc J* 33:280–286, 1986.

13. Thomson I, Putnins CL: Adverse effects of pancuronium during high-dose fentanyl anesthesia for coronary artery bypass grafting. *Anesthesiology* 62:708–713, 1985.

14. Sethna DH, Estafanous FG, Starr NJ, et al: Hemodynamic comparison of neuromuscular blockers in aortic valve disease. *Can J Anaesth* 34:582–588, 1987.

15. Miller RD, Rupp SM, Fisher DM, et al: Clinical pharmacology of vecuronium and atracurium. *Anesthesiology* 61:444–453, 1984.

16. Salmenpera M, Peltola K, Takkunen O, Heinonen J: Cardiovascular effects of pancuronium and vecuronium during high dose fentanyl anesthesia. *Anesth Analg* 62:1059–1064, 1983.

17. George KA, Dundee JW: Relative amnesic actions of diazepam, flunitrazepam and lorazepam in man. *Br J Clin Pharmacol* 4:45, 1977.

18. Reves JG, Fragen RJ, Vinik HR, et al: Midazolam: pharmacology and uses. *Anesthesiology* 62:310–324, 1985.

19. Langdon D: Thrombophlebitis following diazepam. *JAMA* 225:1389, 1973.

20. Kaplan SA, Jack ML, Alexander K, et al: Pharmacokinetic profile of diazepam in man following single intravenous and oral and chronic oral administrations. *J Pharm Sci* 62:1789–1796, 1973.

21. Frumin MJ, Herekar VR, Jarvik ME: Amnesic actions of diazepam and scopolamine in man. *Anesthesiology* 45:406–412, 1976.

22. Tomichek RC, Rosow CE, Philbin DM, et al: Diazepam-fentanyl interaction—hemodynamic and hormonal effects in coronary artery surgery. *Anesth Analg* 62:881–884, 1983.

23. Samuelson PN, Lell WA, Kouchoukos NT, et al: Hemodynamics during diazepam induction for coronary artery bypass grafting. *South Med J* 73:332–334, 1980.

24. Dauchot PJ, Staub F, Berzina L, et al: Hemodynamic responses to diazepam: dependence on prior left ventricular end-diastolic pressure. *Anesthesiology* 60:499–503, 1984.

25. Dundee JW, McGowan WAW, Liburn JK, et al: Comparison of the actions of diazepam and lorazepam. *Br J Anaesth* 51:439–445, 1979.

26. Heikkila H, Jalonen J, Laaksonen V, et al: Lorazepam and high-dose fentanyl anaesthesia: effects on haemodynamics and oxygen transportation in patients undergoing coronary revascularization. *Acta Anaesthesiol Scand* 28:357–361, 1984.

27. Reves JG, Corssen G, Holcomb C: Comparison of two benzodiazepines for anesthesia induction: midazolam and diazepam. *Can Anaesth Soc J* 25:211, 1978.

28. Kanto J, Himburg JJ, Heikkila H, et al: Midazolam kinetics before, during and after cardiopulmonary bypass surgery. *Int J Pharm Res* 2:123–126, 1985.

29. Samuelson PN, Reves JG, Kouchoukos NT, et al: Hemodynamic responses to anesthetic induction with midazolam or diazepam in patients with ischemic heart disease. *Anesth Analg* 60:802–809, 1981.

30. Kawar P, Carson IW, Clarke RSJ, et al: Haemodynamic changes during induction of anaesthesia with midazolam and diazepam (Valium) in patients undergoing coronary artery bypass surgery. *Anaesthesia* 40:767–771, 1985.

31. Marty J, Nitenberg A, Blanchet F, et al: Effects of midazolam on the coronary circulation in patients with coronary artery disease. *Anesthesiology* 64:206–210, 1986.

32. Lepage J-Y, Blanloeil Y, Pinaud M, et al: Hemodynamic effects of diazepam, flunitrazepam and midazolam in patients with ischemic heart disease: assessment with a radionuclide approach. *Anesthesiology* 65:678–683, 1986.

33. Lowry KG, Dundee JW, McClean E, et al: Pharmacokinetics of diazepam and midazolam when used for sedation following cardiopulmonary bypass. *Br J Anaesth* 57:883–885, 1985.

34. White PF: Comparative evaluation of intravenous agents for rapid sequence induction—thiopental, ketamine and midazolam. *Anesthesology* 57:279–284, 1982.

35. Cartwright PD, Pingel SM: Midazolam and diazepam in ketamine anaesthesia. *Anaesthesia* 39:439–442, 1984.

36. Edge KR, Braude BM, Press P, et al: Dissociative anaesthesia for coronary artery bypass surgery using ketamine and midazolam. *S Afr Med J* 70:624–625, 1986.

Section 4
THE EARLY POSTOPERATIVE PHASE: IN THE HOSPITAL

Chapter 11
NORMAL CONVALESCENCE

RICHARD J. GRAY, M.D.

The physiologic impact of cardiac surgery results in changes of cardiac as well as other systemic functions. Optimum patient management requires one to differentiate between changes that represent a true complication and those that are part of normal convalescence. Further, one must recognize derangements that have a benign, self-limited course and those requiring active management. The unique features and common complaints of the normally convalescing cardiac surgery patient are described in this chapter, with commentary on certain aspects that require intervention.

ABNORMAL LABORATORY TESTS

Electrolytes do not often deviate widely from normal, but they may reveal mild metabolic acidosis for the first 12 hr after surgery, particularly as the patient remains hypothermic. Serum bicarbonate levels of 18 to 26 mEq/liter and arterial pH of 7.30 or above are common. With satisfactory renal and cardiac function, no treatment is necessary as long as a trend toward recovery is seen.

Serum potassium levels should be carefully monitored, usually at 4- to 6-hr intervals, for the 1st postoperative day. During this early phase, serum potassium concentration can decrease dramatically and suddenly due to shifts in intravascular volume, rapid diuresis and correc-

tion of acidosis, and transfusion of blood. This, along with the observation that many arrhythmias seem to be related to hypokalemia, has led to the practice of maintaining serum potassium at or above 4.0 mEq/liter. This is often done using a sliding scale for intravenous potassium chloride supplements (Table 12.1)

Serum glucose is almost always elevated, commonly reaching 250 to 400 mg/dl. This is due to the large volume of glucose-containing intravenous solution administered coupled with surgically induced increases in serum catecholamine and cortisol levels. In the nondiabetic patient, insulin therapy is not required because blood glucose returns to normal within 18 to 24 hr. Insulin is required to avoid diabetic ketoacidosis in the insulin-dependent diabetic patient and with the hopes of maintaining white blood cell chemotaxis in others. Because of uncertain cardiac performance and hypothermia-

---

TABLE 11.1

POTASSIUM PROTOCOL

If K^+ is <3.8, give three boluses of 10 mEq of KCl in 50 ml/hr.

If K^+ is 3.9 to 4.2, give two boluses of 10 mEq of KCl in 50 ml/hr.

If K^+ is 4.3 to 4.6, give one bolus of 10 mEq of KCl in 50 ml/hr.

Notify M.D. if K^+ is < 3.6 or >5.2 mEq/100 ml.

---

induced vasoconstriction, the intravenous route is necessary, preferably as a continuous infusion. The goal of therapy should be to achieve a blood sugar of approximately 200 mg/dl during the first 48 hr. Following this, diabetics are usually able to resume their preoperative insulin regimen. Those on oral diabetic agents may require a few extra days of insulin therapy prior to resumption of their oral medication.

Serum total calcium and phosphorus levels are decreased initially and for approximately 24 hr after surgery—the former, often below 7.0 mg/dl, and the latter, often below 1 mEq/liter. These abnormalities are the result of hemodilution arising from the use of non-blood-containing electrolyte solutions to prime the cardiopulmonary bypass pump as well as other intravenous solutions and should not be taken to indicate temporary failure of parathyroid function. Ionized calcium concentration is also decreased, although the impact is lessened by a compensatory shift toward the ionized partition (1). Specific cardiovascular effects have not been attributed to this type of acute hypocalcemia or hypophosphatemia, which, if left untreated, will return to preoperative levels, usually within 24 hr. It should be kept in mind, however, that in the presence of hypotension, a prompt and sustained increase in systolic blood pressure often results from intravenous administration of 0.5 to 1.0 gm of calcium chloride. This approach is often used in weaning from cardiopulmonary bypass and should also be kept in mind for the first few hours postoperatively (2).

Hematologic abnormalities are extremely common and can be profound. Hemoglobin and hematocrit levels vary widely depending on intraoperative transfusion policies and reinfusion of shed blood. Most patients emerge from the operating room anemic, and if (as is the usual policy) they remain untransfused, the blood count returns to normal slowly, often requiring 6 weeks. Blood is lost in the operating room, but the amount is relatively small due to the ability to reinfuse most of the blood from the sterile operative field. In addition, most blood remaining in the pump at termination of cardiopulmonary bypass can be retransfused, depending on the patient's ability to tolerate intravenous volume.

The greatest amount of blood loss, often exceeding 1 liter, occurs via the mediastinal chest tubes during the first 24 hr while the patient is in the intensive care unit. In cases of unusually rapid bleeding a mechanism for sterile collection and reinfusion exists, but in the majority of cases in which bleeding is slower, sterility cannot be ensured and such blood is discarded. An additional cause for blood loss is hemolysis, which results from the mechanical injury of red blood cells within the bubble-type oxygenators used in cardiopulmonary bypass. During bypass, platelets are also damaged, both qualitatively and quantitatively, often resulting in platelet counts below 100,000/ml. Values substantially below this level are not common, but, even in the absence of excessive bleeding, therapy is unnecessary. A follow-up platelet count is initiated to ensure that recovery is under way and, in the absence of other specific defect, should be complete by 3 to 4 days. Thrombocytopenia in the range of 25,000 to 50,000/ml in the absence of intraaortic balloon counterpulsation is abnormal and should stimulate a search for causative factors other than the surgery. Other measures of coagulation status, such as partial thromboplastin time (PTT) and prothrombin time (PT), are often borderline abnormal and, in the absence of bleeding, can be left to self-correct over 1 to 2 days. These tissues are discussed in greater detail in Chapter 17.

HEMODYNAMIC RESPONSE TO CARDIAC SURGERY

As measured by numerous parameters, transient depression of cardiac function is expected, even if normal preoperatively (3). Since heart rate (usually in the 80s), blood pressure, and urine flow are often well maintained, cardiac depression will not be appreciated unless invasive hemodynamic monitoring is performed. In the uncomplicated patient, cardiac index may be as low as 1.5 liters/min/m^2, associated with a diminished stroke volume, stroke work index, and ejection fraction. Often, the cardiac index may be maintained near preoperative levels by sinus tachycardia associated with a marked diminution in stroke volume and stroke work index. In the absence of a perioperative myocardial infarction, these changes in cardiac function have been attributed to incomplete recovery of operative global myocardial ischemia and the effects of hypothermia (4). Management usually consists of optimization of cardiac filling pressures by intravenous fluid administration, with a goal of reaching a pulmonary capillary wedge pressure of 15 mm Hg. Augmentation of the heart rate to 90 beats/min, through the use of epicardial pacemaking wires placed at the time of surgery, and the occasional and brief use of afterload reduction therapy with nitroprusside are also common. Inotropic drug support is rarely needed, as long as a recovery trend begins with reversal of hypothermia, which is usually complete by 6 to 8 hr. It should be particularly noted that, despite emergence from surgery with a positive fluid balance, these patients often tolerate large volumes of intravenous infusate that may be needed to maintain cardiac filling pressures.

HOSPITAL COURSE LANDMARKS

Inasmuch as most patients are transferred directly to an intensive care unit rather than a recovery room, they are rarely extubated in the operating room. Ideally, some formal weaning criteria should be applied, following which extubation usually takes place in the intensive care unit on the evening of surgery or the morning afterward. Mediastinal chest tubes are removed a few hours after bleeding has ceased, usually on the afternoon of the 1st postoperative day; of course, chest tubes should be left in place until after any direct intracavitary pressure-monitoring cannulae have also been safely removed. Pleural chest tubes may also be present, especially after internal thoracic artery bypass, and may have to be left in place for a longer period because of continued hemothorax due to low-grade hemorrhage from the internal thoracic artery removal site. If other hemodynamic monitoring catheters are used, such as pulmonary artery lines, they can also be removed on the afternoon of the 1st postoperative day. This enables the patient to be transferred to a step-down unit or floor care on the afternoon of the 1st postoperative day or the morning of the 2nd day. Because of the high incidence of postoperative arrhythmias, electrocardiographic mon-

itoring is required for a minimum of 2 to 3 days. A normal diet should be tolerated within 36 to 48 hr, and patients can sit on the edge of the bed the day following surgery and begin ambulation with assistance after transfer to floor care (see Chapter 29). Incisional chest discomfort should be only moderate in severity and easily managed with oral analgesics of moderate strength, such as those containing codeine.

Typically, an uncomplicated patient can be discharged from the hospital 7 to 8 days after surgery. Although occasionally warranted symptomatically, earlier hospital discharge, say on day 5 or 6, carries the risk of undetected, potentially serious arrhythmias that may first appear as late as 5 days after surgery. Coincidentally, prolongation of hospital stay is usually due to recurrent arrhythmias or persistent fatigue (see Chapters 28 and 29 for further discussion of discharge planning).

Preexisting Conditions

Although the cardiac surgery itself may be uncomplicated, certain preexisting conditions may alter convalescence, or quiescent diseases may be stirred to activity by the surgical procedure.

A preoperative myocardial infarction, occurring as distantly as several months before surgery, is often associated with recurrent electrocardiographic changes such as S-T segment elevation or T wave inversion in the previously affected leads. Of course, there may be a new perioperative myocardial infarction, but this need not be the case. Such "benign" recurrent electrocardiographic changes should resolve within 3 to 4 days.

Preoperative arrhythmias, both atrial and ventricular, will amost always reappear, sometimes after a 1- to 2-day postoperative hiatus. These arrhythmias may be more aggressive and resistant than they were preoperatively, and consequently more aggressive therapy may be needed (see Chapter 18).

A patient with a remote cerebral vascular accident (CVA) will often exhibit signs of reactivation, even though he or she may have nearly completely recovered in the past. Some or all of the previous CVA symptoms may reappear but are usually milder than they had been initially. Rarely, early preoperative seizure activity can occur. Although the prognosis for recovery is good, several weeks are sometimes needed.

Interestingly, patients with preoperative intermittent claudication due to atherosclerotic peripheral vascular disease often experience a lessening of their claudication symptoms afterward. Although this improvement is often dramatic, it is temporary, rarely lasting more than 3 or 4 months. The mechanism is unknown, but improvements in cardiac performance and diminution in peripheral vascular tone or blood viscosity are possible explanations.

Unfortunately, the syndrome of chronic and recurring low back pain is often worsened during the course of hospitalization because of the prolonged bed rest necessary. This is lessened only slightly by the use of a firm mattress or bedboard. The most important approach is to ambulate the patient as soon as feasible.

COMMON PATIENT COMPLAINTS AND MINOR COMPLICATIONS

Many diverse symptoms and physical findings are seen with enough frequency to warrant specific comment. Many of these occurrences, because of their potential physiologic significance, have been studied extensively; other, more pedestrian complaints, remain part of the practitioner's "lore," often remaining undescribed except possibly in a remote corner of a cardiovascular surgery textbook. Because of the long list of such items they are best catalogued according to the apparent body system of origin and are not necessarily presented in order of their frequency or apparent seriousness.

Cardiac System

Electrocardiographic changes are numerous and sometimes profound, even in the absence of a perioperative myocardial infarction (with its characteristic changes). Certain common but apparently benign electrocardiographic changes can be seen in the patient with a recent preoperative myocardial infarction (see "Preexisting Conditions" above). In this section are described the many additional electrocardi-

ographic changes associated with a generally uncomplicated convalescence.

Sinus Bradycardia or Tachycardia

Perhaps the most frequent finding is either sinus bradycardia or sinus tachycardia. Despite normal preoperative sinoatrial node function, sinus bradycardia, occasionally with sinus arrest and junctional escape, is a relatively common finding during recovery from hypothermia. Benign causes are usually associated with heart rates above 45, however, and generally do not persist beyond the period of hypothermia. More significant bradyarrhythmias are discussed in Chapter 8. After recovery from hypothermia, heart rate is usually in the mid-80s or 90s, but many patients exhibit sinus tachycardia of 100 to 120 beats/min beginning a few hours after surgery. This should lead to an investigation of possible causes, including the adequacy of intravascular volume and blood loss replacement, the presence of infection (even in the absence of fever), low cardiac output syndrome, pericardial effusion or tamponade and, much less likely, occult hyperthyroidism. While relatively uncommon, these causes of sinus tachycardia deserve investigation because of their therapeutic implications.

A common explanation of the sinus tachycardia, but one of exclusion, is withdrawal of preoperative β-blocking agents. The overall clinical picture is often one of hyperdynamic cardiovascular status with systolic hypertension, normal or moderately elevated cardiac output in addition to the tachycardia. Even in the absence of preoperative β-blocker use, sinus tachycardia is relatively common and often persists for 2 to 4 weeks after surgery. Therapy is generally warranted if the patient is symptomatic and is often successful with small doses of β-blocking agents, such as 10 mg of propranolol every 8 hr.

Intraventricular Conduction Delays

Intraventricular conduction delays of all types have been observed after cardiac surgery. Most common are the hemiblocks, left anterior-superior and posterior-inferior (12 to 15%); right bundle-branch block (5%) and right bundle-block with anterior-superior hemiblock (3 to

5%) are also common. Although there is some disagreement (5), most believe that these findings are not associated with postoperative complications or an adverse long-term prognosis (6). There is even more agreement, however, that the occurrence of left bundle-branch block or nonspecific intraventricular conduction delay has adverse prognostic consequences and may be associated with perioperative myocardial infarction (5, 7). The author's experience demonstrates a significant likelihood of cardiac death within the 1st year after surgery if the patient demonstrates either left bundle-branch block or nonspecific intraventricular conduction delay (7). More advanced heart block or need for permanent or even temporary cardiac pacing is not more common in this situation, and the mechanism of cardiac death, when it does appear, does not seem to be specifically related to the conduction defect. Rather, the causes of death encompass the usual cardiac diagnoses, that is, recurrent myocardial infarction, congestive heart failure, or sudden unwitnessed cardiac death (7). This suggests that, as with nonsurgical series of patients, the ill-fated prognosis associated with fascicular conduction defect is a nonspecific indicator of more significant cardiac disease (8–11). New intraventricular conduction delays are usually noted on arrival from the operating room. In the case of right bundle-branch block and the hemiblocks, most are transient; many disappeared within 48 hr and the majority by the time of hospital discharge. Intraoperative myocardial ischemia, inadequate cardioplegia, or retained air in the coronary tree are logical potential explanations, but despite investigation of these and other factors, the mechanism of postoperative fascicular conduction defects remains a puzzle.

Pathologic Q Waves

Appearance or disappearance of pathologic Q waves in the absence of a new perioperative infarction is an intriguing and relatively common occurrence. Naturally, the appearance of new pathologic Q waves should alert one to the possibility of a new infarction, but this need not be the case. Unmasking of previously "silent" inferior wall Q waves has been reported (12), and an even more common occurrence is the pseudo inferior wall infarction picture associated with a marked leftward axis shift, such as occurs with left anterior-superior hemiblock. Conversely, disappearance of anterior wall pathologic Q waves has also been reported (13). The proposed mechanism is that coronary bypass has corrected ischemia that was severe enough to prevent normal electrocardiographic depolarization in an area of viable or nontransmurally infarcted myocardium.

T Wave Flattening

Another common and apparently benign electrocardiographic change is that of progressive T wave flattening or even inversion, most often seen in the lateral precordial leads. This usually appears 3 to 4 days after surgery and progresses for an additional 5 to 7 days. Normalization of these changes often occurs at the time of the 6 week postoperative visit. Although ischemic in appearance, these changes are rarely accompanied by chest pain or other electrocardiographic or enzymatic evidence of myocardial infarction. It is tempting to speculate that they represent resolving localized pericarditis. This explanation is tenuous, because signs and symptoms of pericarditis are often absent.

Pericardial Friction Rub

A diffuse pericardial friction rub is expected early postoperatively while mediastinal (pericardial) chest tubes are still in place. It is usually multicomponent and extremely loud, often obscuring all other cardiac sounds. This is particularly true, as is commonly the case, when air is also in the pericardium, resulting in especially prominent extracardiac sounds. This rub can persist for several hours or even a day after removal of the chest tubes. Persistence longer or the new appearance of a pericardial friction rub later should imply additional pericardial inflammation and is the subject of discussion in Chapter 20. Even in the absence of clinical pericarditis, a small amount of (usually bloody) fluid can be found in the pericardium, almost always detectable echocardiographically. Consequently, this echocardiographic finding is not a specific indicator of postoperative pericarditis.

Hypotension

In certain patients, recurrent and often disabling orthostatic hypotension may occur and persist for up to 2 weeks after surgery. This occurrence should lead to investigation of intravascular volume status, liberalization of salt intake, and reduction or discontinuation of any antihypertensive medications that have been ordered. This syndrome is often seen in a setting of persistent sinus tachycardia. With the heart rate relatively fixed at 100 to 120 beats/min, one potential compensatory mechanism normally able to prevent orthostasis is lost. Well-fitting, thigh-length, venoocclusive stockings or a 6-inch Ace bandage carefully applied to each leg, in addition to instructions to the patients about slowly rising from sitting and lying positions, are occasionally helpful, but most often the syndrome will run a self-limited course. β-blockage is not advised because it may further reduce cardiac output and blood pressure.

Pulmonary System

Postextubation Symptoms

Directly after extubation the patient will normally cough, producing dark brown sputum that contains small amounts of old clotted blood and occasionally even small mucous plugs, the former representing residue of blood from the trauma of intubation or endotracheal suctioning. Directly after extubation many patients have a hoarse or weak voice, and some are almost aphonic. In most cases, even the most severely afflicted will return to normal within 6 weeks. The usual cause for this is edema resulting from vocal chord trauma associated with intubation. If the patient is aphonic or exhibits little or no improvement after 2 weeks, endoscopic examination of the vocal cords is warranted to define the prognosis and rule out other more serious conditions, such as a completely paralyzed vocal cord from recurrent laryngeal nerve damage, vocal cord cyst, or previously unrecognized tumor or occult localized abscess, especially if the paatient was intubated for a prolonged period.

Atelectasis

Atelectasis is extremely common as evidenced by the nearly universal presence of bi-basilar inspiratory crackling rales in the absence of fluid overload or congestive heart failure. Despite the absence of a typical x-ray appearance, a significant pulmonary alveolar-arteriolar oxygen gradient is often noted, requiring supplemental oxygen use. The findings are so common that they are not classified as a complication, but were they so classified, atelectasis would undoubtedly be the most common noncardiac complication of heart surgery. Coughing, deep breathing, and incentive spirometry are usually sufficient, but other measures when needed are more fully discussed in Chapter 23.

Pleural Effusions

Pleural effusion, often bilateral, is expected. Most often, no specific therapy or, at most, gentle diuresis is required and resolution takes place in 2 to 6 weeks. When lasting longer and occupying 25% or more of the hemithorax by x-ray, thoracentesis is commonly performed, depending on pulmonary reserve and individual patient tolerance. With the use of internal thoracic artery revascularization, pleural effusions are more common and often larger. This may neccesitate "prophylactic" placement of a chest tube at surgery that may need to be left in place after the patient is transfered from the intensive care unit. This is discussed in more detail in Chapter 23.

Chest Film Findings

The typical postoperative chest x-ray in an uncomplicated patient has a "wet" look, often exhibiting pulmonary venous redistribution into the middle and upper lobe zones despite normal or even low capillary wedge pressure. This appearance is consistent with the fact that colloid osmotic pressure is reduced (14) and with the reported increase in pulmonary extravascular water (15). If the patient emerges from the operating room with a pneumothorax, it is usually benign and does not require chest tube placement as long as it is small (less than 20%) and as long as arterial blood remains well oxygenated without requiring excessive supplemental oxygen. Pneumothorax appearing later (after 12 hr) is of somewhat greater concern because a continuous air leak is more likely. Although a chest tube may still not be needed, the patient should be observed with more frequent chest x-rays and blood gas determinations. The chest x-ray appearance of air in the pericardium is extremely common, and air entering the abdomen through diaphragm eventration is also common on postoperative chest x-ray. The latter is also benign except when it appears later after surgery in the presence of ongoing abdominal disease.

Hiccups

Persistent hiccups (singultus) are an odd but common occurrence that can first begin 3 days or so after surgery and may persist for several days despite aggressive attempts at medical therapy. They are particularly annoying and even painful because of the sudden and intense diaphragmatic contraction that markedly worsens incisional pain of the sternum. Possible mechanisms include phrenic nerve injury (especially common with the use of pericardial ice solutions), pericarditis, perioperative inferior wall myocardial infarction, and gastric distension. Therapy is usually aimed at correcting any underlying causative condition and often includes periodic administration of dry, granulated sugar swallowed slowly; one-time administration of chlorpromazine tablets 25 to 50 mg; administration of Reglan; administration of small doses of CO_2 by face mask or rebreathing into a paper bag; as well as such physical measures as brief insertion of a soft rubber catheter into the posterior nasopharynx.

Gastrointensinal System

Constipation

Constipation is a nearly universal complaint, often blamed on inactivity, fluid restriction, and little or no dietary fiber. Constipation is often worsened and may itself further aggravate such associated rectal conditions as anal fissure or anal stenosis. Therapy consists of daily use of a stool softener, increased intake of dietary fiber, and liberalization of fluids, occasionally assisted with the administration of Milk of Magnesia, Dulcolax suppository, or Fleets enema. The problem can be severe enough to result in visits to the emergency room or rehospitalization for disimpaction and more definitive therapy of such

associated conditions as hemorrhoids and anal fissure. Proctology consultation is warranted in the presence of severe hemorrhoids or when other rectal pathology is known or suspected.

Appetite

Equally frustrating, but rarely as painful, are the changes in appetite often seen after cardiac surgery. Anorexia can be profound but may respond to discontinuation of certain potentially offending medications, such as potassium chloride supplements, ferrous sulfate, nonsteroidal anti-inflammatory agents, and certain analgesics. In some instances, this condition is accompanied by a distorted sense of taste (dysgeusia). In these cases, zinc sulfate (20 mg orally every 8 hr) may be helpful despite normal zinc levels. Other than as a medication side effect, the mechanism of postoperative anorexia is not known, but if it is severe and persists for 3 days or more, alternative forms of alimentation must be considered, using either nasogastric feeding or peripheral or central venous alimentation.

Genitourinary System

The most common problem in men usually consists of urinary retention due to prostatic hypertrophy. This condition is usually worsened by prolonged bed rest, overdistension of the bladder due to nonrecognition of the obstructed bladder, and the use of diuretics. A prolonged indwelling Foley catheter also leads to diminished bladder tone and can result in edema of the already enlarged prostate gland. Reinsertion of an indwelling Foley catheter, progressive ambulation, retraining of the bladder, and passage of a few days are often successful. Occasionally, however, the Foley catheter cannot be withdrawn, and after suitable further convalescence, prostatectomy must be performed.

Nervous System

Ulnar and Median Neuropathy

Ulnar and median neuropathy are common neurologic sequelae of cardiac surgery (16, 17). Careful protection of the extremities against injury is warranted, but this has not reduced the incidence of ulnar neuropathy, which remains at 3 to 5%. Median nerve involvement occurs less frequently (1 to 3%) (9). Both are the result of brachial plexus injury occasionally associated with rib fractures, thought to be due to excessive retraction of the sternum during surgery (18). It has been pointed out that both brachial plexus injury and rib fractures were more frequent when the chest retractor was placed higher, resulting in more vigorous retraction of the manubrium, clavicles, and scapulae (19, 20).

Symptoms are usually first noted on the 3rd or 4th postoperative day, with involvement of the left side somewhat more common than that of the right. Ulnar involvement follows a typical pattern of sensory distribution of the small finger and medial portion of the ring finger in the affected extremity. The sensation, usually one of numbness, is generally well tolerated. Occasionally, however, disabling painful paresthesia can occur, requiring periodic analgesics or even transcutaneous nerve stimulation therapy. Median neuropathy results in motor weakness to the muscles of the forearm and hand, typically noted when the patient is unable to grasp and hold a coffee cup or eating utensils. The grip strength is distinctly affected, but extensor function of the thumb is preserved (radial nerve). In even the most severely affected cases resolution is seen, but it occasionally takes as long as 2 to 3 months. Often a worsening of paresthesia occurs prior to major improvement or resolution, especially with ulnear neuropathy.

Vision

Visual symptoms are common and often consist of poor visual acuity, blurring, or scotomata. Many patients will describe prominent "floaters" that they had not previously experienced; others report seeing various spots or stripes. In a recent study of neurologic complications of bypass surgery, 17% had evidence of retinal infarction consisting of cotton wool-appearing spots. Of these patients, half were symptomatic; the others complained of visual disturbances, such as reading difficulty or haziness in the peripheral field of vision (17). Experience has taught that, despite the presence of definite pathologic changes, full recovery of visual acuity is the

rule. Because spontaneous recovery may require up to 6 months, it is ill-advised to change eyeglasses during this time in all but the most severely afflicted patients. Cortical blindness can occur and may be missed during brief daily hospital visits with the patient. One should be alerted when the patient appears to stare through rather than focus on the objects of his or her intended vision. When asked, the patient is unable to read or comprehend the content, often turning the reading material in various directions to help clarify his or her confusion. Despite these rather profound derangements, patients rarely spontaneously mention such symptoms and often flatly deny their presence (Anton's syndrome) (21). This condition is a complication and, when it is suspected, a clinical neurologic examination and formal visual field testing are indicated to define the extent of injury and any associated pathology. Computed tomography may be useful in differentiating retinal from cortical causes of visual disturbances (22). The prognosis for symptomatic improvement is good, but detectable visual abnormalities often remain.

Tremor

A transient tremor is extremely common, especially in older patients. This is often first noted as shaky handwriting when corresponding to friends and relatives after surgery. If it was not present before surgery, this too resolves within 6 to 8 weeks postoperatively.

Musculoskeletal and Miscellaneous Generalized Complaints

Pain

Incisional pain is usually not especially severe; if it is, complications of healing, such as sternal infection or nonunion of the sternum, should be ruled out. After the 1st week, the incisional pain is less intense in the midline, but becomes more pronounced in the costochondral cartilage area, with persistent discomfort in this area recurring unpredictably days to weeks after surgery. Poststernotomy pain may also involve the area beneath both axillae, as well as the middle and upper thoracic and cervical spine area. Internal thoracic artery revascularization is associated with somewhat more pronounced chest wall discomfort, often affecting the base of the neck on the side from which the internal thoracic artery was removed. After a week of healing, there is sufficient bone callus formed to result in a raised area of the superior end of the sternum incision. This is often slightly tender and may become reddened. As a result of the inflammation or poor skin healing in this area, localized wound infection is common. In the ensuing months, further molding of the healing sternum results in partial flattening of the area and return of the sternal notch.

Keloids

Occasionally the xiphoid process, usually soft and flexible, calcifies into a hardened, somewhat tender spike of bony tissue that, if extremely annoying to the patient, may require surgical removal. Despite good approximation of skin edges, areas of the middle and lower sternum, as well as the upper thigh, seem prone to keloid formation. This can present as a rather tender, painful, reddened, exuberant scar that may respond to intradermal injections of steroid. Less severely affected individuals, or those contemplating cosmetic plastic surgical repair, should be urged to wait for 6 months or so to allow for possible spontaneous regression.

Fatigue

The most common complaint during convalescence is generalized fatigue and poor exercise tolerance. In the 1st week, these symptoms wax and wane and may be particularly severe on certain days but should not alarm either the patient or the physician. The degree of fatigue is not related to patient age or cardiac function, but is somewhat predictable based on preoperative conditioning and exercise habits.

The symptoms discussed here should not be considered a complete list, but they have many features in common. All are seen in patients who may continue to be classified as uncomplicated or, at worst, exhibiting minor complications; all or most of the aforementioned complaints are transient, requiring no or relatively minor intervention.

References

1. Gray RJ, Braunstein G, Krutzik S, et al: Calcium homeostasis during coronary bypass surgery. *Circulation* 62:I-57–I-61, 1980.
2. Lappas DG, Drop L, Mundth ED, et al: Hemodynamic response to intravenous calcium chloride during coronary artery surgery. *Surg Forum* 26:234–235, 1978.
3. Gray RJ, Maddahi J, Berman D, et al: Scintigraphic and hemodynamic demonstration of transient left ventricular dysfunction immediately after uncomplicated coronary artery bypass surgery. *J Thorac Cardiovasc Surg* 77:504–510, 1979.
4. Czer L, Hamer A, Murphy F, et al: Transient hemodynamic dysfunction after myocardial revascularization: temperature dependence. *J Thorac Cardiovasc Surg* 86(2):226–234, 1983.
5. Zeldis SM, Morganroth J, Horowitz LN, et al: Fascicular conduction disturbances after coronary bypass surgery. *Am J Cardiol* 41:860–864, 1978.
6. O'Connell JB, Wallis D, Johnson A, et al: Transient bundle branch block following use of hypothermic cardioplegia in coronary artery bypass surgery: high incidence without perioperative myocardial infarction. *Am Heart J* 103:85–91, 1982.
7. Bateman TM, Weiss MH, Czer LSC, et al: Fascicular conduction disturbances and ischemic heart disease: adverse prognosis despite coronary revascularization. *J Am Coll Cardiol* 5:632–639, 1985.
8. DePasquale NP, Brune MS: Natural history of combined right bundle branch block and left anterior hemiblock (bilateral bundle branch block). *Am J Med* 54:297–303, 1973.
9. Denes P, Dhingra RC, Wu D, et al: Sudden death in patients with chronic bifascicular block. *Arch Intern Med* 137:1005–1010, 1977.
10. Schneider JF, Thomas HE, Kreger BE, et al: Newly acquired left bundle-branch block: the Framingham study. *Ann Intern Med* 90:303–310, 1979.
11. Schneider JF, Thomas HE, Kreger BE, et al: Newly acquired right bundle-branch block: the Framingham study. *Ann Intern Med* 92:37–44, 1980.
12. Bassan MM, Oatfield R, Hoffman I, et al: New Q-waves after aortocoronary bypass surgery. Unmasking of an old infarction. *N Engl J Med* 290:349–353, 1974.

13. Conde CA, Meller J, Espinoza J, et al: Disappearance of abnormal Q waves after aortocoronary bypass surgery. *Am J Cardiol* 36:889–893, 1975.

14. Gallagher JD, Moore RA, Kerns D, et al: Effects of colloid or crystalloid administration on pulmonary extravascular water in the postoperative period after coronary artery bypass grafting. *Anesth Analg* 64:753–758, 1985.

15. Byrick RJ, Kay C, Noble WH: Extravascular lung water accumulation in patients following coronary artery surgery. *Can Anaesth Soc J* 24:332–345, 1977.

16. Breuer AC, Furlan AJ, Hansen MR, et al: Neurologic complications of open heart surgery. *Clevel Clin Q* 48:205–206, 1981.

17. Shaw PJ, Bates D, Carlidge NEF, et al: Early neurological complications and coronary artery bypass surgery. *Br Med J* 291:1384–1387, 1985.

18. Vandersalm TJ, Cereda JM, et al: Branchial plexus injury following median sternotomy. *J Thorac Cardiovasc Surg* 80:447–452, 1980.

19. Vandersalm TJ, Cutler BS, Okiki ON: Brachial plexus injury following median sternotomy. *J Thorac Cardiovasc Surg* 83:914–917, 1982.

20. Baisden CE, Greenwald LV, Symbus PN: Occult rib fractures and brachial plexus injury following median sternotomy for open-heart operations. *Ann Thorac Surg* 38:192–194, 1984.

21. Meyendorf R: Visual disturbances after open-heart surgery. In Becker R (ed): *Psychopathological and Neurological Dysfunctions following Open-Heart Surgery*. Berlin, New York, Springer-Verlag, 1982, pp 16–31.

22. Smith LA, Cross SA: Occipital lobe infarction after open heart surgery. *J Clin Neuro Ophthalmol* 3:23–30, 1983.

Chapter 12
LOW OUTPUT STATES FOLLOWING CARDIAC SURGERY

MYLES EDWIN LEE, M.D.
RICHARD J. GRAY, M.D.

Modern techniques of cardiopulmonary bypass and perioperative hemodynamic monitoring have extended the safe application of cardiac surgery to high-risk patients. Although diligent assessment of preoperative cardiac and noncardiac risk factors has reduced surgical morbidity and mortality, significant low output states occur nevertheless in 10 to 15% of patients and intraaortic balloon pumping is needed in 2% of patients in the postoperative period (1). Most commonly, this results from impaired myocardial function, but may be caused by pericardial tamponade. The importance of prompt differentiation between these causes cannot be overemphasized, because emergency reoperation in the latter situation can be life saving. Other factors contributing to low output states include residual uncorrected valvular lesions or intracardiac shunts, metabolic abnormalities, anesthetic or cardiac drugs, sepsis, endocrine dysfunction, and central nervous system disorders. This entire spectrum of multisystem disorders must be kept in mind to enable the administration of the appropriate therapy in a timely manner. Treatment of low output is discussed in Chapters 13 and 14.

MYOCARDIAL FACTORS

Preoperative abnormalities of right and left ventricular function may be severe, irreversible, and associated with a prohibitive surgical mortality. It is now recognized, however, that certain akinetic ventricular segments may be viable and can regain contractility after revascularization. This response can be accurately predicted by successful uptake of thallium-201 prior to bypass surgery (2, 3). The predictive value of thallium scintigraphy can be indispensable in assessing preoperative surgical risk.

Postoperative pump failure has been identified in patients with essentially normal preoperative ventricular function. Although transient, some degree of myocardial insufficiency occurs in all patients following cardiopulmonary bypass (4) and may result from intramyocardial edema, myocardial ischemia, or the presence of free oxygen radicals (5). Perioperative myocardial infarction can produce sequential or even global dysfunction of either the right or the left ventricle. Embolic debris from atheromatous lesions in native coronary arteries or from old saphenous vein grafts may cause infarction ex-

147

tensive enough to impair the heart's ability to maintain the circulation (6).

The patient with a large zone of myocardium subtended by a totally occluded artery dependent on intercoronary collaterals for viability may be at increased risk of infarction unless intraoperative strategies are tailored to ensure cardioplegic protection to these areas. There is experimental evidence that the collateral-dependent segment cannot be protected solely by maintenance of high-pressure coronary perfusion and that intramyocardial collaterals cease to function with the onset of cardiopulmonary bypass (7). The loss of these collaterals is accompanied by electrocardiographic evidence of ischemia, ventricular ectopy, ventricular fibrillation, and gross contraction abnormalities in the affected territory.

The potential implications of these changes are further highlighted by the uncertainty of being able to deliver cardioplegic solutions through the aortic root to collateral-dependent myocardial segments. This risk is further increased if the internal thoracic artery has been selected to bypass a collateral-dependent segment because use of this conduit usually commits one to bypass its target last. In this instance, delivery of cardioplegia to a collateral-dependent area may be facilitated by direct infusion through a small arteriotomy at the proposed site of bypass using a 20-gauge catheter. The infusion may be repeated at 30-min intervals until the anastomosis of the internal thoracic artery has been completed. If vein grafts are chosen, they should be anastomosed to collateral-dependent or totally obstructed arteries first, and cardioplegia infused through the completed distal saphenous vein–coronary artery anastomosis. Retrograde delivery of cardioplegia through the coronary sinus has been reported experimentally and clinically as a useful adjunct to the standard route of cardioplegic infusion through the aortic root that may provide additional myocardial protection in patients with diffuse and severely obstructive coronary disease (8).

PERICARDIAL FACTORS

The pericardium is a structure with limited distensibility in which a small increment in in-

trapericardial volume can result in a marked increase intrapericardial pressure. When this pressure equals or exceeds right atrial pressure, the transmyocardial or effective cardiac filling pressure becomes negligible and pericardial tamponade will occur. This diagnosis should be considered in any postoperative patient with unexplained hemodynamic instability in whom acute mediastinal hemorrhage has occurred.

Pericardial tamponade resulting from nonsurgical effusions generally results in uniform compression of the cardiac chambers. Pulsus paradoxus and elevation and equalization of filling pressures require equal compression of both ventricles by a uniformly distributed volume of fluid or clot throughout the inelastic pericardium. In a study of the hemodynamics of patients with pericardial tamponade by effusions largely of uremic or metastatic etiology, Reddy and coworkers demonstrated that right ventricular end-diastolic pressure exceeded 7 mm Hg and was equal to pericardial pressure (9). In the majority of patients, the pulmonary capillary wedge pressure generally equilibrated with pericardial and right atrial pressure.

In an equally distributed tamponade, each ventricle is required to fill against a uniform intrapericardial resistance. During inspiration, the increase in venous return to the right heart limits left ventricular filling within the confines of a fluid- or clot-filled pericardium. This results in a transient decrease in left ventricular output and a decrease in arterial blood pressure. During expiration, pulmonary wedge pressure increases to or above systemic venous pressure, resulting in increased left ventricular filling and stroke volume with an increase in arterial pressure. These changes result in the exaggerated normal response to respiration known as pulsus paradoxus.

Prior to the availability of postoperative hemodynamic monitoring with the Swan-Ganz flotation catheter, Frater measured postoperative intrapericardial pressure with a saline-filled manometer connected to the posterior pericardial chest tube (10). When the intrapericardial pressure equaled the central venous pressure, tamponade was found at reoperation. Weeks and coworkers subsequently used a Swan-Ganz catheter to demonstrate a pressure plateau in postoperative pericardial tamponade with elevation and equalization of the right atrial, pulmonary artery diastolic, and pulmonary capillary wedge pressures (11).

Postoperative tamponade is frequently not uniformly distributed within the pericardium but tends to be localized, often due to blood clots. Asymmetric compression of one or more cardiac chambers is the rule, rather than the exception. The diagnosis may therefore be missed if reliance is placed solely on the identification of the hemodynamic patterns established for nonsurgical uniformly distributed tamponade. Whereas systemic hypotension and depressed cardiac output are common to all forms of tamponade, a spectrum of subtle hemodynamic differences exist depending on which cardiac chamber has been compressed by clot. For example, acute superior vena cava syndrome, consisting of marked cervical venous distension with filling pressures that remain in the normal range despite volume infusion, has been seen at the author's institution. Bateman and coworkers described two cases of right atrial tamponade with distended cervical veins but with right atrial pressures markedly in excess of right ventricular end-diastolic and pulmonary capillary wedge pressures in response to volume infusion (12). Jones and coworkers reported a case of left ventricular tamponade characterized by normal right atrial and right ventricular end-diastolic pressures but with elevation of the pulmonary arterial diastolic and pulmonary capillary wedge pressures (13). Pericardial evacuation was performed successfully in all cases and confirmed the preoperative diagnoses.

Diagnostic Difficulties

The differentiation between hemodynamic instability resulting from myocardial insufficiency and pericardial tamponade can be difficult despite clinical examination, chest x-ray, electrocardiography, echocardiography, and hemodynamic monitoring. Cervical venous distension, for example, can result from biventricular failure or tamponade. Distant heart sounds, commonly observed in nonsurgical tamponade, are typical in postoperative patients without tamponade, due to increased lung volume or mediastinal air or blood. The cardiac silhouette

is almost always enlarged on a postoperative chest roentgenogram because of portable anteroposterior technique, because of heart failure, or because of a pericardial fluid collection. It is important to realize, however, that pericardial tamponade can occur with a posteriorly located clot that will result in no enlargement of the cardiac silhouette and also that tamponade by clot can occur despite freely draining chest tubes.

Electrocardiographic low voltage may not represent a pericardial fluid collection but nontamponading mediastinal clot or overlying lung. Similarly, postoperative echocardiographic assessment is very difficult because of intervening mediastinal air, blood, or clot; the presence of postoperative dressings; and difficulties in positioning an acutely ill patient.

Ventricular Dysfunction versus Pericardial Tamponade

Differentiation between biventricular dysfunction and tamponade on a purely hemodynamic basis may not be possible. Elevation and equalization of filling pressures may occur in both conditions. Right ventricular dysfunction may cause markedly elevated right atrial pressure, mimicking right atrial tamponade.

Technetium-99m tagged RBC radionuclide ventriculography has long been used to assess postoperative ventricular function. The same technique can also be used to help distinguish the various causes for low cardiac output. In a group of 50 patients in whom the etiology of postoperative cardiogenic shock could not be elucidated using conventional means as outlined above, radionuclide ventriculography was able to differentiate between ventricular dysfunction and abnormalities of the pericardial space in 70% of the patients studied: 16 patients had ventricular dysfunction only, and 19 patients had pericardial tamponade only (14). Of the patients with tamponade, nine had a large pericardial region of photon deficiency (Fig. 12.1). This was associated with large pericardial effusion with no evidence of active bleeding. In 10 patients, the abnormal accumulation of radionuclide activity dispersed throughout the pericardium suggested active bleeding associated with generalized tamponade

FIGURE 12.1

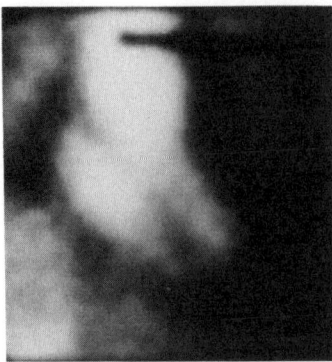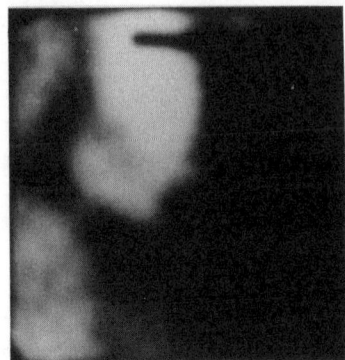

The presence of a photon-free space surrounding the heart indicates the presence of a large pericardial fluid collection.

(Fig. 12.2). The finding of abnormalities in the pericardial space associated with normal biventricular function in patients with postoperative instability influenced the decision to explore the pericardium in 16 patients and resulted in the restoration of normal hemodynamics in all cases.

Localized pericardial bleeding leading to localized tamponade is also discernible with this technique. This will appear as an abnormal accumulation of radioactivity localized within the pericardium. While this can appear in any location, the most common site for a localized blood collection is around the right atrium in the region of the atrial cannulation. This technique requires a specialized approach employing both zoomed and nonzoomed images, as well as delayed imaging (up to 4 hr).

Tamponade can also be precipitated in the postoperative period by chest tube irrigation with saline solution. Chest tubes are invariably surrounded by clot which may act as a ball valve, preventing egress of the irrigant and precipitating tamponade in a patient who may initially have had ventricular failure. This complication can be prevented by using a sterile suction catheter inserted into the chest tube and attempting to aspirate the intraluminal clot.

OTHER MISCELLANEOUS CONDITIONS

Other conditions are known to be associated with a low output state in the postoperative period. Metabolic acidosis resulting from poor tissue perfusion or inadequately treated diabetes mellitus may interfere with the vasomotor re-

FIGURE 12.2

ACTIVE PERICARDIAL BLEEDING

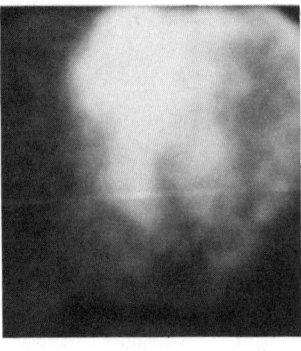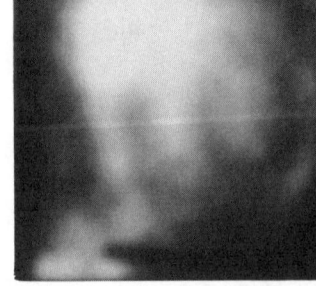

INITIAL   DELAYED

The presence of abnormal radioactivity due to [^{99m}Tc]RBC in the pericardial space indicates the presence of active bleeding in the region of the right atrium.

sponse to endogenous or exogenous catecholamines, resulting in low systemic vascular resistance and hypotension. A similar vasomotor response occurs in septic patients. Depression of myocardial function occurs in both instances. Treatment includes volume replacement, correction of acidosis, and treatment with appropriate antibiotics and interim support of the circulation.

Endocrine dysfunction, especially hypoadrenalism, may be the cause of unexplained hypotension and can result from hemorrhage into the adrenal glands during cardiopulmonary bypass. Similarly, unrecognized, even subclinical, hypothyroidism can result in dependence on pharmacologic circulatory support in the absence of ventricular wall motion abnormalities. Recently, liothyronine sodium has received attention as an agent for restoring hemodynamic stability in patients with postoperative myocardial failure even in the absence of hypothyroidism (15).

References

1. Frazier OH: Mechanical circulatory assistance. In Attar S (ed): *New Developments in Cardiac Assist Devices.* New York, Praeger, 1985, pp 124–139.

2. Rozanski A, Berman D, Gray R, et al: Preoperative prediction of reversible myocardial asynergy by postexercise radionuclide ventriculography. *N Engl J Med* 307:212, 1982.

3. Bateman T, Gray R, Czer L, et al: The severely depressed left ventricle in ischemic heart disease: rest-redistribution Tl-201 imaging predicts improvement after revascularization. *J Nucl Med* 27:933, 1986.

4. Czer L, Hamer A, Murphy F, et al: Transient hemodynamic dysfunction after myocardial revascularization: temperature dependence. *J Thorac Cardiovasc Surg* 86(2):226–234, 1983.

5. Bernard M, Menasche P, Canioni P, et al: Cardioplegic arrest superimposed on evolving myocardial ischemia: improved recovery with the free radical scavenger peroxidase (abstract). *Circulation* 76(IV):116, 1987.

6. FitzGibbon GM, Keon WJ: Atheroembolic perioperative infarction during repeat coronary bypass surgery: angiographic documentation in a survivor. *Ann Thorac Surg* 43:218–219, 1987.

7. Miyamoto A, Robinson L, Matloff J, et al: Perioperative infarction: effects of cardiopulmonary bypass on collateral circulation in an acute canine model. *Circulation* 58(I):1–148, 1978.

8. Partington MT, Acar C, Buckberg GD, et al: Studies of retrograde cardioplegia. *J Thorac Cardiovasc Surg* 97:605–622, 1989.

9. Reddy PS, Curtiss EI, O'Toole JD, et al: Cardiac tamponade: hemodynamic observations in man. *Circulation* 58:265–272, 1978.

10. Frater RWM: Intrapericardial pressure and pericardial tamponade in cardiac surgery. *Ann Thorac Surg* 10:563–565, 1970.

11. Weeks KR, Chatterjee K, Block S, et al: Bedside hemodynamic monitoring; its value in the diagnosis of tamponade complicating cardiac surgery. *J Thorac Cardiovasc Surg* 71:250–252, 1976.

12. Bateman T, Gray R, Chaux A, et al: Right atrial tamponade caused by hematoma complicating coronary artery bypass graft surgery: clinical hemodynamic and scintigraphic correlates. *J Thorac Cardiovasc Surg* 84:413–419, 1982.

13. Jones MR, Vine DL, Attas M, et al: Late isolated left ventricular tamponade: clinical, hemodynamic and echocardiographic manifestations of a previously unreported postoperative complication. *J Thorac Cardiovasc Surg* 77:142–146, 1979.

14. Bateman TM, Czer L, Kass RM, et al: Cardiac causes of shock early after open heart surgery: etiologic classification by radionuclide ventriculography. *Circulation* 71:1153–1161, 1985.

15. Novitzky D, Cooper DKC, Swanepoel A: Initial experience with triiodothyronine (T_3) therapy in patients with low cardiac output following open heart surgery (abstract). *J Am Coll Cardiol* 9(2):7A, 1987.

Chapter 13
PHARMACOLOGIC SUPPORT OF THE CIRCULATION

DHUN H. SETHNA, M.D.
ARNOLD FRIEDMAN, M.D.
RICHARD J. GRAY, M.D.

VASOACTIVE DRUGS

Heart pump function is closely dependent on peripheral vascular function. The major determinants of cardiac function—preload and afterload—are controlled predominantly by the peripheral circulation, and heart rate and myocardial contractility are strongly influenced by peripheral vascular neurohormonal receptors. Hence, effects of drugs on peripheral arteries and veins will influence heart pump function, even without direct actions on the myocardium, and this forms the basis for the perioperative use of vasodilators for the failing heart. Conversely, heart muscle function (contractility) is improved by the positive inotropic agents.

Vasodilators

Capacitance and Impedance Characteristics of Blood Vessels

The walls of blood vessels, with the exception of capillaries and some venules, have vascular smooth muscle which, by contraction, can alter vessel caliber and the viscoelastic properties

(compliance) of the vessel wall. The cardiovascular effects of this response depend on the fluid storage (capacitance) or fluid flow resistance (impedance) properties of the vascular bed involved.

The venous bed, especially the venules and the sinusoids of the liver and spleen, is the principle site of fluid storage, with the small veins and sinusoids containing about 45% of the intravascular volume and the central venous reservoirs of the vena cava and large veins holding about 18%. Steady-state elastic properties of the vascular bed show that most of the blood volume is stored under the minimal hydrostatic pressure that is consistent with the hollow shape of the blood vessel ("unstressed vascular volume"); a smaller component of the stored blood volume pressurizes the vessel apart from pressure associated with flow and constitutes the "stressed vascular volume" (1, 2). The pressure arising from the volume-pressure relationship of the stressed vascular component is the driving pressure (mean circulatory pressure) to venous return.

Reflexogenic or pharmacologic alterations in

venous volume capacity in intact animals result from fluid shifts between the unstressed and stressed components of the total vascular volume (2, 3). Rapid mobilization of up to 10% of intravascular volume can occur into or from the unstressed vascular volume component by subtracting from or adding to the stressed vascular volume. Changes in the latter result in changes in pressure in the vascular system, so that at any level of total vascular volume, the mean circulatory pressure changes when volume is transferred between stressed and unstressed storage. For example, when unstressed vascular volume decreases, as it does with increasing activity of the baroreceptors, stressed vascular volume increases, causing a rise in mean circulatory pressure with enhancement of venous return and cardiac output. When unstressed vascular volume increases, as it does with nitroprusside administration, stressed vascular volume decreases, thus decreasing mean circulatory pressure, venous return, and, ultimately, cardiac output (4).

The property of the pulsatile vascular system to dissipate the energy of fluid flow is called impedance (2). Aortic input impedance involves a pulsatile component determined by arterial compliance, blood inertia, and wave reflection, and a nonpulsatile (static) component which is the peripheral vascular resistance. In the simplest Poiseuille model of steady, nonturbulent flow of fluid down a long, rigid tube, assuming blood viscosity and length of blood vessel are constant, resistance is inversely proportional to the 4th power of the radius. Although blood is a non-Newtonian fluid showing pulsatile flow in elastic blood vessels, the conceptual simplicity of the Poiseuille relationship makes it convenient for clinical use, and it is the systemic vascular resistance measurement rather than aortic impedance that is normally used clinically. Moreover, the small arteries and arterioles, because of their content of vascular smooth muscle and the richness of their innervation and receptors for neurohumoral influences, account for about 60% of the vascular resistance and can produce rapid change in vascular impedance.

Storage and resistance properties of the vascular system are interrelated, such that changes in blood flow distribution, which are a function of resistance and therefore arteriolar tone, can affect blood volume storage, conventionally believed to require changes in venous tone (5).

Peripheral Circulation Effects in Heart Failure

Heart failure usually reduces arterial pressure and cardiac output and increases venous pressure in association with absolute and relative changes in blood flow distribution. These effects may be influenced by compensatory neurohormonal and local tissue metabolic factors, which include activation of the renin-angiotensin-aldosterone system, release of vasopressin, and secretion of epinephrine and norepinephrine from adrenal medullary or peripheral vascular sites. Despite high blood levels at rest in heart failure, exercise usually results in normal or blunted hormonal responses, and the extent of actual tissue activity of these hormones is uncertain (6, 7).

Active vasoconstriction and a limitation of vasodilation are the predominant peripheral vascular compensatory mechanisms that maintain patterns of regional blood flow when cardiac function and output fail (8, 9). If not present at rest, abnormal patterns of vasoconstriction due to increased α-receptor stimulation almost invariably occur with exercise. Coronary, cerebral, and skeletal muscle blood flows are preserved, while splanchnic, renal, and skin flows are decreased. With advancing failure, blood flow is seriously reduced in the latter circulations, especially during exercise. Reduced renal flow stimulates the renin-angiotensin cascade leading to increased circulating levels of angiotensin II, and also allows an intrarenal redistribution of flow to favor sodium retention and plasma volume expansion. This adds to the effects of renin-angiotensin-aldosterone activation leading to increases in vascular sodium content and stiffness of large and medium-sized arteries (8).

At some point, the vasoconstriction associated with congestive heart failure becomes excessive and detrimental. By increasing aortic impedance, a further burden is placed on the already failing heart, and decline in cardiac function in accelerated. Amplifying this response is an attenuation of baroreceptor function, which further enhances sympathetic-mediated vasoconstriction, and a "stiffness" factor in peripheral vessels, which makes them poorly responsive to vasodilator stimuli (8, 10).

Venous capacitance, as examined in limb veins in humans, is markedly reduced with advancing heart failure, although neurohumoral factors that actively stimulate venous smooth muscle probably play only a minor role in the increased venous tone (8). This fall in venous capacitance tends to shift blood from peripheral reservoirs toward the central circulation.

Rationale for Vasodilator Therapy

The rationale of vasodilator therapy derives from the relationship between heart pump function and state of the vascular capacitance and impedance properties (10). When the aortic valve opens, pressure in the left ventricle is a function not only of myocardial fiber shortening but also of impedance to ejection of blood. Arterial compliance and arteriolar resistance to systolic runoff become determinants of the rise of aortic pressure, ejection-phase indices and heart chamber volume during ejection. By relaxing vascular smooth muscle, vasodilators can increase capacitance or reduce impedance. Increasing capacitance with reduced ventricular filling and end-diastolic (presystolic) volume reduces presystolic ventricular wall stress ("preload"). Reducing impedance leads to a greater shortening of contractile elements, and thus to an enhanced fall in end-systolic volume and improved ejection fraction. Effects of improved systolic function on stroke volume depend on concomitant change in left ventricular end-diastolic volume.

Arterial dilator drugs do not acutely alter diastolic ventricular volume, and the improved stroke volume they induce translates to an increased ejection fraction. Venodilator drugs, however, acutely redistribute blood volume into the capacitance vessels and reduce ventricular filling. The fall in ventricular end-diastolic volume may therefore limit the stroke volume increases that result from the lower end-systolic volume. Thus, the net effect of any vasodilator drug on stroke volume reflects the relative changes in capacitance and resistance vessels.

Vasodilator drugs in patients do not only produce direct vasodilation, but also activate counteropposing mechanisms that cause peripheral vasoconstriction and reflex tachycardia via the sympathetic nervous and the renin-angiotensin systems. Thus, hemodynamic responses to vasodilator treatment are the net result of these two interacting forces which can limit the magnitude of therapeutic improvement. This endogenous neurohumoral response is most apparent in normal subjects and hypertensive patients who are not in congestive heart failure, but can be minimal in those with congestive failure in whom the full beneficial effect of vasodilation can occur unopposed. Differences in endogenous neurohumoral responses can explain much of the interpatient variability observed during vasodilator therapy. The extent of the observed improvement in cardiac performance is also limited in patients with valvular obstruction and idiopathic hypertrophic subaortic stenosis, in whom increased forward output is opposed by a mechanical interference to ejection.

The magnitude of the hemodynamic response to vasodilators alone when administered acutely in heart failure is comparable to the response observed when specific inotropic drugs are used alone in the same patients (11). The beneficial effect of reductions in impedance is greatest in the dilated left ventricle, and close correlations have been demonstrated between left ventricular chamber size and improved responses to vasodilation in patients with severe heart failure. In aortic regurgitation, drugs that reduce aortic impedance enhance forward ejection from the left ventricle relative to regurgitant flow. Venodilator drugs can also improve myocardial function by reducing mitral regurgitation. Reductions in ventricular volumes result in an improved function of the papillary muscles and the mitral subvalvular apparatus, with decreases in effective mitral valve area and mitral regurgitation. The systolic pressure gradient between left ventricle and left atrium and the duration of regurgitation are not affected by venodilators.

Specific Vasodilator Drugs

Vasodilators can relax vascular smooth muscle by direct reductions in vascular tone or by activation of receptor-mediated neurohumoral mechanisms. Direct-acting drugs (e.g., hydralazine, nitroprusside, and nitrates) depend on delivery of active drug to the sensitive vascular tissue, and the magnitude of vasodilation is dose dependent. Dose requirements vary and cumulative effects can occur, so careful dose titration is needed. In contrast, receptor-dependent vasodilators require specific pathophysiologic derangements for their responses; that is, increased sympathetic nervous activity or activation of the renin-angiotensin system. Drugs in this group include postsynaptic α-sympathetic blockers (e.g., prazosin) and angiotensin-converting enzyme inhibitors (e.g., captopril). The magnitude of vasodilation is receptor dependent (not dose dependent).

Sodium Nitroprusside. Nitroprusside is a smooth-muscle-relaxing agent that acts directly on arterioles to decrease systemic vascular resistance and on peripheral veins to increase venous capacitance. Venodilation and arteriolar dilation occur to almost the same degree. In the forearm, the rates of reduction in vascular resistance and venous tone approach unity. Both pulsatile and static components of aortic input impedance are lowered. However, animal studies do show variability of response between vascular beds. The drug has no effect on ventricular contractility or compliance when the pericardium is non intact. Vasodilator effects are not mediated by α, β or muscarinic receptors, but are probably related to the ability of the drug to oxidize sulfhydryl groups. The active nitroso molecule of the drug is rapidly metabolized when the ferrous ion in nitroprusside reacts with sulfhydryl groups in red blood cells and tissues. Cyanogen is produced in this reaction and is converted by the liver enzyme rhodanese to thiocyanate, which is excreted by the kidneys with a half-life of 7 days.

Nitroprusside must be administered intravenously with an infusion pump and its action monitored with systemic arterial pressure monitoring. The onset and cessation of action are almost immediate. Standard infusion rates vary from 0.5 to 8 μg/kg/min, using a preparation of 50 mg of the drug dissolved in 250 ml of 5% dextrose in water. The drug must be discontinued gradually to avoid rebound vasoconstriction.

Variability in stroke volume responses occurs in patients given nitroprusside. In those with congestive heart failure and elevated filling pressures, the drug causes significant reductions in these pressures with improvements in stroke volume. Blood pressure and heart rate remain virtually unchanged. In patients with only mild degrees of heart failure and modest elevations in left ventricular filling pressures, nitroprusside produces substantial leftward and downward shifts in the relation between stroke volume and left ventricular filling pressure (12). This observation is consistent with a diminished venous return to the heart resulting from venous capacitance increasing more than the shift in volume from the central to the systemic venous circuit. In such cases, effects of arterial dilation and impedance reduction on stroke volume fail to balance the consequences of lowered preload, and cardiac output falls. With constant nitroprusside infusion, a rapid volume challenge can fill the capacitance bed, thus augmenting venous return and elevating preload to a more favorable point, with increases in stroke volume. These observations emphasize the dynamic nature of the interaction between venodilation and arterial relaxation in modulating cardiac performance, and the critical dependence of the system on blood volume both before and during therapy. Hence, although nitroprusside appears to dilate both precapillary resistance vessels and postcapillary capacitance vessels to approximately equivalent degrees, the net effects on cardiac performance vary widely depending on the initial point of operation and shape of the ventricular function curve.

Several investigators have compared the effects of nitroglycerin and nitroprusside on regional myocardial ischemia. In patients with acute myocardial infarction, the magnitude and extent of S-T segment elevation recorded by precordial S-T segment mapping was shown to worsen when nitroprusside was administered (13). When sublingual nitroglycerin was given to the same patients, S-T segment elevation was reduced. In an animal model using radioactive microspheres to quantify regional myocardial blood flow, epicardial S-T segments in the region of myocardium distal to a coronary ligation became more elevated and regional myocardial flow decreased after nitroprusside infusion. When nitroglycerine was infused and comparable hemodynamic effects obtained, S-T segment elevation in the ischemic region was reduced and myocardial blood flow improved in that region. Thus, nitroprusside appeared to worsen regional ischemia by reducing coronary perfusion pressure without augmenting collateral flow (13, 14). Recently a large multicenter study evaluating nitroprusside infusion in patients with acute myocardial infarctions showed a higher mortality in the first 9 hr in those who were randomized to nitroprusside.

Differences between nitroglycerin and nitroprusside on blood flow to ischemic myocardium may be due to differing effects on the coronary arteries. Nitroglycerin appears to dilate large conductance vessels and to have brief effects on smaller resistance vessels, whereas nitroprusside exerts a major dilating action on resistance vessels. Perfusion of an ischemic zone via collateral channels is dependent on a pressure gradient between the vessel feeding the collateral and vessels within the ischemic zone. Since near maximum dilation is presumed to be present in the ischemic zone, drugs that reduce resistance in vessels of the nonischemic zone may result in a "coronary steal" during which collateral flow to the ischemic zone is reduced in favor of flow to the nonischemic zone. Nitroprusside particularly exacerbates ischemia when given in the absence of congestive heart failure or when excessive hypotension is produced.

In patients with heart failure, nitroprusside increases renal blood flow along with increases in cardiac output. The drug also increases minute urine flow, total cation excretion, and filtration fraction, while total renal resistance is decreased. Reductions in pulmonary artery pressures and pulmonary vascular resistance result in diminished afterload to the right ventricle, but may also cause arterial hypoxemia with significant reductions in arterial PO_2.

Immediate side effects of nitroprusside such as retching, diaphoresis, tachycardia, and hypotension are the results of too-rapid administration. However, if dosage requirements exceed 10 μg/km/min, or if tachyphylaxis develops, the drug should be discontinued. Because cyanide inhibits mitochondrial cytochrome oxidase oxygen transport, effects of cyanogen accumulation (nitroprusside toxicity) include metabolic acidosis, increased mixed venous oxygen ten-

sion, or decreased arterial-venous oxygen difference. Treatment of nitroprusside toxicity includes (*a*) a bolus of thiosulfate 150 mg/kg, to provide a sulfate donor for conversion of cyanide to thiocyanate; (*b*) inhalation of amyl nitrate and infusion of 5 mg/kg of sodium nitrate in 20 ml of water over 3 to 4 min, as nitrites convert hemoglobin to methemoglobin, which in turn converts cyanide to the nontoxic cyanmethemoglobin; (*c*) hydroxycobalamin infusion, which converts the cyanide to cyanocobalamin, which is excreted in the urine.

Nitroprusside in contraindicated in Lebers congenital amaurosis in which there is a deficiency in hepatic rhodanese. It should be used cautiously in patients with hypothyroidism or severe liver or renal disease.

Nitroglycerin. Nitroglycerin is a potent relaxant of vascular, gastrointestinal, and genitourinary smooth muscle. Probable mechanisms include formation of disulfide bonds from reduced sulfhydryl groups on cell membranes; inhibition of calcium mobilization from intracellular sites; and inhibition of platelet aggregation, thereby limiting the production of prostaglandin thromboxane A_2, a potent vascular constrictor. Nitroglycerin is widely distributed in the body and rapidly metabolized in the liver, with an estimated half-life of 2 to 3 min.

At low doses, venodilation predominates with peripheral venous pooling and reduction of left ventricular filling pressure. Venodilation is due to systemic (nonsplanchnic) and pulmonary veins. Maximal venodilator effects occur at low doses, with reductions in ventricular volumes and wall stress. When cardiac preload declines to levels below the point optimal for cardiac performance as determined by the Frank-Starling relation, cardiac output falls. At higher doses, nitroglycerin allows dilation of both venous and arterial smooth muscle in a dose-dependent fashion, with reductions in peripheral resistance and increases in stroke volume. Dilation of extramural coronary arteries and intracoronary collateral channels and redistribution of myocardial blood flow to deeper subendocardial layers have been described (15).

Intravenous nitroglycerin can, in the majority of cases, be as effective as sodium nitroprusside for the treatment of perioperative hypertension. In a randomized, cross-over study design, nitroglycerin and nitroprusside lowered arterial pressure and peripheral vascular resistance equally in 85% of anesthetized patients after myocardial revascularization, when comparable infusion rates were used (16). Nitroglycerin increased cardiac output more than sodium nitroprusside, and showed more potent vasodilating effects on the pulmonary circulation with a greater lowering of mean pulmonary arterial pressure especially in patients with initially elevated pulmonary pressures. In addition, the drug produced smaller increases in the alveolar-arterial oxygen gradient than did nitroprusside, and improved intrapulmonary shunting while nitroprusside worsened it. Some patients, however, failed to respond to nitroglycerine even with high drug doses. Studies in anesthetized patients with coronary artery disease have shown that intravenous nitroglycerin increased coronary sinus oxygen content and reduced myocardial oxygen comsumption (17).

Potential adverse reactions to intravenous nitroglycerin in the anesthetized patient include hypotension, sinus tachycardia, and sinus bradycardia. Drug-induced hypotension is quickly reversed by discontinuing or reducing the rate of infusion. Occasionally, leg elevation is required. Sinus tachycardia or bradycardia might be expected if blood pressure is rapidly lowered with an intravenous bolus of the drug. Reflex effects can be minimized by slow changes of the infusion rate. Methemoglobinemia and uncoupling of oxidative phosphorylation have been reported in patients receiving high doses of intravenous nitroglycerin.

Phentolamine. The predominant action of phentolamine is direct relaxation of vascular smooth muscle, with a somewhat less potent effect as an α-receptor antagonist. A combined pre- and postsynaptic blockage produced by phentolamine at the postganglionic sympathetic nerve terminal with inhibition of presynaptic reuptake results in accumulation of neurotransmitter. As a consequence, phentolamine administration commonly results in tachycardia and positive inotropic cardiac stimulation. In humans, intravenous injection of the drug results in profound reductions of sys-

temic vascular resistance and arterial pressure with increases in heart rate and cardiac output (18). The drug can be given as a single intravenous bolus (1 to 3 mg) or as a continuous infusion (0.1 to 0.5 mg/min) titrated to individual patient responses. The fate of phentolamine in the body is unknown.

INOTROPES

The use of inotropic agents to stimulate depressed myocardium is predicated on the existence of residual myocardial function ("contractile reserve"), which must be of sufficient magnitude to significantly augment global cardiac performance and systemic perfusion. Effectiveness of inotropes may be limited by their relative potency, their toxic:therapeutic ratios, their mechanism of action, and the amount of contractile reserve available. Metabolic effects of inotropic stimulation differ with respect to the etiology and stage of myocardial depression—a drug may directly increase myocardial oxygen demand or may reduce metabolic demands by reduction of heart size and wall tension.

Inotropic stimulation appears to work by increasing the amount of ionic calcium available for the contractile system (19). Stimulation of β_1 receptors by catecholamines activates adenyl cyclase, which catalyzes the conversion of ATP to 3', 5'-cyclic AMP. Protein kinases thus activated allow phosphorylation of membrane systems, resulting in increased availability of ionized calcium to the contractile proteins. Phosphodiesterase inhibitors such as aminophylline, and the newer agents amrinone and milrinone, increase myocardial cellular levels of 3', 5'-cyclic AMP by decreasing the rate of degradation of adenyl cyclase. Direct activation of adenyl cyclase, independent of the β-adrenergic receptor, can be induced by glucagon. The mechanism of action of digitalis glycosides is believed to involve partial inhibition of the Na-K-ATPase located on the sarcoplasmic reticulum. Extrusion of calcium from the myocyte during systole is thereby inhibited, thus increasing intracellular calcium stores available for myocardial tension development.

Catecholamines

Isoproterenol

Isoproterenol is a potent synthetic β-agonist catecholamine that increases heart rate, AV conduction, myocardial contractility, and myocardial oxygen consumption and decreases systemic and pulmonary vascular resistance (20). At infusion rates of 0.025 to 0.05 mg/kg/min, isoproterenol can be used in cardiac surgical patients with low cardiac output and pulmonary hypertension (i.e., after mitral valve replacement for mitral stenosis), recently transplanted heart, significant β-blockade prior to surgery, and hemodynamically significant bradycardia unresponsive to atropine (21–23). At higher doses, the drug can markedly increase myocardial oxygen demand by increasing heart rate and myocardial oxygen consumption and can decrease myocardial oxygen supply by causing hypotension, particularly during hypovolemia, and an intracoronary "steal" (24). Thus, isoproterenol should be used with caution in patients with coronary artery disease because it can cause myocardial ischemia and arrhythmias and increase myocardial infarct size.

Epinephrine

Epinephrine is a potent α- and β-adrenergic receptor agonist. At all doses, $β_1$ stimulation produces positive inotropic and chronotropic effect, and α stimulation causes vasoconstriction of the skin and kidneys. At low doses (1 to 10 μg/min), $β_2$ stimulation also allows vasodilation in the splanchnic and skeletal muscle beds, whereas α vasoconstriction predominates at higher doses (above 10 μg/min). Since vasoconstriction of the kidney increases renal vascular resistance at all doses, patients with marginal renal function may be at risk for further kidney dysfunction.

In a study comparing dopamine, dobutamine, and epinephrine in patients during emergence from cardiopulmonary bypass, epinephrine (0.04 μ/kg/min) increased cardiac index 30%, mean arterial pressure 24%, heart rate 11%, stroke volume index 9%, and left ventricular stroke work index 52%. As opposed to dopamine or dobutamine, there were no instances in which epinephrine failed to increase cardiac index (25).

Because the drug also caused the largest increase in pulse pressure, myocardial ischemia may occur secondary to an increased myocardial oxygen demand. Since improvements in ventricular performance may be overshadowed by tachycardia and increases in myocardial oxygen consumption, an unfavorable myocardial oxygen supply:demand ratio could lead to myocardial ischemia and arrhythmias. Large doses of epinephrine have been associated with premature ventricular contractions, ventricular tachycardia, and ventricular fibrillation, especially in the presence of myocardial ischemia, particularly if sensitized by halothane. Thus, epinephrine is primarily used when the failing myocardium is unresponsive to dopamine or dobutamine, in cardiac arrest, and for anaphylactic drug reaction (e.g., to protamine or antibiotics).

Norepinephrine

Norepinephrine is the principal chemical transmitter released from peripheral adrenergic nerve endings. It has a primary α-agonist effect on the peripheral vasculature causing vasoconstriction and less potent $β_1$-agonist effect producing positive inotropy and chronotropy (26). Since the increased blood pressure is associated with reflex decrease in sinoatrial activity, there are usually no significant changes in heart rate during norepinephrine infusion. $α_1$-Adrenergic receptors are commonly found in the myocardium and cause increased myocardial contraction when stimulated; however, the overall physiologic importance of activating myocardial $α_1$-receptors by norepinephrine infusion remains to be determined.

Phentolamine is often used in combination with norepinephrine to decrease peripheral vasoconstriction and enhance β-agonist activity. In one study of patients with low cardiac output after open-heart surgery, norepinephrine (0.02 to 0.1 μg/kg/min) plus phentolamine (0.05 to 0.25 μg/kg/min) produced increases in systemic and total pulmonary resistances and blood pressure with no changes in cardiac index, stroke volume index, heart rate, and pulmonary capillary wedge and right atrial pressures. Although dopamine and dobutamine both augmented cardiac index and stroke volume index, norepinephrine-phentolamine allowed more predictable vasopressor responses without tachycardia or ventricular irritability (27). Independent titration of norepinephrine and phentolamine after cardiopulmonary bypass increased cardiac index, mean arterial pressure, stroke volume index, and left ventricular stroke work index, and reduced pulmonary vascular resistance and mean left atrial and pulmonary artery pressures without significant changes in heart rate or systemic vascular resistance (28). Norepinephrine with phentolamine should be considered for patients with low systemic vascular resistance, cardiac output, and blood pressure in whom coronary and cerebral perfusion are jeopardized and in patients with low cardiac output who develop tachyarrhythmias when other inotropes are used.

The use of norepinephrine may be limited by increases in myocardial work and decreases in vital organ perfusion. However, an animal model of the low-cardiac-output syndrome demonstrated that infusion norepinephrine plus phentolamine at three doses restored cardiac pump performance and regional blood flow, as determined by tracer-labeled microspheres, without evidence of excessive myocardial oxygen consumption (29). Another study involving simultaneous administration of norepinephrine and phentolamine in optimal ratios showed renal blood flows were maintained near baseline levels (30). Low-dose dopamine (4 μg/kg/min) added to norepinephrine has been shown to significantly increase renal blood flow and decrease renal vascular resistance (31).

Dopamine

Dopamine is a naturally occurring sympathomimetic agent that acts on α, β, and dopaminergic receptors and is a precursor in the synthesis and release of norepinephrine. Since myocardial catecholamine stores may be largely depleted in advanced heart failure, drug effects in these patients may be limited (32). At low doses (1 to 3 μg/kg/min) dopamine acts predominantly on dopaminergic receptors and vasodilates the renal and mesenteric circulations (33, 34). These effects are blocked by butyrophenones and phenothiazines but not by β-adrenoreceptor blockade. Cardiac output is augmented and systemic vascular resistance is re-

duced at this dose with little change in left ventricular filling pressures. At intermediate doses of dopamine (5 to 10 μg/kg/min), β-receptor stimulation becomes predominant and myocardial contractility and cardiac output increase. Concomitant increases in pulmonary capillary pressure have been observed and may be related to increased venous return secondary to venoconstriction (35). Moreover, enhanced myocardial performance and elevated blood pressure can result in increased myocardial oxygen consumption (36). At higher doses (above 10 μg/kg/min), α-adrenergic mediated vasoconstriction predominates and the hemodynamic effects of dopamine resemble those of norepinephrine.

In cardiac surgical patients studied in the intensive care unit, hemodynamic comparison between dopamine and dobutamine in the dose range 5 to 10 μg/kg/min have shown that both drugs produce increases in heart rate, mean arterial pressure, cardiac index, and stroke volume index with reductions in pulmonary and systemic vascular resistances. Similar increases in cardiac index and stroke volume index were produced in the same patient with a smaller dose of dopamine than dobutamine (7.2 versus 11.3 μg/kg/min). However, in 4 of 9 patients, the maximum dose of dopamine (10 μg/kg/min) was discontinued because of arrhythmias, tachycardia, or hypertension (27). In patients studied immediately after cardiopulmonary bypass, dopamine at doses of 5, 10, and 15 μg/kg/min increased cardiac index, mean arterial pressure, heart rate, and stroke volume index and decreased systemic vascular resistance. When compared to dobutamine, dopamine was found to be twice as potent and produced larger increases in cardiac index at each dose (25). Since hemodynamic effects of dopamine at low to moderate doses augment cardiac performance, it is useful in patients with hypotension, low cardiac output, and sinus bradycardia. However, sinus tachycardia and arrhythmias may limit its use in some patients.

In the kidney, dopamine causes vasodilation, increased glomerular filtration, interference with aldosterone synthesis and release, and increased urine flow (34, 37). Since this drug has been shown to enhance diuresis, natriuresis, and kaliuresis by either a direct action on renal tubular solute transport or redistribution of blood flow within the kidney independent of renal and systemic perfusion and glomerular filtration (38), it can be very efficacious in patients with compromised renal function.

Dopamine and dobutamine have been studied after cardiac surgery in patients in whom left ventricular hemodynamics and dimensions and coronary sinus blood flows were measured while heart rates were held constant with atrial pacing. Both drugs increased peak left ventricular contractility (dp/dt) and myocardial oxygen consumption. With dobutamine these increases were matched by similar increases in coronary blood flow; however, failure of the expected increases in coronary blood flow with dopamine suggested altered coronary artery autoregulation and the potential of limiting myocardial oxygen supply during periods of increased myocardial oxygen demand (36).

Dobutamine

Dobutamine is s synthetic catecholamine that exerts predominant β_1-adrenergic receptor stimulation with few effects on heart rate or vascular tone. Inotropic effects of dobutamine result from direct stimulation of myocardial β receptors with secondary increases in cyclic AMP and are not dependent on endogenous norepinephrine stores (39). Recent studies indicate that dobutamine is a racemic mixture that may cause a more complex interaction with α and β adrenergic receptors in both the heart and the peripheral vasculature. The 1-isomer is a potent α_1-adrenergic agonist and a relatively weak β_1 and β_2 agonist, whereas the d-isomer is a potent β_1 and β_2 agonist with only minimal effects on α-adrenergic receptors (40). The cumulative effects of dobutamine at α and β receptors in the myocardium and vasculature may provide an explanation for the predominantly positive inotropic response of this agent. With β-adrenergic blockade, dobutamine fails to increase cardiac output but increases total peripheral resistance, which suggests the drug has modest direct effects on vascular α receptors (41). Because of β_2 and α_1 agonist effects, there may be little net direct effect on systemic vascular resistance. These variable actions of do-

butamine may occur in clinical situations in which α- or β-receptor activity or density is altered, and may partly explain selective tachycardia or blunted positive chronotropic response or the limited inotropic action observed in some patients. Since dobutamine does not release norepinephrine from endogenous stores, it may be effective in situations in which myocardial norepinephrine is depleted or absent (chronic congestive heart failure or cardiac transplantation) and dopamine is ineffective. With continuous infusion of dobutamine, attenuation of hemodynamic effect may occur, presumably on the basis of "down regulation" of myocardial β_1 receptors, and this effect requires upward dose titration (42).

When comparing dobutamine and isoproterenol in cardiac surgical patients immediately after cardiopulmonary bypass, dobutamine seemed to be a more suitable inotrope and was associated with fewer arrhythmias. At 5 and 10 μg/kg/min, dobutamine increased cardiac index 16 and 28%, and heart rate 6 and 15%, respectively. In comparison, isoproterenol at 0.02 μg/kg/min augmented cardiac index 9% while increasing heart rate 44% (43). In another study of cardiac surgical patients weaned from cardiopulmonary bypass, dobutamine at doses of 5, 10 and 15 μg/kg/min increased cardiac index, mean arterial pressure, heart rate, and stroke volume index (25). In patients studied in the intensive care unit 6 hr following open-heart surgery, dobutamine increased heart rate, cardiac index, stroke volume index, and stroke work index without causing significant tachycardia or arrhythmias (44).

Peripheral vascular effects of dobutamine after cardiac surgery are difficult to assess because of drug interactions on vascular receptor activity and density, temperature-dependent alterations in vascular tone, and effects of aging and disease on vascular tone. In patients with aortic valve replacements who were weaned from cardiopulmonary bypass and given calcium chloride, dobutamine at 200 μg/min/m^2 resulted in no significant change in systemic vascular resistance (45). However, in another study following cardiopulmonary bypass, patients with coronary artery bypass grafting and normal ventricular function, and mitral and aortic regurgitation patients with volume-loaded ventricles, when given dobutamine at 2.5 and 5 µg/kg/min showed significant reductions in left ventricular afterload which partially explained their improvements in hydraulic performance (46). Moreover, in coronary artery bypass patients studied with ultrasonic dimension transducers and micromanometers within 24 hr after cardiopulmonary bypass, dobutamine decreased systemic vascular resistance, which probably accounted for partial enhancement of left ventricular contractility without the disadvantage of excess demand on myocardial oxygen reserve (47). These studies suggest that in most cardiac surgical patients, increases in cardiac output are accompanied by a reduction or maintenance of systemic resistance at all dose levels.

In adequately revascularized patients after coronary artery bypass surgery, dobutamine showed increases in myocardial oxygen consumption that were accompanied by larger increases in coronary blood flow. Because coronary sinus content or global myocardial lactate extraction remain unchanged despite an increased metabolic cost, global myocardial ischemia was not observed (48). However, since dobutamine has been shown to produce a maldistribution of coronary blood flow in animals (24) and to cause chest pain with S-T segment depression and adverse changes in myocardial lactate extraction in patients with coronary artery disease (49), myocardial ischemia could occur in incompletely revascularized patients or those who are internal thoracic artery–collateral dependent after cardiac surgery.

Noncatecholamines

Amrinone

Amrinone is a new nonadrenergic, nonglycoside bipyridine drug with potent inotropic and vasodilatory effects. This agent appears to selectively inhibit phosphodiesterase III in myocardial cellular membrane and increase cyclic AMP and availability of ionic calcium to the sarcoplasmic reticulum. Since β-adrenergic agonists stimulate production of adenylate cyclase at the β receptor to increase cyclic AMP, while amrinone increases cyclic AMP by preventing its degradation, inotropic activity of the two

drugs may be additive or synergistic. The loading dose of intravenous amrinone is 0.75 to 3 mg/kg/min given over 3 to 5 min, followed by a maintenance infusion of 5 to 20 µg/kg/min. Since 40% of the drug is excreted unchanged in the urine, infusion rates must be decreased in patients with severe renal insufficiency.

In patients with refractory congestive heart failure, amrinone increased cardiac output, decreased pulmonary capillary wedge pressure and systemic vascular resistance, and maintained heart rate and blood pressure. Myocardial oxygen consumption declined, as did systolic wall tension (50). In patients who had received adrenergic agonists after cardiac surgery, amrinone significantly increased cardiac index and reduced systemic and pulmonary vascular resistances and pulmonary capillary wedge and right atrial pressures (51). Arrhythmias are infrequent compared to other inotropes, but hypotension may limit the use of this agent in patients with coronary artery disease. To minimize hypotension in cardiac surgical patients, norepinephrine can be titrated with amrinone to maintain systemic blood pressure and adequate coronary and cerebral perfusion pressure. Because experience with amrinone is limited in patients requiring inotropes after cardiopulmonary bypass, further studies are needed to determine the role of amrinone during cardiac surgery.

Major complications of oral amrinone therapy in patients with congestive heart failure include thrombocytopenia (3%), hepatocellular damage (1%), arrhythmias (2%), and hypotension (2%). In a prospective study evaluating platelet function in cardiac surgical patients, amrinone in the early postoperative period failed to result in any significant reduction in platelet count or aggregation (52).

SUMMARY

This review provides a conceptual framework for the perioperative intravenous use of vasodilators and inotropes in patients with heart failure. The physiologic and pharmacologic determinants of vasodilator and inotrope responses are discussed, and important characteristics of the commonly used drugs are presented.

References

1. Shoukas AA, Sagawa K: Total systemic vascular compliance measured as incremental volume-pressure ratio. *Circ Res* 28:277–289, 1971.
2. Gow BS: Vascular impedance, resistance and capacity. In Bohr DF, Somlyo AP, Sparks HV (eds): *Handbook of Physiology. The Cardiovascular System*, vol 2. Bethesda, MD, American Physiological Society, 1980, p 353.
3. Shoukas AA, Sagawa K: Control of total systemic vascular capacity by the carotid sinus baroreceptor reflex. *Circ Res* 33:22–33, 1973.
4. Rubin SA, Misbach G, Lekven J, et al: Resistance and volume changes caused by nitroprusside in the dog. *Am J Physiol* 237:H99–H103, 1979.
5. Caldini P, Permutt S, Waddell JA, et al: Effect of epinephrine on pressure, flow, and volume relationships in the systemic circulation of dogs. *Circ Res* 34:606–623, 1974.
6. Thomas JA, Marks BH: Plasma norepinephrine in congestive heart failure. *Am J Cardiol* 41:233–243, 1978.
7. Rutenberg HL, Spann JF Jr: Alterations of cardiac sympathetic neurotransmitter activity in congestive heart failure. *Am J Cardiol* 32:472–480, 1973.
8. Zelis R, Flaim SF: Alterations in vasomotor tone in congestive heart failure. *Prog Cardiovasc Dis* 24:437–459, 1982.
9. Swan HJC, Rubin SA: *Chronic Heart Failure and Vasodilator Therapy*. Bethesda, MD, American College of Cardiology, 1980.
10. Packer M, Le Jemtel TH: Physiologic and pharmacologic determinants of vasodilator response: a conceptual framework for rational drug therapy for chronic heart failure. *Prog Cardiovasc Dis* 24:275–292, 1982.
11. Mikulic E, Cohn JN, Franciosa JA: Comparative hemodynamic effects of inotropic and vasodilator drugs in severe heart failure. *Circulation* 56:528–533, 1977.
12. Miller RR, Vismara LA, Zelis R, et al: Clinical use of sodium nitroprusside in chronic ischemic heart disease: effects on peripheral vascular resistance and venous tone and on ventricular volume, pump and mechanical performance. *Circulation* 51:328–336, 1975.
13. Chiariello M, Gold HK, Leinbach RC, et al: Comparison between the effects of nitroprusside and nitroglycerin on ischemic injury during acute myocardial infarction. *Circulation* 54:766–773, 1976.
14. Mann T, Cohn PF, Holman BL, et al: Effect of nitroprusside on regional myocardial blood flow in coronary artery disease. *Circulation* 57:732–738, 1978.
15. Goldstein RE: Coronary vascular responses to vasodilator drugs. *Prog Cardiovasc Dis* 24:419–436, 1982.
16. Flaherty JT, Magee PA, Gardner TL, et al: Comparison of intravenous nitroglycerin and sodium nitroprusside for the treatment of acute hypertension developing after coronary artery bypass surgery. *Circulation* 65:1072–1077, 1982.
17. Sethna DH, Moffitt EA, Bussell JA, et al: Intravenous nitroglycerine and myocardial metabolism during anesthesia in patients undergoing myocardial revascularization. *Anesth Analg* 61:828–833, 1982.
18. Stern MA, Gohlke HK, Loeb HS, et al: Hemodynamic effects of intravenous pentolamine in low output cardiac failure. *Circulation* 58:157–163, 1978.
19. Storstein L, Taylor SH: New and old inotropic drugs: controversies and challenges. *Eur Heart J* 3(Suppl D):1–157, 1982.
20. Beregovich J, Reicher-Reiss H, Kunstadt D, et al: Hemodynamic effects of isoproterenol in cardiac surgery. *J Thorac Cardiovasc Surg* 62:957–964, 1971.
21. Mentzer RM, Alegre CA, Nolan SP: The effects of dopamine and isoproterenol on the pulmonary circulation. *J Thorac Cardiovasc Surg* 71:807–814, 1976.
22. Stinson EB, Caves PK, Griepp RB, et al: Hemodynamic observations in the early period after human heart transplantation. *J Thorac Cardiovasc Surg* 69:264–270, 1975.
23. Halloway EL, Stinson EB, Derby GC, et al: Action of drugs in patients after early cardiac surgery. *Am J Cardiol* 35:656–659, 1975.
24. Warltier DC, Zyvoloski M, Gross GJ, et al: Redistribution of myocardial blood flow distal to a dynamic coronary arterial stenosis by sympathomimetic amines. *Am J Cardiol* 48:269–279, 1981.
25. Steen PA, Tinker JA, Pluth JR, et al: Efficacy of dopamine, dobutamine, and epinephrine during emergence from cardiopulmonary bypass in man. *Circulation* 57:378–384, 1978.
26. Weiner N: Norepinephrine, epinephrine and the sympathomimetic amines. In Gilman AG, Goodman LS, Gilman A (eds): *The Pharmacological Basis of Therapeutics*. New York, MacMillan, 1980, pp. 151–153.
27. Gray R, Shah PK, Singh B, et al: Low cardiac output states after open heart surgery. *Chest* 80:16–22, 1981.
28. Kirsh MM, Bove E, Detmer M, et al: The use

of levarterenol and phentolamine in patients with low cardiac output following open-heart surgery. *Ann Thorac Surg* 29:26–31, 1980.

29. Lemmer JH, Botham MJ, McKenney P, et al: Norepinephrine plus phentolamine improves regional blood flow during experimental low cardiac output syndrome. *Ann Thorac Surg* 38:108–116, 1984.

30. Cimmino VM, Bove EL, Argenta LC, et al: The effect of simultaneous administration of levarterenol and phentolamine on renal blood flow. *Ann Thorac Surg* 21:158–163, 1976.

31. Schaer GL, Fink MP, Parrillo JE: Norepinephrine alone versus norepinephrine plus low-dose dopamine: enhanced renal blood flow with combination pressor therapy. *Crit Care Med* 13:492–496, 1985.

32. Chidsey CA, Braunwald E, Morrow AG: Catecholamine excretion and cardiac stores of norepinephrine in congestive heart failure. *Am J Med* 39:442–451, 1965.

33. Goldberg LI: Cardiovascular and renal actions of dopamine: potential clinical implications. *Pharmacol Rev* 24:1, 1972.

34. McDonald RM Jr, Goldberg LI, McNay JL, et al: Effects of dopamine in man: augmentation of sodium excretion, glomerular filtration rate and renal plasma flow. *J Clin Invest* 43:1116–1124, 1964.

35. Marino RJ, Romagnoli A, Keats AS: Selective venoconstriction by dopamine in comparison with isoproterenol and phenylephrine. *Anesthesiology* 43: 570–572, 1975.

36. Fowler MB, Alderman EL, Oesterle SN, et al: Dobutamine and dopamine after cardiac surgery: greater augmentation of myocardial blood flow with dobutamine. *Circulation* 70(Suppl I):103–111, 1984.

37. Carey RM, Thorner MO, Ortt EM: Dopaminergic inhibition of metoclopramide-induced aldosterone secretion in man. *J Clin Invest* 66:10–18, 1980.

38. Hilberman M, Maseda J, Stinson EB, et al: The diuretic properties of dopamine in patients after open-heart operation. *Anesthesiology* 61:489–494, 1984.

39. Tuttle RR, Mills J: Dobutamine—development of a new catecholamine to selectively increase cardiac contractility. *Circ Res* 36:185–196, 1975.

40. Ruffolo RR Jr, Spradlin TA, Pollack GD, et al: Alpha and beta adrenergic effects of the stereoisomers of dobutamine. *J Pharmacol Exp Ther* 219:447–452, 1981.

41. Sonnenblick EH, Frishman WH, LeJemtel TH: Dobutamine: a new synthetic cardioactive sympathetic amine. *N Engl J Med* 300:17–22, 1979.

42. Unverferth DV, Blanford M, Kates RE, et al: Tolerance to dobutamine after a 72 hour continuous infusion. *Am J Med* 69:262–266, 1980.

43. Tinker JH, Tarhan S, White RD, et al: Dobutamine for inotropic support during emergence from cardiopulmonary bypass. *Anesthesiology* 44:281–286, 1976.

44. Sakamoto T, Yamada T: Hemodynamic effects of dobutamine in patients following open heart surgery. *Circulation* 55:525–533, 1977.

45. d'Hollander A, Primo G, Hennart D, et al: Compared efficacy of dobutamine and dopamine in association with calcium chloride on termination of cardiopulmonary bypass. *J Thorac Cardiovasc Surg* 83:264–271, 1982.

46. DiSesa VJ, Brown E, Mudge GH Jr, et al: Hemodynamic comparison of dopamine and dobutamine in the postoperative volume-loaded, pressure-loaded, and normal ventricle. *J Thorac Cardiovasc Surg* 83:256–263, 1982.

47. Van Tright P, Spray TL, Pasque Mk, et al: The comparative effects of dopamine and dobutamine on ventricular mechanics after coronary artery bypass grafting: a pressure-dimension analysis. *Circulation* 70(Suppl I):112–117, 1984.

48. Sethna DH, Gray RJ, Moffitt EA, et al: Dobutamine and cardiac oxygen balance in patients following myocardial revascularization. *Anesth Analg* 61:917–920, 1982.

49. Pacold I, Kleinman B, Gunnar R, et al: Effects of low-dose dobutamine on coronary hemodynamics, myocardial metabolism, and anginal threshold in patients with coronary artery disease. *Circulation* 68:1044–1050, 1983.

50. Benotti JR, Grossman W, Braunwald E, et al: Effects of amrinone on myocardial energy metabolism and hemodynamics in patients with severe congestive heart failure due to coronary artery disease. *Circulation* 62:28–34, 1980.

51. Goenen M, Pedemonte O, Baele P, et al: Amrinone in the management of low cardiac output after open heart surgery. *Am J Cardiol* 56:33B–38B, 1985.

52. Hines R, Barash PG: Amrinone associated thrombocytopenia: does it occur with short-term administration? *Abstracts of Ninth Annual Meeting of Society of Cardiovascular Anesthesiologists,* 1987, p 90.

Chapter 14
MECHANICAL SUPPORT OF THE CIRCULATION

MYLES EDWIN LEE, M.D.

Advances in hemodynamic monitoring, vasoactive pharmacologic agents, arrhythmia control, pacing techniques, and myocardial protection have allowed cardiac surgery to be performed safely even in patients with impaired ventricular function. Nevertheless, postoperative ventricular failure refractory to pharmacologic therapy can occur, requiring mechanical circulatory assistance. Of 45,375 patients undergoing cardiopulmonary bypass at the Texas Heart Institute (1), 970 patients (0.02%) required such support: 943 patients (95%) were stabilized with intraaortic balloon counterpulsation and 22 (2%) required a left ventricular assist device (LVAD).

Prolonged postischemic ventricular dysfunction may result from very brief periods of coronary occlusion. Sixty seconds of acute ischemia leads to functional changes from active systolic shortening to passive systolic lengthening (2). Twenty minutes of ischemia at normothermia causes structural, metabolic, and functional abnormalities that may persist for several days before functional recovery (3). Segmental wall motion abnormalities also arise from repetitive ischemia in the same coronary distribution.

Coronary bypass grafting can improve regional coronary perfusion and segmental wall motion; this can be predicted in patients who demonstrate reversal of perfusion defects after exercise thallium scintigraphy (4). Buckberg and coworkers (5), however, found that functional recovery of myocardial segments subjected to more than 6 hr of acute ischemia depends on both the conditions of reperfusion and the composition of the reperfusate (5). Following a period of hypothermic arrest, improved cardiac performance results from reperfusion during cardiopulmonary bypass with a vented, nonworking ventricle, with a perfusate of warm potassium cardioplegic solution containing the Krebs cycle precursors, aspartate and glutamate, which favor production of high-energy phosphates within the myocardial cell. With these nutrients, functional recovery is possible even after prolonged ischemia.

INTRAAORTIC BALLOON COUNTERPULSATION

The postoperative need for circulatory assistance arises when the failing ventricle is unable to maintain adequate tissue perfusion, as demonstrated by systolic pressure below 90 mm Hg, a cardiac index of less than 1.5 liters/min/m^2, persistent lactic acidosis, and mixed venous O$_2$ saturation below 30%. If these parameters can be maintained only with large doses of vasoactive agents, dual-chamber pacing, and continuous correction of acid-base abnormalities, the indications for circulatory assistance exist.

The type of assistance most frequently used

for left ventricular failure is intraaortic balloon counterpulsation (IABC). The concept of counterpulsation was introduced by Harken (6). Subsequently, Clauss and coworkers (7) described a counterpulsator that removed a volume of blood during cardiac systole and reinfused it during diastole through a cannula inserted in the subclavian artery. While reducing left ventricular work and enhancing coronary artery perfusion, the technique caused hemolysis and never received widespread clinical use. Similar physiologic benefits, but with greater ease of application and less hemolysis, were demonstrated by Moulopoulos and coworkers (8) using a carbon dioxide activated intraaortic balloon (IAB) that deflated during cardiac systole and inflated during diastole. After further technical refinements, Kantrowitz and coworkers introduced a helium-driven IAB that was associated with an early survival rate of 81% (9).

Indications for IABC

The most common indication for IABC is left ventricular failure following cardiac surgical procedures. More than 50% of patients who otherwise would not have been separated successfully from cardiopulmonary bypass will survive to be discharged from the hospital (10). Cardiogenic shock resulting from a massive left ventricular infarction is another indication for IABC. However, only about 25% of patients initially stabilized with the IAB and with no subsequent surgery survive to hospital discharge (11).

Survival following surgical intervention in patients with cardiogenic shock depends on the cause of the hemodynamic instability. If cardiogenic shock results from a 30% loss of left ventricular contractility, ultimate survival will depend on the functional recruitment of non-infarcted myocardial segments. If cardiogenic shock results from a mechanical complication of the infarction, such as an acute ventricular septal defect, newer methods of repair may result in long-term survival above 75% (12). Acute rupture of a mitral valve papillary muscle may cause circulatory collapse. IABC with prompt surgical intervention has been associated with survival of 75% of such patients (13). Occasionally, cardiogenic shock results from acute

closure of a coronary artery following percutaneous transluminal coronary angioplasty. IABC may be used in this circumstance if efforts at maintaining distal coronary flow are not successful.

With the advent of thrombolytic therapy and percutaneous transluminal coronary angioplasty for impending infarction, and with intravenous nitroglycerin and heparin for progressive angina thought to result from platelet emboli from ulcerated intracoronary plaques (14), IABC is now used infrequently in patients with unstable angina syndromes. Similarly, malignant ventricular arrhythmias, once treated with IABC (10), can more frequently be controlled with antiarrhythmic agents until electrophysiologic studies define the location of arrhythmogenic focus, providing guidance for more definitive ablative therapy. More recently, IABC has been used successfully as a bridge to cardiac transplantation.

Physiology of IAB

The IAB is inserted percutaneously, usually through the common femoral artery, and advanced retrograde to the descending thoracic aorta. The use of helium as the driving medium permits rapid inflation and deflation of the balloon. During cardiac systole, the balloon deflates. Rapid deflation of the balloon creates a potential space which the column of blood in the aorta proximal to the balloon rushes to fill. As a result, the blood in the ascending aorta is already moving forward when cardiac systole begins. This results in a 10 to 15% decrease in peak aortic systolic pressure and arterial end-diastolic pressure (Fig. 14.1). There is a decrease in peak left ventricular pressure, left ventricular end-diastolic pressure, left ventricular dp/dt, and pulmonary capillary wedge pressure (PCWP) and an increase in left ventricular ejection fraction and in cardiac index.

During cardiac diastole, at the time of closure of the aortic valve, the IAB inflates, causing an increase in aortic volume, augmenting diastolic aortic pressure, and increasing coronary blood flow. Using a coronary sinus catheter during balloon pumping in three patients with cardiogenic shock, Summers and coworkers (15) demonstrated improved myocardial lactate utilization 2 hr after pumping was begun. These

FIGURE 14.1

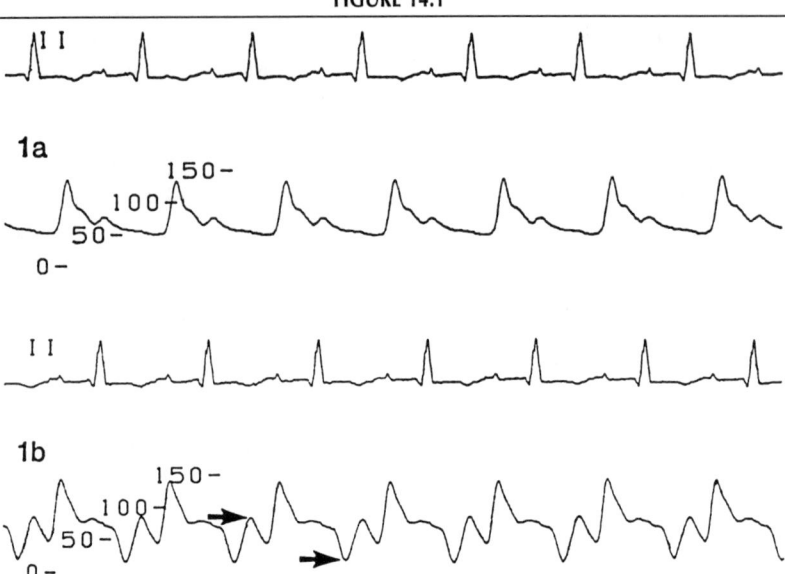

A, ECG and radial arterial pressure tracing. **B**, Radial arterial pressure tracing with 1:1 diastolic augmentation, demonstrating a decrease in peak aortic systolic pressure and arterial end-diastolic pressure (*arrows*).

findings suggested that the IAB is capable of converting anaerobic myocardial metabolism to aerobic metabolism by increasing coronary artery flow. As a clinical correlate, it is rare for the patient with acute reversible ischemia to experience angina during balloon pumping.

Timing of Inflation and Deflation

The timing of inflation and deflation may be accomplished using the electrocardiogram (ECG) or the arterial pressure waveform. With the ECG, balloon inflation is set to occur at the peak of the T wave and deflation within the P-R interval. If the ECG is of poor quality, or if large T waves, pacing spikes, or intraoperative use of the cautery interferes with the sensing mechanism of the balloon console, the timing of inflation can be set at the dicrotic notch of the arterial pressure trace, with deflation completed just before the onset of systole. It is important that the balloon not obstruct the subclavian artery; if it does, it could dampen the pressure trace obtained from the left radial artery. Some balloons now incorporate a lumen that allows direct measurements of central aortic pressure at the balloon tip.

Accurate timing of the inflate-deflate sequence is essential for optimal hemodynamic benefit. If inflation occurs before aortic valve closure, the ventricle will have to eject against both a closed aortic valve and an inflated balloon, increasing left ventricular afterload and work. Late inflation or early deflation will reduce the period of diastolic augmentation. Late deflation will impair left ventricular emptying.

Weaning

Weaning from the IAB may be accomplished by decreasing frequency of counterpulsation (e.g., from 1:1 to 1:2) or by decreasing the volume of helium pumped with each cycle. Before weaning is begun, the amount of pharmacologic circulatory support should be reduced or eliminated. Also, as intrinsic cardiac function improves, equalization of the peak aortic systolic pressure and balloon systole may be observed. If the patient can maintain a cardiac index of 2 liters/min/m^2, a PCWP below 18 mm Hg, and a left ventricular stroke work index above 20 gm-m/m^2, with progressive decreases in the frequency or volume of counterpulsation, weaning will likely succeed.

Methods of Insertion and Removal

Most commonly the IAB is inserted percutaneously through the common femoral artery.

The artery is initially punctured with a needle, a long guide wire is passed retrograde into the descending thoracic aorta, and a dilator is passed over the guide wire followed by a long sheath through which the IAB is inserted to the appropriate level. The tip of the balloon should be 2 cm distal to the origin of the left subclavian artery. Correct positioning is essential to allow optimum benefit and avoid obstruction of the subclavian artery. If fluoroscopy is not available, the proper level may be estimated by placing the IAB on the chest and abdomen with the tip 2.5 cm below the suprasternal notch and noting the point on the shaft adjacent to the femoral puncture site. Once the balloon has been inserted, the sheath is partially withdrawn to be certain that the balloon is free to inflate throughout its length.

Failure to obtain appropriate diastolic augmentation can result from retention of the balloon within the sheath, incomplete inflation resulting from failure of the balloon to unwrap, an empty helium tank, or mechanical failure of the pumping console. Other considerations include perforation of the aorta with retroperitoneal or intraabdominal balloon position or insertion of the IAB into the common femoral vein, in which case balloon systole is recorded in the right atrial pressure measurement. Fluoroscopic examination can readily determine the position of the balloon.

If severe aortoiliac disease precludes passage of the IAB to the descending thoracic aorta, entry into the circulation may be accomplished through the retroperitoneal abdominal aorta, the left axillary artery, or directly through the ascending aorta. The axillary approach should not be used in patients who have had coronary artery bypass grafting with the left internal thoracic artery since the balloon may compromise flow in this vessel as it courses through the subclavian artery. The IAB may also be introduced directly into the ascending aorta during cardiac surgery. This approach usually requires re-sternotomy for removal but can be accomplished without reentering the chest (16, 17).

IAB removal from the common femoral artery may be performed percutaneously. The femoral artery distal to the insertion site should be compressed for 2 or 3 cardiac cycles to permit thrombus that may have formed around the balloon or sheath to be ejected through the puncture site as the device is removed. The puncture site must be compressed for 30 to 60 min to control bleeding from the arteriotomy.

Percutaneous removal of an IAB should not be done if the patient has a coagulopathy or if the IAB has been in place for more than 1 week or has entered an arteriosclerotic vessel. In these instances, it is likely the arteriotomy will not seal with compression and will require surgical closure to prevent formation of a false aneurysm.

Complications

The most frequent complication of the IAB inserted in the femoral artery is ischemia of the lower limb. This results from arterial obstruction or spasm induced by the IAB. The IAB must be removed immediately to prevent irreversible ischemic damage to the lower extremity. If the patient is balloon dependent, the IAB may be inserted into the other femoral artery or blood flow may be restored with a femoral-femoral crossover graft interposed between the uninvolved side and the femoral artery distal to the IAB (18).

A false aneurysm may appear at the puncture site if inadequate compression has been applied or faulty plugging has occurred.

An IAB may be advanced within the vessel wall, causing a retrograde aortic dissection. This should be suspected when unusual difficulty is noted in passing the balloon and is associated with severe back pain. Fluoroscopy will confirm the diagnosis by demonstrating the tip of the IAB to be immobile during pumping, rather than vibrating freely in the aorta with each cycle. A late diagnosis of dissection may be suspected if there is no decrease in the platelet count after several days. Satisfactory augmentation may be achieved with intramural positioning of the IAB and does not rule out this complication. Removal should be accomplished as soon as possible to prevent fixation of the balloon to the aortic wall and possible aortic rupture.

Intraaortic balloon pumping has been associated with atherosclerotic emboli to the gut, kidneys, and rarely to the spinal cord. To prevent thrombus formation and subsequent embolization, patients should receive intravenous heparin or low molecular weight dextran infusion or both, except for the first few postoperative hours. Also, it is important that some motion of the balloon occur during the final stages of weaning to reduce the risk of thrombus formation.

Wound infections are rare with appropriate sterile technique. Though most infections can be anticipated in obese or diabetic patients, all patients should probably receive prophylactic antibiotics while the IAB is in place.

On rare occasions, rupture of the balloon may occur and manifest as the appearance of blood within the shaft of the balloon. Immediate change of the balloon is indicated. The usual causes, tearing of the balloon by an arteriosclerotic plaque or excessive twisting of the balloon, have been virtually eliminated by using the long introducer sheath and prewrapping of the balloon by the manufacturer.

Contraindications

The IAB should not be used in patients who have irreversible incapacitating cerebral dysfunction, nor can it sustain adequate tissue perfusion in patients with severely impaired forward flow (less than 1.5 liters/min/m^2). Aortic insufficiency is a relative contraindication to IAB. If more than 1+ aortic insufficiency exists, balloon inflation may result in acute left ventricular dilation, subendocardial ischemia with left ventricular and subsequent right ventricular failure, and possible tamponade or impairment of right ventricular filling by the acutely dilated left ventricle (19).

VENTRICULAR ASSIST DEVICES

When systolic blood pressures remain below 90 mm Hg, the cardiac index is less than 1.8 liters/min/mm^2, and left atrial pressures are more than 25 mm Hg despite pharmacologic support and balloon counterpulsation, direct ventricular assist is indicated.

The most frequent indications for ventricular assist are ventricular pump failure following open-heart surgery, myocardial infarction or cardiomyopathy, and acute rejection of the transplanted heart.

Ventricular assist devices (VAD) provide temporary support for the failing ventricle or may function as a bridge to cardiac transplantation. In the former instance, return of enough ventricular function to sustain the circulation may be anticipated in 72 hr (20). If this does not occur, or if there is a permanent functional loss of more than 40% of the left ventricle, the VAD functions as a bridge to transplantation. In this instance, it must be capable of nonthrombogenic circulatory support without damage to tissues or organs for periods up to 2 weeks or until a donor heart can be located.

The most common type of VAD is the vortex (centrifugal) pump, which provides long-term asynchronous nonpulsatile flow while minimizing the complications of prolonged roller pumping such as tubing wear, particle generation, and systemic embolization. Asynchronous pulsatile flow is provided by paracorporeal pneumatic pumps. Ventricular output is captured by cannulae placed proximal and distal to the impaired ventricle, with bypass of the left ventricle being accomplished by placement of a drainage cannula in the left atrium either through the right superior pulmonary vein or through the lateral or superior walls of the left atrium. Drainage catheters may also traverse the mitral valve and enter the left ventricle directly, or pass retrograde across the aortic valve or through a stab in the left ventricular apex. The transapical approach is generally not used unless the patient is expected to be a candidate for heart transplantation. Blood from the left ventricle may be returned to the body through the ascending, descending, or intraabdominal aorta or through the femoral artery.

Bypass of the right ventricle may be accomplished by placing a drainage cannula in the right atrium and returning the captured blood into the main pulmonary artery, or the right pulmonary artery lateral to the superior vena cava if access to the main pulmonary artery is impeded by coronary artery bypass grafts crossing over the pulmonary artery.

Left Ventricular Failure

Patients with left ventricular failure who meet the criteria described previously are candidates for left ventricular assist. Left atrial pressure of 10 mm Hg or more is required for effective LVAD output. It is important to determine the optimal flow rate delivered by the LVAD, especially in systems employing the centrifugal pump, because too much suction on the left atrial cannula can cause collapse of the left atrium around the catheter tip, impairing drainage. The goal is to use the least amount of flow that, together with whatever is ejected by the left ventricle, will achieve a total flow rate of 2.5 liters/min/m^2.

Right Ventricular Failure

Patients with severe left ventricular failure are candidates for a right ventricular assist device (RVAD). The diagnosis of right ventricular failure may be made if the cardiac index remains at less than 1.8 liters/min/m^2, the systemic blood pressure less than 90 mm Hg, and the left atrial pressure less than 15 mm Hg despite volume loading to a right atrial pressure of greater than 25 mm Hg. Initial treatment of acute right ventricular failure includes correction of metabolic acidosis and hypoxemia, and infusion of Isuprel into the pulmonary artery in an attempt to increase contractility and reduce pulmonary vascular resistance. Should these interventions fail, right ventricular assist is indicated.

Biventricular Failure

Biventricular failure resulting from ischemia or infarction of both ventricles is an indication for biventricular assist. Right ventricular failure which is thought to be secondary to left ventricular failure may improve with left ventricular assist alone. If it does not improve after a period of observation, intrinsic failure of the right ventricle is present. If the right ventricle is incapable of providing adequate filling of the left atrium with a pressure of 10 mm Hg or more, left ventricular assist will be impossible unless right ventricular assist is instituted.

Right Ventricular Function during Left Ventricular Assist

There is a 23% incidence of right ventricular failure in patients on LVAD support (21). It is clear that mechanical assist of the left ventricle can unmask previously unrecognized borderline dysfunction of the right ventricle. Preexisting disorders such as pulmonary hypertension, right ventricular infarction, right coronary artery disease, or inadequate intraoperative protection of the right ventricle can contribute to right ventricular failure. The effect of an LVAD on right ventricular preload, afterload, and contractility were reviewed by Farrar and coworkers (21) with emphasis on the beneficial and detrimental effects on right ventricular function in each category as summarized below.

Preload. An LVAD will increase preload to the right ventricle, the actual amount being determined by the systemic vascular resistance and LVAD flow. Increases in right ventricular preload can cause increases in right ventricular compliance from leftward shifts of the intraventricular septum during left ventricular unloading. If right ventricular contractility is severely impaired due to infarction or ischemia, however, right ventricular failure will ensue.

Afterload. Right ventricular afterload is a function of pulmonary vascular resistance. In the presence of normal pulmonary vasculature, unloading of the left ventricle by an LVAD lowers pulmonary artery pressure, thereby reducing right ventricular afterload.

Contractility. Right ventricular contractility may be improved by an LVAD if it reverses ischemia by increasing coronary artery perfusion. An extreme degree of left heart bypass, however, has been associated with a decrease in right ventricular dp/dt, probably due to a reduction of intraventricular septal contribution to right ventricular ejection (22). It is important, therefore, that an optimal level of ventricular assist be achieved so that the pump output complements the output of the left ventricle to maintain a total output in the physiologic range.

The study of Baird and coworkers (23), demonstrating the persistence of at transmural myocardial pressure gradient under conditions of total left ventricular unloading, further underscores the need for an optimal level of ventricular assist. In this study, systolic intramyocardial pressure in the inner third of the left ventricle frequently exceeded coronary perfusion pressure, and was also associated with increased myocardial oxygen consumption. Administration of negative inotropic agents such as Ca^{2+} blockers or β-blockers could decrease myocardial contractility and may improve the intramural pressure gradient, thus allowing increased perfusion and oxygenation of ischemic myocardium in a setting of reduced myocardial work. This approach may be appropriate if the goal is to provide temporary assistance to the ventricle in anticipation of ultimate recovery rather than transplantation.

With the onset of right ventricular failure during left ventricular assist, preload to the left atrium diminishes and the left-sided output will fall. Left ventricular assist flow rates must be reduced and pharmacologic methods of treating right ventricular failure instituted. These include increasing right ventricular preload and contractility, reducing right ventricular afterload with pulmonary vasodilators, including O_2 administration, and correcting metabolic acidosis. Should these efforts fail, an RVAD is indicated. When right ventricular failure occurs unexpectedly in a patient on left ventricular assist, right ventricular assist can be performed without opening the chest by cannulation of the right atrium through the right internal jugular vein, followed by oxygenation of the right atrial effluent with a membrane oxygenator discharged in the LVAD return line.

General Considerations

For left ventricular bypass, the aortic valve must be competent to allow appropriate forward flow and prevent left ventricular distension. If a patent foramen ovale is suspected in a patient on an LVAD, arterial desaturation will occur when the left atrial pressure falls below the right atrial pressure; the defect must be recognized and closed at the time of surgery (24). Closed-chest CPR is contraindicated in patients on ventricular assist because it is unnecessary for any cardiac action to maintain the circulation, especially if biventricular assist is employed, and the resuscitation maneuvers can dislodge the cannulas. A rise in both right and left atrial pressures may indicate pericardial tamponade. This assumes importance in univentricular assist because tamponade can interfere with filling of the nonbypassed ventricle and prevent maintenance of the circulation.

Weaning from Ventricular Assist

Weaning from ventricular assist may begin when reductions in pump flow permit mainte-

nance of the cardiac output with physiologic intracardiac pressures. The patient's contribution to the cardiac output is the difference between the measured cardiac output and the pump flow. Ventricular function under varying conditions of preload and afterload can be monitored by transesophageal or transthoracic echocardiography (25), radioisotopic multigated nuclear scanning (26), or epicardial ultrasonic dimension gauges. Intracardiac pressures, as determined by right atrial, pulmonary artery, left atrial, and left ventricular monitoring catheters, as well as determination of mixed venous O_2, provide physiologic correlates to the noninvasive determinants of ventricular contractility. When pump flows can be gradually decreased without sustained elevation on intracardiac pressures (left atrial pressure less than 20 mm Hg) and evidence of adequate systemic perfusion as measured by mixed venous O_2 and cardiac output (more than 2 liters/min/m^2), separation of the patient from the device may be anticipated.

In patients on right ventricular assist alone, reduction in pump flow should result in adequate filling of the left atrium as manifested by a left atrial pressure of 10 mm Hg or more without dilation of the right ventricle or a rise in right atrial pressure.

Contraindications to Ventricular Assist

Infection.   Patients with known systemic infections are not candidates for ventricular assist. Even in the absence of preexistent infection, cannulae passing from cardiac chambers and the great vessels across the mediastinum, through the skin to an external assist device adds to the risk of an infection arising de novo from the device. All patients with an assist device in place should be covered with broad spectrum antibiotics.

Renal Failure.   Acute postoperative renal failure has a high mortality. The associated abnormalities of the clotting mechanism, need of vascular access for dialysis, and risk of gastrointestinal bleeding present a prohibitive risk to the patient on ventricular assist. The resultant morbidity and mortality seriously damage any benefits from ventricular assist.

Multisystem Organ Failure.   The clinical setting of multisystem organ failure precludes successful ventricular assist. Conversely, ventricular assist should be instituted before the effects of hypoperfusion result in irreversible dysfunction of the lungs, liver, and kidneys.

Disseminated Intravascular Coagulopathy. The passage of blood through cannulae and pumping chambers will exacerbate abnormalities of the clotting mechanism, resulting in a recurrent need for blood products and the associated risks of transfusion reaction and transmission of disease (hepatitis, AIDS).

Coma. Except when due to low cardiac output, patients who remain unresponsive despite correction of metabolic abnormalities, and in the absence of alcohol, anesthetics, or neuromuscular blocking agents, are not candidates for ventricular assist.

Complications of Ventricular Assist

The most frequently reported complications of ventricular assist are infection and bleeding. Infections are more frequent in assist devices requiring cannulae that traverse the mediastinum, penetrate the skin, and are connected to an external pumping device. Unfortunately, when a patient acquires an infection, he or she is not a candidate for transplantation even if he or she becomes VAD dependent.

Bleeding frequently accompanies the use of a VAD since its insertion usually begins at the end of a prolonged period of cardiopulmonary bypass which is known to result in altered platelet function. The destruction of platelets by concomitant intraaortic balloon pumping may exacerbate bleeding, as will the need to suture cannulae to the great vessels or the aorta. Bleeding will then occur through the suture lines or through the graft material itself. Particularly brisk bleeding may be encountered if the left ventricle is cannulated directly through the apex. This route is generally chosen only if one intends to commit the patient to cardiac transplantation, because subsequent repair of the apex can be difficult, especially if the apical myocardium has undergone infarction.

Other complications of ventricular assist include cerebrovascular accident from clots forming within either the prosthetic material or the hypokinetic ventricle. Although heparin anticoagulation is advisable during the assist period,

the risks, including mediastinal and intracerebral hemorrhage, have led some investigators to recommend ventricular assist without use of anticoagulants (27).

Results of Ventricular Assist

Penn State. Pae and coworkers (28) reported a series of 15 patients requiring circulatory assistance with the Penn State pneumatic paracorporeal assist device between 1980 and 1985 (1.1% of all patients having cardiac surgery). Of 11 patients requiring an LVAD, eight (73%) were weaned from the device and six (55%) were discharged from the hospital. One patient requiring an RVAD was weaned and discharged. None of three patients requiring a biventricular assist device (BVAD) could be weaned. Causes of death included bleeding, patent foramen ovale, recurrent ventricular septal defect, and VAD dependency with persistent low cardiac output.

Pierce-Donachy. Pennington and coworkers (26) reported a series of 17 patients out of 2192 patients (0.8%) undergoing cardiac surgery between 1982 and 1984 treated with the Pierce-Donachy assist device. Of eight patients requiring an LVAD, three (38%) were weaned, but none survived more than 3 months. Of five patients requiring an RVAD, two (40%) were weaned, surviving 6 and 22 months. Of four patients requiring a BVAD, three (75%) were weaned, with the longest survival being 7 months. Eight patients died from bleeding, multisystem organ failure, or biventricular failure.

Biomedicus (Centrifugal) Pump. Magovern and coworkers (27) reported a series of 21 patients out of 3000 patients undergoing cardiac surgery (0.7%) that required left heart assist with the Biomedicus pump. Of the 21 patients, 10 (48%) were weaned from the device and five patients were discharged from hospital, surviving 1 to 3 years. Hospital deaths were caused by low cardiac output, arrhythmias, septicemia, and pulmonary complications.

Zumbro and coworkers (29) reported a series of 33 patients requiring circulatory assist with Pierce-Donanchy and Biomedicus pumps. Of 21 patients requiring an LVAD, 12 (57%) were weaned and seven patients (33%) discharged. Of two patients requiring an RVAD, two (100%)

were weaned and discharged. Of 10 patients requiring a BVAD, five (50%) were weaned, but only one patient (20%) survived after support was terminated.

A combined registry for the use of ventricular assist pumps and the total artificial heart as bridges to transplantation was established in 1985 (30). From 1984 to 1986, 83 patients were entered in the registry. Of 23 patients requiring an LVAD, 14 of 16 (60.9%) survived, and all subsequently had successful transplantation. The one patient who received an RVAD survived subsequent transplantation. Of 19 patients having received a BVAD, six of 20 (31.6%) survived subsequent transplantation. Of 40 patients having received a total artificial heart, 19 of 31 (47.5%) survived subsequent transplantation.

Improved survival rates have been reported in patients with ventricular failure who were supported with the Jarvik 7R assist device used as a bridge to transplantation (31). As of November 1986, 35 devices had been implanted in 33 patients, with five deaths. Nineteen of 24 patients (57.6%) survived subsequent cardiac transplantation.

CONCLUSIONS

The need for mechanical circulatory support is small in the average practice but can be life-saving and should be instituted promptly if an appropriate hemodynamic profile cannot be maintained by correcting metabolic abnormalities and using pharmacologic support. At this time, the intraaortic balloon pump serves as the initial modality of mechanical circulatory assist because of its ready availability and ease of insertion. Ventricular assist devices must be inserted in the operating room but can provide total circulatory support in patients inadequately maintained with balloon counterpulsation.

The early experience with balloon counterpulsation has demonstrated that, for long-term survival, a definitive corrective surgical procedure is required after the initial period of stabilization. Similarly, in patients requiring an LVAD, about one-half can be weaned from the device, but only one-quarter will be discharged from the hospital. Of patients requiring an RVAD, about 80% can be weaned from the

device and discharged. Of patients requiring a BVAD, 42% can be weaned, but with no long-term survivors. The overall survival for all patients receiving ventricular assist as a bridge to transplantation is about 50%.

It is clear from this limited experience that long-term survival in patients receiving any kind of mechanical assist can be achieved only when these devices are implanted early enough to prevent multisystem organ failure and when a subsequent procedure, such as coronary bypass grafting, repair of mechanical defects (ventricular septal defect, papillary muscle rupture), or cardiac transplantation is performed.

References

1. Frazier OH: Mechanical circulatory assistance. In Attar S (ed): *New Developments in Cardiac Assist Devices*. New York, Praeger, 1985, pp 124–139.
2. Tennant T, Wiggers CJ: Effect of coronary occlusion on myocardial contraction. *Am J Physiol* 112:351–361, 1935.
3. Braunwald E, Kloner RA: The stunned myocardium: prolonged, postischemic ventricular dysfunction. *Circulation* 66:1146–1149, 1982.
4. Rozanski A, Berman D, Gray R, et al: Use of thallium 201 redistribution scintigraphy in the preoperative differentiation of reversible and non-reversible myocardial dysynergy. *Circulation* 64:936–944, 1981.
5. Buckberg GD, et al: Studies of controlled reperfusion after ischemia (Part 2). *J Thorac Cardiovasc Surg* 92:3, 1986.
6. Harken DE: Concept of counterpulsation. Presented at the International College of Cardiology, Brussels, Belgium, 1958.
7. Clauss RH, Birtwell WC, Albertal G, et al: Assisted circulation I. The arterial counterpulsator. *J Thorac Cardiovasc Surg* 41:447–458, 1961.
8. Moulopoulos SD, Topaz S, Kolff WF: Diastolic balloon pumping (with carbon dioxide) in the aorta—a mechanical assist to the failing circulation. *Am Heart J* 63:669–675, 1962.
9. Kantrowitz A, Tjonneland S, Freed PS, et al: Initial clinical experience with intra-aortic balloon pumping in cardiogenic shock. *JAMA* 203:135–140, 1968.
10. McEnany MT, Kay HR, Buckley MJ: Clinical experiences with intra-aortic balloon pump support in 728 patients. *Circulation* 58(Suppl I):1–124, 1978.
11. Scheidt S, Collins M, Goldstein J, et al: Me-

chanical circulatory assistance with the intra-aortic balloon pump and other counterpulsation devices. *Prog Cardiovasc Dis* 25:55–76, 1982.

12. Miyamoto A, Lee ME, Kass R, et al: Post-myocardial infarction ventricular septal defects: improved outlook. *J Thorac Cardiovasc Surg* 86:41–46, 1983.

13. Killen DA, Reed WA, Wathanacharoen S, et al: Surgical treatment of papillary muscle rupture. *Ann Thorac Surg* 35:243–248, 1983.

14. Sherman CT, Litvack F, Grundfest W, et al: Coronary angioscopy in patients with unstable angina pectoris. *N Engl J Med* 315:913–919, 1986.

15. Summers DN, Kaplitt M, Morris J, et al: Intra-aortic balloon pumping—hemodynamic and metabolic effects during cardiogenic shock in patients with triple coronary artery obstructive disease. *Arch Surg* 99:733–738, 1969.

16. McGeehan W, Feroz S, Donahoo JS, et al: Transthoracic intraaortic balloon pump support: experience in 39 patients. *Ann Thorac Surg* 44:26–30, 1987.

17. Lee ME: Method of insertion of intra-aortic balloon through the ascending aorta (Letter to the Editor). *Ann Thorac Surg* 20:237, 1975.

18. Alpert J, Bhaktan EK, Geilchinsky I, et al: Vascular complications of intra-aortic balloon pumping. *Arch Surg* 111:1190–1195, 1976.

19. Lee ME, Neptune WB: Cardiac tamponade complicating closure of a median sternotomy. *Chest* 70:84–86, 1976.

20. Connolly MW, Grossi EA, Rose DM, et al: Early prognostic hemodynamic indices for survival with use of postoperative partial left heart bypass (Abstract). *Circulation* 72(II):111–393, 1985.

21. Farrar DJ, Compton PG, Hershon JJ, et al. Right heart interaction with the mechanically assisted left heart. *World J Surg* 9:89–102, 1985.

22. Miyamoto A, Tanaka S, Matloff J: Right ven-tricular function during left heart bypass. *J Thorac Cardiovasc Surg* 85:49–53, 1983.

23. Baird RJ, Goldbach MM, de la Rocha A: Intramyocardial pressure: the persistence of its transmural gradient in the empty heart and its relationship to myocardial oxygen consumption. *J Thorac Cardiovasc Surg* 64:635–646, 1972.

24. Magovern JA, Pae WE Jr, Richenbacher E, et al: The importance of a patent foramen ovale in left ventricular assist pumping. *Trans Am Soc Artif Int Organs* 32:449–453, 1986.

25. Nakatani T, Takano H, Beppu S, et al: Natural heart recovery under left ventricular assist device pumping studied by echocardiography. *Trans Am Soc Artif Int Organs* 32:461–466, 1986.

26. Pennington DG, Samuels LD, Williams G, et al: Experience with the Pierce-Donachy assist device in postcardiotomy patients with cardiogenic shock. *World J Surg* 9:37–46, 1985.

27. Magovern GJ, Park SB, Maher TD: Use of a centrifugal pump without anticoagulants for postoperative left ventricular assist. *World J Surg* 9:25–36, 1985.

28. Pae WE Jr, Gaines WE, Pierce WS, et al: Mechanical circulatory assistance for postoperative cardiogenic shock. *Surgical Rounds* 49–63, July 1985.

29. Zumbro GL, Kitchens WR, Shearer G, et al: Mechanical assistance for cardiogenic shock following cardiac surgery, myocardial infarction, and cardiac transplantation. *Ann Thorac Surg* 44:11–13, 1987.

30. Pae WE Jr, Pierce WS: Combined registry for the clinical use of mechanical ventricular assist pumps and the total artificial heart: first official report—1986. *J Heart Transplant* 6:68–70, 1987.

31. *A Current Report on Use of the Jarvik 7R (100 cc) and Jarvik 7R (70 cc) as a Bridge to Transplant.* Symbion, Inc., 825 North 300 West, Salt Lake City, UT 84103, November 1986.

Chapter 15
POSTOPERATIVE HYPERTENSION

RICHARD J. GRAY, M.D.

Postoperative hypertension can develop several hours after surgery but is usually established within 1 to 2 hr, and often by the time the patient returns to the intensive care unit. It is a well-established entity occurring in 30 to 60% of patients (1–3). It has been defined variably as an absolute level of mean arterial pressure above 105 mm Hg (4) or a 20 mm Hg increase in mean arterial pressure (5). Because systolic elevations tend to predominate and are especially associated with potentially damaging excessive aortic shear forces, it has also been defined as systolic blood pressure exceeding 140 mm Hg (6). Although common after all types of cardiac operations, its appearance and severity tend to favor cardiac valve surgery, especially surgery for relief of aortic stenosis (7). The hazards of this condition, especially if severe, include cerebral vascular accident, risk of suture line disruption, and dissection of the aorta due to associated aortic pathology. A more subtle risk is imposed as greater cardiac work places heavy metabolic demands on myocardium just recovering from an ishemic insult (8, 9). As one of many possible causes for "nonspecific" S-T segment and T-wave electrocardiographic changes, this problem may go undetected in the intubated and sedated patient.

Additional future risks also include hypertension-mediated intimal damage to saphenous vein graft endothelium, which may contribute to graft closure or premature atherosclerosis (10).

PREDISPOSING FACTORS

Mechanisms that have been implicated include elevated levels of plasma epinephrine and norepinephrine (11–13), renin and angiotensin (14), vasopressin (15), excessive sympathetic nervous system activity (3), and certain reflexes originating in the heart or great vessels (16, 17). While the events of anesthesia, cardiopulmonary bypass, surgical stimulation, and hypothermia have all been associated with increase in catecholamine levels (12, 13, 18, 19), there may be some question as to the causative role of catecholamine excess, inasmuch as plasma catecholamine levels are elevated in most patients irrespective of the presence or absence of hypertension (20). In a broad survey of catecholamine responses to surgery, epinephrine levels are most profoundly elevated (12, 21), but norepinephrine elevations may persist for several days (21). It should be remembered that epinephrine is the consequence of adrenomedullary secretion, and norepinephrine is the neurotransmitter released from sympathetic nerve endings, and its plasma value provides an index of sympathetic nervous system activity. Infusions of the latter result in intense hypertension due to α-adrenergic constriction. Indeed, postoperative hypertension has been linked to a markedly positive peripheral norepinephrine gradient (22). The author also has found that in patients with postoperative hypertension, it was only the norepinephrine level that was consistently and profoundly elevated (two- to sevenfold in all patients), whereas epinephrine and renin levels were normal in some patients and modestly elevated in others (23). This implication of sympathetic nervous system stimulation is consistent with the observation that hypertension is often lessened following extubation and adequate sedation.

Clinically, a preoperative history of hypertension (3) and preoperative use of propranolol (20) have been linked to acute postoperative hypertension. Interestingly, preoperative left ventricular ejection fraction may be lower in patients remaining normotensive than in those who become hypertensive (7). The causal relationship of any of these factors remains speculative, of course. Like its more common counterpart, essential hypertension, the basic mechanisms remain unknown; however, certain physiologic features are common. Current data support the importance of sympathetic nervous system stimulation and elevated norepinephrine levels with varying cardiovascular responses based on preoperative hypertension, β-blocker usage, adequacy of cardiac function, and type of anesthesia, possibly working through alterations in adrenergic receptor number and function.

CLINICAL FEATURES AND TREATMENT

In addition to the hypertension, hemodynamic measurements often reveal normal or slightly reduced cardiac output and moderate to significant elevations of systemic vascular resistance. Because of these features, nitroprusside has been used extensively for treatment (24, 25). Starting at a dosage of 0.5 μg/kg/min, an average effective dose is 1 to 2 μg/kg/min. Nitroprusside allows titration of mean arterial blood pressure to the desired level with significant reductions in systemic vascular resistance and cardiac filling pressures (5). Cardiac output usually increases, but if cardiac filling pressures are

lowered excessively cardiac index may not increase (4).

The guidelines to successful drug therapy in this condition requires an agent that must address the prevailing hemodynamic characteristics, be rapid in onset as well as cessation to allow titration, be easily and safely administered by nursing personnel, and be free of short-term side effects. Nitroprusside is usually well tolerated and has the distinct advantage of rapid onset and cessation of action, allowing for easy titratability. Usually a modest reflex tachycardia occurs in prolonged usage and especially at high dose (generally above 4μg/kg/min). Toxicity can develop, which usually consists of tachyphylaxis, metabolic acidosis, and elevations of sodium thiocyanate and cyanide levels. A potentially serious drawback, especially in older patients and individuals with limited pulmonary function, is the occurrence of marked decrease in PO_2, suggesting ventilation-perfusion mismatch. The mechanism by which nitroprusside worsens intrapulmonary shunting appears to be inhibition of hypoxic vasoconstriction in the pulmonary bed, resulting in increased perfusion of poorly ventilated regions (26, 27). Another potential drawback with nitroprusside is the possibility of worsening myocardial anaerobic metabolism by excessive reduction of diastolic blood pressure and consequent reduction in coronary blood flow despite a decrease in myocardial oxygen consumption (4). For these reasons, the use of intravenous nitroglycerin has been suggested; this was able to achieve blood pressure control equivalent to nitroprusside in 14 of 17 patients in one study, and did not result in worsening of intrapulmonary shunting (5). Patients with chronic congestive heart failure and elevated filling pressures tolerated nitroglycerin particularly well. The average infusion rate of nitroglycerin for successful control of blood pressure is 1 to 2 μg/kg/min.

Postoperative hypertension is often seen in the setting of overall hyperdynamic cardiovascular function with sinus tachycardia and normal or even elevated output with normal or modestly elevated systemic vascular resistance. β-Blocker therapy seems particularly ideal in this type of patient, especially in view of the elevation of catecholamines often seen and the frequent history of preoperative β-blocker use. Intermittent dosing with intravenous propranolol 1 to 5 mg every 6 hr has been successful but is not traditionally used as a continuous infusion. The intravenous ultrashort-acting β-blocker esmolol, given as a continuing infusion, appears to provide effective control of hypertension in a majority of patients with minimum reduction of cardiac function. The principal advantages with this approach are the lack of any deleterious effects on intrapulmonary shunting, titratable onset and cessation of action, and freedom from excessive lowering of diastolic blood pressure (23).

Intravenous labetalol, an α- and β-blocking agent available for use both orally and intravenously, has also been used successfully in early postoperative hypertension. Incremental bolus doses of 10 to 40 mg are associated with reduction in blood pressure and heart rate (28) and appear to be as successful at controlling postoperative hypertension as hydralazine but without the tendency for increased heart rate (29). Continuous intravenous infusion has also been used with similar success at a dosage of 2 mg/min.

A decrease in heart rate with labetalol in this clinical situation is less certain than the blood pressure reduction, but a significant decline in both heart rate and cardiac index with no reduction in systemic resistance has been reported, suggesting that typical β-blockade effects can predominate over α-blocking effects, especially in intravenous form (30).

Calcium channel blocking agents have been used increasingly for control of chronic hypertension, and as intravenous formulations become widely available they are likely to be used for acute hypertension control as well. One such agent, nicardipine, has no discernable negative inotropic or chronotropic effects, and, when given as either an intravenous bolus or an infusion, has rapid enough onset and cessation of action to allow titration of blood pressure. It has shown the ability to control hypertension associated with an increase in cardiac output and heart rate.

Several hours' therapy with an intravenous agent may be sufficient if hypertensive tendencies decrease with extubation and relief of pain and anxiety. Other patients, particularly those with hypertension preoperatively will require longer-term therapy. Successful weaning from intravenous to oral control has been achieved with hydralazine 10 to 50 mg every 6 hr, α-methyldopa 250 to 500 mg every 6 hr, or clonidine 0.1 to 0.2 mg every 6 to 8 hr. More recently, however, nifedipine 10 to 20 mg every 6 hr orally or sublingually has been used with success and is tolerated well.

In general, patients would be wise to resume preoperative antihypertensive regimes that may have been well tolerated; however, daily adjustments in dosage may be necessary, and regimes that include chronic thiazide diuretics should be reevaluated in view of possible rapid changes in electrolytes and intravascular volume early postoperatively, as well as long-term adverse effects on serum lipids.

References

1. Estafanous FG, Tarazi RC, Viljoen JF, et al: Systemic hypertension following myocardial revascularization. Am Heart J 85:732–738, 1972.
2. Hoar PF, Hickey RF, Ullyot DJ: Systemic hypertension following myocardial revascularization. J Thorac Cardiovasc Surg 71:859–864, 1976.
3. Roberts AJ, Niarchos AP, Subramanian VA, et al: Systemic hypertension associated with coronary artery bypass surgery. Predisposing factors, hemodynamic characteristics, humoral profile, and treatment. J Thorac Cardiovasc Surg 74:846–859, 1977.
4. Fremes SE, Weisel RD, Baird RJ, et al: Effects of postoperative hypertension and its treatment. J Thorac Cardiovasc Surg 86:47–57, 1983.
5. Flaherty JT, Magee PA, Gardner TL, et al: Comparison of intravenous nitroglycerin and sodium nitroprusside for treatment of acute hypertension developing after coronary artery bypass surgery. Circulation 65:1072–1077, 1982.
6. Gray RJ, Bateman TB, Czer LSC, et al: Use of esmolol in hypertension after cardiac surgery. Am J Cardiol 56:49F–56F, 1985.
7. Cooper TJ, Clutton-Brock TH, Jones SN, et al: Factors relating to the development of hypertension after cardiopulmonary bypass. Br Heart J 54:91–95, 1985.
8. Kaplan JA, Jones EL: Vasodilator therapy during coronary surgery. Comparison of nitroglycerin

and nitroprusside. *J Thorac Cardiovasc Surg* 77:301–309, 1979.

9. Hilton JD, Weisel RD, Barid RJ, et al: The hemodynamic and metabolic response to pacing after aortocoronary bypass. *Circulation* 64(II):48–53, 1981.

10. Brody WR, Kosek JC, Angell WW: Changes in vein grafts following aorto-coronary bypass induced by pressure and ischemia. *J Thorac Cardiovasc Surg* 64:847–854, 1972.

11. Wallach R, Karp RB, Reves JG, et al: Pathogenesis of paroxysmal hypertension developing during and after coronary bypass surgery: a study of hemodynamic and humoral factors. *Am J Cardiol* 46:559–565, 1980.

12. Reves JG, Karp RB, Buttner EE, et al: Neural and adenomedullary catecholamie release in response to cardiopulmonary bypass in man. *Circulation* 66:49–55, 1982.

13. Hoar PF, Stone JG, Faltas AN et al: Hemodynamic and adrenergic responses to anesthesia and operation for myocardial revascularization. *J Thorac Cardiovasc Surg* 80:242–248, 1980.

14. Taylor KM, Morton IJ, Brown JJ: Hypertension and the renin-angiotensin system following open-heart surgery. *J Thorac Cardiovasc Surg* 74:840–845, 1977.

15. Hawkins SS, Aveling W, Treasure T, et al: Hypertension, vasopressin and renin in coronary artery surgery. *Br J Anesth* 55:1161P, 1983.

16. Fouad FM, Estafanous FG, Bravo EL, et al: Possible role of cardioaortic reflexes in post coronary bypass hypertension. *Am J Cardiol* 44:866–872, 1979.

17. James TN, Hageman GR, Uthaler F: Anatomic and physiologic considerations of a cardiogenic hypertensive chemoreflex. *Am J Cardiol* 44:852–859, 1979.

18. Lillehei RC, Lillehei CW, Grismer JT, et al: Plasma catecholamines in open-heart surgery: prevention of their pernicious effects by pretreatment with dibenzyline. *Surg Forum* 14:269–271, 1963.

19. Chee-Ken T, Glisson SN, El-Etr AA, et al: Levels of circulating norepinephrine and epinephrine before, during and after cardiopulmonary bypass in man. *J Thorac Cardiovasc Surg* 71:928–931, 1976.

20. Whelton PK, Flaherty JT, MacAllister NP, et al: Hypertension following coronary artery bypass surgery. Role of preoperative propranolol therapy. *Hypertension* 2:291–298, 1983.

21. Engleman RM, Haag B, Lemeshaw S, et al: Mechanism of plasma catecholamine increases during coronary artery bypass and valve procedures. *J Thorac Cardiovasc Surg* 86:608–615, 1983.

22. Young YD, Jones M, Hanowell ST, et al: Changes in peripheral vascular and cardiac sympathetic activity before and after coronary artery bypass surgery: interrelationships with hemodynamic alterations. *Am Heart J* 102:972–979, 1981.

23. Gray RJ, Bateman TB, Czer LSC, et al: Comparison of esmolol and nitroprusside for acute post-cardiac surgical hypertension. *Am J Cardiol* 59:887–892, 1987.

24. Estafanous FG, Tarazi RC: Systemic arterial hypertension associated with cardiac surgery. *Am J Cardiol* 46:685–694, 1980.

25. Gall WE, Clarke WR, Dota DB: Vasomotor dynamics associated with cardiac operations. I. Venous tone and the effects of vasodilators. *J Thorac Cardiovasc Surg* 83:724–731, 1982.

26. Colley PS, Cheney FW: Sodium nitroprusside increases Qs/Qt in dogs with regional atelectasis. *Anesthesiology* 47:338–341, 1977.

27. Hill AB, Chir B, Sykes MK, et al: A hypoxic pulmonary vasoconstrictor response in dogs during and after infusion of sodium nitroprusside. *Anesthesiology* 50:484–488, 1979.

28. Morel DR, Forster A, Suter PM: I.V. labetalol in the treatment of hypertension following coronary-artery surgery. *Br J Anaesth* 54:1191–1196, 1982.

29. Gabrielson G, Lingham R, Dimich I, et al: Comparative study of labetalol and hydralazine in the treatment of postoperative hypertension. *Anesth Analg* 66:S63, 1987.

30. Meretoja OA, Allonen H, Arola M, et al: Combined alpha- and beta-blockade with labetalol in post-open heart surgery hypertension. Reversal of hemodynamic deterioration with glucagon. *Chest* 78:810–815, 1980.

Chapter 16
PERIOPERATIVE MYOCARDIAL INFARCTION

TIMOTHY M. BATEMAN, M.D.
RICHARD J. GRAY, M.D.

Acute ischemic insult of the myocardium has been recognized as a nearly inevitable complication of coronary bypass and other open-heart procedures for more than 20 years. Its occurrence reflects limitations in myocardial protection immediately before, during, and after open-heart surgery. It can manifest as transient ventricular dysfunction (1–4), transient or permanent electrocardiographic changes (5, 6), or frank myocardial infarction. The latter has been shown in the past to occur in up to 40% of operated patients (7, 8) with an adverse impact on surgical survival (9). Refinements in technique have resulted in a decline in the incidence of perioperative infarction (10), and a National Institutes of Health consensus meeting has concluded that the current rates of expected perioperative infarction are 5% for stable patients and 10% for those with unstable angina before bypass (11). Nevertheless, the fact that ventricular function is directly related to survival (12) mandates continuing effort in understanding and countering the pathophysiology of perioperative ischemic damage.

MECHANISM AND DIAGNOSIS

Historical Considerations

As in nonsurgical patients, perioperative myocardial infarction occurs when myocardial oxygen demand exceeds its supply for at least 20 min. In the past, perioperative infarctions occurred predominantly because of grossly inadequate metabolic protection of the heart during the entire perioperative period, technical problems such as particulate or air emboli, and, during aortic valve replacement, unrecognized escape of cardioplegia annulae from coronary ostia. Resulting infarctions tended to be large and contributed to poor surgical results. Studies reported in the early 1970s quote relatively high perioperative infarction rates with ensuing mortality exceeding 20% (13, 14). Advances in surgical technique have dramatically decreased the incidence of perioperative infarction due in large part to improved attention to myocardial preservation.

Clinical Risk Factors

Extensive investigation has attempted to identify those patients at higher risk for perioperative infarction. Old age, high left ventricular end-diastolic pressure, unstable angina, left main coronary disease, ventricular dysfunction, long cardiopulmonary bypass time, and large number of grafts inserted have all been shown to correlate with an increased incidence of perioperative infarction. More recently, these have been reexamined as to their relevance with newer methods of cardiopulmonary protection. Again, indices of left ventricular dysfunction (left ventricular end-diastolic pressure; cardiomegaly on the preoperative chest x-ray) and longer operative time (cardiopulmonary pump time; more grafts) (10, 13) occurred more frequently in patients with perioperative infarctions. Not surprisingly, more stenotic vessels and lack of collaterals were also identified as risk factors (14, 15). However, no study has found strong cause-effect relationships and few have identified the same correlates, so that both scientific data and clinical experience suggest that patients destined to have a perioperative infarction cannot be well predicted from commonly known preoperative characteristics.

Mechanism

Myocardial infarction occurring days or weeks after surgery is most often due to bypass graft closure and may be amenable to therapy commonly used for native disease (16). Myocardial infarction noted immediately after coronary artery bypass grafting is often reflective of a different process, however. A variety of causes have been documented in immediate postoperative patients, including both vein graft and native coronary spasm (17), atheroembolism (18), vasoactive effect of pressor drugs (19), and, possibly the most important of all, inadequate myocardial preservation (20). During cardiopulmonary bypass and aortic cross-clamping, coronary flow is nil. Myocardial viability is dependent solely, then, on preexisting energy stores and reduction to near zero of all sources of energy requirement such as those of both mechanical and electrical activity. While potassium-based crystalloid and blood cardioplegia have brought great advances in this area, the technology is not yet perfect, as evidenced by the temporary deterioration of left and right ventricular function as well as by the presence of myocardial-specific creatine kinase (CK) enzyme release in virtually all patients. In addition to these factors, there is also evidence of myocardial ischemia preceeding cross-clamping itself (20). Coupled with the observation that intraoperative infarction is relatively uncommonly associated with bypass graft closure (21), this has led to speculation that infarction occurring during cardiopulmonary bypass is due to

a profound mismatch of myocardial oxygen supply and demand (22). This mismatch in patients with coronary disease and in whom there is already a predisposition to recurrent segmental ischemia explains the transient subclinical signs of ischemia (23) seen nearly universally; when severe enough, this mismatch results in appearance of enzyme, electrocardiographic, and scintigraphic signs typical of frank infarction.

DIAGNOSIS

No single test is highly sensitive and specific for diagnosing perioperative infarction. Further, test results are frequently discordant, leading to disagreement on the specific criteria for diagnosis of perioperative infarction. Most commonly, the clinician must consider the results of a number of diagnostic approaches before he or she can be reasonably certain that an infarction has occurred. The diagnosis should not be made casually, because an erroneous diagnosis could lead to quite different therapy early postoperatively and later may leave the patient with a concern that surgery was not successful, may prevent him or her from obtaining life insurance, and may encourage unnecessarily aggressive follow-up.

Electrocardiogram

The electrocardiogram is relied on more than any other single test. The strongest criteria are the development of new and persistent pathologic Q waves with persistent but evolutionary S-T segment and T wave changes (24). In contrast to traditional nonsurgical infarction, appearance of new Q waves is not an electrocardiographic evolution, but rather these new waves are present upon emergence from the operating room. Furthermore, S-T segment and T wave changes in the absence of Q waves, although of concern, are often present in the absence of confirming enzyme or scintigraphic evidence of infarction, and more commonly are the result of electrolyte shifts or pericarditis, both localized and generalized. Nonpersistent Q waves are often seen early postoperatively and often accompany axis shifts, but also could reflect profound but reversible myocardial ischemia. Therefore, it is important to perform electrocardiography serially for at least 3 days after surgery.

It is well known that abnormal electrocardiographic Q waves are neither highly sensitive nor specific for transmural necrosis. In an autopsy study, 23% of patients with perioperative myocardial infarction had no pathologic Q waves despite the presence of significant transmural necrosis, while 20% of patients without transmural myocardial necrosis did have new Q waves (25). Similarly, contrast ventriculographic studies have demonstrated regional wall motion abnormalities much more frequently than development of Q waves (26–28). Conversely, others have demonstrated the persistence of Q waves despite restoration of normal ventricular contractility after revascularization (29). Adding to the confusion over the meaning of Q waves is the very interesting demonstration that the rate of resolution of QRS changes after perioperative infarction is much more rapid than that of nonoperative myocardial infarction (30).

Myocardial-Specific Enzymes

Total creatine phosphokinase (CPK) and its myocardial-specific band (MB fraction) are routinely elevated in the early postoperative period. This is due to the fact that the atria (incised for cannulation as well as sump placement) and thoracic aorta contain high levels of CPK and MB fraction similar to those found in ventricular myocardium (32). This, in addition to the occurrence of subclinical myocardial injury, accounts for the universal appearance of MB-CK even in the absence of perioperative infarction. As a practical solution, most institutions have established CPK elevations from consecutively operated cohorts of uncomplicated coronary artery bypass graft patients. For example, at the authors' institution, uncomplicated patients who have no postoperative electrocardiographic abnormalities have CPK-MB levels below 80 units/liter (23). Those who have CPK-MB levels above 80 units/liter are more likely to have electrocardiographic Q waves. This enzyme criterion is important in substantiating the significance of new electrocardiographic abnormalities; in allowing the diagnosis of perioperative infarction in the case of new fascicular conduction disturbance; and in diagnosing nontransmural

myocardial infarction. Analyses of CPK release in perioperative myocardial infarction has revealed that levels tend to peak between 16 and 24 hr (33, 34), whereas in patients without perioperative myocardial infarction, CPK is usually elevated immediately after surgery but decreases by 12 to 16 hr. This observation is not of practical assistance in diagnosing or excluding perioperative infarction, however, because of extensive overlap. A recent intriguing discovery in the enzymatic investigation of perioperative infarction patients is the presence of enzyme bands migrating cathodal to CK-MB in creatine kinase isoenzyme electrophoretograms, probably representing adenolate kinase (35); the finding of one or, worse yet, two such bands may be important prognostically, identifying patient groups with greater degrees of myocardial damage.

Technetium-99m Pyrophosphate

A number of studies have compared the electrocardiogram, enzymes, and myocardial pyrophosphate scintigrams for diagnosis of perioperative infarction. A newly positive scintigram is perhaps the most sensitive and specific finding (36, 37). Unfortunately, pyrophosphate scintigraphy must be performed in accordance with certain guidelines to attain high accuracy. Ideally, all patients must have preoperative scintigrams for comparison, because aneurysms, earlier infarction, and valvular or paravalvular calcification can all lead to positive scans in the absence of perioperative infarction. Furthermore, postoperative presentation with unstable angina may result in a high incidence of positive scans as well (38). Postoperative imaging should be done 48 to 72 hr after surgery. Blood pool activity must be differentiated from diffuse pyrophosphate uptake, and rib uptake must be recognized and distinguished from localized myocardial positivity. Inasmuch as it does not seem cost effective to perform pyrophosphate scintigraphy on all preoperative patients in order to detect perioperative infarction in about the 5% in whom this is likely to occur, the value of this test is severely limited. In clinical practice, it has the most use in patients known not to have had previous infarction and in whom the diagnosis postoperatively is complicated by equivocal or difficult-to-interpret enzyme or electrocardiographic data (39).

Regional Wall Motion Analysis

Although not invariably present, new regional wall motion abnormalities often accompany new postoperative findings of perioperative infarction. Unfortunately, analysis of postoperative wall motion is complicated by preoperative wall motion abnormalities, by transient global and widespread segmental postoperative abnormalities even in the absence of perioperative infarction, and also by abnormal movement of the heart in the absence of normal pericardial restraint (1, 2). Nevertheless, both radionuclide and echocardiographic studies are useful in analyzing the significance of Q waves or marked CPK enzyme elevation. For example, diagnostic accuracy for detection of regional wall motion abnormalities using a quantitative echocardiographic technique was markedly enhanced when a special floating-axis analysis was compared to the more traditional fixed-axis analysis. Using the improved axis, regional left ventricular wall motion abnormalities were detected in 88% of patients with new Q waves versus 15% of uncomplicated patients after coronary bypass (40). Parenthetically, the same technique enabled the diagnosis of non-Q wave perioperative myocardial infarction by detection of new regional wall motion abnormality in the presence of CPK elevation without new Q waves (41). Ventriculographic analysis several months after surgery suggests that new and persisting Q waves are virtually always associated with new areas of asynergy, and CPK elevations are often, but not always, associated with such changes; however, nearly one-half of newly asynergic regions will be associated with neither QRS change nor CPK-MB appearance. This indicates that these diagnostic criteria underestimate the true incidence of perioperative infarction. More likely, there are numerous other causes of asynergic changes detected several months after bypass.

Analysis of the intraventricular septum is a potential problem in that as many as two-thirds of patients having bypass surgery will have echo or radionuclide evidence of septal dyskinesis early after bypass. In the great majority of patients

such changes not are not due to perioperative infarction (42).

PROGNOSTIC IMPORTANCE

Early Effects

The early adverse consequences of this complication are well known, as several investigators, including the authors, report a two- to tenfold increase in hospital mortality with this complication (10, 15, 24, 43). Furthermore, several common postinfarction complications have been reported and include ventricular arrhythmias, cardiogenic shock, congestive heart failure, bradyarrhythmias, and supraventricular tachyarrhythmias (43); it should be recognized, however, that rhythm disturbances are common even in uncomplicated noninfarcted patients.

Our investigations have indicated that patients at risk for either death or serious morbidity early after perioperative infarction are relatively homogeneous and hence identifiable: they are older, have had more previous infarctions with poor left ventricular function preoperatively, and have had more complications from their perioperative infarct in the early convalescent period. A model for prediction of death or survival from perioperative infarction with more than 80% probability has been developed based on four factors: the need for intraaortic balloon pump, major intraventricular conduction disturbances (left bundle-branch block and nonspecific intraventricular conduction defect), ventricular tachycardia, and exploratory reoperation (22).

Late Effects

Considerable difference of opinion exists regarding the long-term consequence of perioperative infarction. Adverse long-term consequences have been described (43, 44) with one report (15) suggesting a 5-year survival of only 76% in perioperative infarction patients compared to 90% in those without infarction. Conversely, no adverse effect on long-term prognosis or morbidity after surgery has been reported by many others (45–49). This is consistent with the reported experience at the authors' institution with no adverse consequences at 5 years

(24). A recent reanalysis at 10 years also indicates no adverse impact on survival.

The resolution in this conflict almost certainly lies in the ever more clearly emerging concept that long-term prognosis in ischemic heart disease is related to residual ventricular function. Consequently, any adverse impact from perioperative infarction is likely related to the size of infarction and its effects on ventricular function. This is underscored by one report in which adverse long-term effects on survival were limited to patients with complicated perioperative infarction (43). Persisting deterioration in global left ventricular function is generally related to the magnitude of perioperative CK release and to demonstrably evident perioperative myocardial infarction (50). However, even a small infarction can have long-term deleterious effects if it occurs in the setting of preexistent ventricular dysfunction.

Since most bypass grafts tend to be patent early postoperatively despite perioperative injury (46), perioperative infarctions are probably most commonly of the "reperfusion type"; high levels of cardiac enzymes may occur due to "washout" despite a relatively small degree of necrosis. Other factors including the presence of myocardial hypothermia at the time of ischemic damage, the blunting of sympathetic and adrenal responses to infarction by general anesthesia, and the presence of preexisting coronary and mediastinal collaterals may serve to limit infarction size. For these reasons, the impact on global left ventricular function is often equivocal: the immediate decrease in ejection fraction is greater in the setting of perioperative myocardial infarction, but at 7 days resting left ventricular ejection fraction is no different than that in uncomplicated patients. Exercise increase in ejection fraction months after surgery appears to be blunted in patients with perioperative myocardial infarction (51). Compared to uncomplicated bypass patients, this presumably reflects some degree of myocardial incompetence, but the significance, if any, is unclear.

Thus, while most perioperative infarctions may be small, larger ones obviously can have potential negative impact, and every possible effort should be expended toward prevention.

Avoidance of Perioperative Infarction

It should be clear that the pathophysiology of perioperative myocardial damage is diverse and often difficult to determine precisely. Careful attention to the processes of myocardial oxygen supply and demand are to be emphasized throughout the perioperative period.

Immediately Preoperative

Since anaerobic metabolism has been documented during anesthesia and surgical interventions that precede cardiopulmonary bypass, this is a critical period when appropriate clinical management can prevent myocardial infarction. Careful attention to blood pressure, heart rate, and the electrocardiogram is essential during induction of anesthesia and cannulation. It has been suggested that a rate-pressure product below 12,000 minimizes perioperative myocardial ischemia (52).

In selected patients, pulmonary artery balloon flotation catheters may be useful for avoiding myocardial ischemia. Certainly, in patients with unstable angina, marked left ventricular hypertrophy, and combined valvular and coronary artery disease problems, careful maintenance of cardiac filling pressures can decrease the likelihood of undetected myocardial ischemia.

Intraoperative

Although it is clear that perioperative infarction is less likely with hypothermic cardioplegic cardiac arrest than with aortic cross-clamping, there is no clear-cut benefit to chemical versus blood solutions. Research has shown that multidose hypothermic potassium cardioplegia, hypothermic intermittent cross-clamping, and cold blood cardioplegia can all provide excellent preservation of the left ventricle during routine bypass surgery.

A large number of events can lead to intraoperative myocardial infarction. Fixed coronary artery disease with superimposed coronary spasm, platelet aggregation, and other factors may all contribute. Probably of more importance however, are local myocardial changes in pH, temperature, oncotic pressure, and osmolality, which may adversely affect myocardial energy processes. Hemodynamic disturbances may increase oxygen consumption, adversely influencing myocardial cellular integrity.

Infarction in the perioperative period may also occur because of new perfusion from the bypass grafts. Myocardial reperfusion injury has been postulated to occur when flow is replenished after a period of operative nonperfusion.

Early Postoperative

Treatment of all tachyarrhythmias, including noncompensatory sinus tachycardia, and postoperative hypertension is important, and extremes of hypotension must be avoided. Adequate oxygen delivery must be ensured by maintenance of blood oxygen saturation of well over 90% and prompt replenishment of blood loss. Early postoperative spasm in native coronary, saphenous vein bypass, and internal mammary artery grafts have all been reported and can worsen early postoperative ischemia and potentially contribute to infarction in progress. Treatment with intravenous nitroglycerin or calcium channel blocking agents is indicated whenever this is suspected based on S-T segment elevation.

CONCLUSION

While seemingly decreasing in prevalence and in size, perioperative myocardial infarctions continue to represent one of the most significant threats to patients undergoing open-heart surgical procedures. Large, devastating infarctions have become less common, but even small amounts of myocardial injury can be deleterious in patients with preexisting ventricular dysfunction. Such patients represent an ever-increasing percentage of surgical populations, and this fact underscores the importance of aggressive attempts to better understand and hopefully eliminate perioperative myocardial injury.

References

1. Gray RJ, Maddahi J, Berman DS, et al: Scintigraphic and hemodynamic demonstration of transient left ventricular dysfunction immediately after uncomplicated coronary artery bypass graft surgery. J Thorac Cardiovasc Surg 77:504–510, 1979.

2. Gray RJ, Maddahi J, Raymond M, et al: Noninvasive radionuclide assessment of left ventricular segmental wall motion and global function immediately following coronary artery bypass surgery. Clin Res 27:5a, 1979.

3. Gray RJ, Maddahi J, Raymond M, et al: Cardiac dysfunction and interventricular relationship immediately after coronary bypass. In Roberts A (ed): Coronary Artery Surgery: Application of New Technologies. Chicago, Year Book, 1983, pp 423–435.

4. Czer L, Hamer A, Murphy F, et al: Transient hemodynamic dysfunction after myocardial revascularization: temperature dependence. J Thorac Cardiovasc Surg 86(2)226–234, 1983.

5. Olthof H, Middelhof C, Meijne NG, et al: The definition of myocardial infarction during aortocoronary bypass surgery. Am Heart J 106:631–637, 1983.

6. Sternberg L, Wisneski JA, Ullyot DJ, et al: Significance of new Q-waves after aortocoronary bypass surgery. Circulation 52:1037–1044, 1975.

7. Oldham HN Jr, Roe CR, Young WG Jr, et al: Intraoperative detection of myocardial infarction during coronary artery surgery by plasma creatine phosphokinase isoenzyme analysis. Surgery 74:917–925, 1973.

8. Alderman EL, Matloff JH, Shumway NE, et al: Evaluation of enzyme testing for the detection of myocardial infarction following direct coronary surgery. Circulation 48:135–140, 1973.

9. Gray RJ, Ganz W, Charuzi Y, et al: Morbidity and mortality of perioperative myocardial infarction in coronary bypass surgery. Circulation 58(Suppl II):18, 1978.

10. Chaitman BR, Alderman EL, Sheffield LT, et al: Use of survival analysis to determine the clinical significance of new Q-waves after coronary bypass surgery. Circulation 67(Suppl II):302–309, 1983.

11. National Institutes of Health, Consensus Development Conference Statement: Coronary artery bypass surgery: scientific and clinical aspects. N Engl J Med 304:680–684, 1981.

12. Sanz G, Castaner A, Betriu A, et al: Determinants of prognosis in survivors of myocardial infarction: a prospective clinical angiographic study. N Engl J Med 306(18):1065–1070, 1982.

13. Jarvinen A, Mattila T, Kyosola K, et al: Per-

ioperative myocardial infarction in coronary by-pass surgery. *J Thorac Cardiovasc Surg* 31:147–150, 1983.

14. Schneider RR, Pichard AD, Mindich B: Factors predisposing to intraoperative myocardial infarction during coronary artery bypass surgery. *Mt Sinai J Med* 52:2:123–129, 1985.

15. Namay DL, Hammermeister KE, Zia MS, et al: Effect of perioperative myocardial infarction on late survival in patients undergoing coronary artery bypass surgery. *Circulation* 65:1066–1071, 1982.

16. Slysh S, Goldenberg S, Dervan JP, et al: Unstable angina and evolving myocardial infarction following coronary bypass surgery. Pathogenesis and treatment with interventional catheterization. *Am Heart J* 109:744–752, 1985.

17. Tanimoto Y, Matsuda Y, Kobayaski Y: Coronary spasm as a cause of perioperative myocardial infarction. *Jpn Heart J* 25:275–281, 1984.

18. Keon WJ, Heggtveit HA, Leduc J: Perioperative myocardial infarction caused by atheroembolism. *J Thorac Cardiovasc Surg* 84:849–855, 1982.

19. Jett GK, Arcidi JM, Dorsey LM: Vasoactive drug effects on blood flow in internal mammary artery and saphenous vein grafts. *J Thorac Cardiovasc Surg* 94:2–11, 1987.

20. Gray RJ, Harris WS, Shah PK, et al: Coronary sinus blood flow and sampling for detection of unrecognized myocardial ischemia and injury. *Circulation* 56(Suppl II):58–61, 1977.

21. Brindis RG, Brundage BH, Ullyot DJ, et al: Graft patency in patients with coronary artery bypass operation complicated by perioperative myocardial infarction. *J Am Coll Cardiol* 3:55–62, 1984.

22. Bateman TM, Matloff JM, Gray RJ: Myocardial infarction during coronary artery bypass surgery—benign event or prognostic omen? *Int J Cardiol* 6:259–263, 1984.

23. Gray RJ, Shell WE, Conklin C, et al: Quantification of myocardial injury during coronary artery bypass graft. *Circulation* 58(Suppl I):38–42, 1977.

24. Gray RJ, Matloff JM, Conklin CM, et al: Perioperative myocardial infarction: late clinical course after coronary artery bypass surgery. *Circulation* 66:1185–1190, 1982.

25. Bulkley BH, Hutchins GM: Myocardial consequences of coronary artery bypass graft surgery. *Circulation* 56:906–913, 1977.

26. Lim JS, Proudfit WL, Sheldon WC, et al: Perioperative myocardial infarction related to coronary bypass surgery. *Am Heart J* 96:463–466, 1978.

27. Achuff SC, Griffith LSC, Conti CR, et al: The "angina-producing" myocardial segment: an approach to the interpretation of results of coronary bypass surgery. *Am J Cardiol* 36:723–733, 1975.

28. Warren SG, Wagner GS, Bethea CF, et al: Diagnostic and prognostic significance of electrocardiographic and CPK isoenzyme changes following coronary bypass surgery: correlation with findings at one year. *Am Heart J* 93:189–196, 1977.

29. Bashour T, Goldshlager A: Persistent Q waves with restoration of normal ventricular contractility after emergency coronary reperfusion. *Am Heart J* 110:888–891, 1985.

30. Albert DE, Kaliff RM, LeCocq DA, et al: Comparative rates of resolution of QRS changes after operative and nonoperative acute myocardial infarctions. *Am J Cardiol* 51:378–381, 1983.

31. Bateman TM, Weiss MH, Czer LSC, et al: Fascicular conduction disturbances and ischemic heart disease: adverse prognosis despite coronary revascularization. *J Am Coll Cardiol* 5:632–639, 1985.

32. Lee ME, Sethna DH, Conklin CM, et al: CK-MB release following coronary artery bypass grafting in the absence on myocardial infarction. *Ann Thorac Surg* 35:277–279, 1983.

33. DePuey EG, Aessopos A, Monroe LR, et al: Clinical utility of a two-site immunoradiometric assay for creatine kinase-MB in the detection of perioperative myocardial infarction. *J Nucl Med* 24:703–709, 1983.

34. Graeber GM, Shawl FA, Head HD, et al: Changes in serum creatine kinase and lactate dehydrogenase caused by acute perioperative myocardial infarction and by transatrial cardiac surgical procedures. *J Thorac Cardiovasc Surg* 92:63–72, 1986.

35. Keshgegian AA, Marchant BL: Cathodal bands in electrophoretograms of creatine kinase isoenzymes in serum collected after cardiac surgery: a poor prognostic sign. *Clin Chem* 29:1727–1729, 1983.

36. Raabe DS, Morise A, Sbarbaro JA, et al: Diagnostic criteria for acute myocardial infarction in patients undergoing coronary artery bypass surgery. *Circulation* 62:869–878, 1980.

37. MacGregor GGA, Muir AL, Smith AF, et al: Myocardial infarction related to coronary artery bypass graft surgery. *Br Heart J* 51:339–406, 1984.

38. Klausner SC, Botfinek EH, Shames D, et al: The application of radionuclide infarct scintigraphy to diagnose perioperative myocardial in-

farction following revascularization. *Circulation* 56:173–181, 1977.

39. Li Wei I, Hanelin LG, Riggins RCK, et al: Perioperative ischemic injury after coronary bypass graft surgery. *Am J Surg* 150:122–126, 1985.

40. Force T, Bloomfield P, O'Boyle J, et al: Quantitative two-dimensional echocardiographic analysis of regional wall motion in patients with perioperative myocardial infarction. *Circulation* 70:233–241, 1984.

41. Force T, Kemper A, Bloomfield P, et al: Non-Q wave perioperative myocardial infarction: assessment of the incidence and severity of regional dysfunction with quantitative two-dimensional echocardiography. *Circulation* 72:781–787, 1985.

42. Riberio P, Nihoyannopoulos P, Farah S, et al: Role of transient ischaemia in perioperative myocardial infarction in the genesis of new septal wall motion abnormalities after coronary bypass surgery. *Br Heart J* 54:140–144, 1985.

43. Schaff HV, Gersh BJ, Fisher LD, et al: Detrimental effect of perioperative myocardial infarction and late survival after coronary artery bypass. *J Thorac Cardiovasc Surg* 88:972–981, 1984.

44. Oberman A, Cutter G, Kouchoukos N, et al: Survival following perioperative myocardial infarction. *Circulation* 62(Suppl III):94, 1980.

45. Bonchek LI, Rahimtoola SH, Chaitman BR, et al: Vein graft occlusion: immediate and late consequences and therapeutic implications. *Circulation* 49(Suppl II):84–97, 1974.

46. Assad-Morell JL, Fry RL, Connolly DL, et al: Relation of intraoperative or early postoperative transmural myocardial infarction to patency of aortocoronary bypass grafts and to diseased ungrafted coronary arteries. *Am J Cardiol* 35:767–773, 1975.

47. Burton JR, FitzGibbon GM, Keon WJ, et al: Perioperative myocardial infarction complicating coronary bypass. *J Thorac Cardiovasc Surg* 82:758–764, 1981.

48. Codd JE, Wiess RD, Kaiser GC, et al: Late sequelae of perioperative myocardial infarction. *Ann Thorac Surg* 26:208–214, 1978.

49. Hacker RW, Torca M, Galling FR, et al: Perioperative myocardial infarction in coronary artery bypass surgery. *J Thorac Cardiovasc Surg* 28:96–101, 1980.

50. Melandri G, Maresta A, Contrafgho F, et al: Effects of coronary artery revascularization and perioperative myocardial infarction on left ventricular wall motion. *Int J Cardiol* 15:47–54, 1987.

51. Roberts AJ, Spies SM, Lichtenthal PR, et al: Changes in left ventricular performance related to perioperative myocardial infarction in coronary artery bypass graft surgery. *Ann Thorac Surg* 35:516–522, 1983.

52. Kaplan JA, Dunbar RW, Jones EL: Nitroglycerin infusion during coronary artery surgery. *Anesthesiology* 45:14–21, 1976.

Chapter 17
MEDIASTINAL BLEEDING, BLOOD CONSERVATION TECHNIQUES, AND TRANSFUSION PRACTICES

LAWRENCE S. C. CZER, M.D.

Excessive bleeding necessitates mediastinal exploration in 3 to 14% (average, 6.2%) of patients undergoing cardiac surgery (1–10). These patients experience an increased incidence of heart failure, hypotension, shock, arrhythmias, infection, and mortality (1–3, 5, 8–10). Thus, excessive bleeding is a serious complication of open-heart surgery. The bleeding tendency is related to hemostatic derangements resulting from cardiopulmonary bypass, to vascular trauma from the surgical incisions, and to preoperative and early postoperative factors that increase the risk of bleeding. Recent advances in blood conservation techniques, changes in transfusion practices, and the availability of nonhematogenous therapies have reduced dependence on donor blood and its attendant risks.

CAUSES OF BLEEDING

Cardiopulmonary Bypass

All patients who undergo cardiopulmonary bypass develop a multitude of hemostatic derangements. These derangements are caused by exposure of the blood to artificial surfaces during extracorporeal circulation and oxygenation, by the resultant requirement for high-dose heparinization to prevent clotting in the extracorporeal circuit, and by priming of the extracorporeal circuit with nonblood solutions, resulting in hemodilution.

Platelet functional impairment is the most important hemostatic derangement and is a major cause of excessive bleeding (9–21). Platelet activation occurs during passage of blood through the plastic tubing, roller pumps, oxygenator, cardiotomy suction, and filters of the cardiopulmonary bypass device. This results in a selective depletion of platelet α granules, reduced membrane binding of fibrinogen and α-adrenergic agonists, and increased plasma levels of platelet constituents such as platelet factor 4 and β-thromboglobulin (9–12, 20, 21). As a consequence, there is a prolonged in vivo template bleeding time, defective in vitro aggregation in response to adenosine diphosphate and collagen, and decreased platelet adhesiveness (7, 9–21). The degree of platelet functional impairment is proportional to the duration of bypass and the depth of hypothermia, and is usually reversed within 1 hr after termination of bypass (11, 12, 19). Membrane oxygenators may produce less platelet dysfunction than bubble oxygenators, especially if cardiotomy suction is controlled by minimizing aspiration of air (22).

Persistent platelet dysfunction may occur, manifested by a prolonged template bleeding time more than 1 hr after termination of bypass. These patients often bleed excessively during the early postoperative period (9, 11, 12). Common intraoperative causes of persistent platelet dysfunction include prolonged cardiopulmonary bypass and reinfusion of large volumes of blood from uncontrolled cardiotomy suction (9, 11, 12, 22, 23).

The platelet count declines immediately after institution of cardiopulmonary bypass due to hemodilution from the nonblood pump priming solution, usually to the range of 100,000 to 150,000/μl. Taken alone, this decline in platelet number is not sufficient to produce abnormal hemostasis. The decline in platelet number may be more severe in patients who had a prolonged course of heparin therapy preoperatively (heparin-associated thrombocytopenia) (24, 25) or who require hemodynamic support with intraaortic balloon counterpulsation or a left ventricular assist device.

Complement is activated during cardiopulmonary bypass as a result of contact with the artificial surfaces of pump components (26). The anaphylatoxins C3a and C5a are produced, and microvascular permeability is increased (27). Pore-forming C5b-9 complexes are deposited on red blood cells, causing intravascular hemolysis (28). The C5b-9 complexes also cause platelet activation (28), thus augmenting direct activation of the platelets by pump components.

Coagulation factor levels are reduced by approximately 50% due to hemodilution, except for factors V and VIII (factor V is reduced to 20 to 30% of normal, and factor VIII remains relatively unaffected) (11). However, none of the coagulation factors is reduced to levels that may produce abnormal bleeding (30% or less, except factor V, which demonstrates adequate hemostasis to levels of 10 to 15%) (11). Clotting factor levels return to baseline values within 12 hr after termination of cardiopulmonary bypass.

Plasminogen and fibrinogen levels are reduced by 50% immediately upon institution of bypass, due to hemodilution. Fibrin degradation products do not usually appear during cardiopulmonary bypass, suggesting effective heparin blockade of fibrin formation. Fibrin degradation products appear after termination of bypass, but fibrinogen levels increase and return to normal within 12 hr, and kinetic and total clottable fibrinogen measurements are equivalent, suggesting that activation of the fibrinolytic system does not contribute significantly to abnormal hemostasis (11).

The effectiveness of heparinization can be monitored intraoperatively by measurement of the activated clotting time (ACT) (29–35). The optimal level of anticoagulation appears to be achieved with an ACT of 400 to 480 seconds (33–35). Thrombus deposition, fibrin stranding, and excessive clotting factor consumption occur with an ACT of less than 300 seconds, while excessive bleeding occurs with an ACT over the optimal range (29, 33–35). It has been recommended to monitor ACT every 30 min during cardiopulmonary bypass, and after protamine administration. Significant reductions in heparin and protamine dosage, postoperative bleeding, and transfusion requirements have been reported with use of the ACT in comparison with a fixed schedule of heparinization (29–32).

Harker and coworkers (11) found no evidence for a protamine-induced coagulopathy. In patients with a history of protamine sensitivity, heparin neutralization may be accomplished with hexadimethrine bromide (Polybrene) (36), or may be omitted entirely. when heparin neutralization is omitted, excessive postoperative bleeding often occurs, necessitating multiple transfusions of blood products.

Thus, excessive bleeding after cardiopulmonary bypass is usually not due to reduction in coagulation factor levels, the presence of fibrin degradation products, or excessive protamine administration. Nonetheless, in patients with abnormal baseline hemostasis (for example, due to advanced liver disease), the change in factor levels, fibrinogen, and fibrin degradation products may contribute significantly to postoperative bleeding.

Surgical Trauma

Open-heart surgery results in direct trauma to the tissues of many different structures, including the heart, aorta, coronary arteries, sternum, and skin. Also affected are the thigh and leg (when harvesting the saphenous vein), the parietal pleura and adjacent thoracic structures (during harvesting of the internal thoracic artery), and venous and arterial sites of cannulation for hemodynamic monitoring during anesthesia. The bladder and urethra may become injured during catheterization of the urinary tract. Similarly, the trachea may become traumatized if the patient is a difficult intubation or is not carefully intubated. Recent cardiac catheterization may injure vascular structures in the inguinal area, arm, and neck. All of these structures may become potential bleeding sites during and immediately after cardiac surgery. Extensive adhesions may develop between the sternum and the heart if the patient has had prior cardiac surgery. These adhesions are often quite well vascularized and may bleed excessively after surgical division. In addition, the distortion of normal anatomic relationships (right ventricle in direct contact with posterior table of sternum), the obscuring of surgical landmarks and targets, and the increased difficulty and length of the operation all contribute to an increased risk of bleeding.

When mediastinal exploration is required for excessive postoperative bleeding, the most common localized sites of bleeding have been the bypass graft anastomoses and side branches, the aortic cannulation site, and the sternum. However, any of the structures traumatized may potentially become a bleeding source, and meticulous surgical technique is necessary to prevent hemorrhage.

Preoperative and Early Postoperative Factors

Certain drugs frequently interfere with normal hemostasis and thus predispose to excessive bleeding. These include aspirin and other nonsteroidal anti-inflammatory agents, warfarin, thrombolytic drugs (streptokinase, urokinase, tissue plasminogen activator), antibiotics (especially carbenicillin, ticarcillin, moxalactam, cefamandole, third generation cephalosporins, and most chronically administered antibiotics), dextrans, amrinone, quinidine, cytotoxic drugs, gold, phenylbutazone, ethanol, and fish oils (37–39).

Because aspirin acetylates platelets irreversibly, the drug should be discontinued at least 7 days prior to surgery (40, 41). Warfarin therapy should be discontinued at least 5 days before surgery (41); if necessary (e.g., in a patient with a mechanical valve prosthesis), heparin therapy is initiated within 48 hr of warfarin discontinuation and adjusted according to the prothrombin and partial thromboplastin times. The heparin may then be stopped 4 to 12 hr before the operation without enhancing the risk of mediastinal bleeding (41). Heparin may produce an immune-mediated thrombocytopenia in about 5% of patients (range, 0 to 30%) if used for 6 to 12 days or more (24, 25, 37).

Patients given aspirin preoperatively and early postoperatively to maintain saphenous vein graft patency have increased mediastinal blood loss and a fourfold greater rate of reoperation (6.5%) when compared with patients receiving placebo (reoperation rate, 1.7%) (8).

Hypertension may cause fresh vascular anastomoses to bleed or rupture due to excessive intraluminal pressure; therefore, control of hypertension is important in the early postoperative period (42). Therapy of hypertension can be initially accomplished with the use of intravenous nitroprusside or esmolol (43). The therapeutic goal is generally to achieve a systolic pressure between 110 and 130 mm Hg. A somewhat higher systemic pressure may be appropriate in patients with cerebral, renal, or intestinal arterial disease, to prevent organ hypoperfusion.

Any disease process that affects platelet number or function, coagulation factor activity, or the fibrinolytic system may potentially contribute to a bleeding tendency. These include inherited disorders such as hemophilia and other coagulation factor deficiencies; von Willebrand's disease; certain platelet, membrane, and granule diseases (Bernard-Soullier syndrome, Glanzmann's thrombasthenia, gray platelet and dense granule deficiency); and α 2 antiplasmin deficiency. Many acquired disorders adversely affect normal hemostasis: advanced liver disease, uremia, hypersplenism, malabsorption, severe viral infections, Gram-negative sepsis, certain parasitic infections, massive transfusions, extensive trauma, burns, malignant-hyperthermia, disseminated cancer, giant hemangiomas, systemic lupus erythematosis, vasculitis, acute leukemia, lymphoma, myeloproliferative disorders, myeloma, macroglobulinemia, idiopathic or thrombotic thrombocytopenic purpura, hemolytic-uremic syndrome, microangiopathic hemolytic anemia, disseminated intravascular coagulation, hemolytic transfusion reactions, and circulating coagulation factor inhibitors (37).

The presence of certain structural lesions may predispose to localized extramediastinal bleeding. These include gastrointestinal erosions due to peptic ulcer disease; vascular malformations and well-vascularized neoplasms of the gastrointestinal, genitourinary, or central nervous systems; recent cerebrovascular accidents; recent obstetric delivery; and recent surgery or trauma. Of special note, the possibility of bleeding from gastrointestinal angiodysplasias should be considered in patients undergoing aortic valve replacement for aortic stenosis.

Preoperative Screening

The best preoperative screen for disordered hemostasis remains the clinical history, with special attention to drug or medication usage, and excessive bleeding with prior surgery or trauma. Basic coagulation tests (prothrombin time, partial thromboplastin time, platelet count, and template bleeding time) are often routinely performed to identify unsuspected or previously undiagnosed bleeding disorders. The value of such laboratory screening tests for predicting bleeding or transfusion requirements is controversial. Ramsey and coworkers (44) found that patients with abnormal preoperative tests received no more blood products than those with normal tests and that no individual test predicted excessive bleeding. Conversely, Bachman and coworkers (6) demonstrated that a severely abnormal coagulation profile, while unusual (occurring in 5.6% of patients), conferred a 4.5-fold greater risk of bleeding (13.8%) than if the profile was not severely abnormal

(3.1% risk). Because of these data and the risks associated with excessive bleeding, we perform basic coagulation testing in all patients preoperatively.

If the clinical history or preoperative coagulation screen suggests disordered hemostasis, then additional laboratory tests and consultation with a hematologist should be obtained to precisely define the nature of the disorder and plan a therapeutic approach. Patients with preoperatively disordered hemostasis can usually undergo cardiac surgery safely (45–53), but exquisite attention to intraoperative hemostasis, blood salvage techniques, and appropriate blood product support are required.

Preoperative screening tests for occult bleeding include a complete blood count, stool guaiac test, and routine urinalysis. When anemia is found, bone marrow aspiration is indicated; if iron deficiency is documented, then a further workup to identify the source of bleeding is mandatory.

EVALUATION OF MEDIASTINAL BLEEDING

Suspected or apparent mediastinal bleeding in the early postoperative period requires evaluation of chest tube drainage, hemodynamics, imaging of the heart and surrounding structures, and a careful hemostatic and hematologic assessment. The purpose of the evaluation is to identify surgically treatable causes of bleeding (hemorrhage, cardiac tamponade) and hemostatic defects amenable to medical therapy.

Chest Tube Drainage and Hematocrit

Excessive mediastinal bleeding is readily apparent when the chest tube drainage surpasses 250 to 300 ml/hr during the first 2 hr after termination of cardiopulmonary bypass, or 100 to 150 ml/hr thereafter (5, 9). Bleeding rates exceeding these limits suggest the presence of a surgically correctable lesion, and surgical exploration is required in 36 to 100% of patients (3, 5, 6, 9) to prevent cardiac tamponade or hemorrhagic shock. A substantial fall in hematocrit (3% or more) or hemoglobin concentration (1 gm/dl or more) is usually observed. Recognition of excessive bleeding is more difficult when the chest tube drainage is minimal (less than 50 ml/hr). Drainage may be impeded by clotted blood within the chest tubes, or by adhesions or loculations around the site of bleeding. A relatively small amount or short duration of bleeding may produce cardiac tamponade. There may be no significant change in hematocrit or hemoglobin concentration. Alternatively, there may be substantial bleeding into an extramediastinal structure not drained by the chest tubes (e.g., the pleural space). Hemodynamic monitoring and cardiac imaging techniques are especially helpful under these circumstances.

With moderate rates of bleeding (50 to 150 ml/hr), there may be generalized oozing from multiple small bleeding sites or a surgically correctable lesion with partial blockage of chest tube drainage. Since generalized oozing is more often responsible for the bleeding, hemostatic evaluation is particularly important. A surgically correctable lesion is less likely, and can be evaluated by hemodynamics and cardiac imaging techniques if the hemostatic evaluation is normal.

Active bleeding and drainage of old blood can be distinguished by color (old blood is dark) and by comparison of the hematocrit of the chest tube drainage to that of the peripheral blood. If the hematocrit ratio (chest tube to peripheral blood) is 0.9 or greater, active bleeding is suggested. The bleeding rates mentioned above exclude dark, old blood which may suddenly drain when the patient sits up for a portable chest x-ray or other procedure; this does not constitute active bleeding.

Hemodynamics

Pulmonary artery catheterization is essential for complete hemodynamic characterization of mediastinal bleeding, especially when hypotension and tachycardia are present. Low filling pressures with a low cardiac output less than 2.0 liters/min/m^2) indicate significant intravascular volume depletion. An elevated right atrial to pulmonary capillary wedge pressure ratio and low cardiac output suggest generalized pericardial tamponade. However, these findings are not specific to cardiac tamponade. Right ventricular dysfunction, biventricular failure, per-

ioperative infarction involving the right ventricle, inadequate myocardial preservation, residual hypothermia, and severe tricuspid regurgitation may produce a similar clinical picture during the early postoperative period (54–56). Further, single-chamber tamponade may occur, and its presentation is frequently atypical (57, 58). Thus, despite hemodynamic monitoring, cardiac tamponade may be difficult to diagnose and to differentiate from other commonly occurring syndromes during the early postoperative period.

Cardiac Imaging Techniques

Chest Radiography.   A portable chest radiograph may suggest the presence of mediastinal bleeding if enlargement of the cardiac silhouette is observed in comparison with prior chest films. Portable studies should not be compared with prior PA films, since the cardiac silhouette will always appear larger on the portable film.

A useful radiographic sign relates to the position of the pulmonary artery catheter. The distance between the right heart border (adjacent to the right atrium) and the pulmonary artery catheter (as it passes through the right atrium) is measured. If this is less than 5 mm at any point below the level of the pulmonary artery, then the finding is normal (Fig. 17.1). Otherwise, pericardial effusion, hematoma, or active bleeding should be suspected along the right cardiac silhouette (Fig. 17.2).

Cardiac Scintigraphy.   Portable cardiac blood pool scintigraphy (radionuclide ventriculography) is extremely useful for differentiating the various causes of low cardiac output with hypotension and elevated filling pressures after open-heart surgery (55, 59, 60). Because red blood cells are labeled with ^{99m}Tc, the location and extent of active pericardial bleeding can be directly imaged as an area of brightness outside the cardiac blood pool (Figs. 17.3 and 17.4). By means of nonzoomed images, active extramediastinal thoracic bleeding can also be detected (55, 60). Pericardial effusion appears as an exaggerated area of photon deficiency surrounding the ventricles. Pericardial hematoma without active bleeding appears as a localized area of photon deficiency. Because wall motion can be evaluated, global and segmental dys-

FIGURE 17.1

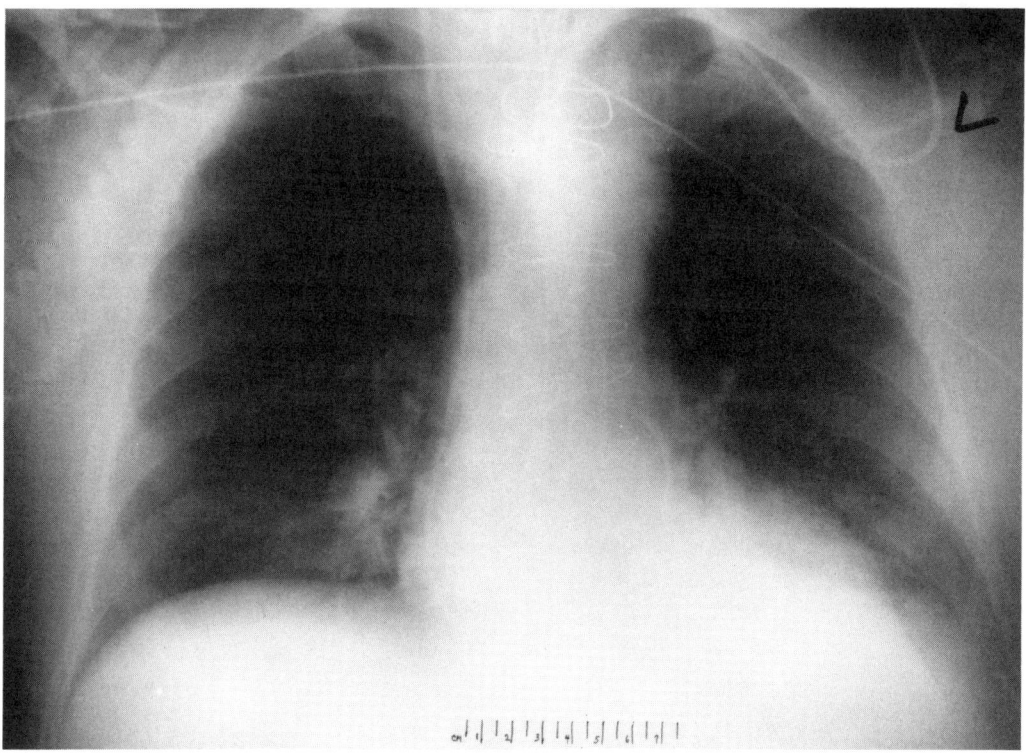

Portable chest radiograph demonstrating normal relationship between pulmonary artery catheter and right heart border. There was no evidence of mediastinal bleeding in this patient. The width of the mediastinum is normal.

function of the right or left ventricle is readily diagnosed. Thus, the presence of active pericardial or thoracic bleeding, pericardial effusion, pericardial hemotoma without active bleeding, and ventricular dysfunction can be accurately determined and differentiated with a single diagnostic test.

Echocardiography. While echocardiography can provide diagnostic information regarding the presence of pericardial effusion, hematoma, or ventricular dysfunction, technical considerations limit its usefulness in the early postoperative period (55, 61–63). In our experience, 31% of postoperative echocardiographic studies have been technically inadequate, due to the presence of mediastinal air, the location of the chest tubes, and the placement of bandages on the chest (55). By comparison, technically inadequate radionuclide ventriculographic studies have been rare (55). Additionally, echocardiography cannot reliably distinguish pericardial effusion from active pericardial bleeding.

For these reasons, radionuclide ventriculography has greater diagnostic usefulness than echocardiography during the early postoperative period.

Computed Tomography (CT) and Magnetic Resonance Imaging (MRI). Pericardial effusion, hematoma, and ventricular dysfunction are readily detected by CT and MRI. However, because images cannot be obtained portably, these techniques are usually not appropriate for critically ill patients, and their application during the early postoperative period has been limited

Hemostatic Evaluation

Abnormal hemostasis may cause or contribute to excessive postoperative bleeding when there are major deviations from the expected pattern of hemostatic recovery after termination of cardiopulmonary bypass.

Expected postoperative values for many coagulation parameters have been published (11,

FIGURE 17.2

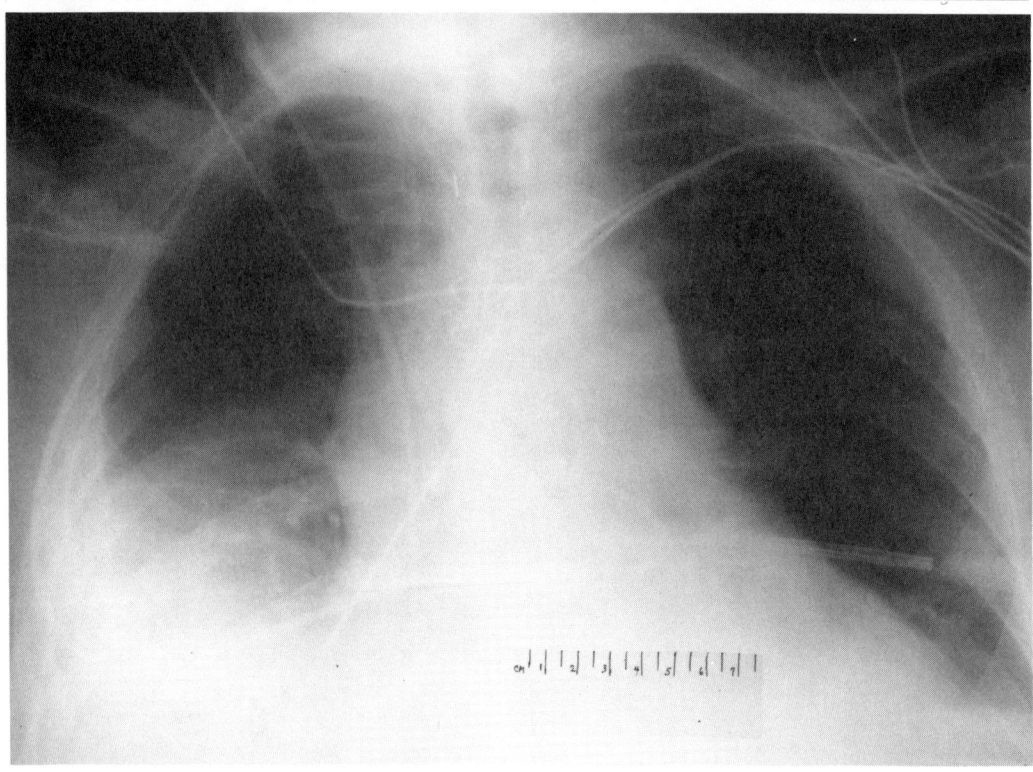

Portable chest film of patient with mediastinal bleeding and increased distance between pulmonary artery catheter and right heart border, suggesting blood clot or loculated fluid accumulation along right cardiac silhouette. Note the widened mediastinum and right pleural fluid or blood collection.

14, 64), and selected data are summarized in Tables 17.1 and 17.2. It should be noted that the expected values vary as a function of time, generally being most different from normal early postoperatively, then trending toward normal as time progresses. These expected values also vary somewhat among the reported series, principally due to differences in patient populations, protocols for antiplatelet or anticoagulant therapy before surgery, and technique and length of cardiopulmonary bypass.

Early postoperative screening tests for disturbed hemostasis should include at least a platelet count, template bleeding time, prothrombin time, and partial thromboplastin time (or ACT). The results of these tests are then compared with the expected values (Tables 17.1 and 17.2). Alternatively, simplified guidelines have been formulated at our institution to indicate the presence of severely disturbed hemostasis (Table 17.3).

Additional tests may be indicated when conditions that predispose to abnormal bleeding exist prior to, or shortly after, surgery. The presence of high levels of fibrinogen-fibrin degradation products, D-dimers, a shortened euglobulin clot lysis time, and an abnormally depressed fibrinogen level suggest accelerated fibrinolysis, which may be caused by disseminated intravascular coagulation or residual effects from prior therapy with thrombolytic drugs.

Use of Tests to Guide Therapeutic Approach

If the hemostatic screening tests are outside the expected range but there is no evidence for clinically apparent or occult mediastinal bleeding, no therapy is indicated. Hemostatic abnormalities should be treated (*a*) in the presence of excessive bleeding, as suggested by 50 ml/hr or greater mediastinal tube output, or (*b*) if there is evidence for significant occult bleeding (car-

FIGURE 17.3

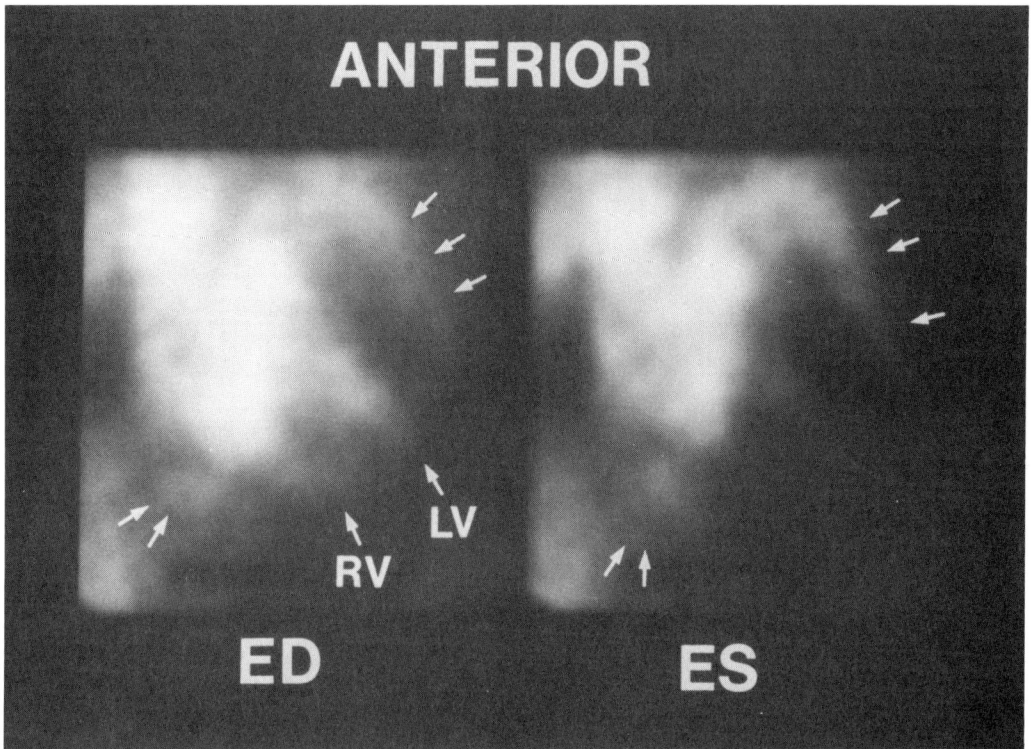

Cardiac scintigraphy with ^{99m}Tc-labeled red blood cells (anterior view) (55, 59, 60). There are two areas of brightness (*double and triple arrows*) located outside the cardiac blood pool, along the diaphragmatic and anterolateral surfaces of the heart, respectively. There is also an exaggerated area of photon deficiency around the entire heart, suggesting prior pericardial accumulation of blood or fluid. *RV*, right ventricular blood pool; *LV*, left ventricular blood pool; *ED*, end diastole, *ES*, end systole. (Images courtesy of Timothy M. Bateman, M.D.)

diac tamponade or extramediastinal bleeding) from hemodynamics, chest radiography, or radionuclide studies. Hemostatic tests should be repeated at least every 4 hr if mediastinal bleeding continues.

Specific targets should be set for hemostatic therapy. Ideally, the platelet count should be brought above 100,000/mm^3, the template bleeding time below 10 min, and the prothrombin time and partial thromboplastin time less than 1.2 times the control value.

Surgical exploration of the mediastinum is indicated when bleeding results in cardiac tamponade, when bleeding is massive (more than 400 ml during any hour) (9), or when it persists despite correction of disturbed hemostasis by appropriate medical therapy (more than 1200 ml cumulative over 8 to 12 hr, or exceeds 100 to 150 ml/hr). Cardiac scintigraphy with ^{99m}Tc-

labeled red blood cells may be helpful in localizing the source of occult bleeding within the mediastinum prior to operative exploration, and in distinguishing tamponade from ventricular dysfunction (55).

Many patients with excessive mediastinal bleeding and severely disturbed hemostasis do not require operative exploration. In our experience, the bleeding pattern in these patients consists of generalized oozing or multiple small-caliber bleeding sizes, and the bleeding significantly slows or ceases with appropriate hemostatic therapy.

MEDICAL TREATMENT OF BLEEDING

The goals of medical therapy are (*a*) prevention of severe anemia, (*b*) maintenance of intravascular volume, and (*c*) elimination of palliation of

FIGURE 17.4

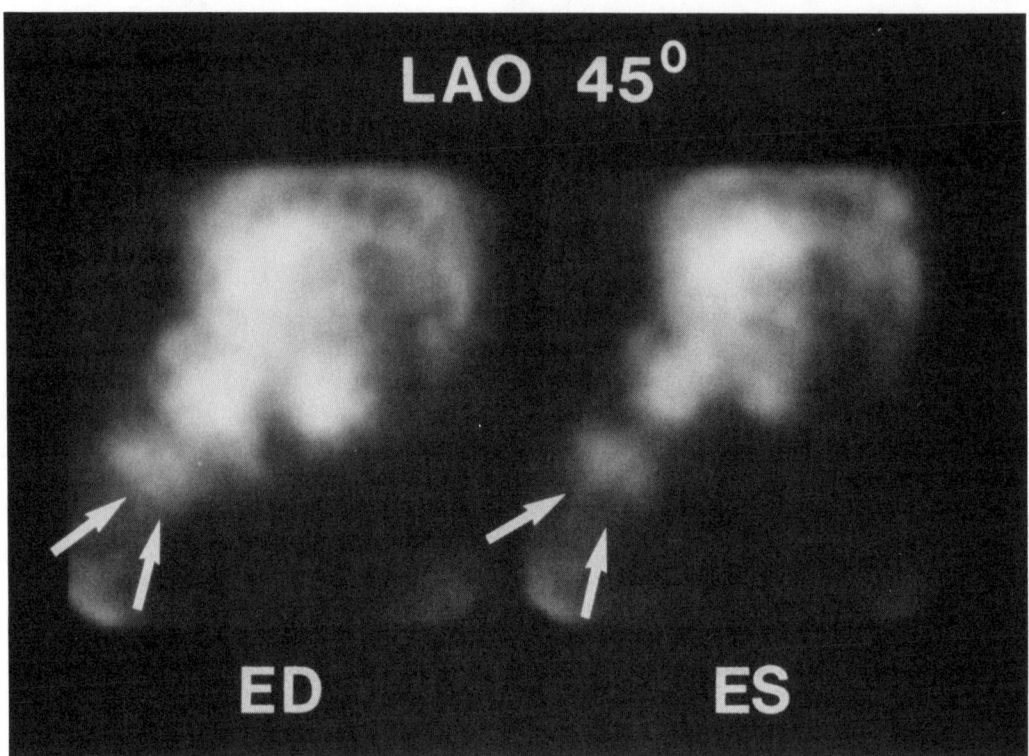

Cardiac scintigraphy with ^{99m}Tc-labeled red blood cells (LAO 45° view; same patient as in Fig. 17.3) (55, 59, 60). In this view, the diaphragmatic area of brightness (*double arrows*) is seen to originate from the inferior surface of the right ventricle. (The anterolateral area of brightness seen in Fig. 17.3 is obscured by the great vessels.) An exaggerated area of photon deficiency is seen around the entire heart. Note the excellent ventricular function (difference between end-diastolic and end-systolic frames). *ED*, end diastole; *ES*, end systole. (Images courtesy of Timothy M. Bateman, M.D.)

the hemostatic defect. While blood components can achieve all of these goals, there has been increasing recognition of the potential for infectious complications from donor blood (65–78) (Table 17.4). Serologic testing of donor blood is currently performed only for syphilis, hepatitis B, and human immunodeficiency virus type I (HIV-I). Nevertheless, cases of hepatitis B and HIV-I transmission have occurred despite screening (66–68). No specific screening test currently exists for non-A, non-B hepatitis, the major cause of post-transfusion hepatitis, which develops in 7.7% of all blood recipients (66). Screening for non-A, non-B hepatitis by use of surrogate markers is performed at many centers but is neither sensitive nor specific. Screening for human T cell lymphotropic virus type I (HTLV-I) is not yet widely employed. Many other infectious agents and diseases are transmissible by blood transfusions (Table 17.4). Thus, current screening methods for blood-borne infectious agents are incomplete and imperfect, and until screening methods improve it is prudent to use blood conservation techniques whenever possible.

Blood Conservation Techniques

The main components of a blood conservation program include autologous blood donation preoperatively or during induction of anesthesia, intraoperative and postoperative salvage and transfusion of shed mediastinal blood, acceptance of normovolemic anemia, and the use of nonhematogenous therapies to improve hemostasis (79–83). Also important are proper

TABLE 17.1

EXPECTED VALUES OF SELECTED COAGULATION PARAMETERS BEFORE AND AFTER OPEN-HEART SURGERY, FROM PUBLISHED STUDIES[a]

	Harker[b]				Milam[c]			Mammen[d]		
	Preop Baseline	Postop 10 min	Postop 2–4 hr	Postop 19–24 hr	Preop Baseline	Postop 1 hr	Postop 24 hr	Pre-pump	Postop Protamine	Postop ICU
Platelets (conc × 10^{-3} mm^{-3})	225 ± 22	116 ± 18	132 ± 16	114 ± 17	194 ± 58	144 ± 50	156 ± 51	243 ± 63	118 ± 69	120 ± 82
Factor II (% activity)	94 ± 7	44 ± 4	73 ± 8	74 ± 7	81 ± 14	71 ± 13	74 ± 12	102 ± 17	67 ± 15	39 ± 5
Factor V (% activity)	105 ± 8	51 ± 9	85 ± 13	86 ± 8	88 ± 8	62 ± 15	84 ± 16	59 ± 32	34 ± 15	10 ± 13
Factor VII (% activity)	114 ± 9	58 ± 5	115 ± 10	83 ± 11	94 ± 31	79 ± 24	55 ± 23	—	—	—
Factor VIII:C (% activity)	113 ± 10	84 ± 21	151 ± 40	145 ± 32	89 ± 42	120 ± 59	159 ± 73	78 ± 55	58 ± 29	70 ± 19
Factor IX (% activity)	106 ± 7	82 ± 9	102 ± 8	101 ± 10	77 ± 25	87 ± 27	93 ± 31	—	—	
Factor X (% activity)	97 ± 3	53 ± 8	73 ± 9	68 ± 6	83 ± 19	71 ± 16	71 ± 17	93 ± 13	53 ± 15	58 ± 29
Fibrinogen (mg/dl)	313 ± 22	145 ± 9	234 ± 20	322 ± 12	282 ± 76	237 ± 62	411 ± 86	262 ± 79	173 ± 48	125 ± 127
Fibrin split products[e] (μg/ml)					3 ± 3	7 ± 7	14 ± 37			
Prothrombin time					12 ± 1	14 ± 2	12 ± 1			
Partial thromboplastin time (sec)					35 ± 6	33 ± 5	33 ± 4			

[a]Data expressed as mean ± SD.

[b]Data from Harker LA, Malpass TW, Branson HE, et al: Mechanism of abnormal bleeding in patients undergoing cardiopulmonary bypass: acquired transient platelet dysfunction associated with selective alpha-granule release.

[c]Data from Milam JD, Austin SF, Martin RF, et al: Alteration of coagulation and selected clinical chemistry parameters in patients undergoing open heart surgery without transfusions. Am J Clin Pathol 76:155–162, 1981.

[d]Data from Mammen EF, Koets MH, Washington BC, et al: Hemostasis changes during cardiopulmonary bypass surgery. Semin Thromb Hemost 11:281–292, 1985.

[e]Tanned erythrocyte hemagglutination inhibition immunoassay (normal, 2–10).

TABLE 17.2

EXPECTED VALUES OF TEMPLATE BLEEDING TIME BEFORE, DURING, AND AFTER SURGERY[a]

	Bleeding Time
	min
Preoperative	4.8 ± 0.1
Cardiopulmonary bypass	
10 min	19.0 ± 0.8
1 hr	25.0 ± 1.0
2 hr	>30
After termination of bypass	
Protamine administration	15.2 ± 0.6
2–4 hr postoperatively	8.9 ± 0.6
6–8 hr postoperatively	8.3 ± 1.8

[a]Modified from Harker LA, Malpass TW, Branson HE, et al: Mechanism of abnormal bleeding in patients undergoing cardiopulmonary bypass: acquired transient platelet dysfunction associated with selective alpha-granule release. *Blood* 56:824–834, 1980. Data summarized as mean ± SD.

TABLE 17.3

SIMPLIFIED GUIDELINES INDICATING SEVERELY DISTURBED POSTOPERATIVE HEMOSTASIS

Platelet count less than 100,000/mm³
Template bleeding time more than 10 min[a]
Prothrombin time more than 1.2 times control
Partial thromboplastin time more than 1.2 times control

[a]More than 2 hr after termination of cardiopulmonary bypass.

hemostatic preparation (e.g., preoperative discontinuation of aspirin or warfarin and correction of preexisting hemostatic defects), the use of intraoperative techniques to limit blood loss, and the avoidance of prophylactic administration of banked blood components (79–83).

Blood conservation techniques are especially appropriate in elective procedures. In a study of elective myocardial revascularization at the Cleveland Clinic, more than 90% of patients received no banked blood during their hospital stay (82). In patients undergoing urgent or emergent operations, there may not be sufficient time for preoperative donation of autologous blood and proper hemostatic preparation. Nevertheless, by enactment of the other elements of a blood conservation program, as many as 40% of these patients can be managed without the use of banked blood (84).

Autologous Blood Donation. With daily oral iron supplementation, phlebotomy for autologous blood can be performed at 4- to 7-day intervals up to 72 hr preoperatively (85–88).

Usually, a total of 2 to 4 units of such "predeposited" blood is obtained, but as many as 8 units can be removed, depending on the time interval to surgery, the type of surgical procedure, and the anticipated requirements for blood (81). After collection, the units may be stored as whole blood, erythrocytes, plasma, or platelets (85) for later transfusion into the same patient.

Autologous blood can be safely donated by potentially "high-risk" patients such as the elderly, those with coronary artery disease, children, and pregnant women (86). Most programs require a hemoglobin above 11 gm/dl or hematocrit greater than 34% before phlebotomy (81, 85, 87, 88), and no more than 10% of the estimated blood volume is removed at a single donation. The donated blood is usually subjected to ABO and Rh typing and antibody screening; in addition, screening for HIV-I, hepatitis B, and syphilis is performed. If not used by the donor, the blood can be released by the blood bank for homologous use.

Alternatively, phlebotomy for autologous blood can be preformed after induction of anesthesia on the day of surgery (82, 83, 85). Hemodynamic stability is maintained by simultaneous infusion of crystalloid or colloid solution, resulting in normovolemic hemodilution. Usually, this normovolemic hemodilution is well tolerated (81, 82); whether it is beneficial or harmful in patients with resting myocardial ischemia has been debated (81, 89). Up to 15% of the patient's blood volume can be removed and stored with citrate-phosphate-dextrose-adenine-1 (or heparin) at room temperature and reinfused as whole blood after termination of cardiopulmonary bypass (83).

A distinct advantage of autologous blood donation preoperatively or after induction of anesthesia is that the blood has not been exposed to cardiopulmonary bypass, damaged tissue, or air, and their deleterious effects on formed blood elements, clotting factors, fibrinogen, and complement (4, 6, 7, 9–35, 81). Thus, the levels of platelets and clotting factors are maintained (81, 83), and transfusion of whole blood, platelets, or plasma can be achieved in an autologous manner, in addition to the transfusion of red cells.

TABLE 17.4

INFECTIOUS COMPLICATIONS OF TRANSFUSION THERAPY

Disease	Infectious Agent
Hepatitis B	Hepatitis B virus (65, 66)
Non-A, non-B hepatitis	Non-A, non-B hepatitis viruses (66, 67)
Infectious mononucleosis syndrome	Cytomegalovirus, Epstein-Barr virus (65)
Acquired immunodeficiency syndrome (AIDS)	Human immunodeficiency virus I (HIV-I) 66–71)
Variant form of immunodeficiency syndrome	Human immunodeficiency virus II (HIV-II) (72)
Adult T-cell leukemia	Human T-cell lymphotropic virus (HTLV-I) (73, 74)
Tropical spastic paraparesis	Human T-cell lymphotropic virus (HTLV-I) (73, 75)
Transient aplastic crisis	Parvovirus B19 (75a)
Erythema infectiosum (fifth disease)	Parvovirus B19 (75a)
Creutzfeld-Jakob disease	Slow virus (77, 78)
Septic shock	*Yersinia enterocolitica* (76)
Syphilis	*Treponema pallidum* (65)
Malaria	*Plasmodium vivax* and others (65)
Toxoplasmosis	*Toxoplasma gondii*
Babesiosis	*Babesia microti*
Brucellosis	*Brucella*

Predeposit autologous blood programs have been shown to eliminate exposure to homologous blood in two-thirds of participants, and to reduce exposure in the remainder (87, 90, 91). As a result, the risks of infectious disease transmission, transfusion reactions, and alloimmunization are reduced or eliminated (91). An additional benefit is that unused predeposit autologous units can be released for homologous use, thus increasing the hospital's supply of banked blood (87).

Salvage and Transfusion of Shed Mediastinal Blood. During the course of surgery and early postoperatively, blood and blood-containing fluids are shed in the operative field or into the chest tubes that drain the mediastinum. This material, which would otherwise be discarded, can be salvaged in two ways (81, 85, 92–100): (*a*) by collection, filtration, and reinfusion as shed blood; or (*b*) by collection, processing, and reinfusion as washed red blood cells.

Devices that employ the first technique are simpler, faster, and less expensive (81, 85). Examples (92–97) include the modified cardiotomy reservoir (many manufacturers) (95–97), the Pleur-evac autotransfusion system, the Sorenson system, and the Bentley roller-pump device (now discontinued). The modified cardiotomy reservoir is attached to a standard intravenous infusion pump and offers the advantages of continuous transfusion of shed blood

and maintenance of a closed system, thus reducing the risks of contamination (95). Other devices (Pleur-evac and Sorenson systems) require periodic transfusion at least every 4 hr to prevent septic complications (96). All of the devices use a filter (which varies in size from 20 to 170 μm) to screen out particulate debris.

Shed mediastinal blood is hemostatically abnormal, due to exposure to cardiopulmonary bypass, injured tissue, air, and the collection system. Studies by Schaff, Hauer, Thurer, Hartz, and others (81, 92–97) have demonstrated that shed mediastinal blood, in comparison with circulating peripheral blood, has lower fibrinogen and factor levels (except possibly factors VIII and IX), elevated fibrinopeptide A and B β 15–24 levels, a lower platelet count, greater platelet dysfunction, a lower hematocrit, and a variable amount of free hemoglobin. These abnormalities are most pronounced with slow bleeding, presumably due to prolonged tissue contact and extensive defibrinogenation. As a result, shed mediastinal blood usually does not clot. With rapid bleeding, clotting can occur, and anticoagulation with citrate-phosphate-dextrose-adenine-1 is necessary. Despite these hematologic abnormalities, transfusion of shed mediastinal blood can be safely performed without producing fibrinolysis or disseminated intravascular coagulation, and may reduce use of banked blood by as much as 50% (92–97).

Cell-washing devices include the Haemonetics Cell-Saver and similar devices manufactured by COBE, Shiley, and Electromedics; the IBM blood cell processor can be modified to wash red blood cells. Blood is collected in a cardiotomy reservoir, Sorenson system, or other suitable device and is anticoagulated with citrate-phosphate-dextrose-adenine-1 or heparin. The blood is then transferred to a rigid Latham bowl (Haemonetics) or disposable plastic bag, and a saline solution is added to wash the cells. The process is repeated several times, after which the washed red blood cells can be transferred to a standard blood bag for transfusion into the patient. The final product has a hematocrit of 55 to 80% (81).

Red blood cells processed by the Cell Saver have normal in vivo survival as measured by a dual isotope-labeling technique (98). The concentration of 2,3-diphosphoglycerate in washed autologous erythrocytes is higher than in banked blood (99). Hyperkalemia and hypocalcemia occur less frequently with washed autologous than with banked blood (96). Washing eliminates many potentially deleterious substances that may be infused with unprocessed shed mediastinal blood, such as free hemoglobin, activated clotting factors, fibrin degradation products, and anticoagulants (81, 85). The volume of erythrocytes recovered after washing is comparable to that obtained from unprocessed blood (100, 101). These cell-washing devices are therefore used in many operating rooms, despite the longer time, greater expense, and increased expertise required to operate them.

Contamination of the operative site by bacteria or malignant cells is a contraindication to the use of any form of blood salvage, since these are not completely removed even if the blood is washed (81, 85). Complications of blood salvage include hemolysis, which can be minimized by reducing suction pressure and avoiding aspiration of air during salvage; formation of microaggregates and debris, which can be removed by in-line micropore filters (size 20 to 170 μm); blood clotting, which can be prevented by anticoagulation with citrate-phosphate-dextrose-adenine-1 (preferred because systemic effects are minimal) or heparin; and air embolism, due to operator inattention and

associated with the use of the Bentley roller-pump device (81, 85). With massive transfusion of shed mediastinal blood (3000 ml or more) or washed red blood cells (6 to 8 units or more), a dilutional coagulopathy may occur; this can be treated by supplemental component therapy with fresh frozen plasma and platelets.

Normovolemic Hemodilution. Acceptance of normovolemic anemia in the postoperative period enhances blood conservation, because crystalloid or colloid solutions can be used for volume replacement rather than blood or blood products.

Hemodilution is accompanied by a compensatory increase in cardiac output in response to decreases in blood viscosity and systemic vascular resistance (102–104). Consequently, oxygen delivery is maintained within a narrow range at hematocrit values between 20 and 50% (105), assuming normal cardiac reserve; the optimal hematocrit may be 30% (104–106). In the clinical practice of normovolemic hemodilution, the hematocrit is usually not permitted to be below 25 or 30%, to allow for some limitation of cardiac reserve. In patients at risk for postoperative ischemic injury (low cardiac output, incomplete revascularization, perioperative infarction or ischemia), a higher hematocrit may be advisable (89).

Colloids may be preferable to crystalloid solutions for normovolemic hemodilution. Weisel and coworkers (89) demonstrated that patients receiving crystalloids require twice as much fluid to maintain normovolemia; as a result, anemia is more severe, and peripheral edema occurs more commonly. Crystalloid use was associated with a delayed postoperative recovery of myocardial oxygen and lactate extraction; atrial pacing and volume loading reduced myocardial lactate extraction to ischemic levels (89). These findings were not observed with colloid use, possibly because oxygen delivery was better maintained with colloids than with crystalloids. Nevertheless, the delay in myocardial metabolic recovery associated with crystalloid use did not increase the incidence of perioperative mortality or infarction (89).

Colloid solutions include albumin, plasma protein fraction, hetastarch, and the dextrans. Albumin and plasma fraction are derived from pooled human plasma which is heat treated (60°C for 10 hr) and negative for hepatitis B surface antigen; transmission of hepatitis has not been reported (107). Neither preparation contains clotting factors. Plasma protein fraction contains both albumin (at least 83%) and globulin (no more than 17%); severe bradykinin-induced hypotension has been much less frequent since prekallikrein activator levels were reduced (107, 108).

Hetastarch is a synthetic carbohydrate polymer that closely resembles glycogen. The 6% solution has osmotic properties similar to 5% albumin. Plasma volume is increased slightly in excess of the volume infused, and the volume expansion persists for 24 to 36 hr (107, 109). Hetastarch has proved to be safe and effective for volume replacement after cardiac surgery, with no adverse impact on coagulation parameters or blood loss (110–112); it has also been used successfully as a pump prime (113, 114). Nevertheless, hetastarch is contraindicated in patients with severe bleeding disorders, because of possible worsening of the coagulopathy (115–117). Anaphylactoid reactions (118) may occur rarely (incidence 0.006%). The major route of elimination is renal, by which 40% of the administered dose is removed within 24 hr; therefore, hetastarch is contraindicated in oliguric renal failure (107). A significant proportion of the administered dose is distributed to the liver and spleen, from which the elimination half-life is 17 days (107). Because of this, long-term administration is not recommended, and the total dose in a 24-hr period usually does not exceed 1500 ml (20 ml/kg). Nevertheless, larger volumes (up to 3000 ml in 24 hr) have been administered in cardiac surgical patients without adverse effects (111).

Dextrans 40, 70, and 75 are biosynthetic glucose polymers with average molecular weights of 40,000, 70,000, and 75,000, respectively. Low-molecular-weight dextran (dextran 40) remains in the intravascular space for 2 to 4 hr, and the high-molecular-weight preparations (dextrans 70 and 75) for 12 hr (107). Dextrans have been used in cardiac surgery as volume expanders and as a priming fluid for cardiopulmonary bypass. A prominent side effect has been an antiplatelet action, resulting in a prolonged bleeding time and clinical bleeding. Hypersensitivity reactions occur more commonly than with hetastarch (118), and can be life-threatening. Dextran 70 causes red cell agglutination and interferes with cross-matching procedures performed by the blood bank. Therefore, with the availability of hetastarch, the use of dextrans for volume expansion after cardiac surgery should be avoided, if possible.

Experimental approaches to volume therapy include the use of oxygen-carrying solutions such as Fluosol-DA and stroma-free hemoglobin. Fluosol-DA is a perfluorocarbon emulsion with a linear oxygen-dissociation curve (119); it achieves significant dissolved oxygen concentrations only at arterial oxygen tensions close to 1 atmosphere (i.e., at 100% FiO_2). It has been used in patients with severe anemia who refuse blood, in the emergency treatment of patients with rare blood types, and in organ preservation (107, 120). Concerns regarding the stability of the emulsion, tissue uptake and storage, the long elimination time, and effects on the microcirculation have prevented general approval by the FDA; however, Fluosol remains available for investigational use. Stroma-free hemoglobin is devoid of red cell membrane components that may cause nephrotoxicity and coagulation disorders. The oxygen-dissociation curve is sigmoid but is shifted to the left, significantly impeding oxygen unloading at the tissue level (121, 122). Pyridoxylated stroma-free hemoglobin is a chemically altered hemoglobin that has a more normal oxygen dissociation curve; it can unload oxygen more readily under physiologic conditions and shows promise as a red cell substitute in animals (123, 124).

Nonhematogenous Therapies for Improvement in Hemostasis. Desmopressin acetate (DDAVP) reduces blood loss in transfusion requirements when administered intraoperatively or early postoperatively (125–127). It is given intravenously at a dose of 0.3 µg/kg in 30 ml normal saline infused over 30 min (126). It is especially useful in bleeding patients with severe platelet dysfunction after prolonged cardiopulmonary bypass or complex cardiac surgery (126, 127); it is less effective in uncomplicated cardiac surgical procedures with short pump times (128). Desmopressin shortens the template bleeding time and improves platelet function by increasing circulating levels of von Willebrand factor, thereby augmenting platelet adhesion to injured surfaces (126). Desmopressin also increases factor VIII:C levels, thereby shortening the partial thromboplastin time.

Protamine is useful in patients with prolonged partial thromboplastin or activated clotting times; usually these patients have received an inadequate neutralization dose of protamine upon termination of cardiopulmonary bypass, or have developed heparin rebound. An empiric dose of 25 to 50 mg of protamine sulfate is administered by slow intravenous infusion over 10 to 30 min. The drug should be avoided or used very cautiously in insulin-dependent diabetics who have taken NPH insulin, and in patients with a history of fish allergy, because of an increased risk of protamine sensitivity (129).

Aminocaproic acid (Amicar) is an antifibrinolytic agent that produces a small but significant decrease in postoperative bleeding after routine, elective coronary artery bypass grafting (130). It inhibits conversion of plasminogen to plasmin. It should not be used if there is evidence of disseminated intravascular coagulation, because of an increased risk of thrombus formation. A loading dose of 5 gm is administered intravenously over 5 min, followed by a 6-hr infusion (at 1 gm/hr).

Aprotinin (Trasylol) is an experimental drug that has been demonstrated to reduce bleeding and transfusion requirements when given as a continuous infusion during cardiopulmonary bypass (131, 132). It preserves platelet function by inhibition of kallikrein and plasmin, thus preventing platelet activation and thromboxane release (132). Dipyridamole also reduces postoperative bleeding by preserving platelet function during cardiopulmonary bypass when administered by intravenous infusion preoperatively, intraoperatively, and for 36 hr postoperatively (133). Prostacyclin infusion during cardiopulmonary bypass has been shown to reduce bleeding and improve platelet number and function, but the benefit has been small in some studies, and side effects have limited its use (134–136). Aprotinin, dipyridamole, and prostacyclin remain investigational drugs when ad-

ministered as intravenous infusions during cardiac surgery.

Aspirin may be withheld when postoperative hemostasis is severely disturbed. When the mediastinal bleeding has been controlled by appropriate therapy, it is our practice to reinstitute aspirin administration after a "safety" interval of 8 hr, during which time the bleeding should be minimal (less than 50 ml/hr).

Transfusion Practices

Transfusion therapy with donor blood is indicated if blood conservation methods fail to prevent severe anemia or if severe hemostatic defects persist with continued bleeding. Component therapy is favored because the optimal storage requirements vary for each of the blood components; stored whole blood is relatively deficient in platelets and in factors V and VIII (65, 137). Nevertheless, component therapy should be used judiciously, to minimize transfusion-associated complications and infectious disease transmission (Table 17.4). It should be remembered that a single unit of donor platelets or plasma carries as much risk of disease transmission as a unit of erythrocytes (79). Elimination of one of two exposures in a patient receiving 10 or fewer units of donor blood components achieves a substantial reduction in infectious risk, since the risk of transmitting non-A, non-B hepatitis peaks at 10 to 15 exposures (79).

Red Blood Cells.   Transfusion of banked red blood cells is indicated when the hematocrit is less that 25% (hemoglobin less than 8.3 gm/dl). A moderate degree of anemia is usually well tolerated in the postoperative period, as long as normovolemic conditions are maintained (83, 138). However, in patients with very limited cardiac reserve, those at risk for perioperative ischemic injury, or in very elderly patients, a higher hematocrit of 30% (hemoglobin 10 gm/dl) may be advisable (89).

The preferred component preparation is packed red blood cells in most instances (65, 137). Each unit of packed red blood cells should raise an average adult's hematocrit by 3% or hemoglobin by 1 gm/dl. The absence of such a rise indicates active bleeding, hemodilution from concomitant fluid administration, or hemolysis due to a transfusion reaction. Washed red blood cells are used in multiply transfused patients who have antibodies to donor immunoglobulin, and leukocyte-poor erythrocytes are used in multiply transfused patients who have been sensitized to HLA or cell-type specific antigens on leukocytes or platelets. Because of their expense, frozen red blood cells are principally used for rare blood types.

Platelets. Transfusion of platelets is indicated when the platelet count is less than 100,000/mm^3 in the presence of excessive mediastinal bleeding (139). Platelet transfusion is also indicated (regardless of platelet count) in actively bleeding patients with severe platelet dysfunction as manifested by a prolonged template bleeding time (more than 10 min if it is more than 2 hr after termination of cardiopulmonary bypass; see Tables 17.2 and 17.3). In patients without excessive bleeding, prophylactic platelet transfusion is unwarranted unless the platelet count is 20,000/mm^3 or lower (140). Massively transfused patients develop a dilutional thrombocytopenia which should be treated according to the aforementioned criteria and the presence or absence of continued bleeding. It should be noted that these recommendations differ from guidelines published for platelet transfusion in other settings (140, 141), due to the unusually complex nature of the platelet dysfunction resulting from cardiopulmonary bypass and the morbidity associated with continued mediastinal bleeding.

In general, 4 to 6 platelet packs are infused. Each platelet pack should raise the platelet count by 10,000/mm^3 for each square meter of body surface area; if this rise does not occur within 1 h after platelet infusion, then alloimmunization to random donor platelets or platelet consumption (e.g., due to disseminated intravascular coagulation) should be suspected. When alloimmunization occurs, platelet transfusions from HLA-matched donors or siblings may be given.

Fresh Frozen Plasma. Transfusion of fresh frozen plasma is indicated in patients with significant mediastinal bleeding who experience excessive consumption or dilution of coagulation factors (such as after prolonged cardiopul-

monary bypass or with the use of ventricular assist devices) (139). These patients typically have prolongation of both the prothrombin and partial thromboplastin times in excess of 1.2 times the control value despite protamine reversal of heparin effect. There may also be evidence of excessive fibrinolysis, with appearance of D-dimers, fibrinogen-fibrin degradation products, a shortened euglobulin clot lysis time, and a low fibrinogen level. An isolated prolongation of the partial thromboplastin time (more than 1.2 times control) with a normal postoperative prothrombin time (less than 1.2 times control) suggests heparin rebound or inadequate neutralization of heparin. Treatment with protamine (25 to 50 mg intravenously over 15 to 30 min) effectively neutralizes the residual heparin, and administration of fresh frozen plasma is often not necessary.

Transfusion of fresh frozen plasma is also indicated for patients with preexisting factor deficiencies, regardless of bleeding status. However, in several preexisting disorders, alternative therapies are available and may be tried first. These disorders include vitamin K deficiency, which is suggested by a compatible history (malabsorption, malnutrition, warfarin effect, prolonged antibiotic therapy) and confirmed by a prolonged prothrombin time. If the bleeding is not rapid, subcutaneous or intravenous administration of vitamin K may be effective. Patients with mild to moderate hemophilia A or von Willebrand's disease may respond to treatment with intravenous desmopressin.

Prophylactic administration of fresh frozen plasma is rarely indicated in nonbleeding patients, unless a preexisting factor deficiency has been identified. In massively transfused patients, the platelet concentrates that are usually administered for a dilutional thrombocytopenia contain approximately 50 ml of fresh plasma, so that routine use of fresh frozen plasma is frequently not necessary (142). Fresh frozen plasma is not indicated for use as a volume expander or as a nutritional source (142–144).

When indicated, 2 to 4 units of plasma are usually administered. It should be remembered that two forms of human plasma are available from the blood bank (143, 144). Fresh frozen plasma is derived from 1 unit of blood by centrifugation, separation, and freezing at $-18°C$ within 6 hr of collection. Single-donor plasma is prepared from whole blood up to 5 days after its expiration date, and also from outdated fresh frozen plasma; it is deficient in the labile clotting factors V and VIII. It is also deficient in fibrinogen if cryoprecipitate has been removed (142). Single-donor plasma is less expensive than fresh frozen plasma and is an acceptable substitute for fresh frozen plasma in many instances (e.g., liver disease, warfarin effect, massive transfusion, factor deficiencies except V and VIII) (142).

Cryoprecipitate. Cryoprecipitate contains factor VIII and fibrinogen. It may be used to treat excessive bleeding in patients with von Willebrand's disease, hemophilia A, uremia, and fibrinogen depletion states. Desmopressin is an alternative therapy for bleeding in the first three conditions because of its effect in releasing factor VIII from storage sites. Commercially produced factor VIII concentrates are also available for treatment of hemophilia.

References

1. Gomes MM, McGoon DC: Bleeding patterns after open heart surgery. *J Thorac Cardiovasc Surg* 60:87–97, 1970.
2. Craddock D, Logan A, Fodali A: Re-operation for hemorrhage following cardiopulmonary bypass. *Br J Surg* 55:17–20, 1968.
3. Verska J, Lonser E, Brewer L: Predisposing factors and management of hemorrhage following open-heart surgery. *J Cardiovasc Surg* 13:36–38, 1972.
4. Porter JM, Silver D: Alterations in fibrinolysis and coagulation associated with cardiopulmonary bypass. *J Thorac Cardiovasc Surg* 56:869–878, 1968.
5. Michelson EL, Torosian M, Morganroth J, et al: Early recognition of surgically correctable causes of excessive mediastinal bleeding after coronary artery bypass graft surgery. *Am J Surg* 139:313–317, 1980.
6. Bachmann F, McKenna R, Cole ER, et al: The hemostatic mechanism after open-heart surgery. I. Studies on plasma coagulation factors and fibrinolysis in 512 patients after extracorporeal circulation. *J Thorac Cardiovasc Surg* 70:76–85, 1975.
7. McKenna R, Bachmann F, Whittaker B: The hemostatic mechanism after open-heart surgery. II. Frequency of abnormal platelet functions during and after extracorporeal circulation. *J Thorac Cardiovasc Surg* 70:298–308, 1975.
8. Goldman S, Copeland J, Moritz T, et al: Improvement in early saphenous vein graft patency after coronary artery bypass surgery with antiplatelet therapy: results of a Veterans Administration Cooperative Study. *Circulation* 77:1324–1332, 1988.
9. Czer LSC, Bateman TM, Gray RJ, et al: Treatment of severe platelet dysfunction and hemorrhage after cardiopulmonary bypass: reduction in blood product usage with desmopressin. *J Am Coll Cardiol* 9:1139–1147, 1987.
10. Salzman EW, Weinstein MJ, Weintraub RM, et al: Treatment with desmopressin acetate to reduce blood loss after cardiac surgery. A double-blind randomized trial. *N Engl J Med* 314:1402–1406, 1986.
11. Harker LA, Malpass TW, Branson HE, et al: Mechanism of abnormal bleeding in patients undergoing cardiopulmonary bypass: acquired transient platelet dysfunction associated with selective alpha-granule release. *Blood* 56:824–834, 1980.
12. Harker LA: Bleeding after cardiopulmonary bypass. *N Engl J Med* 314:1446–1448, 1986.
13. Friedenberg WR, Myers WO, Plotka ED: Platelet dysfunction associated with cardiopulmonary bypass. *Ann Thorac Surg* 25:298–305, 1978.
14. Mammen EF, Koets MH, Washington BC, et al: Hemostasis changes during cardiopulmonary bypass surgery. *Semin Thromb Hemost* 11:281–292, 1985.
15. Salzman EW: Blood platelets and extracorporeal circulation. *Transfusion* 3:274–277, 1963.
16. de Leval M, Hill JD, Mielke H, et al: Platelet kinetics during extracorporeal circulation. *Trans Am Soc Artif Intern Organs* 18:355–358, 1972.
17. Umlas J: In vivo platelet function following cardiopulmonary bypass. *Transfusion* 15:596–599, 1975.
18. Hennessy VL, Hicks RE, Niewiarowski S, et al: Function of human platelets during extracorporeal circulation. *Am J Physiol* 232:622–628, 1977.
19. Beurling-Harbury C, Galvan CA: Acquired decrease in platelet secretory ADP associated with increased postoperative bleeding in post-car-

diopulmonary bypass patients and in patients with severe valvular heart disease. *Blood* 52:13–23, 1978.

20. Musial J, Niewiarowski S, Hershock D, et al: Loss of fibrinogen receptors from the platelet surface during simulated extracorporeal circulation. *J Lab Clin Med* 105:514–522, 1985.

21. Wachtfogel YT, Musial J, Jenkin B, et al: Loss of platelet α-adrenergic receptors during simulated extracorporeal circulation: prevention with prostaglandin E$_1$. *J Lab Clin Med* 105:601–607, 1985.

22. Boonstra PW, van Imhoff GW, Eysman L, et al: Reduced platelet activation and improved hemostasis after controlled cardiotomy suction during clinical membrane oxygenator perfusions. *J Thorac Cardiovasc Surg* 89:900–906, 1985.

23. Okies JE, Goodnight SH, Litchford. B, et al: Effects of infusion of cardiotomy suction blood during extracorporeal circulation for coronary artery bypass graft surgery. *J Thorac Cardiovasc Surg* 74:440–444, 1977.

24. King DJ, Kelton JG: Heparin-associated thrombocytopenia. *Ann Int Med* 100:535–540, 1984.

25. Cines DB, Tomaski A, Tannenbaum S: Immune endothelial-cell injury in heparin-associated thrombocytopenia. *N Engl J Med* 316:581–589, 1987.

26. Kirklin JK, Westaby S, Blackstone EH, et al: Complement and the damaging effects of cardiopulmonary bypass. *J Thorac Cardiovasc Surg* 86:845–857, 1983.

27. Smith EEJ, Naftel DC, Blackstone EH, et al: Microvascular permeability after cardiopulmonary bypass. An experimental study. *J Thorac Cardiovasc Surg* 94:225–233, 1987.

28. Salama A, Hugo F, Heinrich D, et al: Deposition of terminal C5b-9 complement complexes on erythrocytes and leukocytes during cardiopulmonary bypass. *N Engl J Med* 318:408–414, 1988.

29. Niinikoski J, Laato M, Laaksonen V, et al: Use of activated clotting time to monitor anticoagulation during cardiac surgery. *Scand J Thorac Cardiovasc Surg* 18:57–61, 1984.

30. Preiss DU, Schmidt-Bleibtreu H, Berguson P, et al: Blood transfusion requirements in coronary artery surgery with and without the activated clotting time (ACT) technique. *Klin Wochenschr* 63:252–256, 1985.

31. Babka R, Colby C, El-Etr A, et al: Monitoring of intraoperative heparinization and blood loss

following cardiopulmonary bypass surgery. *J Thorac Cardiovasc Surg* 73:780–782, 1977.

32. Verska JJ: Control of heparinization by activated clotting time during bypass with improved postoperative hemostasis. *Ann Thorac Surg* 24:170–173, 1977.

33. Bull BS, Huse WM, Brauer FS, et al: Heparin therapy during extracorporeal circulation. II. The use of a dose-response curve to individualize heparin and protamine dosages. *J Thorac Cardiovasc Surg* 69:685–689, 1975.

34. Bull BS, Korpman RA, Huse WM, et al: Heparin therapy during extracorporeal circulation. I. Problems inherent in existing heparin protocols. *J Thorac Cardiovasc Surg* 69:674–684, 1975.

35. Young JA, Kister CT, Doty DB: Adequate anticoagulation during cardiopulmonary bypass determined by activated clotting time and the appearance of fibrin monomer. *Ann Thorac Surg* 26:231–240, 1978.

36. Campbell FW, Goldstein MF Atkins PC: Management of the patient with protamine hypersensitivity for cardiac surgery. *Anesthesiology* 61:761–764, 1984.

37. Schrier SL: Disorders of hemostasis and coagulation. In Rubenstein E, Federman DD (eds): *Scientific American Medicine* New York, Scientific American, 1988, 5 Hematology, pp 1–49.

38. Sattler FR, Weitekamp MR, Ballard JO: Potential for bleeding with the new beta-lactam antibiotics. *Ann Intern Med* 105:924–931, 1986.

39. Abramowicz M (ed): *Handbook of Antimicrobial Therapy*, New York, The Medical Letter, 1986, p 8.

40. Michelson EL, Morganroth J, Torosian M, et al: Relation of preoperative use of aspirin to increased mediastinal blood loss after coronary artery bypass graft surgery. *J Thorac Cardiovasc Surg* 76:694–697, 1978.

41. Torosian M, Michelson EL, Morganroth J, et al: Aspirin- and Coumadin-related bleeding after coronary-artery bypass graft surgery. *Ann Intern Med* 89:325–328, 1978

42. Gray RJ, Bateman TM, Czer LSC, Conklin C, Matloff JM: Use of esmolol in hypertension after cardiac surgery. *Am J Cardiol* 56: 49F–56F, 1985.

43. Gray RJ, Bateman TM, Czer LSC, Conklin C, Matloff JM: Comparison of esmolol and nitroprusside for acute post-cardiac surgical hypertension. *Am J Cardiol* 59:887–891, 1987.

44. Ramsey G, Arvan DA, Stewart S, et al: Do preoperative laboratory tests predict blood transfusion needs in cardiac operations? *J Thorac Cardiovasc Surg* 85:564–569, 1983.

45. Rodewald G, Mathey D, Krebber H-J: Bypass surgery following thrombolytic therapy. *Z Kardiol* 74(Suppl 6):143–146, 1985.

46. Holub PA, Norman JC, Cooley DA: Successful aortocoronary bypass surgery for a patient with classical hemophilia A. *Cardiovasc Dis* 5:229–234, 1978.

47. Aris A, Pisciotta AV, Hussey CV, et al: Open-heart surgery for Von Willebrand's disease. *J Thorac Cardiovasc Surg* 69:183–187, 1975.

48. de Leval MR, Taswell HF, Bowie EJW, et al: Open heart surgery for patients with inherited hemoglobinopathies, red cell dyscrasias, and coagulopathies. *Arch Surg* 109:618–622, 1974.

49. Gagliardi C, D'Aviaro R, Stassamo P, et al: Open-heart surgery with factor VII deficiency. *J Cardiovasc Surg* 24:172–174, 1983.

50. Leggett PL, Doyle D, Smith WB, et al: Elective cardiac operation in a patient with severe hemophilia and acquired factor VIII antibodies. *J Thorac Cardiovasc Surg* 87:556–560, 1984.

51. Tourbaf KD, Bettigole RE, Zizzi JA: Coronary bypass in a patient with hemophilia B, or Christmas disease. Case report. *J Thorac Cardiovasc Surg* 77:562–569, 1979.

52. Brunken R, Follette D, Wittig J: Coronary artery bypass in hereditary factor XI deficiency. *Ann Thorac Surg* 38:406–408, 1984.

53. Kelly JP, Thomas L, Moulder PV, et al: Coronary bypass surgery in patients with circulating lupus anticoagulant. *Ann Thorac Surg* 40:261–263, 1985.

54. Czer L, Hamer A, Murphy F, et al: Transient hemodynamic dysfunction after myocardial revascularization. Temperature dependence. *J Thorac Cardiovasc Surg* 86:226–234, 1983.

55. Bateman TM, Czer LSC, Kass RM, et al: Cardiac causes of shock early after open-heart surgery: etiologic classification by radionuclide ventriculography. *Circulation* 71:1153–1161, 1985.

56. Gray R, Maddahi J, Berman D, et al: Scintigraphic and hemodynamic demonstration of transient left ventricular dysfunction immediately after uncomplicated coronary artery bypass grafting. *J Thorac Cardiovasc Surg* 77:504–510, 1979.

57. Bateman T, Gray R, Chaux A, et al: Right atrial tamponade complicating cardiac operation: clinical, hemodynamic and scintigraphic correlates. *J Thorac Cardiovasc Surg* 84:413–419, 1982.

58. Weiss MH, Bateman TM, Kass RM, et al: Extravascular obstruction of the superior vena cava by hematoma after open-heart surgery and diagnosis by scintigraphy. *Am J Cardiol* 51:1229–1231, 1983.

59. Bateman TM, Massumi R, Gray RJ, et al: Noninvasive detection of active pericardial bleeding using cardiac blood pool scintigraphy. *Am J Cardiol* 51: 329–331, 1983.

60. Bateman TM, Czer LSC, Gray RJ, et al: Detection of occult pericardial hemorrhage early after open-heart surgery using technetium-99m red blood cell radionuclide ventriculography. *Am Heart J* 108: 1198–1206, 1984.

61. Kronzon I, Cohen ML, Winer H: Cardiac tamponade by loculated pericardial hematoma: limitations of M-mode echocardiography. *J Am Coll Cardiol* 1:913–915, 1983.

62. Gondi B, Nanda NC: Two-dimensional echocardiographic diagnosis of mediastinal hematoma causing cardiac tamponade. *Am J Cardiol* 53:974–976, 1984.

63. Fyke FE III, Tancredi RG, Shub C, et al: Detection of intrapericardial hematoma after open heart surgery. The roles of echocardiography and computed tomography. *J Am Coll Cardiol* 5:1496–1499, 1985.

64. Milam JD, Austin SF, Martin RF, et al: Alteration of coagulation and selected clinical chemistry parameters in patients undergoing open heart surgery without transfusions. *Am J Clin Pathol* 76:155–162, 1981.

65. Schrier SL: Transfusion therapy. In Rubenstein E, Federman DD (eds): *Scientific American Medicine*. New York, 1985 5 Hematology X, pp 1–10.

66. Bove JR: Transfusion-associated hepatitis and AIDS. *N Engl J Med* 317:242–245, 1987.

67. Shorey J: Southwestern internal medicine conference: the current status of non-a non-B viral hepatitis. *Am J Med Sci* 289(6):251–261, 1985.

68. Ward JW, Holmberg SD, Allen JR, et al: Transmission of human immunodeficiency virus (HIV) by blood transfusions screened as negative for HIV antibody. *N Engl J Med* 318:473–478, 1988.

69. Scheinberg DA: Human immunodeficiency virus infection in transfusion recipients and their family members. *Morbidity and Mortality Weekly Report* 36:137–140, 1987.

70. Blomback M: Survey of non-U.S. Hemophilia treatment centers for HIV seroconversions fol-

lowing therapy with heat-treated factor concentrates. *Morbidity and Mortality Weekly Report* 36:121–124, 1987.

71. Burke DS, Brundage JR, Redfield RR, et al: Measurement of the false positive rate in a screening program for human immunodeficiency virus infections. *N Engl J Med* 319:961–964, 1988.

72. Weiss SH: AIDS due to HIV-2 infection—New Jersey. *Morbidity and Mortality Weekly Report* 37:33–35, 1988.

73. Williams AE, Fang CT, Slamon DJ, et al: Seroprevalence and epidemiological correlates of HTLV-I infection in U.S. blood donors. *Science* 240:643–646, 1988.

74. Larson CJ, Taswell HF: Human T-cell leukemia virus type I (HTLV-I) and blood transfusion. *Mayo Clin Proc* 63:869–875, 1988.

75. Bhagavati S, Ehrlich G, Kula RW, et al: Detection of human T-cell lymphoma/leukemia virus type I DNA and antigen in spinal fluid and blood of patients with chronic progressive myelopathy. *N Engl J Med* 318:1141–1147, 1988.

75a. Center for Disease Control. Risks associated with human parvovirus B19 infection. *Morbidity and Mortality Weekly Report* 38:81–97, 1989.

76. Davis JP: Yersinia enterocolitica bacteremia and endotoxin shock associated with red blood cell transfusion—United States, 1987–1988. *Morbidity and Mortality Weekly Report* 37:577–578, 1988.

77. Manuelidis EE, Kim JH, Mericangas JR, et al: Transmission to animals of Creutzfeldt-Jakob disease from human blood (letter). *Lancet* 2:896, 1985.

78. Jenike MA: Risk of using blood products from patients with dementia defined. In Rubenstein E, Federman DD (eds): *Scientific American Medicine*, New York, Scientific American, 1988, 13 Psychiatry, VII Alzheimer's Disease, p 2.

79. Thurer RL: Blood conservation in cardiac operations. *Mayo Clin Proc* 63:292–293, 1988.

80. McCarthy PM, Popovsky MA, Schaff HV, et al: Effect of blood conservation efforts in cardiac operations at the Mayo Clinic *Proc* 63:225–229, 1988.

81. Thurer RL, Hauer JM: Autotransfusion and blood conservation. In Ravitch MM (ed): *Current Problems in Surgery*. Chicago, Year Book, 1982, pp 100–156.

82. Cosgrove DM, Thurer RL, Lytle BW, et al: Blood conservation during myocardial revascularization. *Ann Thorac Surg* 28:184–189, 1979.

83. Kaplan JA, Cannarella C, Jones EL, et al: Au-
tologous blood transfusion during cardiac surgery. A re-evaluation of three methods. *J Thorac Cardiovasc Surg* 74:4–10, 1977.

84. Loop FD: Transfusion requirements of patients undergoing cardiovascular surgery. Lecture delivered during Symposium on Transfusion Therapy for the Surgical Patient, Cedars-Sinai Medical Center, Los Angeles, CA, February 20, 1987.

85. Council on Scientific Affairs: Council report. Autologous blood transfusions. *JAMA* 256:2378–2380, 1986.

86. Mann M, Sacks HJ, Goldfinger D: Safety of autologous blood donation prior to elective surgery for a variety of potentially "high-risk" patients. *Transfusion* 23:229–232, 1983.

87. Kruskall MS, Glazer EE, Leonard SS, et al: Utilization and effectiveness of a hospital autologous preoperative blood donor program. *Transfusion* 26:335–340, 1986.

88. Haugen RK, Hill GE: A large-scale autologous blood program in a community hospital. A contribution to the community's blood supply. *JAMA* 257:1121–1211, 1987.

89. Weisel RD, Charlesworth DC, Mickleborough LL, et al: Limitations of blood conservation. *J Thorac Cardiovasc Surg* 88:26–38, 1984.

90. Toy PTCY, Strauss RG, Stehling LC, et al: Predeposited autologous blood for elective surgery. A national multicenter study. *N Engl J Med* 316:517–520, 1987.

91. Surgenor DM: The patient's blood is the safest blood. *J Engl J Med* 316:542–544, 1987.

92. Schaff HV, Hauer JM, Bell WR, et al: Autotransfusion of shed mediastinal blood after cardiac surgery: a prospective study. *J Thorac Cardiovasc Surg* 75:632–641, 1978.

93. Thurer RL, Lytle BW, Cosgrove DM, et al: Autotransfusion following cardiac operations: a randomized, prospective study. *Ann Thorac Surg* 27:500–507, 1979.

94. Schaff HV, Hauer J, Gardner TJ, et al: Routine use of autotransfusion following cardiac surgery: experience in 700 patients. *Ann Thorac Surg* 27:493–499, 1979.

95. Cosgrove DM, Amiot DM, Meserko JJ: An improved technique for autotransfusion of shed mediastinal blood. *Ann Thorac Surg* 40:519–520, 1985.

96. Jacobs LM, Hsieh JW: A clinical review of autotransfusion and its role in trauma. *JAMA* 251:3283–3287, 1984.

97. Hartz RS, Smith JA, Green D: Autotransfusion after cardiac operation. Assessment of hemo-

static factors. *J Thorac Cardiovasc Surg* 96: 178–182, 1988.

98. Ansell J, Parrilla N, King M, et al: Survival of autotransfused red blood cells recovered from the surgical field during cardiovascular operations. *J Thorac Cardiovasc Surg* 84:387–391, 1984.

99. Orr M: Autotransfusion: The use of washed red cells as an adjunct to component therapy. *Surgery* 84:728–730, 1978.

100. Breyer RH, Engleman RM, Rousou JA, et al: A comparison of Cell Saver versus ultrafilter during coronary artery bypass operations. *J Thorac Cardiovasc Surg* 90:736–740, 1985.

101. Ottesen S, Froysaker T: Use of Haemonetics Cell Saver for Autotransfusion in cardiovascular surgery. *Scand J Thorac Cardiovasc Surg* 16:263–268, 1982.

102. Michalski AH, Lowenstein E, Austen WG, et al: Patterns of oxygenation and cardiovascular adjustment to acute, transient, normovolemic anemia. *Ann Surg* 168:946–956, 1968.

103. Messmer K, Lewis DH, Sunder-Plassman L, et al: Circulatory significance of hemodilution: rheologic changes and limitations. *Adv Microcir* 4:1, 1972.

104. Laks H, O'Connor NE, Pilon RN, et al: Acute normovolemic hemodilution; effects on hemodynamics, oxygen transport, and lung water in anesthetized man. *Surg Forum* 34:201, 1973.

105. LeVeen HH: Normovolemic hemodilution and autotransfusion in surgery. In Hauer JM (ed): *Autotransfusion.* New York, Elsevier/North Holland, 1981, p 71.

106. Czer LSC, Shoemaker WC: Optimal hematocrit value in critically ill postoperative patients. *Surg Gynecol Obstet* 147:363–368, 1978.

107. Bennett DR: Blood, blood components, and blood substitutes. In Bennett DR (ed): *AMA Drug Evaluations,* ed 5. Chicago, American Medical Association, 1983, pp 837–853.

108. Alving BM, et al: Hypotension associated with prekallikrein activator (Hageman-factor fragments) in plasma protein fraction. *N Engl J Med* 299:66–70, 1978.

109. Lazrove S, Waxman K, Shippy C, et al: Hemodynamic, blood volume, and oxygen transport responses to albumin and hydroxyethyl starch infusions in critically ill postoperative patients. *Crit Care Med* 8:302–306, 1980.

110. Diehl JT, Lester JL III, Cosgrove DM: Clinical comparison of hetastarch and albumin in postoperative cardiac patients. *Ann Thorac Surg* 34:674–679, 1982.

111. Kirklin JK, Lell WA, Kouchoukos NT: Hydroxyethyl starch versus albumin for colloid infusion following cardiopulmonary bypass in patients undergoing myocardial revascularization. *Ann Thorac Surg* 37:40–46, 1984.

112. Hicks GL Jr, Jensen LA, Norsen LH, et al: Platelet inhibitors and hydroxyethyl starch: safe and cost-effective interventions in coronary artery surgery. *Ann Thorac Surg* 39: 422–425, 1985.

113. Palanzo DA, Parr GVS, Bull AP, et al: Hetastarch as a prime for cardiopulmonary bypass. *Ann Thorac Surg* 34:680–683, 1982.

114. Sade RM, Crawford FA Jr, Dearing JP, et al: Hydroxyethyl starch in priming fluid for cardiopulmonary bypass. *J Thorac Cardiovasc Surg* 84:35–38, 1982.

115. Belcher P, Lennox SC: Avoidance of blood transfusion in coronary artery surgery: a trial of hydroxyethyl starch. *Ann Thorac Surg* 37:365–370, 1984.

116. Strauss RG: Review of the effects of hydroxyethyl starch on the blood coagulation system. *Transfusion* 21:299–302, 1981.

117. Strauss RG, Stump DC, Henriksen RA: Hydroxyethyl starch accentuates von Willebrand's disease. *Transfusion* 25:235–237, 1985.

118. Ring J, Messmer K: Incidence and severity of anaphylactoid reactions to colloid volume substitutes. *Lancet* 1:466–469, 1977.

119. Mitsuno C, Ohyanagi H, Naito R: Clinical studies of a perflurorochemical whole blood substitute (Fluosol-DA). *Ann Surg* 195:60–69, 1982.

120. Tremper KK, Friedman AE, Levine EM, et al: The preoperative treatment of severely anemic patients with a perfluorochemical oxygen-transport fluid, Fluosol DA. *N Engl J Med* 307:277–283, 1982.

121. Dudziak R, Bonhard K: The development of hemoglobin preparations for various indications. *Anaesthetist* 29:181, 1980.

122. Gould SA, Rosen S, Sehgal LR, et al: The effects of altered hemoglobin oxygen affinity on oxygen transport by hemoglobin solution. *J Surg Res* 28:246–251, 1980.

123. Greenburg AG, Schooley M, Ginsburg KA, et al: Pyridoxalated stroma-free hemoglobin in resuscitation of hemorrhagic shock. *Surg Forum* 29:44, 1978.

124. Sehgal LR, Rosen A, Noud G, et al: Large volume preparation of pyridoxalated hemoglobin with high in vivo P_{50}. *Eur Surg Res* 11(Suppl 2):43, 1979.

125. Czer L, Bateman T, Gray R, et al: Prospective trial of DDAVP in treatment of severe platelet dysfunction and hemorrhage after cardiopulmonary bypass (abstract). *Circulation* 72(Suppl III):130, 1985.

126. Czer LSC, Bateman TM, Gray RJ, et al: Treatment of severe platelet dysfunction and hemorrhage after cardiopulmonary bypass: reduction in blood product usage with desmopressin. *J Am Coll Cardiol* 9:1139–1147, 1987.

127. Salzman EW, Weinstein MJ, Weintraub RM, et al: Treatment with desmopressin acetate to reduce blood loss after cardiac surgery. A double-blind randomized trial. *N Engl J Med*, 314:1402–1406, 1986.

128. Rocha E, Llorens R, Paramo JA, et al: Does desmopressin acetate reduce blood loss after surgery in patients on cardiopulmonary bypass? *Circulation* 77:1319–1323, 1988.

129. Stewart WJ, McSweeney SM, Kellett MA, et al: Increased risk of severe protamine reactions in NPH insulin-dependent diabetics undergoing cardiac catheterization. *Circulation* 70:788–792, 1984.

130. Vander Salm TJ, Ansell JE, Okike ON, et al: The role of epsilon-aminocaproic in reducing bleeding after cardiac operation: a double-blind randomized study. *J Thorac Cardiovasc Surg* 95:538–540, 1988.

131. Royston D, et al: Effect of aprotinin on need for blood transfusion after repeat open-heart surgery. *Lancet* 2:1289–1291, 1987.

132. van Oeveren W, Jansen NJG, Bidstrup BP, et al: Effects of aprotinin on hemostatic mechanisms during cardiopulmonary bypass. *Ann Thorac Surg* 44:640–645, 1987.

133. Teoh KH, Christakis GT, Weisel RD: Preoperative dipyridamole reduces postoperative bleeding. *J Am Coll Cardiol* 7:139A, 1986.

134. Aren C, Feddersen K, Radegran K: Effects of prostacyclin infusion on platelet activation and postoperative blood loss in coronary bypass. *Ann Thorac Surg* 36:49–54, 1983.

135. DiSesa VJ, Huval W, Lelcuk S, et al: Disadvantages of prostacyclin infusion during cardiopulmonary bypass: a double-blind study of 50 patients having coronary revascularization. *Ann Thorac Surg* 38:514–519, 1984.

136. Fish KJ, Sarnquist FH, van Steennis C, et al: A prospective, randomized study of the effects of prostacyclin on platelets and blood loss during coronary bypass operations. *J Thorac Cardiovasc Surg* 91:436–442, 1986.

137. Myhre BA (ed): *Blood Component Therapy, a Physician's Handbook*, ed. 3. Washington, DC, American Association of Blood Banks, 1977, pp 1–55.

138. Consensus conference: perioperative red blood cell transfusion. *JAMA* 260:2700–2703, 1988.

139. Copeland JG, Harker LA, Joist JH, DeVries WC: Bleeding and anticoagulation. *Ann Thorac Surg* 47:88–95, 1989.

140. Consensus conference: platelet transfusion therapy. *JAMA* 257:1777–1780, 1987.

141. McCullough J, Steeper TA, Connelly DP, et al: Platelet utilization in a university hospital. *JAMA* 259:2414–2418, 1988.

142. Oberman HA: Inappropriate use of fresh-frozen plasma. *JAMA* 253:556–558, 1985.

143. Consensus conference: fresh-frozen plasma. Indications and risks. *JAMA* 253:551–553, 1985.

144. Bove JR: Fresh frozen plasma: too few indications—too much use. *Anesth Analg* 848–850, 1985.

Chapter 18
MANAGEMENT OF COMMON POSTOPERATIVE ARRHYTHMIAS

RICHARD J. GRAY, M.D.
WILLIAM J. MANDEL, M.D.

RHYTHM DISTURBANCES

An appreciation of postoperative rhythm disturbances paralleled the emerging specialty of cardiac surgery in the 1950s (1, 2). It is interesting to note that the spectrum of atrial and ventricular arrhythmias has not materially changed since the pre-coronary bypass, pre-cardiac valve prosthesis era described in an excellent 1961 review (3). This is despite significant changes in patient age, etiology of disease and indications for surgery, and advancements in understanding of myocardial preservation, surgical technique, and postoperative care.

ATRIAL ARRHYTHMIAS

Incidence and Natural History

The incidence of supraventricular tachyarrhythmias approximates 30% following coronary bypass operations. It is even higher in valve-related surgery, particularly in elderly patients undergoing valve replacement for aortic stenosis, in whom the incidence is reported to be as high as 60% (4). Atrial fibrillation is by far the most common arrhythmia observed, fol-

lowed in order by atrial flutter and paroxysmal atrial tachycardia, and, lastly, various junctional rhythms.

Although atrial tachyarrhythmias can occur at any time for up to 2 to 3 weeks during convalescence, the peak incidence is between postoperative days 3 and 5 (5). There is also a tendency for these arrhythmias to be associated with certain discrete elements of the surgical procedure, such as induction of anesthesia, atrial cannulation, and attempts to wean from cardiopulmonary bypass. An interesting and not unusual finding is that of atrial fibrillation occurring during the initial phases of rewarming from hypothermia. The ventricular response rate is often somewhat slower, generally 100 to 120 beats/min, most always followed by spontaneous conversion to sinus rhythm during the later phases of rewarming.

The clinical consequences of atrial tachyarrhythmias vary tremendously. When they occur in the more common setting 4 or 5 days postoperatively, many patients are asymptomatic and demonstrate no hemodynamic consequences. More commonly, a sense of chaotic palpitations is readily apparent, but blood pressure and cardiac output are maintained at slightly lower levels than usual, even during bed rest. Significant reductions in blood pressure and cardiac output ensue, mostly in patients whose tenuous cardiac reserve depends heavily on the atrial contribution to cardiac filling. This is particularly true of such occurrences in the operating room. Another special circumstance in which rapid atrial fibrillation is likely to be poorly tolerated is a patient with partial or incomplete myocardial revascularization. Here, the increase in myocardial oxygen consumption and reduction of diastolic coronary filling time act functionally as a stress test, occasionally producing ischemic chest pain.

The appearance of frequent premature atrial complexes is considered to be a good predictor for the development, within hours, of atrial fibrillation or flutter. Patients attempting to remember an event that may have triggered such an occurrence often recall a coughing bout or sneezing or undergoing respiratory therapy just prior to the development of an atrial tachyarrhythmia. Whether inhalation therapy or use of bronchodilators is causally linked to atrial fibrillation is difficult to determine since both are very common, even in the absence of each other.

Etiology

At present, the mechanism responsible for postoperative atrial tachyarrhythmias is not known. It is tempting to speculate that pericarditis, so common at this time in convalescence, plays an important role; however, this has not been convincingly demonstrated.

The clinical correlates have been analyzed extensively, and it appears that myocardial ischemic time may be related to atrial fibrillation (6). In this same study, age, sex, severity of symptoms, cardiomegaly, heart failure, previous myocardial infarction, and number of bypass grafts were not significantly related to the occurrence of postoperative atrial fibrillation. In a group of individuals having valve replacement for aortic stenosis, age (over 70 years) was a factor, as well as the coexistence of mitral regurgitation or stenosis with significantly elevated pulmonary artery pressures (4).

The possible role played by the well-described elevation in serum catecholamines and possible

changes in β-adrenergic receptor function must also be considered. Evidence for this includes the documentation of elevated norepinephrine and epinephrine levels that may persist up to several days after surgery, the coexistence of sinus tachycardia in other patients, and demonstration, at least in several studies, that β-blockade is successful in preventing supraventricular tachyarrhythmias, especially in patients medicated preoperatively with such agents (7, 8).

Preservation of cardiac structure and function is heavily dependent on hypothermia during cardiopulmonary bypass. Inadequate preservation of the atrium has come under suspicion as a cause of postoperative atrial fibrillation. Atrial hypothermia is less profound, due in part to differential delivery of cardioplegic solution via the coronary circulation and the less effective means of achieving atrial hypothermia by topical cooling of the heart (9). These findings were confirmed in an experimental animal model that demonstrated that ischemic injury of the supraventricular conduction system during hypothermic cardiopulmonary bypass primarily caused delay within the AV node. This delay was prevented in the experimental setting by better atrial hypothermia using intracavitary and specialized topical techniques (10). Other investigators have been able to corroborate the inadequacy of atrial preservation by demonstrating persistence of electrical activity within the AV junctional area, and markedly improved the likelihood of early postoperative sinus rhythm in the animals in which persistent electrical activity was abolished with special ice lavage in the right atrioventricular junction area (11).

Management

Prophylaxis

Preoperative digitalization (1 to 1.5 mg orally beginning 2 to 3 days prior to surgery) resulted in a much lower incidence of supraventricular tachyarrhythmias (5.5%) than in a control group (26%) (12). A similar reduction in the incidence of supraventricular tachyarrhythmia was noted with postoperative digitalization (2% versus 15%) (13). Others using preoperative digitalization were unable to confirm this benefit; in fact, one study demonstrated a higher incidence of postoperative tachyarrhythmia in the treated group (27.8%) versus that of the untreated group (11.4%) (14).

Many other attempts at prevention of postoperative atrial arrhythmias have included various β-blocking agents. Actually, the benefits of propranolol in postoperative atrial tachycardias had been appreciated more than 2 decades ago (15). There have been numerous studies demonstrating successful prevention of postoperative supraventricular tachyarrhythmias using propranolol begun postoperatively (7, 8, 16, 17), and one study using preoperative administration of propranolol (18). The results and dosages used are summarized in Table 18.1 (19). This otherwise successful picture is clouded somewhat by the finding, in one double-blind randomized study, that 80 mg daily of propranolol was not effective in reducing the incidence of supraventricular tachyarrhythmia (19) despite the fact that the dosage employed in this latter study was larger than in the other studies that demonstrated efficacy of propranolol. Similar efficacy for prevention of postoperative tachyarrhythmias was demonstrated for timolol (0.5 mg intravenously twice daily) (20), as well as acebutolol, a cardioselective β-blocker (21). Combinations of postoperative digoxin and propranolol were also found to be effective in reducing the incidence of postoperative supraventricular tachyarrhythmia in two studies (22, 23).

TABLE 18.1

SUMMARY OF EFFECTS OF PROPRANOLOL ON POSTOPERATIVE SUPRAVENTRICULAR TACHYARRHYTHMIAS (SVT)[a]

Drug	Time Started	Incidence of SVT	
		Control Group	Treatment Group
		%	%
Propranolol (40 mg)	18 hr postop	18	8
Propranolol (20–40 mg)	6 hr postop	40	5
Propranolol (60 mg)	2 days postop	28	2.2
Digoxin	1 day preop		

[a]Modified from Ivey MF, Ivey TD, Bailey WW, et al: Influence of propranolol on supraventricular tachycardia early after coronary artery revascularization. *J Thorac Cardiovasc Surg* 85:214–218, 1983.

Verapamil 40 mg three times daily begun postoperatively was not successful in prevention of supraventricular arrhythmias (5), whereas in a separate study 80 mg every 6 hr was beneficial but resulted in an unacceptably high incidence of hypotension, pulmonary edema, or cardiogenic shock (24).

The majority of studies, however, favor the use of small doses of propranolol as an agent for prophylaxis of supraventricular arrhythmias in the postoperative cardiovascular surgical patient. This is especially true in individuals taking β-blocking agents preoperatively.

The authors' experience with arrhythmia prophylaxis using both pre- and postoperative digitalization regimens as well as postoperative propranolol has been very disappointing. Consequently, it is our policy to begin medical therapy only at the development of the arrhythmia or at the appearance of frequent atrial premature complexes.

Medical Management

Digitalization is the first line of therapy and is indicated at the time of appearance of frequent atrial premature complexes or the appearance of atrial tachyarrhythmias if the ventricular response rate is faster than 100 beats/min. The dosing regimen depends on initial heart rate, the urgency of conversion, patient age, body size, and renal function. With moderately rapid ventricular response rates (130 to 150 beats/min) in a patient aged 60 to 70 years with normal renal function, 1.0 to 1.5 mg administered over 24 hr is often successful. During the loading phase the intravenous route is recommended to ensure rapid and more complete absorption. By the end of the loading phase, conversion to sinus rhythm usually has occurred; but if not, additional incremental doses of digoxin (total 0.5 mg) can be administered up to a total of 2.0 mg in 36 hr. The end point of digoxin administration, in addition to return to sinus rhythm, will be to control heart rate (i.e., 100 to 110 beats/min or less). Additional supplementation with intravenous propranolol in 1-mg doses is occasionally needed for more complete slowing of the heart rate. Verapamil in the dosage of 5 to 10 mg intravenously has demonstrated effectiveness in slowing the ventricular response rate in most patients and is associated with return to sinus rhythm is approximately 20% of patients (25). Intravenous verapamil has been associated with hypotension occasionally, which is lessened by a slower infusion rate and can be aborted by previous administration of calcium chloride (26). Diltiazem has also demonstrated efficacy in reduction of the ventricular response rate in atrial tachyarrhythmias via inhibition of AV node conduction (27).

More recently, esmolol, an ultrashort-acting intravenous β-blocking agent, has demonstrated effectiveness in controlling the heart rate of postoperative supraventricular tachyarrhythmia (28). The incidence of conversion to sinus rhythm with esmolol is better than placebo and possibly superior to other agents such as verapamil and diltiazem.

If, after these measures have been used, return to sinus rhythm has not occurred, the next step is selection of a type I antiarrhythmic such as quinidine sulfate or procainamide hydrochloride. Oral quinidine sulfate 200 to 300 mg every 2 to 6 hr has been a traditional approach to the medical conversion of supraventricular tachyarrhythmias, particularly atrial fibrillation. Intravenous procainamide hydrochloride has demonstrated effectiveness in acute termination of atrial fibrillation and flutter when given as a 10 to 20 mg/kg loading dose followed by a maintenance infusion of 2 to 4 mg/min (29).

Intravenous amiodarone in the dosage of 2.5 to 5 mg/kg (via central intravenous line) has been moderately successful in conversion to sinus rhythm and slowing of the ventricular response rate but, because of concern over side effects, is not a first-line drug (30).

The above comments apply to the management of atrial fibrillation, while therapy directed toward control of common atrial flutter may require a different response. Digoxin remains indicated as the drug of first choice; however, doses similar to those effective for atrial fibrillation do not often appreciably increase AV blockade. The initial AV conduction ratio is commonly 2:1, resulting in a ventricular response of 150 beats/min. In the presence of AV nodal conduction abnormalities or pretreatment with digoxin, the ventricular rate may be slower as a result of a 3:1 or 4:1 conduction ratio. Loading dosages of digoxin varying from 1.5 to 2.0 mg are often necessary, and even then may result in unpredictable and often disappointingly minor slowing of ventricular response rate. By the time AV blockade occurs, patients may exhibit signs or symptoms suggestive of digoxin toxicity. Consequently, β-blockers and calcium channel blockers such as esmolol, verapamil, and diltiazem have an important role in slowing the ventricular response. Once an arbitrary initial digitalization dosage has been reached (generally 1.5 to 2.0 mg), or when the clinical picture suggests digoxin toxicity, esmolol in the dosage of 0.5 mg/kg over 1 min with a titrated maintenance infusion, or verapamil in the dosage of 5 to 10 mg given intravenously over 1 min is indicated; verapamil may also be used as a constant infusion. These pharmacologic maneuvers are extremely successful in rapidly slowing the ventricular response rate. The results may be transient, thereby requiring repeat administration or constant infusion. Moreover, conversion to sinus rhythm in a relative minority of cases occurs. β-Blockade using intravenous propranolol (0.05 to 0.10 mg/kg) given in increments of 1 mg by slow intravenous bolus injection may also slow the ventricular response rate.

Paroxysmal atrial tachycardia generally related to AV nodal reentry or ectopic atrial rhythms is less common. Traditionally, the first steps include sedation if agitated, often followed by carotid sinus massage. As in the nonsurgical variety, management usually includes intravenous verapamil or digitalization, which results in a high likelihood of conversion to sinus rhythm. Preliminary experience with intravenous adenosine triphosphate has been highly encouraging (31, 32). This naturally occurring high-energy phosphate, when given as a rapid bolus of 20 mg intravenously, blocked the antegrade slow pathway through the AV node, rapidly terminating paroxysmal atrial tachycardia in all patients tested.

Elective Cardioversion

This treatment is reserved for drug treatment failures. It is uncommon for post-coronary bypass patients with no previous history of atrial arrhythmias to require this modality. Cardioversion is more commonly used in patients undergoing valve surgery, especially mitral valve replacement, in whom atrial fibrillation, once established, becomes difficult to revert medically.

If atrial fibrillation is chronic and has been established for more than 1 year preoperatively, aggressive attempts inlcuding cardioversion are not generally recommended because of the high likelihood of relapse to atrial fibrillation. An exception to this is the patient who exhibits several hours of sinus rhythm immediately after return from the operating room. Elective cardioversion may be used if aggressive medical measures fail, including digoxin (if indicated by the presence of a rapid ventricular respnose rate) and quinidine or procainamide or both.

The principal risk of cardioversion, that is, thromboembolism, is approximately 0.5%. In our institution this procedure is performed in a unit equipped for bedside electrocardiographic monitoring. That morning's digoxin dose is held and, if toxicity is clinically suspected, a serum digoxin level is obtained. A serum potassium level should be obtained the morning of cardioversion, and the patient given nothing by mouth for at least 6 hr prior to the procedure. A well-running intravenous tube is inserted. Oxygen 4 to 6 liters by mask is used, and a "crash cart" with intubation equipment and ambu bag is in the patient's room. We prefer the extremely short-acting, but profound effects of brevitol, and arrange to have the patient's anesthesiologist available for administration of the sedative and analgesic and for management of the airway. The safety factor thus provided more than outweighs the small added inconvenience of arranging for an additional physician. Anterior and posterior paddles (placed just beneath the tip of the left scapula) are preferred for conversion of atrial fibrillation. Atropine and lidocaine are available for immediate use. The synchronization circuit is carefully checked.

Direct current shocks are then delivered in a stepwise fashion. Initial shocks are in the low range (i.e., 10 to 30 W) to assess possible induction of ventricular arrhythmias. If atrial fibrillation does not convert at the maximum power setting, anterior paddles are then used at the maximum power setting.

Anticoagulation for cardioversion to terminate a brief period (days) of postoperative atrial fibrillation is not routinely practiced.

Overdrive Pacing

Atrial flutter and paroxysmal supraventricular tachycardia are readily terminated by rapid stimulation of the atrium, using surgically implanted epicardial pacemaker wires. Atrial flutter must be differentiated from atrial fibrillation that is not amenable to overdrive pacing. Two types of atrial fibrillation can be recognized by atrial bipolar electrocardiograms. Type I atrial fibrillation has discrete but irregular atrial activity on epicardial right atrial bipolar recordings interspersed with an isoelectric baseline. Type II fibrillation has similar discrete atrial activity but with no isoelectric portion. The term atrial flutter-fibrillation usually refers to an atrial flutter wave on surface electrocardiogram, but with irregular ventricular conduction as opposed to the predictable conduction ratio (2:1, 3:1, or 4:1) seen in typical atrial flutter. Flutter-fibrillation is not amenable to overdrive pacing; it either represents a form of type I or type II atrial fibrillation or, as has been witnessed in the operating room and in the experimental animal, flutter of the right atrium and fibrillation of the left atrium.

Overdrive pacing should always be performed using a bedside monitor and with a rhythm strip (with multiple leads of possible, i.e., I, aVF, V) to determine the success of atrial capture and termination of the arrhythmia.

The pacing rate is selected to be just below the spontaneous rate and is increased by increments of 10 beats/min until capture is obtained. Capture of the atrium usually requires a rate 10 beats faster than the spontaneous atrial rate, and successful entrainment of the flutter rhythm requires a gradual increase in rate until the flutter waves become positive in orientation as monitored in standard ECG lead 2 (fig. 18.1) (33). Once atrial flutter has been entrained, sinus rhythm will ensue following abrupt cessation of pacing. If atrial flutter has been intermittently recurrent, control of the atrial mechanism may require short-term continuous

FIGURE 18.1

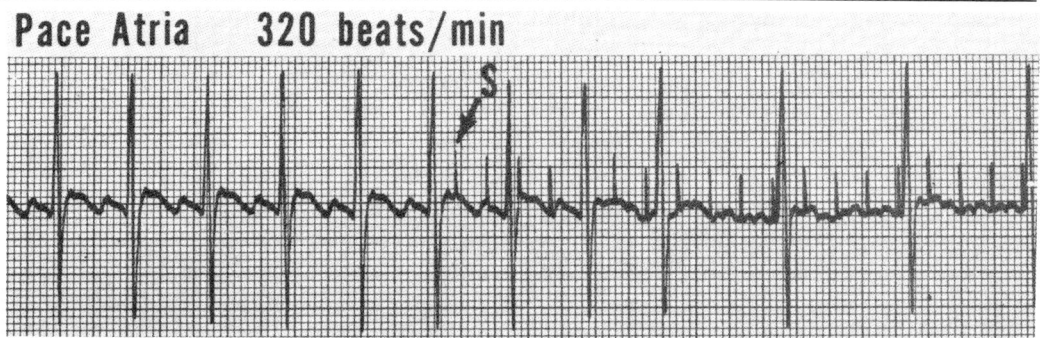

Pace Atria   320 beats/min

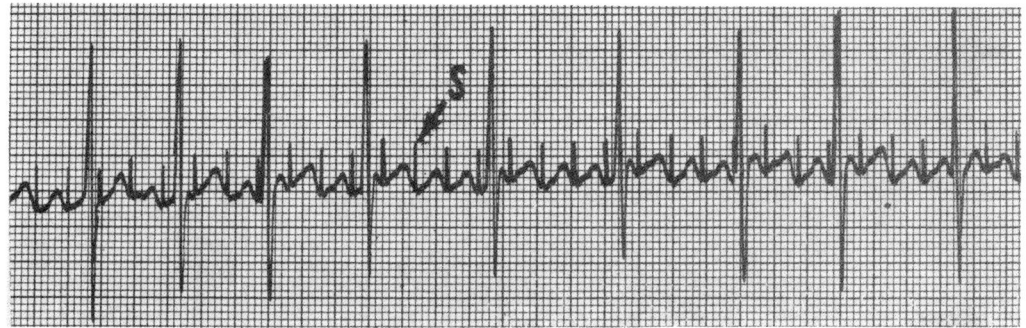

ECG lead II recorded in a patient following open heart surgery. In the top trace, atrial pacing at a rate of 320 beats/min was initiated. The atrial complexes in the ECG that had been predominantly negative became somewhat positive and notched. The bottom trace was recorded several seconds after the top trace. Note that now, although the atrial pacing rate remained 320 beats/min, the atrial complexes have become markedly positive. In fact, their configuration is what one would expect when pacing from the region of the sinus node. *S*, stimulus artifact. (From Cooper TB, MacLean WAH, Waldo AL: Overdrive pacing for supraventricular tachycardia. A review of theoretical implications and therapeutic techniques. *PACE I*:196–221, 1978, with permission.)

atrial pacing, which can be achieved by gradual reduction of the atrial pacing rate to the appropriate physiologic level for that patient. Continuous atrial pacing in this mode over several hours may prevent the recurrence of atrial flutter or even fibrillation.

Failure to convert atrial flutter can be due to a number of factors. First, if the ventricular response rate is irregular, the diagnosis is not typical type I atrial flutter and overdrive pacing usually will not succeed. A broken pacemaker wire or loss of contact with the epicardial surface will also result in failure, but if only one such wire is broken unipolar pacing can be attempted using an electrode patch close to the functional wire exit on the skin surface. Insufficient stimulus strength is occasionally a problem because the threshold for capture may have risen to high levels, especially sev-

eral days after surgery. The threshold will occasionally be above 20 mA, which is the capacity of most commercially available pacemakers. A standard commerically available rapid atrial stimulator (e.g., Medtronics model 5375/2312) can be modified to deliver 25 to 28 mA. It should be noted that stimulus strength above 20 mA almost always results in symptomatic awareness, although this is usually tolerable for brief periods of time once the rationale has been explained to the patient. Finally, a weak pacemaker battery or inadequate contact between the leads and pacemaker must also be excluded.

Often additional dosing with digoxin, quinidine, or procainamide, or simply the passage of time, will ensure greater success. Consequently, repeated attempts at overdrive pacing should be tried until successful. The atrial arrhythmia will likely continue or recur as long as the stimulus responsible for it continues. Thus, it is almost always necessary to continue therapy with digoxin, and occasionally with β-blockers or type I antiarrhythmics as well, despite the success or failure of overdrive pacing.

Rapid atrial overdrive may occasionally precipitate atrial fibrillation. Because the ventricular response rate is often slower than in atrial flutter, this may be a desirable alternative and can usually be achieved by pacing the atria at rates of 450 beats/min or higher for 10 to 20 seconds. Atrial overdrive can be used to reduce the ventricular response in atrial flutter despite failure to reach sinus rhythm. With rapid overdrive pacing at 400 beats/min, for instance, the atrial conduction can be reduced from 2:1 at 150 beats/min to 4:1 at 100 beats/min.

Bipolar atrial electrograms can be recorded by attaching one epicardial lead to each of the two arm leads of the ECG patient cable using an alligator clip. By recording standard lead I on the lead selector, the bipolar atrial electrogram is recorded, since standard lead I records between right and left arm leads. By selecting lead II or III, unipolar atrial electrograms can be recorded. Similarly, unipolar electrograms can be recorded by attaching the patient cables to the appropriate limbs, but attaching the atrial electrodes to the precordial patient lead and recording with the selector in the V lead. Since bipolar atrial electrograms record electrical activity only within the tissue subtended between their positions on the heart, limited or no ventricular activity will be seen in such a recording. Since the unipolar technique records the potential difference between a single atrial electrode and an indifferent electrode distant from the heart, both atrial and ventricular electrical activity will be recorded. This type of recording is preferable when the relationship between atrial and ventricular events is useful. The bipolar electrogram technique, when viewed with a simultaneous surface electrocardiogram, is the preferred technique since it allow clear-cut differentiation of the atrial and ventricular origin of signals and their relationship with each other (Fig. 18.2) (34).

VENTRICULAR ARRHYTHMIAS

Ventricular ectopy, including nonsustained ventricular tachycardia, requiring at least a short course of therapy is seen early in the convalescence in up to 50% of patients after open-heart surgery. As with atrial tachyarrhythmias, the incidence is particularly high in the operating room during induction of anesthesia, cannulation for cardiopulmonary bypass, early weaning from bypass, and the rewarming period. An especially high incidence is also noted beginning on the 3rd and 4th postoperative days. The reported incidence varies with the intensity of monitoring employed; a 57% incidence of complex ventricular arrhythmias (Lown grades 4 and 5) was detected in one study using continuous ambulatory monitoring (35). Although the mechanism and prognosis of postoperative ventricular arrhythmias are not well understood, those occurring in the setting of ischemic heart disease and coronary bypass surgery have been studied to a slightly greater degree.

In a given patient, ventricular arrhythmias are more frequent after surgery, at least within the first 6 or 8 weeks, than they were preoperatively. Furthermore, exercise-induced ventricular ectopy is not reduced, but in fact appears to increase, despite successful revascularization (36). Exercise ventricular ectopy is particularly associated in the patient with extensive coronary disease, a lower resting ejection fraction, and more than 2 mm of ischemic S-T segment depression (37). Similarly, after apparently successful revascularization, continuation or new appearance of exercise-induced ventricular arrhythmias is associated with previous myocardial infarction (34), as well as severe wall motion abnormalities and residual postoperative ischemic S-T segment depression (35).

Potential mechanisms that must be considered include the impact of the elevation in circulating catecholamines known to persist for several days after surgery, the occurrence of clinical or subclinical myocardial necrosis, and the effects of electrolyte abnormalities and postoperative digitalis administration. Studies on the natural history of these arrhythmias are conflicting, one study finding that even single premature ventricular contractions on a resting

FIGURE 18.2

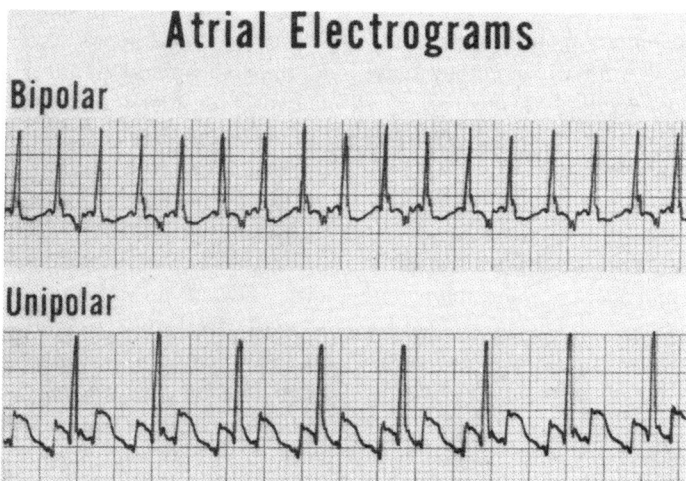

Atrial Electrograms

Bipolar

Unipolar

Simultaneous recording of bipolar and unipolar atrial electrograms using a two-channel ECG machine with the standard arm leads of the ECG patient cable attached and showing the recording selector on the standard lead I (bipolar atrial electrogram) and standard lead II (unipolar atrial electrogram) positions. The rhythm disorder is type I (classical) atrial flutter at a rate of 280 beats/min with 2:1 A-V conduction. (From Waldo AL, MacLean WAH (eds): *Diagnosis and Treatment of Cardiac Arrhythmias following Open Heart Surgery*. Mount Kisco, NY, Futura, 1980, p 25.)

electrocardiogram was a prediction of poor outcome after bypass (38), whereas a more recent study showed no difference in survival based on the presence or absence of complex ventricular ectopy on ambulatory monitoring in a postbypass population carefully selected for normal preoperative ventricular function (35).

Signal-averaged electrocardiography ("late potentials") is believed to have prognostic value in the nonsurgical patient with respect to future occurrence of serious ventricular arrhythmias, and shows promise in the postoperative patient as well (39).

Until more conclusive data emerge, a responsible approach to treatment should be based on lessons learned from a nonsurgical population and individualized based on known or suspected risk factors and the patient's medical history. For instance, high-grade ventricular ectopy in the presence of ventricular dysfunction or segmental wall motion defects, recent myocardial infarction, or recent appearance of ectopy would all suggest a higher risk of untoward outcome. Similarly, a history of sudden cardiac death, sustained ventricular tachycardia, or fibrillation would also impose higher risk and warrant more aggressive therapy.

Persistent frequent ventricular ectopy of 6/min or more should begin to arouse concern. Often this activity can be suppressed by atrial pacing. This is accomplished by progressively increasing the rate until the desired level of suppression is seen. However, it is rare to see benefits with pacing rates above 110 beats/min.

With the new appearance of ventricular ectopy, surveillance for a metabolic or other inciting cause should be routine and initiated promptly. This would include, at minimum, measurement of serum potassium and blood count and assessment of oxygenation status, using either arterial blood gas or noninvasive oximetry (ear lobe or fingertip). The yield in this endeavor will be low, but it should be kept in mind that in comparison with the nonsurgical patient, such abnormalities are much more common and are more poorly tolerated in the post-cardiac surgical patient, and the potential risk of missing such eminently treatable abnormalities can be high.

The decision to use intravenous lidocaine is based on the occurence of frequent or high-grade ventricular ectopy (usually more than 6 premature ventricular contractions per min, R-on-T phenomenon, frequent couplets, or multiform ectopy) or when therapy is likely to be needed for only a short duration. For instance, even in the absence of metabolic factors, brief periods of high-grade ventricular ectopy may occur within the first 4 or 5 days after surgery. Intravenous therapy for as little as 12 hr may be followed by complete freedom from serious ventricular ectopy for the remainder of the hospital course.

Initiation of intravenous lidocaine with changeover to an oral agent is indicated when ventricular ectopy persists despite continued lidocaine, or when preoperative high-grade ectopy returns and therapy with an oral agent alone is not sufficient.

Lidocaine is traditionally administered as a bolus (1 mg/kg) followed by a 2 to 4 mg/min maintenance infusion. Dosing and pharmacology are clinically similar to those of the nonsurgical patient. The principal side effect is disorientation and agitation typically seen in older individuals and those with diminished liver function, usually in the setting of low cardiac output and diminished liver blood flow.

As an alternative, or in addition to lidocaine when it alone is not successful in ectopy suppression, intravenous pronestyl hydrochloride can also be used. An initial loading dose of 5 to 10 mg/kg (30 to 50 mg/min infusion rate) is followed by a maintenance infusion of 2 to 3 mg/min.

Initiation of therapy with an oral agent alone is indicated when the initial presentation is noncomplex ectopy such as frequent singular ectopics or bigeminy, and when therapy is likely to be long-term such as with the history of preoperative arrhythmia. When antiarrhythmic therapy had been used prior to surgery, it is wise to restart the same agent as long as it was well tolerated and seemingly effective. Although many newer agents are now available for oral use, procainamide and quinidine preparations remain extremely popular. Table 18.2 summarizes prescribing indications, dosages, and side effects of these and the newer antiarrhythmics. It should be noted that amiodarone, because of its potential serious side effects, is usually reserved for life-threatening arrhythmias refractory to other agents.

Treatment of ventricular tachycardia is often initiated with lidocaine, especially if nonsustained. Sustained ventricular tachycardia will also respond and lidocaine can be used as long as relative hemodynamic stability is maintained. If resistant or recurrent ventricular tachycardia occurs despite lidocaine, bretylium may be used. Therapy is begun with a loading dose of 5 to 10 mg/kg given over 30 min, followed by an infusion of 1 to 4 mg/min. As with procainamide hydrochloride, hypotension is the major side effect, in this case resulting from the vasodilating properties of bretylium. Polymorphic ventricular tachycardia, a particularly resistant form of ventricular tachycardia known as torsade de pointes, is characterized by a QRS pattern that meanders above and below the baseline. It is occasionally seen after surgery and is most commonly the result of toxicity or adverse reaction to a drug, usually an antiarrhythmic such as quinidine sulfate or procainamide. The initial approach is to stop any offending medication. The usual therapy for ventricular tachycardia is suggested but may be ineffective. Ventricular pacing at a rapid rate is most often helpful, and the addition of intravenous isoproterenol infusion is also indicated if other therapy fails. Bolus injection of intravenous magnesium sulfate (500 to 1000 mg) has also been helpful.

Therapy for ventricular fibrillation begins with rapid defibrillation followed by CPR measures if needed.

Conduction Disturbances

Intraventricular (Fascicular) Conduction Defects

The early postoperative appearance of fascicular conduction defects, including right bundle-branch block, left anterior superior fascicular block (and combinations of the two), as well as left bundle-branch block and interventricular conduction delay of unspecified type, occurs with moderate frequency (3 to 5%). Although long-term adverse prognosis is ascribed to left bundle-branch block and nonspecific interventricular conduction delay, postoperative bundle-branch block has no immediate clinical impact and specific treatment is not needed. These findings are discussed more fully in Chapter 11.

TABLE 18.2

INDICATIONS, DOSAGES, AND SIDE EFFECTS OF ANTIARRHYTHMIC DRUGS

Drug	Dose	Effective Serum Concentration	Side Effects	Route of Metabolism
Quinidine sulfate	200 to 700 mg every 6 hr	2 to 6 µg/ml	Diarrhea, cramps, thrombocytopenia, fever, CNS depression, proarrhythmia	Hepatic primary, renal secondary
Quinidine gluconate	330 to 660 mg every 6 to 8 hr	2 to 6 µg/ml	Similar to quinidine sulfate	Hepatic primary, renal secondary
Procainamide	250 to 1000 mg every 4 hr	4 to 10 µg/ml	Gastric upset, fever, arthralgias, lupus-like syndrome, proarrhythmia agranulocytosis	Hepatic primary, renal secondary
Procan SR	500 to 2000 mg every 6 hr	4 to 10 mg/100 ml	Similar to procainamide, agranulocytosis	Hepatic primary, renal secondary
Mexiletine	150 to 300 mg every 8 hr	0.5 to 2.0 mg/100 ml	Gastric upset, confusion, agitation, CNS depression, nausea	Hepatic
Tocainide	200 to 800 mg every 8 hr	3.5 to 10 mg/100 ml	Gastric upset, confusion, CNS depression, nausea	Renal primary, hepatic secondary
Flecainide	50 to 200 mg every 12 hr	200 to 1000 mg/ml	Blood dyscrasias, bone marrow depression	——
Amiodarone	200 to 800 mg per day	1.0 to 2.5 mg/100 ml	Pulmonary fibrosis, hypo- and hyperthyroidism, skin pigmentation, corneal deposits, myocardial depression, neurologic symptoms	Unknown

Heart Block

Sinus Node Exit Block

Sinus node exit block is the result of inability of the electrical impulse to reach the atrium despite normal formation within the sinus node. This is recognized by failure of the P wave to appear at the anticipated time, resulting in a dropped P wave. This may occur either in a random manner or in a recurring pattern. Observation of a dropped P wave is consistent with SA block if the P-P interval is a multiple of the P-P wave in normal sinus rhythm. For instance, a pause of exactly twice the usual P-P interval identifies a 2:1 SA exit block. Wenckebach periodicity of sinus node exit block may also occur. This is also identified by the dropping of the P wave with progressively shortening P-P intervals preceding the longest P-P interval that includes the dropped P wave. Possible causes of this condition include intrinsic disease of the sinus node; traumatic injuury of this region during surgery; increased vagal tone; and excessive drug effect due to digoxin, β-block, and calcium channel blocker therapy, as well as type I antiarrhythmic agents. If these drugs are present, blood level assessment is indicated. Treatment would consist of reduction in dosage or discontinuation, if possible, of any offending agents. Epicardial atrial pacing is needed only in the unlikely event of frequent dropped beats; permanent pacemaker implantation is rarely needed.

Atrioventricular Conduction Disturbances

First-Degree Block

This is identified when the P-R interval exceeds the upper limits of normal, which for adults is 0.20 second, 0.18 second for adolescents, and 0.16 second for young children and infants. Possible causes include internodal delay, AV node delay, and delay through the bundle of His. These changes can be due to fibrosis of the AV node, as well as toxicity or excessive effect with agents such as digoxin, β-blocking and calcium channel blocking agents, as well as quinidine and pronestyl. When seen after cardiac surgery, it is rarely the result of the surgical anatomic disruption and is much more commonly a feature noted preoperatively. Specific therapy is rarely, if ever, needed. Aortic and mitral valve replacement may result in edema of the AV node region, resulting in an increase in AV conduction delay.

Second-Degree AV Block

Mobitz type I, or Wenckebach phenomenon, is recognized as progressive prolongation of the P-R interval until AV conduction fails, resulting in the absence of a QRS following a normal P wave, following which the P-R interval is again short with repetition of the same sequence. This repetitious process can be recognized by a pattern of QRS appearance referred to as "group beating." Although the P-R interval progressively lengthens, the R-R interval decreases, resulting in a progressively shorter R-R interval just preceding the dropped ventricular beat.

Mobitz Type II Block

This refers to failure to conduct electrical impulse through the AV node not preceded by a progressive lengthening of the P-R interval. This may be represented by sporadic dropped single beats or a predictable pattern of block in which the dropped beats occur as a multiple of the atrial rate (e.g., 2:1, 3:1, or 4:1). Both Mobitz type I and type II AV block are not rare in the immediate postoperative period, especially following valve replacement. Parenthetically, it is extremely common to see all forms of AV blockade in the minutes following intraoperative washout of hyperkalemic myocardial preservation solution.

A vigorous search for offending drug effects or toxicity is in order with discontinuation of any but the most essential ones. Depending on the degree of AV blockade and the consequent heart rate, as well as the potential adequacy of lower escape rhythms, pacing may be needed. Since the condition is often transient, this is an ideal indication for epicardial ventricular pacing.

Complete AV Block

This condition is recognized by atrial activity that is faster than ventricular activity, in the absence of any predictable relationship between the two. As noted above, this is the expected consequence of cardioplegia washout during the first postoperative minutes, and occasionally is the consequence of antiarrhythmic drug therapy or toxicity from such drugs. When noted as a specific result of the surgical procedure itself it most often follows valve replacement and is transient in a majority of such patients. When due to trauma of surgical manipulation in the area of the AV node or bundle of His, the condition may be temporary but often lasts several days. Inadvertent surgical transection of conduction tissue during valve excision and repair is also a well-known complication, obviously leading to permanent AV blockade.

Varying degrees of AV block are more common after aortic valve replacement than with other types of cardiac surgery. The initial observation reported complete heart block in 13% (40). A clinical-pathological study of these cases demonstrated that, due to the proximity of the main bundle of His, a "danger zone" exists in the region of the noncoronary cusp and its adjacent portion of right coronary artery above the junction of the membranous and muscular septum below. Calcium débridement or deep suture placement in this zone was more likely to produce complete heart block (40). On a more positive side, improvement in preoperative AV blockade after aortic valve replacement has also been described in over 20% of patients (41). Improvement seen as late as 18 months after surgery is largely associated with improvement in left ventricular performance, implying that stretching of conduction tissue may have been the instigating mechanism (41). Another important cause is that of inadequate atrial preservation during cardiopulmonary bypass. This has been suggested by the finding in animals of conduction delay, primarily in the AV node area, reversed by careful atrial preservation.

As with incomplete AV block, therapy depends on the underlying heart rate and adequacy of ventricular escape mechanism (a narrow-complex, rapid rate being preferable to a wide-complex, slower rate). Discontinuation of all potentially offending drugs is indicated, including digitalis even when used in small maintenance dosage; and epicardial ventricular pacing is usually instituted when wires are present if the underlying heart rate is inadequate.

The need for a permanent pacemaker is predicated on the severity and permanence of any surgical trauma to the conduction system. The likelihood of recovering sinus rhythm is difficult to predict, but factors weighing against recovery include a heavily calcified AV node or aortic valve ring with extension into septum, appearance of AV block hours (or days) after surgery, and, to a lesser degree, significant preoperative conduction defect. In the absence of excessive calcification, optimism is usually warranted, especially if the escape rhythm exhibits a narrow QRS complex with good rate. Under these conditions it is realistic to wait for up to 2 weeks before implanting a permanent pacemaker.

EPICARDIAL PACEMAKER ELECTRODES

Operative insertion of temporary epicardial or pacemaker electrodes is a commonly used technique. Paired placement on the right atrium and right ventricle enhances diagnostic capability and allows pacing of any type of hemodynamically important bradycardia as well as performance of overdrive atrial pacing. When their value is fully appreciated they are used sufficiently often to warrant routine use in all cases, especially in valve replacement, in which they are often life saving (34).

Care and Handling

Although electrical hazard remains a potential problem with epicardial pacemaking wires, in the authors' experience with over 6000 such patients, this has never actually been identified as a complication. When unused, they are kept wrapped in a clean, dry, electrically isolated dressing, using the cap from a hypodermic needle.

Removal is usually planned for the day prior to discharge and is accomplished using gentle, steady traction. Resistance to removal is often overcome by leaving the wire on gentle traction for 1 to 2 hr. On the occasions when removal is not possible, the wire is pulled as far outward as possible and under sterile conditions is cut and allowed to retract deeply beneath the skin. Rare instances of late, recurrent infection due to a retained electrode have been identified as a consequence of incomplete retraction.

For patients medicated with Coumadin, cessation of therapy to allow the prothrombin time to reach 50% activity prior to wire removal is suggested. All patients should be kept at bed rest for 2 hr after removal.

References

1. MacCuish RK: Cardiac arrhythmias following mitral valvulotomy. *Acta Med Scand* 160:125–134, 1958.
2. Burback B, Schwedel JB, Young D: The role of digitalis in mitral valvuloplasty. *Am Heart J,* 54:863–874, 1957.
3. Rabino MD, Dreifus S, Likoff W: Cardiac arrhythmias following intracardiac surgery. *Am J Cardiol* 7:681–689, 1981.
4. Douglas P, Hirshfeld JW, Edmunds LH: Clinical correlates of postoperative atrial fibrillation. *Circulation* 70(Suppl II):165, 1984.
5. Smith EEJ, Shore DF, Monro JJ, et al: Oral verapamil fails to prevent supraventricular tachycardia following coronary artery surgery. *Int J Cardiol* 9:37–44, 1985.
6. Ormerod OJM, McGregor CGA, Stone DL, et al: Arrhythmias after coronary bypass surgery. *Br Heart J* 51:618–621, 1984.
7. Mohr R, Smolinsky A, Goor DA: Prevention of supraventricular tachyarrhythmia with low-dose propranolol after coronary bypass. *J Thorac Cardiovasc Surg* 81:840–845, 1981.
8. Matangi MF, Neutze JM, Graham KJ, et al: Arrhythmia prophylaxis after aorto-coronary bypass. *J Thorac Cardiovasc Surg* 89:439–443, 1985.
9. Smith PK, Buhrman WC, Levett JM, et al: Supraventricular conduction abnormalities following cardiac operations. *J Thorac Cardiovasc Surg* 85:105–115, 1983.
10. Smith PK, Buhrman BA, Ferguson TB, et al: Conduction block after cardioplegic arrest: prevention by augmented atrial hypothermia. *Circulatation* 68(Suppl II):41–48, 1983.
11. Magilligan DL, Vij D, Peper W, et al: Failure of standard cardioplegic techniques to protect the conducting systems. *Ann Thorac Surg* 39:403–408, 1985.
12. Johnson LW, Dickstein RA, Fruehan T, et al: Prophylactic digitalization for coronary artery bypass surgery. *Circulation* 53:819–822, 1976.
13. Csicsko JF, Schatzlein MH, King RD: Immediate postoperative digitalization in the prophylaxis of supraventricular arrhythmias following coronary artery bypass. *J Thorac Cardiovasc Surg* 81:419–422, 1981.
14. Tyras DH, Stothert JC, Kaiser GC, et al: Supraventricular tachyarrhythmias after myocardial revascularization: a randomized trial of prophylactic digitalization. *J Thorac Cardiovasc Surg* 77:310–314, 1979.
15. Matloff JM, Solfson S, Gorlin R, et al: Control of postcardiac surgical tachycardias with propranolol. *Circulation* 37(Suppl II):133–138, 1968.

16. Stephenson LW, MacVaugh H, Tomasello DN, et al: Propranolol for prevention of postoperative cardiac arrhythmias: a randomized study. *Ann Thorac Surg* 29:113–116, 1980.

17. Williams J, Stephenson LW, Holford FD, et al: Arrhythmia prophylaxis using propranolol after coronary artery surgery. *Ann Thorac Surg* 34:435–438, 1982.

18. Hammon JW, Wood AJJ, Prager RL, et al: Perioperative beta blockade and propranolol: reduction in myocardial oxygen demands and incidence of atrial and ventricular arrhythmias. *Ann Thorac Surg* 38:363–367, 1984.

19. Ivey MF, Ivey TD, Bailey WW, et al: Influence of propranolol on supraventricular tachycardia early after coronary artery revascularization. *J Thorac Cardiovasc Surg* 85:214–218, 1983.

20. White HD, Antman EM, Glynn MA: Efficacy and safety of timolol for prevention of supraventricular tachyarrhythmias after coronary artery bypass surgery. *Circulation* 70:479–484, 1984.

21. Daudon P, Gandjbakhch I, Corcos T, et al: Prevention of atrial arrhythmias after coronary bypass surgery by acebutolol, a cardioselective beta-blocker. *J Am Coll Cardiol* 5(Suppl):437, 1985.

22. Roffman JA, Fieldman A: Digoxin and propranolol in the prophylaxis of supraventricular tachydysrhythmias after coronary artery bypass surgery. *Ann Thorac Surg* 31:496–501, 1981.

23. Mills SA, Poole GV, Breyer RH, et al: Digoxin and propranolol in the prophylaxis of dysrhythmias after coronary artery bypass grafting. *Circulation* 68(Suppl II):222–225, 1982.

24. Davison R, Hartz R, Kaplan K, et al: Prophylaxis of supraventricular tachyarrhythmia after coronary bypass surgery with oral verapamil: a randomized, double-blind trial. *Ann Thorac Surg* 39:336–339, 1985.

25. Gray R, Conklin C, Sethna D, et al: The role of intravenous verapamil in supraventricular tachyarrhythmias after open-heart surgery. *Am Heart J* 104(4):799–802, 1982.

26. Haft JI, Habbab MA: Treatment of atrial arrhythmias. *Arch Intern Med* 146:1085–1089, 1986.

27. Betriu A, Chaitman BR, Bourassa MG, et al: Beneficial effect of intravenous diltiazem in the acute management of paroxysmal supraventricular tachyarrhythmias. *Circulation* 67:88–94, 1983.

28. Gray RJ, Bateman TM, Czer LSC, et al: Esmolol: a new ultrashort-acting beta-adrenergic blocking agent for rapid control of heart rate in postoperative supraventricular tachyarrhythmias. *J Am Coll Cardiol* 5:1451–1456, 1985.

29. Halpern S, Ellrodt AG, Singh BN, et al: Efficacy of intravenous procainamide infusion in converting atrial fibrillation to sinus rhythm. Relation to left atrial size. *Br Heart J* 44:589–595, 1980.

30. Installe E, Schoevaerdts JC, Gadisseux PH, et al: Intravenous amiodarone in the treatment of various arrhythmias following cardiac operations. *J Thorac Cardiovasc Surg* 81:302–308, 1981.

31. DiMarco JP, Sellers D, Belardinelli L: Rapid termination of supraventricular tachycardia by intravenous adenosine. *Circulation* 68(Suppl III):358, 1983.

32. Belhassen B, Pelleg A, Shoshani D, et al: Electrophysiologic effects of adenosine triphosphate in AV reentrant tachycardia. *Circulation* 68(Suppl III):358, 1983.

33. Cooper TB, MacLean WAH, Waldo AL: Overdrive pacing for supraventricular tachycardia. A review of theoretical implications and therapeutic techniques. *PACE* 1:196–221, 1978.

34. Waldo AL, MacLean WAH (eds): *Diagnosis and Treatment of Cardiac Arrhythmias following Open Heart Surgery.* Mount Kisco, NY, Futura, 1980, p 25.

35. Rubin DA, Nieminski KE, Monteferrante JC, et al: Ventricular arrhythmias after coronary artery bypass surgery: incidence, risk factors and long-term prognosis. *J Am Coll Cardiol* 6:307–310, 1985.

36. Huikuri HV, Korhonen UR, Takkunen T: Ventricular arrhythmias induced by dynamic and static exercise in relation to coronary artery bypass grafting. *Am J Cardiol* 55:948–951, 1985.

37. Weiner DA, Levine SR, Klein MD, et al: Ventricular arrhythmias during exercise testing: mechanism, response to coronary bypass surgery and prognostic significance. *Am J Cardiol* 53:1553–1557, 1984.

38. Hammermeister KE, DeRouen TA, Dodge HT: Variables predictive of survival in patients with coronary disease. *Circulation* 59:421–430, 1979.

39. Marcus NH, Falcone RA, Harken AH, et al: Body surface late potentials: effects of endocardial resection in patients with ventricular tachycardia. *Circulation* 70:632–637, 1984.

40. Gannon PG, Sellers RD, Kanjuh VI, et al: Complete heart block following replacement of the aortic valve. *Circulation* 33-34(Suppl I):152–262, 1966.

41. Thompson R, Mitchell A, Ahmed M, et al: Conduction defects in aortic valve disease. *Am Heart J* 98:3–10, 1979.

Chapter 19
ANTITHROMBOTIC THERAPY AFTER CARDIAC SURGERY

STEVEN S. KHAN, M.D.
LAWRENCE S.C. CZER, M.D.

Anticoagulants are probably the most common type of drug used for therapy following open-heart surgery, yet there exist many areas of controversy in the usage of these drugs and their indications. In this chapter we will attempt to briefly outline the essential details of their pharmacology and then present specific recommendations for anticoagulation following both valve replacement and coronary artery bypass surgery.

WARFARIN SODIUM (COUMADIN)

History

The anticoagulant potential of warfarin type agents was first discovered in the early 1920s when it was observed that cattle fed sweet clover hay that had been "damaged" (improperly cured) developed a profound bleeding tendency (1, 2). The causative agent was subsequently isolated, and the first clinical uses of oral anticoagulants in humans began in the early 1940s (3–6). These initial reports were soon followed by an abundance of publications on the use of anticoagulants in all aspects of clinical medicine. The number of different agents has since

been narrowed, and warfarin sodium (Coumadin, Panwarfin) is now the only oral anticoagulant in widespread use in the United States.

Mechanism of Action

Coumadin inhibits the synthesis of the vitamin K dependent factors (factors II, VII, IX, and X) and related proteins (C and S). It does this by blocking the carboxylation of these factors prior to their release into the circulation, which prevents the binding of calcium ions and activation by phospholipid. Although this effect on vitamin K dependent factors is felt to be the primary mechanism of action of Coumadin, other mechanisms have also been postulated. For example, Coumadin causes proteins deficient in γ-carboxyglutamic acid to be released, and experimentally these proteins have been shown to retard thrombin production. The clinical effects of these other mechanisms have not been established, however.

Measurement of Prothrombin Time

The dose of Coumadin is regulated using the prothrombin time (or protime); however, there are several potential difficulties to be aware of when interpreting prothrombin time results. First, the prothrombin time may be affected by the method of collection and transportation. If blood is collected in improperly prepared glass containers, the measured prothrombin time may be reduced, resulting in excessive Coumadin doses. This reduction in the prothrombin time is dependent on the time interval between blood collection and the sample processing and can be reduced either by collecting blood in plastic tubes or by transferring the sample to plastic tubes within 1 hr of collection (7).

An additional problem is the use of different reagents in different countries, resulting in varying recommendations for the optimal prothrombin time ratio. Laboratories in the United States and North America have typically used rabbit brain or lung thromboplastins, which are less sensitive to changes in the vitamin K dependent clotting factors than the human or bovine thromboplastins used in Europe and the United Kingdom. To standardize measurement of the prothrombin time, the World Health Organization has established a standard reference thromboplastin. Any commercially available thromboplastin can be calibrated against this reference and assigned an international normalized ratio (INR). Using this standard, it has become possible to compare test results from different laboratories and to develop standard recommendations for the optimum prothrombin time.

Dosing Regimens

Coumadin is usually begun with a loading dose (typically 10 mg/day) for 2 to 3 days, followed by maintenance doses that are adjusted to regulate the patient's prothrombin time within the desired range (usually on the order of 2 to 12 mg/day). In patients who are already on heparin, the heparin should be continued for at least 2 days after the first dose of Coumadin is given because of the delay in the response to Coumadin. Additionally, abrupt cessation of heparin therapy may cause a hypercoagulable state for 2 to 3 days due to heparin-induced suppression of antithrombin III by heparin and suppression of protein C by warfarin in the first 12 to 24 hrs of administration, while levels of factors II, V, and X are nearly normal.

The prothrombin time can be expressed in several ways for monitoring purposes: as a time in seconds, as a percentage of the control prothrombin time, or as a ratio of the patient's prothrombin time to a control prothrombin time. The latter method (the ratio of patient's prothrombin time: laboratory control prothrombin time) is the preferred way of evaluating the prothrombin time and is the way international standards are expressed.

There has been a general trend toward a reduction in the recommended level of anticoagulation over the past few years. Previously, in the United States, texts have recommended that the prothrombin time be maintained at 1.5 to 2.5 times the control value. Development of a reference standard for measurement of prothrombin time (the INR) has shown, however, that the upper limit of these recommendations is higher than those used in Europe or Great Britain, where a more typical upper range would be 2 times control.

A statement by the American College of Chest Physicians and the National Heart, Lung and Blood Institute has addressed the issue of optimal Coumadin dosing (8). This committee found that the use of higher prothrombin time ratios (2.0 to 2.5) lacked a scientific basis, and recommended that prothrombin time ratios be maintained between 1.2 and 1.5 times control (based on the standard rabbit brain assay used in the United States) for prophylaxis of venous thromboembolism; treatment of venous thrombosis; and prevention of embolism in patients with atrial fibrillation, valvular heart disease, acute myocardial infarction, or bioprosthetic heart valves. Patients with mechanical prosthetic heart valves and patients with recurrent systemic embolism have a significantly higher risk of embolism, however, and the committee recommended that the prothrombin time ratio be maintained between 1.5 and 2.0 times control in these patients.

In summary, the prothrombin time should be maintained between 1.2 and 1.5 times the control value for most uses of Coumadin. The exception is in patients with mechanical prosthetic valves and in patients with recurrent embolism on therapy in whom prothrombin time ratios of 1.5 to 2.0 times control should be used. Prothrombin time ratios higher than 2.0 times the control value are associated with an excessive risk of bleeding complications and should be avoided. Our experience with the St. Jude valve has confirmed an excessive hemorrhagic tendency with protime ratios greater than 2.0 (9).

Drug Interactions

The effect of Coumadin can be altered by a large number of drugs and dietary changes that affect either the availability of vitamin K or its metabolism, or that interact directly with Coumadin. Dietary changes can affect vitamin K availability and, although there is no need to restrict intake of any specific foods, patients should be advised not to make major changes in their diets without consulting their physician. Foods that contain significant amounts of vitamin K include broccoli, Brussels sprouts, asparagus, leafy green vegetables, bacon, and beef liver; sudden changes in the consumption of these foods should be avoided.

Drugs that interact with Coumadin are listed in Table 19.1. As the size of Table 19.1 indicates, it would be unreasonable to list every possible drug interaction for patients. The best approach is to instruct patients to call their physician if any new drugs are taken (including over-the-counter drugs) or if there are any major dietary changes so that the prothrombin time can be monitored more frequently after the change.

ASPIRIN

History

Aspirin, or acetylsalicylic acid, has a surprisingly ancient history. It was probably first used for fever control in the form of willow bark, which contains salicin (10). This compound was first isolated in 1827 by Leroux, and salicylic acid was made from it in 1838 by Piria. Salicylic acid was later made from oil of wintergreen and from phenol. It was first used in the treatment of rheumatic fever in 1875 by both Stricker and MacLagan, working independently, and in the treatment of gout in 1879 by Campbell. Acetylsalicylic acid (aspirin) was first used in clinical applications in 1899 by Dresser. Interestingly, aspirin was originally the

brand name for acetylsalicylic acid produced by Bayer. Over time, however, all acetylsalicylic acid preparations came to be called aspirin and the term became generic.

Mechanisms of Action

The antithrombotic properties of aspirin are primarily due to irreversible inactivation of both platelet and megakaryocyte cyclooxygenase (11–13). This enzyme is responsible for synthesis of thromboxane A_2 in platelets, a substance that induces platelet aggregation and vasoconstriction. Cyclooxygenase is also responsible for the synthesis of PGI_2, a vasodilator, by the endothelial cells of blood vessel walls. Cyclooxygenase inhibition, therefore, also has the potential to increase vasoconstriction.

It should be noted that aspirin does not block all platelet function. For example, smooth muscle cell proliferation can still be induced by platelets since the release of platelet-derived growth factor is not inhibited (14). Similarly, aspirin does not prevent the adherence of the initial layer of platelets to vascular endothelium (15). These effects may be important in saphenous vein graft occlusion. In summary, aspirin reduces thromboxane A_2 mediated platelet aggregation and vasoconstriction but potentially can also increase vasoconstriction by its effect on vascular endothelium.

Dosing

There is still considerable controversy regarding the optimal aspirin dose. Low-dose aspirin (between 80 and 325 mg/day) appears to have fewer side effects than higher-dose aspirin (900 mg/day and higher) and has been shown to be effective in preventing early (in less than 1 year) closure of coronary bypass grafts (100 mg/day) by Lorenz and coworkers (16). Low doses of aspirin have also been shown by Lewis and coworkers (17) to reduce death and myocardial infarction in patients with unstable angina (325 mg/day) without any increase in side effects. In this latter study, aspirin was administered as Alka-Seltzer due to evidence that this form of aspirin can significantly reduce the incidence of gastrointestinal bleeding (18). Several studies using more than 900 mg/day of aspirin

TABLE 19.1

AGENTS INTERACTING WITH COUMADIN[a]

Drug/Agent	Effect on Protime	Onset	Severity	Evidence
Acetaminophen (Tylenol)	Prolonged	Delayed	Moderate	Possible
Allopurinol	Prolonged	Delayed	Major	Possible
Aminoglutethamide	Decreased	Delayed	Moderate	Possible
Amiodarone	Prolonged	Delayed	Major	Established
Androgens (17-alkyl derivatives)	Prolonged	Delayed	Major	Established
Androgens (non-17-alykl derivatives)	Prolonged	Delayed	Moderate	Possible
Barbiturates	Decreased	Delayed	Major	Established
β-Adrenergic blockers	Prolonged	Delayed	Moderate	Possible
Carbamazepine	Decreased	Delayed	Moderate	Suspected
Cephalosporins (parenteral with methyltetrazolethiol chain)[b]	Prolonged	Delayed	Major	Suspected
Cephalosporins (parenteral without methyltetrazolethiol chain)[c]	Prolonged	Delayed	Moderate	Possible
Chloral hydrate	Prolonged	Rapid	Moderate	Probable
Chloramphenicol	Prolonged	Delayed	Major	Possible
Cholestyramine	Decreased	Delayed	Moderate	Suspected
Cimetidine	Prolonged	Delayed	Major	Established
Clofibrate	Prolonged	Delayed	Major	Established
Oral contraceptives	Decreased	Delayed	Moderate	Possible
Corticosteroids	Mixed[d]	Delayed	Moderate	Possible
Cyclophosphamide	Decreased	Delayed	Moderate	Possible
Dextrothyroxine	Prolonged	Delayed	Major	Established
Dicloxacillin	Decreased	Delayed	Major	Unlikely
Diflunisal	Prolonged	Delayed	Moderate	Possible
Disopyramide	Mixed[d]	Delayed	Moderate	Unlikely
Disulfiram	Prolonged	Delayed	Major	Established
Erythromycin	Prolonged	Delayed	Major	Suspected
Estrogens	Mixed[d]	Delayed	Moderate	Possible
Ethacrynic acid	Prolonged	Delayed	Major	Possible
Ethanol	Mixed[d]	Delayed	Moderate	Possible
Ethchlorvynol (Placidyl)	Decreased	Delayed	Moderate	Probable
Fenoprofen (Nalfon)	Prolonged	Delayed	Moderate	Possible
Glucagon	Prolonged	Delayed	Major	Probable
Glutethimide	Decreased	Delayed	Moderate	Probable
Griseofulvin	Decreased	Delayed	Moderate	Probable
Ibuprofen (Motrin)	Mucosal[e]	Delayed	Moderate	Possible
Influenza virus vaccine	Prolonged	Delayed	Major	Possible
Isoniazid	Prolonged	Delayed	Major	Possible
Ketoconazole	Prolonged	Delayed	Major	Possible
Ketoprofen	Prolonged	Delayed	Major	Possible
Meclofenamate	Prolonged	Delayed	Moderate	Possible
Methylpenidate (Ritalin)	Prolonged[f]	Delayed	Minor	Unlikely
Metronidazole (Flagyl)	Prolonged	Delayed	Major	Established
Miconazole (Monistat i.v.)	Prolonged	Delayed	Major	Possible
Mineral oil	Variable	Delayed	Moderate	Unlikely
Nalidixic acid	Prolonged	Delayed	Major	Possible
Naproxen	Prolonged/mucosal	Delayed	Moderate	Possible
Penicillins, parenteral	Prolonged	Delayed	Major	Possible
Phenylbutzones	Prolonged	Delayed	Major	Established
Piroxicam	Prolonged	Delayed	Moderate	Possible
Propoxyphene (Darvon)	Prolonged	Delayed	Major	Possible

TABLE 19.1   (Continued)

Drug/Agent	Effect on Protime	Onset	Severity	Evidence
Quinine derivatives (Quinidine, quinine)	Prolonged	Delayed	Major	Suspected
Ranitidine (Zantac)	Prolonged	Delayed	Moderate	Possible
Rifampin	Decreased	Delayed	Moderate	Established
Salicylates (aspirin)	Prolonged	Delayed	Major	Established
Spironolactone	Decreased	Delayed	Minor	Possible
Sucralfate	Decreased	Delayed	Moderate	Possible
Sulfamethoxazole/trimethoprim (Bactrim, Septra)	Prolonged	Delayed	Major	Established
Sulfinpyrazone	Prolonged	Delayed	Major	Established
Sulfonamides	Prolonged	Delayed	Major	Possible
Sulindc	Prolonged	Delayed	Major	Possible
Tamoxifen	Prolonged	Delayed	Major	Possible
Tetracyclines	Prolonged	Delayed	Major	Possible
Thiazide-type diuretics	Decreased	Delayed	Minor	Possible
Thioamines (propylthiouracil)	Variable	Delayed	Major	Suspected
Thiopurines (azathioprine)	Decreased	Delayed	Moderate	Possible
Thyroid hormones	Prolonged	Delayed	Major	Probable
Tolmetin	Mucosal[e]	Delayed	Moderate	Possible
Trazodone (Desyrel)	Decreased	Delayed	Moderate	Possible
Tricyclic antidepressants	Prolonged	Delayed	Major	Suspected
Vitamin E	Prolonged	Delayed	Major	Possible
Vitamin K	Decreased	Delayed	Moderate	Established

[a]Adapted from Tatro DS (ed): *Drug Interaction Facts and Facts and Comparisons*. St. Louis, JB Lippincott, April 1988.
[b]Cefamandol, cefoperazone, cefotetan, moxalactam.
[c]Cefazolin, cefoxitin, ceftriaxone.
[d]Both increases and decreases in bleeding tendency have been reported with this agent.
[e]There does not appear to be any significant kinetic interaction between Coumadin and this agent; however, this drug may have effects on gastric mucosa which would tend to increase the bleeding tendency and should be used with great caution in patients on Coumadin.
[f]A small amount of data suggests that this agent may reduce elimination of ethyl biscoumacetate. There is no evidence that Coumadin is affected, however.

have all reported an increase in aspirin side effects (19–22).

In contrast to the difference in side effects between low- and high-dose aspirin, there is no clinical evidence that high doses of aspirin provide greater efficacy (23). Experimental evidence in baboons, however, suggests that aspirin may have antithrombotic effects independent of cyclooxygenase inhibition at high doses (24). The clinical significance of this effect is unclear, but at least one recent review has suggested restraint in accepting the efficacy of extremely low-dose aspirin regimens (25). Because of the lower incidence of side effects and lack of clinical evidence of greater efficacy of higher doses at the authors' institution, it is customary to use 80 mg twice a day. The American College of Chest Physicians and National Institutes of Health (ACCP/NIH) consensus committee has recommended that aspirin be used at a dose of 325 mg/day, except for treatment of patients with cerebrovascular disease, in whom the lowest dose evaluated has been 1 gm/day (23).

OTHER ANTIPLATELET AGENTS

Dipyridamole

Dipyridamole inhibits cyclic AMP phosphodiesterase and can prolong platelet survival, especially in settings where prosthetic surfaces are involved. In particular, dipyridamole has been shown to normalize platelet survival in patients with artificial heart valves (26, 27). Experimentally, it has also been shown that aspirin may potentiate the antithrombotic effects of dipyridamole (24).

Clinically, dipyridamole has been reported to reduce the incidence of thromboembolism in patients with prosthetic valves who are also on

Coumadin (28, 29), and to reduce progression of peripheral arterial disease when given with aspirin (30). The use of dipyridamole in coronary bypass surgery will be reviewed in detail later in this chapter.

Sulfinpyrazone

Although sulfinpyrazone was initially introduced as a uricosuric and mild anti-inflammatory agent for the treatment of gout, it has found its widest use as an antiplatelet agent. Sulfinpyrazone may work at high doses by inhibiting platelet aggregation and secretion, but its full mechanism of action remains to be fully defined.

Clinically, sulfinpyrazone has been shown to prolong platelet survival in patients with prosthetic mitral valves (31) and to prolong the patency of hemodialysis shunts (32). Trials in other settings where biologic surfaces are involved have either been less convincing, such as following myocardial infarction (33) and coronary bypass surgery (34), or were negative, as in studies in unstable angina (35) and stroke (36).

Ticlopidine

Ticlopidine is a newer oral antiplatelet agent that inhibits platelet aggregation and prolongs shortened platelet survival (37). Its effects appear to be delayed for 24 to 48 hr after initial administration but, like aspirin, last for several days after the drug is discontinued (38). The mechanism of action of ticlopidine is unknown but it is clear that it is neither a prostaglandin synthetase inhibitor nor a cyclic AMP phosphodiesterase inhibitor. Although the clinical indications for this drug are currently being investigated, ticlopidine appears to be an extremely potent platelet inhibitor.

Anagrelide

Anagrelide is another new oral antiplatelet agent that is an inhibitor of platelet cyclic AMP phosphodiesterase. It is also a nonspecific vasodilator that causes reflex increases in heart rate and cardiac output. Animal studies have shown that anagrelide inhibits platelet aggregation and at high doses can prolong the bleed-

ing time (39). In humans, anagrelide has been shown to produce dose-dependent inhibition of plate aggregation and hypotension at high doses. No prolongation of the bleeding time was seen, however. Anagrelide also has been reported to cause a significant (35%) drop in platelet levels by inhibiting bone marrow production of platelets. There is no clinical data on the use of anagrelide for specific diseases at present.

PATIENTS WITH PROSTHETIC VALVES

Patients who have had prosthetic valves implanted have a lifelong risk of thromboembolism, which has been thought to be greatest in the first few months after surgery. The risk of embolism is strongly correlated with the type of valve implanted (bioprosthetic or mechanical), its location (aortic, mitral, or combined), the presence of atrial fibrillation, prior history of thromboembolism, and the adequacy of anticoagulation. Mechanical and bioprosthetic valves will be discussed separately since the recommendations for anticoagulation differ significantly.

Mechanical Valves

The incidence of thromboembolism in patients with caged-ball type valves has been reported to be as high as 69% in 1 year in patients who are not receiving anticoagulant therapy (40). In patients receiving full doses of anticoagulants, the thromboembolic rate may be reduced to 1.2 to 9.3 events per 100 patient-years (41–44) with this same type of valve. For the Bjork-Shiley disc valve, thromboembolic rates of 0.7 to 5.6% have been reported for patients treated with Coumadin (45, 46). The St. Jude bileaflet valve has been reported to have even lower thromboembolic rates, with 0.6 to 0.7 events per 100 patient-years for aortic valves and 0.9 to 3.9 events per 100 patient-years for mitral valves (47–49).

Antiplatelet agents, when given alone, clearly do not provide enough protection against thromboemboli in patients with mechanical valves (44, 50–52). They are most effective when given with Coumadin. Aspirin has been shown to reduce the incidence of thromboemboli when given with Coumadin (45, 46, 53), but this combination results in an unacceptable incidence of bleeding (28). Dipyridamole has also been shown to reduce the incidence of thromboembolism when given with Coumadin (54–56), but without an increase in perioperative blood loss. Thus, antiplatelet agents provide additional protection against emboli when used with full oral anticoagulation in patients with mechanical valves.

Taken together, the data strongly suggest that all patients who have had mechanical prosthetic valves implanted in either the aortic or the mitral position be placed on full oral anticoagulant therapy. The prothrombin time should be adjusted to between 1.5 and 2.0 times the control value and should be evaluated at least monthly. At the authors' institution, all patients are also placed on oral dipyridamole 75 mg three times a day. This recommendation is supported by several studies, as noted above (28, 44, 46). The ACCP/NIH consensus panel suggests that routine dipyridamole use in this setting is optional (57).

Management of Problems

In patients who have thromboembolism on adequate doses of Coumadin, dipyridamole should be added to the regimen (57). If patients on Coumadin with therapeutic prothrombin times develop significant bleeding clinically, their target prothrombin time should be reduced to 1.2 to 1.5 times control (57), and the addition of dipyridamaole should be considered.

Bioprosthetic Valves

Although bioprosthetic valves are significantly less thrombogenic than mechanical valves, there is still a measurable risk of embolism, and all of these patients should be placed on antiplatelet or anticoagulant therapy at least early postoperatively.

The risk of thromboembolism appears to be significantly time dependent and to be highest in the first 2 to 3 months after valve implantation (58–60), particularly in patients with mitral bioprostheses. It should be noted, however, that this has recently been challenged by Magilligan and coworkers (61), who found a linear incidence of thromboembolic complications over

time in a retrospective study of porcine valves. The consensus of most authors and of the ACCP/NIH committee, however, is that patients with mitral bioprosthetic valves are at a higher risk early after surgery and should be treated for 3 months following implantation.

Certain patient subgroups appear to be particularly at risk for thromboembolic complications. In patients with bioprosthetic valves who are in atrial fibrillation, the incidence of thromboemboli has been reported to be as high as 16% (62, 63). High rates of embolism have also been reported in patients with left atrial thrombi found at surgery and in those with a prior history of embolism (63). There is a consensus that all of these patient subgroups should be treated with oral anticoagulation indefinitely. Although the level of anticoagulation is still debated, most authors recommend that the low range of prothrombin time be used (1.2 to 1.5 times control). There is little current data indicating that an enlarged left atrium is associated with an increased risk of thromboembolism; however, the association of left atrial enlargement with atrial fibrillation has resulted in some authors also including left atrial enlargement as a risk factor for thromboembolism. It should be noted that the ACCP/NIH committee did not recommend that patients with isolated left atrial enlargement be treated with long-term oral anticoagulation.

In summary, all patients with bioprosthetic mitral valves should be placed on Coumadin for the first 3 months after surgery. In patients with aortic bioprosthetic valves, the early risk is lower and the anticoagulant therapy is optional. Subgroups of patients—those in atrial fibrillation, those with a history of prior thromboembolism, and those with left atrial thrombus documented at surgery—should receive long-term oral anticoagulants. Patients in sinus rhythm without any of these risk factors can optionally receive antiplatelet therapy with aspirin 80 mg twice a day or 325 mg/day.

Saphenous Vein Bypass Graft Surgery

In the past decade it has become clear that saphenous vein coronary bypass grafts provide palliation of coronary artery disease and not cure. The recurrence of atherosclerosis in bypass grafts appears to develop by the same mechanisms as atherosclerosis in native coronary arteries, but at a greatly accelerated rate.

Most investigators believe that some form of vascular endothelial injury is the initiating process in coronary atherosclerosis. In bypass grafts, this injury begins abruptly when the vein is harvested from the leg. Handling of the vein by the surgeon, delays between harvesting and implantation, and the demodynamic stress of sudden exposure to high arterial pressures may all play a role in the initial vascular damage of vein grafts. In addition, as soon as blood flow through the graft begins, a layer of platelets is deposited on the endothelium, releasing platelet factors into the vessel wall. This initial layer of platelets begins a series of events that can result in either (a) abrupt closure of the graft by thrombus (the most common cause of graft occlusion in the 1st month after bypass surgery); (b) intimal hyperplasia (a common mechanism of graft narrowing during the 1st year after surgery); or (c) localized smooth muscle proliferation eventually resulting in a recurrence of atherosclerosis in the vein grafts (after the 1st year).

It has been suggested that smooth muscle proliferation is caused by the release of platelet-derived growth factor from platelets deposited on the endothelium. After the 1st year, these areas of smooth muscle proliferation begin to develop lipid accumulations and eventually become indistinguishable from classical atherosclerotic lesions (64). Factors that reduce the deposition of platelets on graft endothelium may attenuate this process and could prolong graft patency on a long-term basis. Since the initial layer of platelets attaches to graft endothelium during surgery, the consensus has been that antiplatelet therapy should be started preoperatively. There is also substantial clinical evidence to support the importance of early antiplatelet therapy in patients underoing saphenous vein bypass surgery.

It should be clear from this discussion that platelets play a key role in both early and possibly late bypass graft closure, and the use of antiplatelet agents has therefore become routine after coronary artery bypass surgery. The most convincing demonstration of the benefits

of these agents was a large, randomized, double-blind, placebo-controlled study from the Mayo Clinic (65). These investigators began dipyridamole 100 mg orally, four times daily, 2 days prior to surgery, with a dose of 100 mg 2 hours prior to surgery and again 1 hour after surgery through the nasogastric tube. Seven hours after surgery, aspirin (325 mg) and dipyridamole (75 mg) were begun three times daily. This study showed a marked reduction in the occlusion of vein grafts early after surgery, with only 5% of treated patients having an occluded graft at 10 days versus 22% of untreated patients ($P<.000001$). These investigators found no increase in bleeding or blood transfusion requirements in the treated group, suggesting that aspirin and dipyridamole can be used safely. A follow-up study from the same group documented a continuing benefit at 1 year (66). Other trials in which these agents were begun within 48 hr of surgery have also documented their efficacy (67, 68), although several trials in which therapy was begun after 48 hr have not shown any benefit (69–71).

Although prior studies have been heavily oriented toward the combined use of aspirin and dipyridamole, Lorenz and coworkers reported a beneficial effect of aspirin alone when begun within 24 hr of surgery in 1984 (16). This question was addressed by a Veterans Administration cooperative study, which demonstrated no additional benefit from adding dipyridamole to aspirin (72). In this study, aspirin 325 mg once daily was compared to aspirin 325 mg three times a day, aspirin 325 mg with dipyridamole 75 mg three times a day, sulfinpyrazone 267 mg three times daily, and placebo. All of the aspirin-treated groups showed significant improvement compared to placebo ($P<.05$), but there was no difference between the groups treated with aspirin alone, once a day (93.5% patency), aspirin three times daily (92.3%), and aspirin with dipyridamole (91.9%). These investigators concluded that there was no additional benefit from the addition of dipyridamole to aspirin in patients following coronary artery bypass surgery with saphenous veins.

These results deserve further comment, however. All of the aspirin regimens included a preoperative dose of aspirin, and, perhaps for this reason, all of the aspirin groups had a significant increase in perioperative blood loss as measured by chest tube drainage (P<.02), and an increased rate of reoperation (P<.01). The authors therefore stop short of recommending the aspirin regimens without dipyridamole used in their study. Instead, they conclude that, "in view of the previous reports showing that preoperative dipyridamole (100 mg daily for 2 days) followed by postoperative aspirin and dipyridamole improved early graft patency without increased blood loss, this preoperative regimen could continue to be used at present. . . ." Thus, due to the general agreement that preoperative therapy is necessary, and the fact that preoperative aspirin therapy increases both postoperative bleeding and the risk of reoperation, preoperative dipyridamole should continue to be given.

In summary, platelets play an important role in both early and late graft occlusion. Early bypass graft patency for saphenous vein grafts has been shown to be improved using perioperative antiplatelet therapy, and this effect has been shown to persist for at least 1 year. Dipyridamole does not appear to provide any additional benefit to aspirin alone but does cause less bleeding than aspirin when given preoperatively. Patients undergoing bypass surgery should therefore receive dipyridamole 100 mg orally each day for 2 days preoperatively followed by aspirin 325 mg orally each day afterward. This postoperative regimen should probably be continued indefinitely.

References

1. Schofield FW: A brief account of a disease of cattle simulating hemorrhagic septicaemia due to feeding sweet clover. *Can Vet Rec* 3:74, 1922.
2. Schofield FW: Damaged sweet clover: the cause of a new disease in cattle simulating hemorrhagic septicaemia and blackleg. *J Am Vet Med Assn* 64:53–575, 1924.
3. Bingham JB, Meyer OO, Pohle FJ: Studies on the hemorrhagic agent 3,3' methylenebis (4-hydroxycoumarin). I. Its effect on the prothrombin and coagulation time of the blood of dogs and humans. *Am J Med Sci* 202:563–578, 1941.
4. Butt HR, Allen EV, Bollman JL: A preparation from spoiled sweet clover [3,3' methylene-bis-

(4-hydroxycoumarin)] which prolongs coagulation and prothrombin time of blood. *Proc Staff Meet Mayo Clin* 16:388–395, 1941.
5. Meyer OO, Bingham JB, Axelrod VH: Studies on the hemorrhagic agent 3-3' methylenebis (4-hydroxycoumarin). II. The method of administration and dosage. *Am J Med Sci* 024:11–21, 1941.
6. Prandoni A, Wright I: The anti-coagulants: heparin and the dicoumarin-3,3' methylene-bis-(4-hydroxycoumarin). *Bull NY Acad Med* 18:433–458, 1942.
7. Palmer RN, Kessler CM, Gralnick HR: Warfarin anticoagulation: difficulties in interpretation of the prothrombin time. *Thromb Res* 25:125–130, 1982.
8. Hirsh J, Deykin D, Poller L: "Therapeutic range" for oral anticoagulant therapy. *Chest* 89:11S–15S, 1986.
9. Czer LS, Matloff J, Chaux A, et al: The St. Jude valve: analysis of thromboembolism, warfarin-related hemorrhage, and survival. *Am Heart J* 114:389–397, 1987.
10. Woodbury DM, Fingl E: Analgesics-antipyretics, anti-inflammatory agents, and drugs employed in the therapy of gout. In Goodman LS, Gilman A, (eds): *The Pharmacological Basis of Therapeutics*, ed. 5. New York, Macmillan, 1975, pp 326–339.
11. Roth GL, Majerus PW: The mechanism of the effect of aspirin on human platelets. I. Acetylation of a particulate fraction protein. *J Clin Invest* 56:624–632, 1975.
12. Demers LM, Budin R, Shaikh B: The effects of aspirin on megakaryocyte prostaglandin production. *Blood* 50:239–247, 1977.
13. Burch JW, Stanford N, Majerus PW: Inhibition of platelet prostaglandin synthetase by oral aspirin. *J Clin Invest* 61:314–319, 1978.
14. Clowes AW, Kanovsky MJ: Failure of certain antiplatelet drugs to affect myointimal thickening following arterial endothelial injury in the rat. *Lab Invest* 36:452–464. 1977.
15. Tschopp TB: Aspirin inhibits platelet aggregation on but not adhesion to collagen fibrils: an assessment of platelet adhesion and deposited platelet mass by morphometry and 51-Cr-labeling. *Thromb Res* 11:619–632, 1977.
16. Lorenz RL, Weber M, Kotzur J, et al: Improved aortocoronary bypass patency by low-dose aspirin (100 mg daily): effects on platelet aggregation and thromboxane formation. *Lancet* 1:1261–1264, 1984.
17. Lewis HD, Davis JW, Archibald DG, et al: Pro-

tective effects of aspirin against acute myocardial infarction and death in men with unstable angina. *N Engl J Med* 309:396–403, 1983.

18. Leonards JR, Levy G: Reduction or prevention of aspirin induced occult gastrointestinal blood loss in man. *Clin Pharmacol Ther* 10:571–575, 1969.

19. Elwood PC, Sweetnam PM: Aspirin and secondary mortality after myocardial infarction. *Lancet* 2:1313, 1979.

20. Aspirin Myocardial Infarction Study Research Group. A randomized controlled trial of aspirin in persons recovered from myocardial infarction. *JAMA* 243:661, 1980.

21. Breddin K, Loew D, Lechnew K, et al: Secondary prevention of myocardial infarction: comparison of acetylsalicylic acid, phenoprocoumon, and placebo: a multi-centre two year prospective study. *Thromb Haemost* 4:225, 1979.

22. Persantine-Aspirin Reinfarction Study Research Group. A randomized controlled trial of aspirin in persons recovered from myocardial infarction. *JAMA* 243:661, 1980.

23. Hirsh J, Fuster V, Salzman E: Dose antiplatelet agents; the relationship among side effects and antithrombotic effectiveness. *Chest* 89 (Suppl):5–10, 1986.

24. Hanson SR, Harker LA, Bjornsson TD: Effects of platelet-modifying drugs on arterial thromboembolism in baboons. Aspirin potentiates the antithrombotic actions of dipyridamole and sulfinpyrazone by mechanisms independent of platelet cyclooxygenase inhibition. *J Clin Invest* 75:1591–1599, 1985.

25. Harker LA, Fuster V: Pharmacology of platelet inhibitors. *J Am Coll Cardiol* 8:21B–32B, 1986.

26. Harker LA, Slichter SJ: Studies of platelet and fibrinogen kinetics in patients with prosthetic heart valves. *N Engl J Med* 283:1302–1305, 1970.

27. Wiely HS, Steele PP, Davies H, et al: Platelet survival in patients with substitute heart valves. *N Engl J Med* 290:534–536, 1974.

28. Chesebro JH, Fuster V, Elveback LR, et al: Trial of combined warfarin plus dipyridamole or aspirin therapy in prosthetic heart valve replacement: danger of aspirin compared with dipyridamole. *Am J Cardiol* 51:1537–1541, 1983.

29. Sullivan JM, Harken DE, Gorlin R: Pharmacologic control of thromboembolic complications of cardiac valve replacement. *N Engl J Med* 284:1391, 1971.

30. Hess H, Mietaschk A, Deichsel G: Drug-induced inhibition of platelet function delays progression of peripheral occlusive arterial disease:

a prospective double-blind arteriographically controlled trial. *Lancet* 1:416–419, 1985.

31. Weily HS, Genton E: Altered platelet function in patients with prosthetic mitral valves: effects of sulfinpyrazone therapy. *Circulation* 42:967, 1970.

32. Kaegi A, Pineo GF, Shimizu A, et al: Arteriovenous-shunt thrombosis: prevention by sulfinpyrazone. *N Engl J Med* 290:304, 1974.

33. Report from the Anturane Reinfarction Study: Sulfinpyrazone in post myocardial infarction. *Lancet* 1:237–242, 1982.

34. Bauer HR, Van Tassel RA, Pierach CA, et al: Effects of sulfinpyrazone on early graft closure after myocardial revascularization. *Am J Cardiol* 49:420–424, 1982.

35. Cairns JA, Gent M, Singer J, et al: Aspirin, sulfinpyrazone, or both in unstable angina: results of a Canadian multicenter trial. *N Engl J Med* 313:1369–1375, 1985.

36. Canadian Cooperative Study Group. A randomized trial of aspirin and sulfinpyrazone in threatened stroke. *N Engl J Med* 299:53–59, 1978.

37. Wilkinson AR, Hawker RJ, Hawker JM: The influence of antiplatelet drugs on platelet survival after aortic damage or implantation of a Dacron arterial prosthesis. *Thromb Res* 15:181–189, 1979.

38. O'Brien JR: Ticlopidine: a promise for the prevention and threat of thrombosis and its complications. *Haemostasis* 13:1–54, 1983.

39. Fleming JS, Buyniski JP: A potent new inhibitor of platelet aggregation and experimental thrombosis, anagrelide (BL-4162A). *Thromb Res* 15:373–388, 1979.

40. Stein DW, Rahimtoola SH, Kloster FE, et al: Thrombotic phenomena with nonanticoagulated composite strut aortic prostheses. *J Thorac Cardiovasc Surg* 71:680–684, 1976.

41. Yeh TJ, Anabtawi IN, Cornett VE, et al: Influence of rhythm and anticoagulation upon the incidence of embolization associated with Starr-Edwards prostheses. *Circulation* 35–36 (Suppl I):177–181, 1967.

42. Dale J: Arterial thromboembolic complications in patients with Starr-Edwards aortic ball valve prostheses. *Am Heart J* 91:653–659, 1976.

43. Moggio RA, Hammond GL, Stansel HC Jr, et al: Incidence of emboli with cloth-covered Starr-Edwards valve without anticoagulation and with varying forms of anticoagulation: analysis of 183 patients followed for 3½ years. *J Thorac Cardiovasc Surg* 75:296–299, 1978.

44. Dale J, Myhre E: Can acetylsalicylic acid alone

prevent arterial thromboembolism? A pilot study in patients with aortic ball valve prostheses. *Acta Med Scand* 645:73–78, 1981.

45. Bjork VO, Henze A: Ten years experience with the Bjork-Shiley tilting disc valve. *J Thorac Cardiovasc Surg* 9:183–191, 1975.

46. Dale J, Myhre E, Storstein O, et al: Prevention of arterial thromboembolism with acetylsalicylic acid. A controlled clinical study in patients with aortic ball valves. *Am Heart J* 94:101–111, 1977.

47. Horstkotte D, Korfer R: The influence of prosthetic valve replacement on the natural history of severe acquired heart valve lesions. In DeBakey ME (ed): *Advances in Cardiac Valves, Clinical Perspectives.* New York: Yorke Medical Books, 1983, pp 47–86.

48. LeClerc JL, Wellens F, Deuvert FE, et al: Long term results with the St. Jude medical valve. In DeBakey ME (ed): *Advances in Cardiac Valves, Clincal Perspectives.* New York, Yorke Medical Books, 1983, pp 33–41.

49. Chaux A, Czer LS, Matloff JM, et al: The St. Jude medical bileaflet valve prosthesis. A 5-year experience. *J Thorac Cardiovasc Surg* 88:706–717, 1984.

50. Bjork VO, Henze A: Management of thromboembolism after aortic valve replacement with the Bjork-Shiley tilting disc valve. *Scand J Thorac Cardiovasc Surg* 9:183–191, 1975.

51. Moggio RA, Hammond GL, Stansel HC Jr, et al: Incidence of emboli with cloth-covered Starr-Edwards valve without anticoagulation and with varying forms of anticoagulation: analysis of 183 patients followed for 3½ years. *J Thorac Cardiovasc Surg* 75:296–299, 1978.

52. Chaux A, Gray RJ, Matloff TM, et al: An appreciation of the new St. Jude valvular prosthesis. *J Thorac Cardiovasc Surg* 81:202–211, 1981.

53. Altman R, Boullon F, Rouvier J, et al: Aspirin and prophylaxis of thromboembolic complications in patients with substitute heart valves. *J Thorac Cardiovasc Surg* 72:127–129, 1976.

54. Sullivan JM, Harken DE, Gorlin R: Effect of dipyridamole on the incidence of arterial emboli after cardiac valve replacement. *Circulation* 39–40 (Suppl I):149–153, 1969.

55. Rajah SM, Sreeharan N, Joseph A, et al: Prospective trial of dipyridamole and warfarin in heart valve patients (abstract) *Therapeutica (Brussels)* 6:6–54, 1980.

56. Kasahara T: Clinical effect of dipyridamole ingestion after prosthetic heart valve replacement—especially on the blood coagulation sys-

tem. *Nippon Kyobu Geka Gakkai Zasshi (J Jpn Assoc Thorac Surg)* 25:1007–1021, 1977.

57. Stein PD, Collins JJ, Kantrowitz A: Antithrombolitic therapy in mechanical and biological prosthetic heart valves and saphenous vein bypass grafts. *Chest* 89(2):46S–53S, 1986.

58. Hetzer R, Topalidis T, Borst HG: Thromboembolism and anticoagulation after isolated mitral valve replacement with porcine heterograft. In Cohn LH, Gallucci V (eds): *Proceedings, Second International Symposium on Cardiac Bioprostheses.* New York, Yorke Medical Books, 1982, pp 170–172.

59. Ionescu MI, Smith DR, Hasan SS, et al: Clinical durability of the pericardial xenograft valve: ten years experience with mitral replacement. *Ann Thorac Surg* 34:265–277, 1982.

60. Oyer PE, Stinson EB, Griepp RB, et al: Valve replacement with the Starr-Edwards and Hancock prostheses: comparative analysis of late morbidity and mortality. *Ann Surg* 186:301–309, 1977.

61. Magilligan DJ Jr, Lewis JW, Tilley B, et al: The porcine bioprosthetic valve—twelve years later. *J Thorac Cardiovasc Surg* 89:499–500, 1985.

62. Williams JB, Karp RB, Kirklin JW, et al: Considerations in selection and management of patients undergoing valve replacement with glutaraldehyde fixed porcine bioprostheses. *Ann Thorac Surg* 32:247–258, 1980.

63. Gonzalez-Lavin L, Tandon AP, Chi S, et al: The risk of thromboembolism and hemorrhage following mitral valve replacement. *J Thorac Cardiovasc Surg* 87:340–351, 1984.

64. Lie JT, Lawrie GM, Morris GC: Aortocoronary bypass saphenous vein graft atherosclerosis. *Am J Cardiol* 40:906–914, 1977.

65. Chesebro JH, Clements I, Fuster V, et al: A platelet inhibitor drug trial in coronary artery bypass operations: benefit of perioperative dipyridamole and aspirin therapy on early postoperative vein graft patency. *N Engl J Med* 307:73–78, 1982.

66. Chesebro JH, Fuster V, Elveback LR, et al: Effect of dipyridamole and aspirin on late vein graft patency after coronary bypass operations. *N Engl J Med* 310:209–214, 1984.

67. Mayer JE Jr, Lindsay WG, Castaneda W, et al: Influence of aspirin and dipyridamole on patency of coronary artery bypass grafts. *Ann Thorac Surg* 31:204–210, 1981.

68. Rajah SM, Salter MCP, Donaldson DR, et al: Acetylsaalicylic acid and dipyridamole improve

the early patency of aorta-coronary bypass grafts. *J Thorac Cardiovasc Surg* 90:373–377, 1985.

69. Sharma GVRK, Khuri SF, Josa M, et al: The effect of antiplatelet therapy on saphenous vein coronary artery bypass graft patency. *Circulation* 68(Suppl II):218–221, 1983.

70. Brown BG, Cukingham RA, Goede L, et al: Improved graft patency with antiplatelet drugs in patients treated for one year following coronary bypass surgery (abstract). *Am J Cardiol* 47:494, 1981.

71. Panteley GA, Goodnight SH Jr, Rahimtoola SH, et al: Failure of antiplatelet and anticoagulant therapy to improve patency of grafts after coronary artery bypass. A controlled randomized study. *N Engl J Med* 301:962–966, 1979.

72. Goldman S, Copeland J, Mortiz T, et al: Improvement in early saphenous vein graft patency after coronary artery bypass surgery with antiplatelet therapy: results of a Veterans Administration Cooperative Study. *Circulation* 77:1324–1332, 1988.

Chapter 20
PERICARDITIS

RICHARD J. GRAY, M.D.

BENIGN PERICARDIAL FRICTION RUB

During normal convalescence from open-heart surgery, pericardial friction rubs are heard under a variety of circumstances. While the mediastinal (pericardial) chest tubes are still in place most patients exhibit a prominent multicomponent rub, which usually disappears immediately or shortly after chest tube removal on the 1st or 2nd postoperative day. It is unusual for this rub to persist beyond a day after chest tube removal. Since there are numerous other reasons for the variety of chest pains experienced at this early time (mostly incisional) and because both low-grade fever and white blood count elevation are common after uncomplicated surgery, it is unlikely that any physiologic consequences can be directly attributed to this particular type of pericardial rub. As noted in an earlier section, the electrocardiogram may exhibit diffuse or even localized S-T segment elevation characteristic of pericarditis, but this phenomenon is more commonly seen in the presence of pericardial friction rub than in its absence. Therefore, the pericardial rub is considered at most to represent mild mechanical irritation from the surgical manipulation of the pericardium and epicardial surface of the heart and the continued presence of the chest tube. It is not a complication and requires no specific therapy.

The next appearance of a new pericardial rub is usually 4 to 6 days after surgery, although persistence of the immediate postoperative rub more than 24 hr after chest tube removal or its reappearance a day or more later should be considered in the same context. It is rarely associated with malaise, typical pericardial chest pain, fever, or elevated white blood cell count. The pericardial rub is seldom as loud as that associated with the chest tube, but it is often multicomponent. Occasionally it has more harmonic qualities and can be confused with a murmur. In a patient with known valvular heart disease or with newly implanted prosthetic valves this latter feature often raises the question of valvular or prosthetic insufficiency. Proper differentiation can be made by careful timing of cardiac events, changing the patient's position (which will alter the characteristics of a rub), and, when all else fails, patiently waiting or actively treating presumed pericarditis and observing for any changes in physical findings. It is not likely that this type of friction rub, in the absence of other physiologic alterations, represents postpericardiotomy syndrome with any of its potential sequelae. At the author's center, it is not treated medically.

On occasion, however, there is chest pain with pericardial features, or perhaps a slightly elevated temperature or white blood cell count. Rarely are any of these features profound, nor are many of the additional characteristics of postpericardiotomy syndrome present. On the grounds that certain of these cases represent milder forms of postpericardiotomy syndrome, most individuals are treated. The finding of an echocardiographically small pericardial effusion is of little help since most unaffected patients will also have this finding. A moderate to large effusion, however, is an obvious indication for therapy. Excepting the case of a large pericardial effusion, we have not used enforced bed rest and have not found salicylate therapy to be particularly beneficial; instead, we advise nonsteroidal anti-inflammatory agents or steroids. Indomethacin, 25 to 50 mg every 6 hr, is a popular nonsteroidal therapy, but it should be avoided in individuals with chronic renal insufficiency (creatinine above 1.7) due to adverse renal vascular effects. Sulindac, 150 mg every 12 hr, has also been used with success and is believed to have less profound adverse renal effects. A combination of steroidal and nonsteroidal therapy that the author has found particularly satisfactory consists of dexamethasone, 4 mg orally every 8 hr for 2 days, followed by indomethacin, 25 to 50 mg every 6 hr. High-dose, steroid-only therapy is generally reserved for more definitive postpericardiotomy syndrome.

POSTPERICARDIOTOMY SYNDROME

Because most early cardiac surgery consisted of commissurotomy for rheumatic mitral valve disease, this syndrome, recognized as early as 1952 (1), was initially termed postcommissurotomy syndrome and was thought to represent reactivation of rheumatic heart disease (2). The same clinical features were soon recognized following surgery for nonrheumatic diseases, and it was then that the current name, postpericardiotomy syndrome, was first used (3). Most investigators believe that this entity is identical to that described by Dressler in 1956 following acute myocardial infarction (4). Although the syndrome is now known not to be rheumatic in origin (3, 5, 6), controversy still exists over the etiology of this interesting condition. Although antiheart antibodies are present in lower titer in many unaffected postsurgery patients, their high titer prevalence (in virtually all cases in some studies) in association with the syndrome has strongly implicated some form of autoimmune response (7, 8). Such a reaction is believed to be possible from postoperative hemopericardium, traumatic pericarditis, or denatured myocardium (9, 10). Additional support for this proposed mechanism is found in the ability to reproduce a similar condition in the animal model by intrapericardial injection of blood as well as subcutaneous fat (11). Furthermore, some degree of success was achieved in preoperatively "desensitizing" patients by intravenous injections of homogenized atrial myocardium in anticipation of mitral commissurotomy (12). The high incidence of heart antibodies in the sera of patients with differing forms of heart disease (7), including myocardial infarction (13), has resulted in limited specificity of this finding for diagnostic confirmation of postpericardiotomy syndrome.

A distinctive spring and summer occurrence pattern (14, 15), and the presence of elevated titers of various viruses known to produce pericarditis (16), led to speculation that this was a viral-mediated condition. Based on persevering work by Engle and associates, who found frequent coprevalence of high-titer antiheart antibody in all patients with postpericardiotomy syndrome, as well as a 4-fold increase in antibody to adenovirus or coxsackie B1 to B6 virus in 70% of affected patients, the present belief is that this is an immunologic reaction triggered by acute or latent virus infection (17). Figure 20.1 illustrates the relationship of antibody to these viruses and the respective incidence of postpericardiotomy syndrome (17). Injured myocardium, pericardial irritation, or hemopericardium appears to play some role, possibly by rendering the pericardium more susceptible to the effect of viral infection.

The most common surgical approach to the pericardium, at least in adults, is to leave it widely open to promote postoperative drainage and hopefully avoid pericardial temponade. The implications of this decision as it may relate to postpericardiotomy syndrome, as well as tamponade, have been investigated with somewhat conflicting results. An early report by Baue and Blakemore suggested that postpericardiotomy

FIGURE 20.1

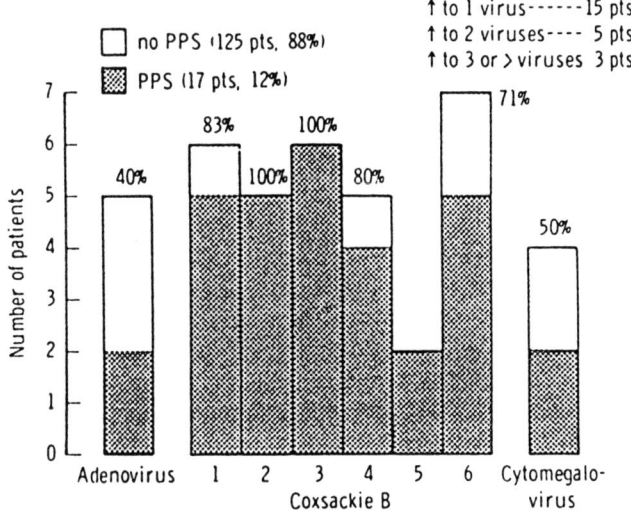

INCIDENCE OF POSTPERICARDIOTOMY SYNDROME FOR EACH VIRUS
WITH RISE IN TITER OR ANTIVIRAL ANTIBODY IN 23 OF 142 ADULTS

The number of adults with a 4-fold or greater rise in antibody is shown for each agent tested, together with the incidence of clinical postpericardiotomy syndrome (*PPS*) among those with a significant rise (23 of 142 adults). (From Engle MA, Gay WA, McCabe J, et al: Postpericardiotomy syndrome in adults: incidence, autoimmunity and virology. *Circulation* 64:[Suppl II]:58–60, 1981.)

syndrome was lessened when the pericardium was left open (18). However, Cunningham and associates reported a 4-fold higher incidence of postpericardiotomy syndrome when the pericardium was left open (10.7% versus 2.8%), compared to patients in whom it was carefully closed (19). Perhaps the best study was that of Asanza and coworkers, which randomly allocated patients to the practice of closing the pericardium or leaving it open (100 in each group). They found postpericardiotomy syndrome in three patients with closed pericardium and one patient with open pericardium, not believed to be a significant difference. Interestingly, pericardial friction rub was more frequent with closed pericardium (14 patients) than with open pericardium (three patients) (20). In summary, it is not clear how leaving the pericardium open influences the incidence of postpericardiotomy syndrome, and it may be most prudent to decide on closure of the pericardium based on greater ease of reoperation and potential need for such a repeat surgery (19, 20).

The incidence of postpericardiotomy syndrome is less in adults than in children, with reports varying from 1 to 40%. The incidence, even within an adult population, varies according to age, from 28.5% for patients under age 40, 19.7% for ages 40 to 59 years, 14.2% for ages 60 to 69, and 10% for 70 years and older (17). Seasonal variation notwithstanding, an incidence of between 10 and 20% should be expected at present.

The symptoms and signs have been well described and vary from low-grade fever, with or without white blood count elevation, to a profound illness with pericardial and pleuritic pain, myalgias, lassitude with fever (up to 104°F), and diaphoresis (21). A pericardial friction rub, often a pleural rub with pericardial and pleural effusions (occasionally left-sided only) and occasionally pulmonary infiltrate are common. Nonspecific laboratory features include elevated white blood count with leftward shift and elevated sedimentation rate.

Table 20.1 illustrates the relative frequency of typical symptoms and physical findings in a group of 45 patients with postpericardiotomy syndrome (22). Fever, chest discomfort, and pleural pericardial rub are present in the over-

TABLE 20.1

TYPICAL SIGNS AND SYMPTOMS IN POSTPERICARDIOTOMY SYNDROME PATIENTS[a]

Sign or Symptom	No. of Patients	Incidence
		%
Fever	45	100
Increased incisional pain	43	95
Pericardial or pleural rub	43	95
Malaise and weakness	31	69
Increased white blood cell count	38	84
Increased erythrocyte sedimentation rate	36	80
Pericardial or pleural fluid	30	67
Asymptomatic	2	4

[a]Modified from Urschel HC, Razzuk MA, Gardner M: Coronary artery bypass occlusion secondary to postcardiotomy syndrome. *Ann Thorac Surg* 22:528–531, 1976.

whelming majority of cases. Chest x-ray findings or cardiomegaly or pleural effusion are helpful but nonspecific. Likewise, the electrocardiogram, if demonstrating diffuse S-T segment elevation, may be helpful, but T wave changes alone are not specific and very often the electrocardiogram will be completely normal despite florid clinical involvement. The echocardiographic finding of a small pericardial effusion is likewise not specific, and its absence need not rule the condition out, as two-thirds of patients may have no pleural or pericardial fluid (22). While antiheart and antiviral antibodies are present in a majority of affected patients, in reality this type of serologic confirmation is rarely obtained, and treatment is based on the clinical diagnosis alone. It appears, for instance, that technetium pyrophosphate imaging is not successful in detecting acute pericarditis (23).

While the syndrome can appear as early as 1 week after surgery, it most commonly appears 2 to 3 weeks postoperatively (21). In the author's experience, delayed appearance for up to 2 months has not been rare. In mild or less obvious cases, it should be suspected in the presence of fever appearing after 6 or 7 days postoperatively, when early postoperative "surgical" pericarditis (as described above) does not disappear after 1 week or reappears after the 1st postoperative week.

Feared consequences include tamponade, aortocoronary bypass graft closure, pericardial constriction and, less well-documented, arrhythmias.

Although pericardial tamponade both early and late in the course has been reported (24, 25), in the author's experience this is uncommon. When examined, the pericardial fluid is usually serosanguinous. Patients with echocardiographically moderate or even large pericardial effusions can be managed conservatively if they remain symptomatically well compensated and physiologic evidence of tamponade is absent. Systolic blood pressure, for instance, should be above 100, pulse pressure greater than 30 mm Hg, and the heart rate no greater than 110 beats/min. In addition, the patient should be examined daily for increasing pulsus paradoxus or decreased urine output. If any of these factors indicated deterioration, pericardiocentesis is recommended. Because of the potential risk of damage to anterior-placed saphenous vein or internal mammary grafts, pericardiocentesis in this setting poses special problems and, unless emergent, should be performed in an intensive care unit by a very experienced physician, preferably one with knowledge of the location of bypass grafts in the patient. Because of the possibility of loculated fluid, it probably should not be attempted unless there is two-dimensional echocardiographic evidence of fluid anteriorly or around the apex of the heart. It should not be attempted without electrocardiographic or echocardiographic monitoring of the probing needle. The anatomic approach used should be either the left parasternal fourth or fifth interspace or the left subcostal approach, and should be chosen based on the operator's experience with this approach and, most importantly, knowledge of bypass graft position. Special care must be taken in skin preparation because of the potential of bacteriologic skin contamination in postoperative patients after several days of hospitalization.

Bypass graft occlusion has been reported as a consequence of uncomplicated postpericardiotomy syndrome (22, 26), and possibly may occur after postpericardiotomy syndrome complicated by constriction (27). Urschel and coworkers reported graft occlusion in 85% of patients with postpericardiotomy syndrome whose therapy consisted of symptomatic relief of pain.

A subsequent group of 31 patients with post-pericardiotomy syndrome all received salicylates, as well as prednisone (in tapering doses for as long as 6 weeks), with an associated graft occlusion rate of 15% (22). Roses and associates reported a bypass patency rate of 50% in three patients with postpericardiotomy syndrome, compared to a patency rate of 79% in eight patients without this complication (26). While the association with graft occlusion is not clearly established, this, in addition to the goal of symptomatic relief, should constitute a potential benefit of aggressive medical therapy.

Although an early review suggested that constrictive pericarditis had not been reported (21), it is now clear that constriction can occur as a result of open-heart surgery, and a significant number of such patients had evidence of preceding postpericardiotomy syndrome. Rice and associates reported that 4 of 5 patients with pericardial constriction had had postpericardiotomy syndrome (28), 7 of 11 patients with postoperative constriction reported by Kutcher and associates had postpericardiotomy syndrome (29), and it preceded constriction in 11 of 19 patients reported by Miller et al (30) and in 4 of 12 patients reported from the Cleveland Clinic (31). While these data strongly suggest that postpericardiotomy syndrome is frequently in the background and is possibly a causative factor in postoperative constriction, it does not allow establishment of the incidence of constriction following postpericardiotomy syndrome. It seems to be rare in view of the low incidence of reported constriction (0.2%) and the relatively common occurrence of postpericardiotomy syndrome (29).

Recurrence of clinical symptoms or pericardial fluid is difficult to establish from the literature, but early reports indicate that the incidence varies from 13% in a pediatric age group (24) to almost 50% in adults (32). At the author's center, recurrence is seen in no more than 10% of cases and is more likely in individuals whose initial presentation is associated with more profound symptoms.

Although arrhythmias in patients with pericarditis are common, a causal relationship assumed by many investigators and clinicians (33–35) may not be warranted. Both pro-spective (36) and retrospective (37) electrocardiographic data, as well as Holter monitoring data (38), indicate that pericarditis per se is not arrhythmogenic and that significant arrhythmias in a patient with pericarditis imply additional cardiac abnormality. Interestingly, in the study employing a Holter monitor in 50 patients with acute pericarditis, all significant arrhythmias were infrequent (there were four episodes of intermittent supraventricular tachycardia). In only four patients with ventricular ectopic beats were arrhythmias judged to be frequent (38).

POSTOPERATIVE CONSTRICTIVE PERICARDITIS

The relationship of cardiac surgery to later constrictive pericarditis has been recognized since 1967 (39). Although constriction is reported to occur as early as 2 weeks (29) and as late as several years (28) after surgery, the majority of cases appear between 3 and 12 months postoperatively (29–31). Symptoms and signs are similar to those of other causes of pericardial constriction. Dyspnea is invariably present, and chest pain is a common but not invariable symptom. Virtually all patients will have distended neck veins and peripheral edema, and most will have ascites and hepatosplenomegaly (29, 31). Prominent X or Y descent is common, but paradoxical pulse is virtually never present. Pericardial knock or pericardial rub is variably present (29). Neither chest x-ray nor electrocardiogram will provide definitive diagnosis. Chest x-ray, if abnormal, may show nonspecific cardiac silhouette widening (29, 31). The most common electrocardiographic findings are nonspecific S-T segment and T wave changes (seen in less than half of patients), and low voltage will be seen in only a small proportion. Echocardiographic findings may include a small pericardial effusion in some patients. Thickening of the pericardium may be helpful, if present. The finding of flattening of left ventricular posterior wall endocardium on M-mode echocardiography distinguished 11 of 12 patients as reported by Voelkel et al (40). Definitive noninvasive diagnosis of constrictive pericarditis has also been reported using standard computed tomography of the thorax (41). More recently, rapid cine-mode tomography has been successfully used to diagnose this condition, providing high-quality tomographic images in the moving picture format (42). The traditional hallmarks of diagnosis have been hemodynamic features that consist of equalization of right and left ventricular filling pressures and a characteristic dip and plateau (square root sign) during diastole in both ventricular chambers and equalization of diastolic pressures in virtually all cardiac chambers. In patients in whom constriction is strongly suspected but cannot be confirmed by equalized diastolic pressures, rapid intravenous volume infusion may unmask the true hemodynamic features of constriction (43).

Aside from severe intercurrent illness or extremely advanced age, most patients will require surgery, which may consist of either localized or radical pericardiectomy (29–31). A trial of medical therapy consisting of diuretics and steroids is warranted by is unlikely to obviate the eventual need for surgery, with the exception of patients presenting relatively early (within 2 months of surgery). The rationale for optimism is based on the higher likelihood of an inflammatory component with less well established fibrosis during this early period (29). The surgical outcome is good with symptomatic relief, resolution of hemodynamic abnormalities, and low operative mortality (29–31).

The suggested mechanisms for this complication include, most prominently, postpericardiotomy syndrome, the use of povidone-iodine pericardial irritation solution, and the late effects of postoperative hemopericardium (29, 31). Interestingly, a condition histologically identical to constrictive pericarditis has been produced by hypothermia in the canine model by exposure of the pericardium to $1\frac{3}{4}$ hr of slush at $-0.5°C$ (44). This seems to be an unlikely cause of the human cases of constrictive pericarditis reported to date in view of the relatively infrequent contemporary use of pericardial slush as a means of attaining hypothermia. In other experimental animal studies pericardial adhesions required only the contact of spilled blood on an injured serosal surface (45).

References

1. Janton OH, Glover RP, O'Neill TJE, et al: Results of the surgical treatment of mitral stenosis. *Circulation* 6:321–333, 1952.
2. Soloff LA, Zatuchni J, Janton OH, et al: Reactivation of rheumatic fever following mitral commissurotomy. *Circulation* 8:481–493, 1953.
3. Ito, T, Engle MA, Goldberg HP: Postpericardiotomy syndrome following surgery for nonrheumatic heart disease. *Circulation* 17:549–556, 1958.
4. Dressler W: Idiopathic recurrent pericarditis. Comparison with the post-commissurotomy syndrome, consideration of etiology and treatment. *Am J Med* 18:591–601, 1955.
5. Epstein S: Is the postcommissurotomy syndrome of rheumatic origin? *AMA Arch Intern Med* 99:253–259, 1957.
6. Larson DL: Relation of the postcommissurotomy syndrome to the rheumatic state. *Circulation* 15:203–209. 1957.
7. Gery I, Davies AM, Ehrenfeld EN: Heart-specific autoantibodies. *Lancet* 1:471–472, 1960.
8. Engle MA, McCabe JC, Ebert PA, et al: The postpericardiotomy syndrome and antiheart antibodies. *Circulation* 49:401–406, 1974.
9. Dressler W: The post-myocardial-infarction syndrome: a report on forty-four cases. *AMA Arch Intern Med* 103:28–42, 1959.
10. Holswade GR, Engle MA, Redo SF, et al: Development of viral diseases and a viral disease-like syndrome after extracorporeal circulation. *Circulation* 27:812–815, 1963.
11. Ehrenhaft JL, Taber RE: Hemopericardium and constrictive pericarditis. *J Thorac Surg* 24:355–368, 1952.
12. Corday E: The nature and management of the post-commissurotomy syndrome. *Dis Chest* 39:222, 1961.
13. Heine WI, Friedman H, Mandell MS, et al: Antibodies to cardiac tissue in acute ischemic heart disease. *Am J Cardiol* 17:798–803, 1966.
14. Cohen G, Dardick I, Greenblatt J: Pleurisy and pericarditis complicating myocardial infarction: the so-called post-myocardial infarction syndrome. *Can Med Assoc J* 82:123–130, 1960.
15. Drusin LM, Engle MA, Hastrom JWC, et al: The postpericardiotomy syndrome. A six-year epidemiologic study. *N Engl J Med* 272:597–602, 1965.
16. Lerner MA, Wilson FM, Reyes MD: Enteroviruses and the heart (with special emphasis on the probable role of coxsackie viruses, group B, types 1–5). II. Observations in humans. *Mod Conc Cardiovasc Dis* 44(3):11–15, 1975.

17. Engle MA, Gay WA, McCabe J, et al: Post-pericardiotomy syndrome in adults: incidence, autoimmunity and virology. *Circulation* 64 (Suppl II):58–60, 1981.
18. Baue AE, Blakemore WS: The pericardium. *Ann Thorac Surg* 14:81–106, 1972.
19. Cunningham JN Jr, Spencer FC, Zeff R, et al: Influence of primary closure of the pericardium after open-heart surgery on the frequency of tamponade, postcardiotomy syndrome, and pulmonary complications. *J Thorac Cardiovasc Surg* 70:119–125, 1975.
20. Asa.:za L, Rao G, Violeti C, et al: Should the pericardium be closed after an open-heart operation? *Ann Thorac Surg* 22:532–534, 1976.
21. Kirsh MM, McIntoch K, Kahn DR, et al: Post-pericardiotomy syndromes. *Ann Thorac Surg* 9:158–179, 1970.
22. Urschel HC, Razzuk MA, Gardner M: Coronary artery bypass occlusion secondary to postcardiotomy syndrome. *Ann Thorac Surg* 22:528–531, 1976.
23. Fleg JL, Siegel BA, Williamson JR et al: 99mTc-pyrophosphate imaging in acute pericarditis: a clinical and experimental study. *Radiology* 126:727–731, 1978.
24. Engle MA, Ito T: The postcardiotomy syndrome. *Am J Cardiol* 7:77–82, 1961.
25. Engle MA, Marx NR: The postpericardiotomy and perfusion syndromes. *Heart Bull* 14:33–36, 1965.
26. Roses DF, Rose MR, Rapaport FT: Febrile responses associated with cardiac surgery. Relationships to the postpericardiotomy syndrome and to altered host immunologic reactivity. *J Thorac Cardiovasc Surg* 67:251–257, 1974.
27. Kabbani SS, Bashour T, Ellertson DG, et al: Constrictive pericarditis following myocardial revascularization: a possible cause of graft occlusion. *Am Heart J* 110:493–495, 1985.
28. Rice PL, Pifarre R, Montoya A: Constrictive pericarditis following cardiac surgery. *Ann Thorac Surg* 31:450–453, 1981.
29. Kutcher MA, King SB, Alimurung BN, et al: Constrictive pericarditis as a complication of cardiac surgery: recognition of an entity. *Am J Cardiol* 50:742–748, 1982.
30. Miller JI, Mansour KA, Hatcher CR: Pericardiectomy: current indications, concepts and results in a university center. *Ann Thorac Surg* 34:40–45, 1982.
31. Ng SH, Dorosti K, Sheldon WC: Constrictive pericarditis following cardiac surgery—Cleveland Clinic experience: report of 12 cases and review. *Cleve Clin Q* 51:39–45, 1983.
32. Larson DL: Relation of the postcommissurotomy syndrome to the rheumatic state. *Circulation* 15:203–209, 1957.
33. Savage DD, Garrison RJ, Brand F, et al: Prevalence and correlates of posterior extra echocardiographic spaces in a free living population based sample (the Framingham Study). *Am J Cardiol* 51:1207–1212, 1983.
34. Mancini GB, Goldberger AC: Cardioversion of atrial fibrillation: consideration of embolization, anticoagulation, prophylactic pacemaker, and long-term success. *Am Heart J* 104:617–621, 1982.
35. Braunwald E: *Heart Disease*, Philadelphia, WB Saunders, 1980, p 1526.
36. Spodick DH: Arrhythmias during acute pericarditis: a prospective study of one hundred consecutive cases. *JAMA* 235:39–41, 1976.
37. Bruce MA, Spodick DH: Atypical electrocardiogram in acute pericarditis: characteristics and prevalence. *J Electrocardiol* 13:61–66, 1980.
38. Spodick DH: Frequency of arrhythmias in acute pericarditis determined by Holter monitoring. *Am J Cardiol* 53:842–845, 1984.
39. Lange RL: Compressive cardiac and circulatory disorders, clinical and laboratory correlation. *Am Heart J* 74:419–430, 1967.
40. Voelkel AG, Pietro DA, Folland ED, et al: Echocardiographic features of constrictive pericarditis. *Circulation* 58:871–875, 1978.
41. Ribeiro P, Sapsford R, Evans T, et al: Constrictive pericarditis as a complication of coronary artery bypass surgery. *Br Heart J* 51:205–210, 1984.
42. Bateman TM, Gray RJ, Whiting JS, et al: Cine-computed tomography evaluation of aorto-coronary bypass graft patency. *J Am Coll Cardiol* 8:693–698, 1986.
43. Bush, CA, Stang JM, Wolley CF, et al: Occult constrictive pericardial disease: diagnosis by rapid volume expansion and correction by pericardiectomy. *Circulation* 56:924–930, 1977.
44. Speicher CE, Ferrigan L, Wolfson SK, et al: Cold injury of myocardium and pericardium in cardiac hypothermia. *Surg Gynecol Obstet* 114:659–665, 1962.
45. Cliff, WJ, Groberty J, Ryan GB: Postoperative pericardial adhesions. The role of mild serosal injury and spilled blood. *J Thorac Cardiovasc Surg* 65:774–750, 1973.

Chapter 21
WORKUP OF POSTOPERATIVE CHEST PAIN

RICHARD J. GRAY, M.D.

Naturally, chest discomfort is expected to occur after sternotomy but occasionally its features may seem more ominous. The purpose of this chapter is to suggest an approach to chest pain occurring during early convalescence (while in the hospital). It is not intended to be a complete discussion of the late reappearance of angina and closure of coronary bypass grafts, which is covered in Chapter 31.

CAUSES OF EARLY POSTOPERATIVE CHEST PAIN

Incisional Pain

This is by far the most common cause of postoperative chest discomfort. Typically, incisional pain is mid- and parasternal and is worse with coughing, deep breathing, and sneezing, but it can also be manifest as shoulder, axillary, or neck pain not specifically related to physical activity or movement. Internal mammary (thoracic) artery bypass is associated with somewhat more severe chest wall pain than that of the typical sternotomy alone. The pain is often worse on the side of the mammary artery takedown, if unilateral, and anterior chest wall numbness is also common. Persistent, nonexertional discomfort at the base of the neck frequently results from mammary artery usage. Usually, incisional pain is severe enough to require par-

enteral analgesics only for the first 2 days, and particularly severe pain after that should trigger a more complete examination of the incisional site. Fracture of the sternum and dehiscence or disruption of the sternum closure are other causes of unusually severe incisional pain. Such occurrences should arouse suspicion of mediastinal infection. It should also be kept in mind that rib fracture, usually of the first or second rib, has been reported after sternotomy. Differentiation between incisional pain and ischemic cardiac pain is often necessary because of the frequency with which preoperative angina was the indication for surgery and because of the therapeutic implications if this does represent ischemic cardiac pain.

Diagnostic features include the reproduction of pain with deep breathing, coughing, or palpation of the area. Lateral compression of the thoracic cage from beneath the axilla and anterior-posterior compression on both sides of the sternum are good tests for rib fracture. Rib series x-ray with special views of the sternum may be useful.

Once assured that incisional discomfort is the cause, most patients feel quite relieved. This, along with a reevaluation of analgesic needs, is often sufficient. In cases of recurrent severe pain, such as in the costochondral cartilage region, local blockade by injection of a combination of a local anesthetic and corticosteroid mixture can provide good temporary relief, but is only useful if a trigger point can be found. One approach is to draw up 12 ml of 0.5% Marcaine and 20 to 30 mg Depo-Medrol in a syringe. This will be sufficient to inject the costochondral cartilage at 3 to 4 levels.

Pericardial Pain

Next in order of frequency is pain originating from the pericardium. The location may be substernal or precordial, but a diagnostic tipoff may be the relationship to moderately deep breathing or even swallowing. The unique feature of nonoperative pericarditis, namely worsening with recumbency and relief with assumption of upright position, may be present or absent. While as many as 30 to 40% of patients will have a pericardial friction rub even after chest tube removal, it is asymptomatic in most. When chest discomfort is associated with a pericardial friction rub, pericarditis is almost certainly the cause. This diagnosis is even more convincing if there is low-grade fever (up to 101.5°) and leukocytosis. Echocardiography is often performed and in this setting usually demonstrates a small pericardial fluid collection. This may be of little diagnostic benefit, however, because the extremely high frequency of pericardial effusion, even in the absence of pericarditis, makes this finding of low specificity. A more complete discussion of postoperative pericarditis is found in Chapter 20.

Ischemic Cardiac Pain

This kind of pain is of great concern, not because of its severity but because of its significance. In the setting of bypass surgery, the concern is obviously that of bypass graft narrowing or closure or, much less likely, closure of a particularly narrowed section of native vessel. In the presence of valve replacement or repair, especially when atrial fibrillation is present, coronary embolism is an additional concern.

The patient will usually remember his or her preoperative angina well enough for comparison. Although postoperative angina when present is almost always similar to its preoperative counterpart, noncardiac causes for pain can also seem remarkably like preoperative angina to the patient. This factor can be especially confounding to the diagnosis. Although diaphoresis can occur with severe pain of any origin, its presence should arouse particular concern over the possibility of cardiac ischemia. Electrocardiograhic changes may be helpful if present but will be misleading if several days have lapsed from a previous tracing, inasmuch as benign repolarization changes will often have occurred in the interim. This is especially common during the latter 4 or 5 days of the hospital course. Although exertional features are helpful, true ischemia certainly can occur at rest in this setting. Likewise, a beneficial response to nitroglycerin is helpful only if the response is rapid and typical of the expected time course. Interestingly, one or two relatively brief periods of ischemic-type pain may occur and not be seen again.

Pain that is long lasting (generally longer than 15 min), similar to preoperative angina, and associated with electrocardiographic changes is suspicious of acute graft closure and may represent a serious threat to the patient. Stat cardiac enzymes and serial electrocardiograms are indicated to determine the presence of infarction. Because of the potential danger posed by graft occlusion, immediate, aggressive treatment is usually based on an index of suspicion and should precede a definitive workup. Immediate therapy with nitroglycerin or even morphine is indicated and, depending on hemodynamic status, intravenous nitroglycerin may be used. Although longer-acting nitrates and calcium channel blocking agents are highly useful in this setting, the acuity of the situation usually demands intravenous therapy. Based on the knowledge that much early graft occlusion is thrombotic in nature, intravenous heparin is often added to the regimen. Dosing must be carefully controlled to avoid pericardial hemorrhage, however.

In the presence of objective evidence of cardiac involvement, such as with electrocardiographic changes, a strategic approach to the patient should be outlined by both the cardiologist or internist and the cardiac surgeon. For instance, intraoperative knowledge about the downstream condition of vessels and anastomotic sites may greatly aid in understanding the likelihood and potential consequences for specific graft closure. Such information is critical to the diagnostic and therapeutic plan. Coronary and graft angiography, if performed, must be predicated on a reasonable certainty that an especially important bypass is in jeopardy and on the expectation that surgery should have been successful, and a secondary attempt at revascularization is likely to succeed. Most important, all parties, including surgeon, internist, and patient, must agree that if the clinical impression is confirmed, interventional therapy will be undertaken. Such intervention will involve either angioplasty or urgent reoperation inasmuch as thrombolysis is not indicated because of the high likelihood of catastrophic hemorrhage due to recent surgery. Such an aggressive interventional approach is rarely undertaken because early bypass closure usually occurs in the setting of poor runoff due to distal coronary disease, and an encore performance is likely to be similarly fated.

Relatively mild pain in the absence of electrocardiographic changes, especially that which occurs with exertion, can be approached much more electively. Diagnostic aids include performance of a bedside atrial pacing study using the surgically implanted epicardial atrial pacemaker wires. One such approach involves pacing for 90-second intervals at heart rates of 70, 90, 110, 130, and 150 beats/min. Reproduction of the chest pain syndrome is of significance, although the test is positive only with the presence of greater than 1 mm S-T segment depression as recorded as 12-lead echocardiography at the end of the pacing. AV Wenckebach after a heart rate of 130 beats/min is common during this type of pacing. Atrial pacing can be very effectively combined with thallium-201 scintigraphy (1–3). Another diagnostic test is a low-level exercise test with or without thallium imaging. Here the end point of testing is the achievement of a heart rate of 120 beats/min, appearance of typical chest pain, or fatigue. The test is interpreted as positive with greater than 1 mm S-T segment depression. Positive responses to either of these tests might indicate the need for a modification of the convalescent activities or addition of antianginal therapy, but

are not usually followed by a more aggressive interventional approach.

The occurrence of even several episodes of ischemic-like pain in the absence of a bona fide myocardial infarction may still be associated with a benign course. Generally, such patients are managed throughout the hospital course on antianginal therapy but are often able to stop all such therapy shortly because the pain may not recur.

Pulmonary Causes

The diagnosis of greatest concern here is that of pulmonary embolism, which appears uncommonly after this type of surgery. This is due to the profound heparin anticoagulation used during the procedure itself, the platelet dysfunction seen in the early postoperative period, and the frequent early application of other antithrombotic therapy such as subcutaneous heparin and oral aspirin and Persantine. Nevertheless, pulmonary embolism can occur, and any appearance of severe pleuritic left or right lateral chest discomfort, tachycardia, or unexplained hypoxemia should cause concern.

Confounding the picture is the fact that all of these features are common in the postoperative patient. A normally convalescing patient may have an aterial PO_2 as low as 55 or 60 mm Hg on room air. Administration of oxygen often helps to differentiate this normal response, because the PO_2 often rises to 85 or 90 mm Hg or more in the absence of pulmonary embolism.

Any suspicion of pulmonary embolism should prompt a rapid workup with a low threshold for initiation of therapy while the remainder of the workup proceeds. Immediate blood gas analysis, electrocardiogram, chest x-ray, and ventilation-perfusion imaging are indicated. The frequency with which basilar atelectasis and even pulmonary infiltrates are seen in this population make refined chest x-ray interpretation and even ventilation-perfusion imaging difficult to interpret. Because of this, it is rare to see a ventilation-perfusion scan read as "normal" or "matching perfusion ventilation defects" or "low likelihood of pulmonary embolism." Instead, the reading in even the most benign of patients is often that of "equivocal" or "cannot rule out pulmonary embolism." The presence of multiple, especially bilateral, nonmatching perfusion defects is a strong indication of pulmonary embolism even when symptoms may be atypical. In this circumstance, rapid institution of intravenous heparin is indicated, and a search for possible embolic sites should begin. Because of the early postoperative status of the patient, there is an increased risk of bleeding; therefore, heparin therapy should be carefully monitored, and the maximum end point of therapy should be prolongation of the baseline partial thromboplastin time to two times normal. Pulmonary angiography is usually reserved for the circumstances in which heparin therapy is at especially high risk and the diagnosis must be confirmed, or when apparent recurrent embolism occurs on seemingly adequate anticoagulation therapy and inferior vena cava interruption is contemplated.

An equivocal ventilation-perfusion scan or one interpreted as "intermediate likelihood" for pulmonary embolism in the presence of unconvincing symptoms should probably not be treated with heparin.

Profound and typical symptoms of pulmonary embolism should prompt immediate heparin therapy, and it is doubtful if further diagnostic testing is necessary.

References

1. Weiss AT, Tzivoni D, Sagie A, et al: Atrial pacing thallium scintigraphy in the evaluation of coronary artery disease. *Isr J Med Sci* 19:495–503, 1983.
2. Stratmann HG, Mark AL, Walter KE, et al: Atrial pacing and thallium 201 scintigraphy: combined use for diagnosis of coronary artery disease. *Angiology* 807–814, Nov 1987.
3. David YB, Shefer A, Weiss AT, et al: Early postoperative assessment of coronary artery bypass surgery using nuclear left ventriculography and atrial pacing. *Thorac Cardiovasc Surg* 31:377–381, 1983.

Chapter 22
WORKUP AND TREATMENT OF POSTOPERATIVE FEVER AND INFECTION

STEPHEN J. UMAN, M.D.

Infections are a major spoiler of most surgical treatments. This is perhaps even more so in cardiovascular surgery because of the involvement of a particularly vital organ, the frequent use of prosthetic materials that are resistant to therapy when infected, and, increasingly, the treatment of elderly patients with multiple medical problems which make the likelihood of postoperative infections greater. The physical and personal effects of infectious complications are obvious. The financial effects, of increasing importance in this era of shrinking monetary resources, have also been documented (1). Efforts to prevent these problems are of paramount importance; early diagnosis and treatment is a necessary alternative if they become established.

OVERVIEW OF POSTOPERATIVE FEVER

Although studies (2–4) have shown that there may be poor correlation between fever and infection after cardiovascular surgery, fever is still the most common initial warning sign that an infectious complication may be present. The level of hyperpyrexia may not be critical since some elderly patients are not able to mount a febrile response and endotoxemia associated with

Gram-negative infection may initially induce hypothermia.

Fever appearing very early in the postoperative period (that is, within the first 12 to 18 hr) is rarely due to infection, unless preexisting. Noninfectious causes of such immediate fevers include drug or transfusion reactions, malignant hyperpyrexia, or aspiration of gastric contents (which may later lead to actual infection). Such problems should be easily recognizable clinically or by review of past personal or family histories or operative occurrences.

Fever presenting in the first 1 to 2 days postoperatively is often due to infection with *streptococci*, which may present and spread particularly rapidly. Atelectasis is also very common during this period.

The majority of fevers due to infection present after the 2nd postoperative day. The main sites of concern for infection after nearly any surgery include the lungs due to intubation and regional hypoventilation thereafter, the urinary tract due to bladder catheterization, and, of course, the operative sites due to the introduction of abnormal flora into previously sterile tissues and the effects of surgical trauma on blood flow and local host defenses. The common feature of each of these problems is the breaching of normal anatomic barriers that normally keep microorganisms away from the anatomic area.

The most common pulmonary complication is pneumonia, usually due to aspiration of bacteria. Although normal upper respiratory flora are well described as a cause of infection in patients soon after admission to a medical institution, very quickly thereafter patients become colonized with abnormal hospital flora, especially Gram-negative bacilli, which tend to be more resistant to antibiotic treatment and more rapidly damaging once infection becomes established. This must be taken into account when planning empiric antibiotic therapy for these patients. Occasionally, bacteremic pneumonia may present with multicentric involvement, often in cases of endovascular infection such as endocarditis. Other common pulmonary causes of fever include atelectasis, pulmonary embolus (which tends to occur later), and, more rarely, empyema.

Urinary tract infections due to bacteria may be expected when they occur early in the postoperative period, especially enterococci and Gram-negative bacilli. Colonization of the bladder with yeast is often seen later, most often in patients requiring long-term catheterization and prolonged antibiotic therapy. Yeasts rarely lead to invasive infection as such, and usually do not require specific treatment. The patient with a prosthetic heart valve presents a special problem, however (5), since even a transient fungemia may lead to prosthetic valve infection, which is usually impossible to cure medically. In these patients, the presence of fungal bladder colonization can usually be successfully treated with 5-fluorocytosine (6).

Surgical site infections present the greatest threat to undoing the accomplishments of the surgical procedure and will be discussed separately.

Fever presenting late in the postoperative period, after the first 4 to 5 days, is frequently due to noninfectious causes such as atelectasis and retained secretions, pulmonary emboli, drug reactions, intravenous line phlebitis, and the very special entities of postcardiotomy syndrome and postperfusion syndrome.

Aside from fever, infection may also be suggested by leukocytosis, wound drainage, and specific organ dysfunction. Any such clues must be sought and investigated fully since early detection and treatment of infection will ensure the best possible outcome.

SPECIAL SYNDROMES AFTER CARDIOVASCULAR SURGERY

Pyogenic infection of the heart itself is quite uncommon (7–9). Suture site infections are usually fatal when they occur, virtually always being discovered postmortem. Pyogenic pericarditis is less rare but still uncommon.

Endocarditis

Endocarditis may be seen more frequently and may be divided into that occurring "early," in the first 4 to 6 weeks postoperatively, and that occurring "late," or thereafter (10). The involvement of natural versus prosthetic valves bears greatly on the treatment and expectations from treatment (11).

Early endocarditis tends to be due to hospital-acquired organisms, notably coagulase positive and negative *staphylococci* and Gram-negative bacilli. These become established during a period of increased susceptibility due to endocardial disruption from the surgery itself, from indwelling vascular catheters, or a prosthetic heart valve. The presence of continuous bacteremia (i.e., the great majority of blood cultures obtained are positive) in the postoperative period makes it very difficult to rule out endocarditis even if another primary source of infection can be found. Treatment includes aggressive use of intravenous antibiotics, often requiring synergistic combination of two or more antibiotics to achieve adequate killing of involved microorganisms (12–14) for 4 to 6 or more weeks. Surgical intervention will be necessary if blood cultures remain positive despite antibiotics, major emboli continue to occur, valve failure with congestive heart failure is seen, or nonbacterial infection is diagnosed (15–18). New valve placement after adequate débridement of the infected area and continued postoperative antibiotic therapy is virtually always successful if enough heart tissue remains to give the new valve a good seat (19).

Late endocarditis, if related to cardiac surgery, involves prosthetic valves. By the time this occurs, the threat from hospital-acquired bacteria is passed and the base of the valve has become sufficiently healed and epithelialized so that the endocarditis is more characteristic of natural valve infection. Symptoms are more subacute and *Streptococcus viridans* is the most commonly occurring organism. Treatment also mirrors that given for natural valve infection—penicillin, with or without an aminoglycoside, is fully adequate, and cure rates approach those for natural valve disease. Culture-negative prosthetic valve endocarditis usually implies fungal infection, with poor prognosis (20, 21).

Mediastinal Infection

Sternal and mediastinal infections are probably the most common serious infectious complications (22–26). These often present after initial discharge from the hospital up to several weeks after surgery. The history commonly includes minimal wound drainage or low-grade fever that was thought to be inconsequential. Symptoms may be subacute, with low-grade fever, persistent wound drainage, and mild pain, or the presentation may be acute, with fever and rigors, gross purulent drainage, and marked pain. In all cases the likelihood of extensive sternal involvement is great, eventually leading to instability and dehiscence, and retrosternal spread of infection. Evaluation must include culture of blood and any drainage for bacteria (if cultures are negative, additional specimens should be submitted for anaerobic and acid-fast bacteria and fungal culture) and computed tomographic scanning to assess the extent of involvement of the sternum and to detect any retrosternal abscess (27). The wound should be opened and débrided as necessary to allow drainage of any loculated infected material. Intravenous antibiotics should be administered to treat the offending organism, usually *Staphylococcus aureus*, although other organisms seen may include enterococcus and aerobic Gram-negative rods and yeast. Mediastinal tubes should be left in place to allow irrigation with antiseptic solutions such as povidone-iodine. If little sternal tissue has been destroyed, rewiring and primary closure is usually successful. If a significant amount of tissue has been lost, plas-

tic surgical evaluation and intervention should be requested early to help plan a means of closing the defect (28–31). Failure to achieve a microbiologic cure is not uncommon, particularly if a nonbacterial infection is present. Sternal instability is not uncommon even if microbiologic sterilization has been achieved.

Pacemaker Infection

Pacemaker infections may occur in the pocket holding the pacemaker, along the route of the leads, or at the site of implantation in the heart itself (32, 33). Inflammation and drainage may be visible in the first two instances. Pacemaker tip infection will almost always be associated with bacteremia (34, 35), usually continuous, but bacteremia may not occur with pocket or tunnel infections. Antibiotic treatment should be based on results of cultures but may be begun initially directed at the Gram-positive cocci, staphylococci and streptococci, which cause the majority of these infections. Vancomycin is the most likely agent to cover these completely until final culture reports are available (36). Surgical intervention is usually necessary as well, to drain any loculated purulence in the pocket (37, 38) or to remove the hardware altogether if cure cannot be achieved at the other sites with antibiotics alone, as is often the case (39–42). Infections at the tip of an old pacemaker wire may be the most easily cured with antibiotics alone, which is fortunate since a long-implanted wire may be most difficult to remove (43). Infections of newly implanted temporary pacemakers are relatively unusual and can be easily resolved by removal of the unit.

Leg Wound Infection

Acute leg wound infections are more common and usually much less serious problems (44). These may appear early or late postoperatively, usually with wound erythema and drainage, often with pain and fever. Aerobic bacteria (*staphylococci, streptococci,* and Gram-negative bacilli) are most often responsible. Etiologic diagnosis can usually be readily made by culturing the wound drainage. Initially, antibiotic treatment can be chosen based on Gram stain of this material and later refined on the basis of culture results. Wound débridement is often necessary, especially in advanced cases. Plastic surgical repair is occasionally needed, usually when there has been sloughing of nonviable skin. These infections lead to increased morbidity and prolonged hospital stay. Rarely these may be implicated as primary sources of infections at distant anatomic sites, presumably via bacteremic spread. Thus, aggressive early attention to these processes is essential.

Well-described over the past few years, but poorly understood, is the syndrome of recurrent bacterial cellulitis of the vein-donor leg (45). This may appear months to years after the vein harvesting. Typical evidence of cellulitis is seen, and, as such, this syndrome is not separable from a common case of cellulitis except by the history of preceding vein harvesting for bypass grafting and, often, its recurrent nature. These infections respond rapidly to antibiotics directed against the *streptococci*, the most common cause, and, less often, *staphylococci*. Episodes must be treated individually, but if recurrences occur frequently a trial of long-term prophylaxis, usually with penicillin VK on a regular basis, may be successful. These episodes, even when recurrent, usually occur for 6 to 18 months and then disappear as mysteriously as they appeared. Other prophylactic measures that may be of use include the use of elastic hose to prevent ventostasis and edema, and meticulous care of any inflammations of the toes and toe webs that may cause skin breaks which, in turn, may allow entry of cutaneous bacteria into normally sterile tissue planes (46).

Postcardiotomy Syndrome

The postcardiotomy syndrome is akin to the postmyocardial infarction syndrome described by Dressler, an allergic pericarditis presenting with fever, pericardial friction rub, and sometimes pain (47). The presence of antiheart antibodies may not be specific (48). This can occur quite early (49, 50) but is most often seen after the 7th postoperative day. Even if a rub is heard early, postcardiotomy syndrome cannot be presumed to be present, and a full evaluation for other causes of fever must be undertaken. However, if no other explanation can be found, a course of anti-inflammatory therapy (indomethacin and corticosteroids are used most fre-

quently) may be given both therapeutically and for diagnosis. The response to indomethacin is characteristically quite prompt with a dramatic defervescence of temperature to the normal range. Indeed, if this type of response is not seen, it has been the author's experience that another explanation for the patient's fever should be sought promptly. Since postcardiotomy inflammation has been associated with premature bypass graft closure, diagnosis and treatment are indicated for more than just the comfort afforded to both the patient and the physicians by the resolution of these fevers.

Postperfusion Syndrome

This is a febrile syndrome presenting 4 or more weeks postoperatively, often with hepatitis and arthralgias, due to the development of a *cytomegalovirus* (CMV) infection acquired at the time of surgery from transfusions given perioperatively. This was commonly seen after the use of 6 or more units of transfused blood but is seen much less frequently at present, perhaps due to the use of less blood products than was previously the norm. Treatment is solely symptomatic once the diagnosis can be established, usually via serologic testing (a high IgM anti-CMV antibody titer or a rising IgG titer) coupled with a compatible clinical picture and a lack of other explanations. Under very special conditions such as in the care of heart transplantation where such infections pose a greater threat, special CMV-negative blood can be made available.

FACTORS PREDISPOSING TO INFECTION AFTER CARDIOVASCULAR SURGERY

The complex nature of cardiovascular surgery increases the risk of surgical infectious complications beyond that which might be seen with more simple procedures (51–53).

The patients undergoing those operations are frequently elderly and bring with them coexisting medical problems that increase the risk of infection. Of these, diabetes and ischemic peripheral vascular disease are probably the most important. Male patients may have preexisting prostatic problems which predispose to urinary infections due to the need for prolonged bladder catheterization. Chronic lung disease leading to the need for prolonged intubation and mechanical ventilatory support is often associated with pneumonia. Limited venous access and decreased integumental flexibility may increase the risk of infections related to intravascular access lines.

A variety of host-defense abnormalities have been described as a consequence of the surgery and cardiopulmonary bypass (54–57).

The nature of the surgery itself is complex. The separate activities of vein harvesting, sternal opening and cardiac preparation, and then the delayed insertion of the harvested vein into the open chest presents many exposures to potential contamination (58, 59). Indeed, it is surprising that infection does not occur more commonly in this setting. The prolonged duration of these surgeries and the occasional need for reoperation to treat complications such as delayed bleeding are other well-recognized factors that lead to an increased risk of infection. The increasingly frequent use of internal mammary arteries in bypass surgery may increase the risk of infection by inducing sternal ischemia (60).

Postoperative care of these patients is also complex and requires invasive monitoring with devices that must breach the normal protective functions of the skin, epiglottis, and the urethral epithelium. Spread of contamination via respiratory therapy, contaminated intravenous solutions and cannulae, and, very importantly, medical staff who do not follow routine methods of infection control, including simple hand washing, are important factors (61).

DIAGNOSTIC EVALUATION OF THE PATIENT SUSPECT FOR INFECTION

The presence of fever (62) or other potential signs of infection such as leukocytosis, unexpected wound drainage, or organ-specific dysfunction should lead to a rapid assessment for demonstrable infection. A routine must be established to aid in the prompt yet complete evaluation of patients to determine whether and in what way they are in fact infected.

Needless to say, a complete review of the patient's past and recent history, followed by a complete physical examination including visual examination of all wounds is necessary. Special attention must be given to factors that might increase the risk of infection such as central intravenous catheters, bladder catheters, pacemakers, chest tubes, and intubation. Any obvious sites of inflammation must be examined in greater detail.

Blood cultures must be obtained in sufficient quantities (four to six sets) to avoid missing a transient bacteremia and to determine whether a positive culture represents a continuous bacteremia (suggestive of an endovascular infection) or discontinuous bacteria (suggestive of a source such as an abscess or a urinary tract infection which would be expected to produce bacteremia only on an intermittent basis). For example, a single positive culture for coagulase-negative *staphylococci* with four or five negative cultures could reliably be disregarded as a contaminant, but four or five positive sets out of five or six submitted would be very hard to disregard as such.

Urinalysis, and in most cases urine culture, should be obtained routinely because of the frequent occurrence of urosepsis in this situation. Any abnormal drainage should likewise by cultured and examined by the Gram method.

Examination of the chest x-ray is necessary to assess for infiltrates, effusions, atelectasis, mediastinal widening, or sternal dehiscence (the so-called "median stripe" sign) (63). This examination may not only give valuable information regarding the site of potential infectious complications but may also guide further workup such as thoracentesis or fiber optic bronchoscopy to obtain or remove secretions that may be causing infection or bronchial obstruction, and secondary atelectasis.

Liver function tests and amylase should be measured because of the not-infrequent development of biliary tract disease. Acalculous cholecystitis has occurred frequently in the author's experience, as have hepatitis (more often due to drug reactions in the acute setting than due to infectious agents) and occasionally pancreatitis. Hepato-iminodiacetic acid (HIDA) scanning and ultrasonography have been of particular value in evaluating this area.

Baseline erythrocyte sedimentation rate, *cytomegalovirus* serologies, and rheumatoid factor should be checked routinely for their initial diagnostic value and also for future comparative use should the inflammatory syndrome continue without explanation.

Once this evaluation has been done, therapeutic intervention can be initiated appropriately.

THERAPY OF THE POSTOPERATIVE PATIENT WITH SUSPECTED INFECTION

If a specific infectious syndrome is apparent after initial examination, an empiric course of therapy can be chosen directed toward the problem which has been discovered. Fortunately, it is rare that more than one such complication appears at one time. Frequently, an etiologic agent cannot be determined immediately, and a course of therapy must be chosen empirically. Sometimes the patient appears comfortable, without any sign of distress or organ dysfunction, and it is possible to delay therapy until a specific diagnosis can be made. More often, however, the patient is in distress, and patients with new prosthetic valves cannot be afforded the luxury of such procrastination since even a very minor, distant infection can give rise to a bacteremia, no matter how transient, which could seed a new valve and produce infection. This is far better prevented than treated.

A basic precept of antibiotic choice in postoperative infections in this author's experience is that when these infections occur they are almost always due to flora that is resistant to the prophylactic antibiotic that was given perioperatively. Therefore, the prophylactic antibiotic, if still being administered, should be discontinued. This also eliminates the possibility of drug fever from that antibiotic.

Any suggestion of bacteremia, such as inflammation around an intravenous device or embolic skin lesion, calls for broad coverage, in particular for skin flora, especially coagulase-negative *staphylococci* and *Staphylococcus aureus*. In most institutions, vancomycin is the drug of choice for this purpose because of the frequent penicillin or semisynthetic penicillin resistance of these organisms, especially of coagulase-negative *staphylococci*. Gram-negative coverage is best added initially since additional processes may as yet be unappreciated. A third-generation cephalosporin is ideal for this purpose, but

may add the risk of drug fever. An aminoglycoside may also be used. Once positive cultures are obtained, this regimen should be tailored to the recovered organisms.

Evidence of urosepsis will most often reveal Gram-negative bacillary infection. An aminoglycoside or third-generation cephalosporin will usually be adequate therapy. Addition of enterococcal coverage with ampicillin or vancomycin is also reasonable unless bacilli are visible on urinalysis and other sites of infection can be reliably ruled out.

Initial therapy of wound infections should be guided by results of Gram stain of the drainage, which is best done by a treating physician experienced with evaluation by this method. If no organisms are visible, broad coverage must be started as suggested above for infections involving intravascular devices. In this case, also, nonbacterial infection might be suggested (though even then these are rare), and specific cultures for acid-fast bacilli and fungi should be submitted. Noninfectious causes of wound drainage such as allergy to suture material, necrotic fat, and exudation of bone wax in the case of the sternum may be present, but the risk of untreated infection dictates that antibiotic coverage be started at least until a negative culture is returned.

Evidence of hepatobiliary dysfunction would indicate the need for antibiotics directed against flora normally found in this anatomic area, including *streptococci* and Gram-negative aerobic bacilli. In patients with prior biliary problems or biliary surgery, anaerobic flora are more frequent agents of disease in this locale and may require additional coverage. In most cases, ampicillin plus an aminoglycoside is a reasonable first choice for coverage of this problem. Of course, further workup to evaluate the underlying pathology is necessary also. If this workup proves positive for biliary disease, general surgical consultation is a necessity since these patients may deteriorate quickly, and urgent surgical intervention may be life saving.

As already noted, a patient may appear unstable, or "septic," yet without focal evidence of disease. In these cases broad empiric coverage is needed for all possible infecting flora that may be reasonably expected. A single antibiotic cannot be relied on for this purpose (though imipenem-cilastatin comes close). Combinations such as vancomycin plus an aminoglycoside or ampicillin plus oxacillin and an aminoglycoside may be chosen. The sensitivity profiles of organism vary in different institutions, but usually gentamicin is fully adequate as the aminoglycoside of choice, and it is much less expensive and no more toxic than other representatives of this group. In many instances, a third-generation cephalosporin may be substituted for an aminoglycoside with a greater margin of safety but somewhat reduced spectrum of coverage and much greater cost.

Another important factor to keep in mind is the presence of drug fever. Any drugs suspected of producing such a reaction should be considered for discontinuation as a therapeutic trial. Antibiotics, diphenylhydantoin, and certain antiarrhythmics, especially procainamide and quinidine, are the most frequent offenders in this regard.

Since postcardiotomy syndrome must also be considered, anti-inflammatory drugs may be of use, especially if the patient does not appear toxic and workup is negative for other diagnoses, especially if a pericardial rub is heard. In most situations a trial of these agents is of little risk and much potential benefit, both diagnostic and therapeutic, but should not be substituted for appropriate empiric antibiotic therapy. The potential for the development of nephrotoxicity must be kept in mind when nonsteroidal anti-inflammatory drugs are prescribed.

Possibly the most difficult infection to treat in the postoperative patient is endocarditis. The presence of multiple positive blood cultures and a clinical setting suitable for endocarditis make it impossible to rule out this type of infection. Patients at special risk are those undergoing prosthetic cardiac valve replacement or valve repair and those with unrepaired native valve deformity or disease. In the absence of these factors, isolated coronary bypass does not confer any special risk of endocarditis. Since blood cultures are usually positive, the choice of antibiotics is made based on these cultures. Adequate doses of antibiotics are needed to ensure effective killing of the organisms without assistance from the host's humoral or cell-mediated immune functions. This choice may be assisted by testing of minimum inhibitory and bacter-

iocidal concentrations (MIC and MBCs) of the candidate antibiotic, and the eventual testing of serum bacteriocidal titers to assess the effect of the antibiotic in vitro against the actual bacteria for which the patient is being treated. A prolonged course of antibiotic therapy is almost always needed, with 6-week courses being the norm. Certain etiologic agents such as *staphylococci* and Gram-negative bacilli pose even grater risk due to their invasiveness, frequency of abscess formation, and high relapse rate with early prosthetic valve endocarditis. With such infections longer therapy may be needed, including chronic oral antibiotic use in some cases.

PREVENTION OF INFECTION

Obviously, any of these syndromes is best avoided rather than dealt with when active.

Prevention must begin preoperatively by ensuring that active infection, if present, is cleared before the patient goes to the operating room. Evaluation for pulmonary and urinary tract infection is usually straightforward. Evidence of significant dental infection can usually be found by clinical examination or historical questioning; sometimes dental x-rays and consultation may be necessary. This is most essential in patients who are to receive new prosthetic valves. Active skin sepsis must also be treated.

Preoperative preparation is important. Removal of hair from the areas of incision should be done with minimal trauma and as close to the time of surgery as possible to prevent induction of active infection with skin bacteria which may then cause transfer of large numbers of bacteria to subcutaneous sites at the time of incision. This may be achieved by either using depilatory agents or shaving, each technique has its own relative merits. Antiseptic skin preparation must be used according to well-established techniques (64).

Probably the area of greatest controversy regards the prophylactic use of antibiotics. Adherence to criteria developed by John Burke (65) requires administration of an antibiotic that will be effective against flora likely to be introduced into the wound at surgery, given at sufficient time preoperatively to be present in the wound when contamination may occur (i.e., it must be given before the incision is made), but not too early preoperatively as to change the patient's own flora which would cause the introduction of other flora resistant to the antibiotic being used for prophylaxis. In most cases a first-generation cephalosporin fulfills these criteria, with minimum risk of toxicity and minimum cost as well (66–70).

Typically, 1 gm of intravenous cefazolin is given on-call to the operating room, or in the preoperative holding area, and is repeated at 8-hr intervals into the postoperative period. For the penicillin-allergic patient, vancomycin is the alternative drug of choice, though clindamycin may also be effective (71).

The subsequent course is actively debated. Several studies (72, 73) suggest that a postoperative therapy ranging from one dose to a 1- to 2-day course is efficacious and would minimize the risk of toxicity and the acquisition of new, resistant flora. The purpose of prophylaxis is to have antibiotic present in the tissues when contamination occurs so as to inactivate such contaminating bacteria at that time. After this scenario has transpired, further therapy is unlikely to have effect since factors such as decreased local wound-edge circulation will decrease the delivery of additional antibiotic to the wound edges, and residual blood and dead space in the wound will decrease the activity of antibiotics as well.

Nevertheless, many physicians working in this field feel ill at ease in using these brief courses of anitbiotics and extend their use, often for many days. Although it would be misleading to claim that this often leads to significant problems, misused drug therapy does finitely increase risk and substantially increases cost.

Other generally accepted factors that may help to prevent development of infection postoperatively also include minimal use of catheters, both intravenous and intrabladder, frequent changing of peripheral intravenous lines, and extubation as rapidly as possible. These efforts will reestablish the normal host mechanisms that prevent acquisition of abnormal flora into normally sterile body sites.

References

1. Nelson RM, Dries DJ: The economic implications of infection in cardiac surgery. *Ann Thorac Surg* 42:240–246, 1986.
2. Bell DM, Goldmann DA, Hopkins CC, et al: Unreliability of fever and leukocytosis in the diagnosis of infection after cardiac valve surgery. *J Thorac Cardiovasc Surg* 75:87–90, 1978.
3. Pien FD, Ho PWL, Furgusson DJG: Fever and infection after cardiac operation. *Ann Thorac Surg* 33:382–384, 1982.
4. Wilson APR, Treasure T, Gruneberg RN, et al: Should the temperature chart influence management in cardiac operations? Result of a prospective study in 314 patients. *J Thorac Cardiovasc Surg* 96:518–523, 1988.
5. Evans EGV: The incidence of pathogenic yeasts among open-heart surgery patients—the value of prophylaxis. *J Thorac Cardiovasc Surg* 70:466–470, 1975.
6. Bennett JE: Flucytosine. *Ann Intern Med* 86:319–322, 1977.
7. Bulkley BH, Hutchins GM: Acute postoperative graft phlebitis: a rare cause of saphenous vein–coronary artery bypass failure. *Am Heart J* 95:757–760, 1978.
8. Douglas BP, Bulkley BH, Hutchins GM: Infected saphenous vein coronary artery bypass graft with mycotic aneurysm. Fatal dehiscence of the proximal anastomosis. *Chest* 75:76–77, 1979.
9. Looser KG, Allmendinger PD, Takata H, et al: Infection of cardiac suture line after ventricular aneurysmectomy. Report of two cases. *J Thorac Cardiovasc Surg* 72:280–281, 1976.
10. Dismukes WE, Karchmer AW, Buckley MJ, et al: Prosthetic valve endocarditis. Analysis of 38 cases. *Circulation* 48:365–377, 1973.
11. Quenzer RW, Edwards LD, Levin S: A comparative study of 48 host valve and 24 prosthetic valve endocarditis cases. *Am Heart J* 92:15–22, 1976.
12. Mayer KH, Schoenbaum SC: Evaluation and management of prosthetic valve endocarditis. *Prog Cardiovasc Dis* 25:43–54, 1982.
13. Pankey GA: The prevention and treatment of bacterial endocarditis. *Am Heart J* 98:102–118, 1979.
14. Wilson WR, Nichols DR. Thompson RL, et al: Infective endocarditis: therapeutic considerations. *Am Heart J* 100:689–704, 1980.
15. Mills SA: Surgical management of infective endocarditis. *Ann Surg* 195:367–383, 1982.
16. Rocchiccioli C, Chastre J, Lecompte Y, et al: Prosthetic valve endocarditis. The case for prompt surgical management. *J Thorac Cardiovasc Surg* 92:784–789, 1986.

17. Saffel JR, Gardner P, Schoenbaum SC, et al: Prosthetic valve endocarditis. The case for prompt valve replacement. *J Thorac Cardiovasc Surg* 73:416–420, 1977.

18. Stinson EB: Surgical treatment of infective endocarditis. *Prog Cardiovasc Dis* 22:145–168, 1979.

19. Calderwood SB, Swinski LA, Karchmer AW, et al: Prosthetic valve endocarditis. Analysis of factors affecting outcome of therapy. *J Thorac Cardiovasc Surg* 92:776–783, 1986.

20. Chaudhuri MR: Fungal endocarditis after valve replacements. *J Thorac Cardiovasc Surg* 60:207–214, 1970.

21. Rudd RM, Hill PR, Kopelman P, et al: Fungal endocarditis after homograft valve replacement: difficulties in diagnosis and treatment. *Thorax* 35:686–689, 1980.

22. Engleman RM, Williams D, Gouge TH, et al: Mediastinitis following open-heart surgery. Review of two years' experience. *Arch Surg* 107:772–778, 1973.

23. Grossi EA, Culliford AT, Krieger KH, et al: A survey of 77 major infectious complications of median sternotomy: a review of 7,949 consecutive operative procedures. *Ann Thorac Surg* 40:214–223, 1985.

24. Newman LS, Szczukowski LC, Bain RP, et al: Suppurative mediastinitis after open heart surgery. A case control study of risk factors. *Chest* 94:546–553, 1988.

25. Ottino G, DePaulis R, Pansini S, et al: Major sternal wound infection after open-heart surgery: a multivariate analysis of risk factors in 2,579 consecutive operative procedures. *Ann Thorac Surg* 44:173–179, 1987.

26. Sarr MG, Godd VL, Townsend TR: Mediastinal infection after cardiac surgery. *Ann Thorac Surg* 38:415–423, 1984.

27. Kay HR, Goodman LR, Teplick SK, et al: Use of computed tomography to assess mediastinal complications after median sternotomy. *Ann Thorac Surg* 36:706–714, 1983.

28. Jurkiewicz MJ, Bostwick J III, Hester R, et al: Infected median sternotomy wound. Successful treatment by muscle flaps. *Ann Surg* 191:738–744, 1980.

29. Lee AB Jr, Schimert G, Shatkin S: Total excision of the sternum and thoracic pedicle transposition of the greater omentum; useful strategems in managing severe mediastinal infection following open heart surgery. *Surgery* 80:433–436, 1976.

30. Pairolero PC, Arnold PG: Management of recalcitrant median sternotomy wounds. *J Thorac Cardiovasc Surg* 88:357–364, 1984.

31. Pearl SN, Dibbell DG: Reconstruction after median sternotomy infection. *Surg Gyn Obstet* 159:47–52, 1984.

32. Choo MH, Holmes DR Jr, Gersh BJ: Permanent pacemaker infections: characterization and management. *Am J Cardiol* 48:559–564, 1981.

33. Lewis AB, Hayes DL, Holmes DR Jr, et al: Update on infections involving permanent pacemakers. *J Thorac Cardiovasc Surg* 89:758–763, 1985.

34. Corman LC, Levison ME: Sustained bacteremia and transvenous cardiac pacemakers. *JAMA* 233:264–266, 1975.

35. Morgan G, Ginks W, Siddons H, et al: Septicemia in patients with an endocardial pacemaker. *Am J Cardiol* 44:221–224, 1979.

36. Hermans PE, Wilhelm MP: Vancomycin. *Mayo Clin Proc* 62:901–905, 1987.

37. Boncheck LI: New methods in the management of extruded and infected cardiac pacemakers. *Ann Surg* 176:686–689, 1978.

38. Golden GT, Lovett WL, Harrah JD: The treatment of extruded and infected permanent cardiac pulse generators: application of a technique of closed irrigation. *Surgery* 74:575–579, 1973.

39. Mansour KA, Kauten JR, Hatcher CR Jr: Management of the infected pacemaker: explantation, serilization, and reimplantation. *Ann Thorac Surg* 40:614–619, 1985.

40. Bryan CS, Sutton JP, Saunders DE Jr, et al: Endocarditis related to transvenous pacemakers. Syndromes and surgical implications. *J Thorac Cardiovasc Surg* 75:758–762, 1978.

41. Choo MH, Holmes DR Jr, Gersh BJ, et al: Infected epicardial pacemaker systems. Partial versus total removal. *J Thorac Cardiovasc Surg* 82:794–796, 1981.

42. Firor WB, Lopez JF, Nanson EM, et al: Clinical management of the infected pacemaker. *Ann Thorac Surg* 6:431–436, 1968.

43. Bilgutay AM, Jensen NK, Schmidt WR, et al: Incarceration of transvenous pacemaker electrode. Removal by traction. *Am Heart J* 77:377–379, 1969.

44. LeLaria GA, Hunter JA, Goldin MD, et al: Leg wound complications associated with coronary revascularization. *J Thorac Cardiovasc Surg* 81:403–407, 1981.

45. Baddour LM, Bisno AL: Recurrent cellulitis after saphenous venectomy for coronary bypass surgery. *Ann Int Med* 97:493–496, 1982.

46. Baddour LM, Bisno AL: Recurrent cellulitis after coronary bypass surgery. *JAMA* 251:1049–1052, 1984.

47. Kirsh MM, McIntosh K, Kahn DR, et al: Post-

pericardiotomy syndromes. *Ann Thorac Surg* 9:158–179, 1970.

48. Baker JR Jr, Cohen DJ, Head HD, et al: Development of circulating antiheart antibodies as a result of coronary bypass surgery. *Ann Thorac Surg* 41:507–510, 1986.

49. Livelli FD Jr, Johnson RA, McEnany MT, et al: Unexplained in-hospital fever following cardiac surgery. Natural history, relationship to postpericardiotomy syndrome, and a prospective study of therapy with indomethacin versus placebo. *Circulation* 57:968–975, 1978.

50. Roses DF, Rose MR, Rapaport FT: Febrile responses associated with cardiac surgery. Relationships to the postpericardiotomy syndrome and to altered host immunologic reactivity. *J Thorac Cardiovasc Surg* 67:251–257, 1974.

51. Calerwood SB, Swinski LA, Waternaux CM, et al: Risk factors for the development of prosthetic valve endocarditis. *Circulation* 72:31–37, 1985.

52. Conklin CM, Gray RJ, Neilson D, Et al: Determinants of wound infection incidence after isolated coronary artery bypass surgery in patients randomized to receive prophylactic cefuroxime or cefazolin. *Ann Thorac Surg* 46:172–177, 1988.

53. Miholic J, Hudec M, Domanig E, et al: Risk factors for severe bacterial infections after valve replacement and aortocoronary bypass operations: analysis of 246 cases by logistic regression. *Ann Thorac Surg* 40:224–228, 1985.

54. Hammerschmidt DE, Stroncek DF, Bowers TK, et al: Complement activation and neutropenia occurring during cardiopulmonary bypass. *J Thorac Cardiovasc Surg* 81:370–377, 1981.

55. Roth JA, Golub SH, Cukingnan RA, et al: Cell-mediated immunity is depressed following cardiopulmonary bypass. *Ann Thorac Surg* 31:350–356, 1981.

56. Silva J Jr, Hoeksema H, Fekety FR Jr: Transient defects in phagocytic functions during cardiopulmonary bypass. *J Thorac Cardiovasc Surg* 67:175–183, 1974.

57. van Velzen-Blad H, Dijkstra YK, Schurink GA, et al: Cardiopulmonary bypass and host defense functions in human beings: I. Serum levels and role of immunoglobulins and complement of phagocytosis. *Ann Thorac Surg* 39:207–217, 1985.

58. Kluge RM, Calia FM, McLaughlin JS, et al: Sources of contamination in open heart surgery. *JAMA* 230:1415–1418, 1974.

59. Rosendorf LL, Daicoff G, Baier H: Sources of Gram-negative infection after open-heart surgery. *J Thorac Cardiovasc Surg* 67:195–201, 1974.

60. Seyfer AE, Shriver CE, Miller TR, et al: Sternal blood flow after median sternotomy and mobilization of the internal mammary arteries. *Surgery* 104:899–904, 1988.

61. Ferrazzi P, Allen R, Crupi G, et al: Reduction of infection after cardiac surgery: a clinical trial. *Ann Thorac Surg* 42:321–325, 1986.

62. Roe CF: Surgical aspects of fever. In Ravitch MM, Ellison EH, Julian OC, et al (eds): *Current Problems in Surgery*. Chicago, Year Book, 1968, pp 2–43.

63. Escovitz ES, Okulski TA, Lapayowker MS: The midsternal stripe: a sign of dehiscence following median sternotomy. *Radiology* 121:521–524, 1976.

64. Polk HC Jr, Simpson CJ, Simmons BP, et al: Guidelines for prevention of surgical wound infection. *Arch Surg* 118:1213–1217, 1983.

65. Burke J: The effective period of preventive antibiotic action in experimental incisions and dermal lesions. *Surgery* 50:161–168, 1961.

66. Bryan CS, Smith CW Jr, Sutton JP, et al: Comparison of cefamandole and cefazolin during cardiopulmonary bypass. *J Thorac Cardiovasc Surg* 86:222–225, 1983.

67. Fekety FR Jr, Cluff LE, Sabiston DC, et al: A study of antibiotic prophylaxis in cardiac surgery. *J Thorac Cardiovasc Surg* 57:757–763, 1969.

68. Fong IW, Baker CB, McKee DC: The value of prophylactic antibiotics in aorta-coronary bypass operations. A double-blind randomized trial. *J Thorac Cardiovasc Surg* 78:908–913, 1979.

69. Kini PM, Fernandez J, Causay RS, et al: Double-blind comparison of cefazolin and cephalothin in open-heart surgery. *J Thorac Cardiovasc Surg* 76:506–509, 1978.

70. Farber BF, Karchmer AW, Buckley MJ, et al: Vancomycin prophylaxis in cardiac operations: determination of an optimal dosage regimen. *J Thorac Cardiovasc Surg* 85:933–940, 1983.

71. Pien FD, Michael NL, Mamiya R, et al: Comparative study of prophylactic antibiotics in cardiac surgery. Clindamycin versus cephalothin. *J Thorac Cardiovasc Surg* 77:908–913, 1979.

72. Goldmann DA, Hopkins CC, Karchmer AW, et al: Cephalothin prophylaxis in cardiac valve surgery. A prospective, double-blind comparison of two-day and six-day regimens. *J Thorac Cardiovasc Surg* 73:470–479, 1977.

73. Hillis DJ, Rosenfeldt FL, Spicer WJ, et al: Antibiotic prophylaxis for coronary bypass grafting. Comparison of a five-day and a two-day course. *J Thorac Cardiovasc Surg* 86:217–221, 1983.

Chapter 23
PULMONARY CARE

MYLES EDWIN LEE, M.D.

Cardiopulmonary bypass superimposes pathophysiologic changes on baseline pulmonary function in patients who may already have impaired intrapulmonary gas exchange. These changes include intrapulmonary aggregation of leukocytes and platelets, increased pulmonary vascular resistance, and increased capillary permeability, all of which have been associated with postoperative hypoxemia. Sequestration of leukocytes and platelets within the pulmonary vasculature with damage to endothelial cells and type I and II pneumocytes is one mechanism that results in increased capillary permeability and decreased pulmonary compliance (1, 2). Activation of the C5a fraction of complement is probably responsible for intrapulmonary leukocyte aggregation, and anaphylatoxins produced by C3 and C5 activation have been associated with histamine release from mast cells as well as lysosomal enzyme release resulting in increased vascular permeability to fluid and protein (3, 4). This has been attenuated in animal models with the free radical scavenger superoxide dismutase, suggesting that the generation of superoxide anions by aggregated intrapulmonary leukocytes may be the initiating event in vascular endothelial injury (5). The role of these events in initiating hypoxemia has not been conclusively established. Intrapulmonary aggregation of leukocytes and platelets can be substantially reduced by incorporating filters on

the arterial and venous sides of cardiopulmonary bypass circuits (6).

Increased surfactant removal during bypass also results in decreased pulmonary compliance (7) and has been associated with atelectasis and hypoxemia in the postoperative period.

Superimposed on these events is the obligatory increase in total body water experienced by all patients undergoing cardiopulmonary bypass resulting from crystalloid infusion to maintain hemodynamic stability during the induction and maintenance of anesthesia, as well as the priming volume of the heart-lung machine. This volume averages 4 to 5 liters in normal adults. Additional problems include a reduced ability of patients to cough effectively because of incisional discomfort, leading to retained secretions and subsequent atelectasis or pneumonia.

PREOPERATIVE ASSESSMENT OF PULMONARY RISK

Because of the effects of cardiopulmonary bypass on basal pulmonary function, it is necessary to identify those patients especially at risk for postoperative pulmonary complications. If surgery is elective, a history of smoking, especially associated with chronic obstructive pulmonary disease or emphysema, should suggest treatment with expectorants, bronchodilators, and mucolytic agents delivered with a heated aerosol or intermittent positive-pressure breathing (IPPB), as well as incentive spirometry for 1 or 2 weeks preoperatively to clear the airways of retained secretions. Certain patients with bronchial asthma may benefit from steroids in the perioperative period, though sufficiently high doses that lead to immunosuppression may facilitate the development of mediastinal infections. The potential contribution of congestive heart failure should be evaluated before instituting steroid therapy in patients with poorly controlled asthma.

Patients with gastroesophageal reflux frequently suffer from bronchiectasis as a result of aspiration of gastric contents. If this is known, vigorous pulmonary toilet as outlined above and sputum culture with appropriate antibiotic therapy are indicated. In addition, strict antireflux measures should be observed, including frequent small meals, elevation of the head of the bed in the reverse Trendelenburg position, and the use of antacids and H_2 blockers such as ranitidine to reduce gastric acidity. Patients who have a large portion of the stomach in the retrocardiac position, whether or not they have gastroesophageal reflux, are at risk for aspiration if the intrathoracic stomach is not decompressed postoperatively. Two or more liters of gastric fluid can be sequestered in the stomach, and care should be taken to ensure that a functioning nasogastric tube is positioned in this segment of the stomach (and confirmed by chest x-ray) until postoperative ileus has resolved. The dilated stomach, aside from presenting a risk for aspiration, can also compress the left lower lobe of the lung, preventing effective ventilation in this area.

Use of the antiarrhythmic drug amiodarone has introduced a spectrum of new pulmonary dysfunctions in postoperative patients. This drug is slowly absorbed, is protein bound, and has an elimination half-life of 30 to 40 days. Pulmonary abnormalities appear to be dose or duration related, or both, in patients receiving daily maintenance doses of greater than 400 mg over a mean period of 14 months, and are more common in those with preexistent pulmonary functional abnormalities. Clinically, patients may experience dyspnea with leukocytosis, an increase in erythrocyte sedimentation rate, and

hypoxemia. Radiologic findings include interstitial or alveolar infiltrates which may progress to a sometimes fatal acute respiratory distress syndrome, especially after cardiopulmonary bypass. Cavitary pleural-based nodules have also been described (8). Treatment of amiodarone-induced pulmonary toxicity involves cessation of the drug and the institution of steroid therapy (the true efficacy of which remains to be documented) (9). Avoidance of an FiO_2 exceeding 0.5 for more than 48 hr is preferable to reduce the additional insults of interstitial or intraalveolar edema, hemorrhage, and hyaline membrane formation associated with oxygen excess (10). Since the mortality from pulmonary insufficiency in patients with known spirometric or diffusion abnormalities resulting from amiodarone has been approximately 50% in the author's institution (11), these patients are no longer accepted for surgical intervention.

Protamine sulfate, a low-molecular-weight polypeptide extract of salmon or other fish sperm, is used to neutralize the heparin employed during cardiopulmonary bypass. Protamine reactions may occur from a few minutes to several hours following its administration and are characterized by hypotension, noncardiac pulmonary edema, and profound hypoxemia. Anaphylactic reactions have been also reported in noncardiac surgical patients, especially leukophoresis donors. Diabetics using NPH or protamine zinc insulin, patients with allergy to fish, or patients having had prior vasectomy appear to be at higher risk. Twenty-nine percent of cardiac patients who develop anaphylaxis have had previous exposure to protamine. The mortality rate can be as high as 30% despite the use of inotropes, intraaortic balloon pumping, and volume replacement (12). Because of the possible role of intrapulmonary mast cell degranulation when the drug is given intravenously, intraarterial protamine administration has been proposed; however, hemodynamic abnormalities have been reported with this route as well. Reactions have not been observed in animals receiving protamine before prior heparinization, suggesting that the phenomenon may be related to a heparin-protamine reaction, perhaps with complement activation (13). Pretreatment with steroids or H_2 receptor agonists such as ranitidine is of questionable benefit but probably should be given to patients who have the identifiable risk factors. In such patients, protamine should be administered with the cardiopulmonary bypass cannulae in place to enable rapid reinstitution of bypass, if necessary, for circulatory support.

Pulmonary function testing may be useful to screen patients suspected of having pulmonary dysfunction. In adults, a vital capacity of less than 1.5 liters, a forced expiratory volume in 1 second of less than 2 liters, a maximum breathing capacity of less than 50% of predicted, a PaO_2 of less than 50 mm Hg, and a $PaCO_2$ greater than 45 mm Hg have been shown to be associated with prolonged ventilatory support in the postoperative period (14).

Reversible pulmonary dysfunction can also be caused by mechanical cardiac dysfunction. Correction of mitral stenosis or insufficiency may reduce pulmonary wedge and pulmonary arterial pressures, allowing resolution of biventricular failure and the symptoms of cardiogenic pulmonary insufficiency. Left ventricular failure caused by myocardial ischemia can be improved with coronary bypass grafting in certain patients. Decision-making in patients with combined pulmonary and cardiac disease is difficult and based on the assumption that correction of the cardiogenic pulmonary dysfunction will permit easier control of any primary pulmonary dysfunction. This assumes, however, that the pulmonary insult resulting from cardiopulmonary bypass itself can be controlled effectively. Simple measures taken intraoperatively, such as maintenance of 5 cm of positive end-expiratory pressure (PEEP) during bypass (15), followed by diuresis, can reduce the incidence of miliary atelectasis and ameliorate the effects of increased pulmonary capillary permeability.

In general, pulmonary function testing should be performed in patients with a history of heavy smoking, chronic obstructive pulmonary disease, emphysema, bronchial asthma, gastroesophageal reflux with bronchiectasis, or large intrathoracic hiatus hernias, and in those who have been on chronic amiodarone therapy. If the results suggest significant impairment of pulmonary function, the patient should be placed on expectorants, mucolytic agents, and bronchodilators delivered with heated aerosols. Antibiotics should be added as indicated. Patients with bronchial asthma should be stabilized with bronchodilators and possibly steroids. Treatment with IPPB or incentive spirometry, coupled with vigorous chest physiotherapy, should likewise be instituted. If possible, these measures should be carried out for 1 or 2 weeks. If there is no improvement in the measured parameters, pulmonary risk may be prohibitively high, precluding surgical intervention.

ROUTINE POSTOPERATIVE MANAGEMENT

Patients are maintained on ventilatory support until they have awakened from anesthesia. Weaning is initiated by changing from assist control to intermittent mandatory ventilation (IMV). The rate of awakening is determined by the elimination of anesthetic agents, which is initially depressed from hypothermia and postpump myocardial dysfunction. Arterial blood gases are obtained hourly for the first 6 hr, during which time the FiO_2 should be progressively decreased, but sufficient to allow a PaO_2 of 100 mm Hg or higher. Prolonged exposure to an FiO_2 of greater than 0.5 should be avoided. When the patient has demonstrated a negative inspiratory force of -25 to 30 cm of water, and a vital capacity of 12 to 15 ml/kg, he or she is tested on a T-tube with or without continuous positive expiratory pressure (CPAP) for 30 to 60 min, and the arterial gases are repeated. If PaO_2 remains greater than 80 mm Hg and $PaCO_2$ less than 40 mm Hg, with an unlabored respiratory rate of less than 18 breaths/min, extubation is recommended. Extubation may not be recommended even with these parameters if a patient is hemodynamically unstable, has life-threatening arrhythmias, or has sustained neurologic damage rendering him or her comatose, or if reoperation is anticipated to control postoperative hemorrhage.

Once the patient has been extubated, pulmonary toilet is encouraged by coughing, incentive spirometry, chest physiotherapy, and early ambulation. Patients with chronic obstructive pulmonary disease may require mucolytic agents and bronchodilators with heated aerosols.

POSTOPERATIVE PULMONARY PROBLEMS

Persistent hypoxemia in the immediate postoperative period demands relentless investigation as to etiology and prompt treatment to prevent irreversible multisystem organ failure. A chest roentgenogram is frequently diagnostic. While awaiting the x-ray, the ventilator settings and oxygen delivery system must be checked. The tip of the endotracheal tube should be 22 to 24 cm from the incisors. Intubation of the right mainstem bronchus by a tube that may have slipped into this position during transfer from the operating table to the bed can cause a profound increase in dead space and a large intrapulmonary shunt because the left lung is perfused but not ventilated. This may be suspected by the absence of breath sounds and ventilatory excursions of the left chest. The condition is simply corrected by withdrawing the endotracheal tube until breath sound reappear on the left side. An abrupt rise in peak inspiratory pressure can result from a kink in the endotracheal tube, by the patient biting on the tube, or by a mucus plug.

Persistent absence of breath sounds, once the correct positioning of the endotracheal tube has been ensured, may arise from atelectasis or tension pneumothorax. Atelectasis of lobar proportions may be recognized clinically by absent breath sounds and decreased ventilatory excursion of the chest on the affected side. Tension pneumothorax may be recognized by absent breath sounds and hyperinflation of the chest on the affected side, and is frequently accompanied by hypotension caused by a massive mediastinal shift with impairment of venous return to the heart. Both atelectasis and tension pneumothorax are readily diagnosed by a chest roentgenogram. The former is treated by vigorous endotracheal suctioning and PEEP or by fiber optic bronchoscopy through the endotracheal tube, and the latter by emergency needle aspiration of the chest followed by tube thoracostomy.

Pleural effusions occurring within the first 12 hr postoperatively are usually the result of bleeding from the mediastinum into the pleural space through an opening in the mediastinal pleura. Such effusions are more frequently seen in patients who have undergone dissection of the internal mammary artery pedicle for coronary artery bypass grafting. Patients with postoperative bleeding diatheses should be monitored with frequent chest x-rays to detect accumulation of blood in the pleural space, especially if a pleural tube was not placed at operation. Persistent bleeding usually requires reoperation if a major coagulopathy has been ruled out, at which time the pleural space must be drained.

Pulmonary artery catheterization has allowed more precise monitoring of hemodynamics during the induction of anesthesia and the postoperative period (16) but has been associated with severe, sometimes life-threatening intrapulmonary hemorrhage before, during, or after the institution of cardiopulmonary bypass (17). The most frequent causes of this are overwedging of the catheter, with placement of the tip in the tertiary branches of the pulmonary artery; overinflation of the wedging balloon, especially in patients with pulmonary hypertension; and manipulation of the heart during cardiac surgery. In the last instance, the catheter becomes stiff from the hypothermia induced during cardiopulmonary bypass. If it is not withdrawn so that the tip lies in the main pulmonary artery, elevation of the heart out of the pericardium to bypass a circumflex coronary artery, for example, may force the tip of the catheter through the pulmonary artery, resulting in intrapulmonary hemorrhage. This may be confined to a parenchymal hematoma or result in catastrophic hemorrhage either into the pleural space or the major airways, requiring emergency pulmonary lobectomy. Bleeding is intensified if it occurs after the patient has been heparinized in preparation for cardiopulmonary bypass, especially in the presence of pulmonary hypertension. Institution of cardiopulmonary bypass may actually decrease or eliminate the bleeding because most of the blood entering the right side of the heart will be diverted into the heart-lung machine (18). Once bypass has been terminated and protamine has been administered, bronchoscopy may be necessary to confirm the cessation of bleeding and to evacuate clots from the tracheobronchial tree. Hemoptysis may also occur in the intensive care unit before or after surgery as well. The diagnosis of pulmonary artery rupture may be suspected from the peripheral position of the catheter tip and a new radiographic density in the same area. Initial treatment should consist of bronchoscopy with balloon occlusion of the bronchus from which the blood is issuing to prevent flooding of the remainder of the airways, correction of any coagulopathy, control of pulmonary hypertension with preload-reducing agents such as intravenous nitroglycerin, and pulmonary arterial repair or emergency lobectomy if hemorrhage continues.

Pulmonary embolism may occur in the postoperative period and, in fact, should be anticipated in patients with a history of prior pulmonary emboli, thrombophlebitis, prolonged bed rest, obesity, congestive heart failure, or hypercoagulability. Unless embolism involves 60 to 70% of the pulmonary vascular bed, acute cor pulmonale usually does not occur (19). In its typical form, the primary symptoms may be pleuritic chest pain, associated with a pleural friction rub and signs of a pleural effusion. These features may be absent or be overshadowed by incisional pain or narcotics. Dyspnea with tachypnea resulting in respiratory alkalosis, but not necessarily hypoxemia, may be seen. Whereas the electrocardiogram and chest x-ray may be normal, a ventilation-perfusion scan may demonstrate diagnostic segmental perfusion defects; however, the diagnosis may be further obscured by false-positive or indeterminate ventilation-perfusion scanning due to the high frequency of coexistent pleural effusion and atelectasis.

Pulmonary angiography needs to be performed only when there is a contraindication to anticoagulation or when recurrent emboli are suspected on effective anticoagulant therapy.

Massive pulmonary embolus with acute cor pulmonale is associated with tachypnea, tachycardia, and systemic hypotension secondary to acute right ventricular failure and subsequent decreased cardiac output. Initially the lungs may be clear or may demonstrate rales if left ventricular failure ensues. Jugular venous distension

and a parasternal heave with a prominent P_2 may be detectable. The patient will be hypoxemic and hypocapneic with marked elevation in central venous or right atrial pressures. Chest x-ray may show a relatively radiolucent area in the embolized segments. If the patient has a patent foramen ovale, intracardiac shunting from the right atrium to the left atrium may compound the pulmonary causes of persistent hypoxemia. Contrast echocardiography or color flow Doppler echocardiography done at the bedside can diagnose this condition. Superimposition of right ventricular ischemia caused by coronary artery disease can exacerbate right ventricular failure if the right ventricular free wall has not been adequately revascularized or protected with cardioplegia during surgery.

If the patient is hemodynamically stable, the diagnosis may be confirmed by a ventilation-perfusion scan and treatment begun with heparin. If recurrent emboli are suspected despite anticoagulation, the diagnosis must be confirmed by pulmonary angiography and caval interruption performed with either a Greenfield filter or a Mobin-Uddin umbrella. Patients who remain hypotensive despite pressors and who have massive, often bilateral emboli are candidates for pulmonary embolectomy by surgical means or by suction through a percutaneously introduced catheter (20). Persistent hypotension after surgical embolectomy suggests residual acute or chronic pulmonary emboli or persistent acute right ventricular failure secondary to subendocaridal ischemia resulting from right ventricular dilation. Mechanical assist of the failing right ventricle, such as right atrial-pulmonary artery bypass or intrapulmonary balloon pumping, has been well described but is not part of the generally available therapeutic armamentarium.

PROLONGED VENTILATORY INSUFFICIENCY

Patients who do not meet the criteria for early extubation should be sedated, unless this is contraindicated to assess evolving neurologic deficits. Occasionally, paralysis of the patient's voluntary ventilation with neuromuscular blocking agents will be required if asynchronous ventilatory efforts interfere with the ability of the ventilator to effect proper gas exchange. In particular, elderly patients require careful management of fluid balance owing to increased pulmonary capillary permeability and marked increases in total body water following cardiopulmonary bypass. Crystalloid or saline-containing colloid solutions may be needed for hemodynamic stability, but when interstitial pulmonary edema and impaired gas exchange are present, the administration of packed red blood cells is probably the best way to expand volume without contributing to the patient's "third space." Furthermore, once extubated, the elderly patient, because of a higher hematocrit, may be able to participate better in coughing, ambulation, and eating. Many surgical programs have adopted autologous and donor-directed transfusion programs to reduce the transmission of transfusion-mediated diseases such as hepatitis and acquired immunodeficiency syndrome (AIDS).

If intubation is required for more than 10 days, tracheostomy should be considered. Tracheostomy should be avoided earlier because of the risk of contaminating the unhealed upper sternotomy incision with endotracheal secretions and producing mediastinitis. Tracheostomy facilitates endotracheal suctioning and bronchoscopy, and the patient can be moved about more freely without risking damage to the vocal cords due to pressure from an indwelling endotracheal tube.

Since stress gastritis is common in these circumstances, an H_2 receptor blocking agent such as ranitidine (50 mg intravenously every 8 hr) should be combined with antacids and nasogastric tube feedings to reduce the risk of upper gastrointestinal bleeding and to provide nutritional support. The risk of aspiration of liquid tube feedings may be reduced by administering them as a continuous drip, frequently turning the patient to the right lateral decubitus position to facilitate gastric emptying, withholding feedings if the gastric residual checked every 2 hr exceeds 150 ml maintaining the patient in reverse Trendelenburg position, and by sustained inflation of the endotracheal tube or tracheostomy cuff. Once oral intake is possible, solid food reduces the risk of aspiration (which

can be retrieved from the airway more easily than liquids). If a tracheostomy tube is present, the cuff should be deflated during oral feedings, because an inflated cuff can project posteriorly and push the membranous portion of the trachea against the adjacent esophagus, causing partial esophageal obstruction.

In patients with depressed cardiac function (cardiac index less than 1.5 liters/min/m^2), respiratory mangement using high peak inspiratory pressures, large tidal volumes, and PEEP (all of which interfere with venous return and right ventricular ejection) may severely reduce the cardiac output further. In this situation, high-frequency jet ventilation may provide adequate arterial oxygenation and CO_2 clearance, with minimal peak inspiratory tracheal pressure and minimal effects on lung volume (21). This technique delivers small tidal volumes at rates between 60 and 2400 breaths/min. The mechanisms of alveolar gas exchange with jet ventilation are not completely understood but include diffusion and coaxial gas flow, with gases in the center of the airway moving distally and CO_2 moving proximally at the edge of the airway (22). The hemodynamic advantages of such a system include minimal effects on cardiovascular function with enhancement of the cardiac index.

Extracorporeal membrane oxygenation (ECMO) may be used for partial ventilatory support in patients with severe impairment of diffusion capacity. Arteriovenous perfusion techniques have been described which, without anticoagulation or pumps, can provide up to 50% of the basal metabolic need for oxygen at flow rates corresponding to 35% of the cardiac output. While ECMO cannot support the circulation, the delivery of oxygenated blood at low flow rates to the lungs allows for pulmonary arteriolar vasodilation and maintenance of baseline right artial, pulmonary arterial, and pulmonary capillary wedge pressures, as well as cardiac output (23).

References

1. Jorgensen L, Hoving T, Rowsell HC, et al: Adenosine diphosphate–involved platelet aggregation and vascular injury in swine and rabbit. *Am J Pathol* 61:161–176, 1970.

2. Ratliff NB, Young WG, Hackel DB, et al: Pulmonary injury secondary to extracorporeal circulation. An ultrastructural study. *J Thorac Cardiovasc Surg* 65:425–432, 1973.

3. Fountain SW, Martin BA, Musclow CE: Pulmonary leukostasis and its relationship to pulmonary dysfunction in sheep and rabbits. *Circ Res* 46:175–180, 1980.

4. Chenowith DE, Cooper SW, Hugli TE, et al: Complement activation during cardiopulmonary bypass: evidence for generation of C3a and C5a anaphylatoxins. *N Engl J Med* 304:497–503, 1981.

5. Perkowski SJ, Havill AM, Flynn GT, et al: Role of intrapulmonary release of eicosanoids and superoxide anion as mediators of pulmonary dysfunction and endothelial injury in sheep with intermittent complement activation. *Circ Res* 53:574–583, 1983.

6. Connell RS, Page US, Bartley TD, et al: The effect on pulmonary ultrastructure of Dacron-wool filtration during cardiopulmonary bypass. *Ann Thorac Surg* 15:217–229, 1973.

7. Morgan TE: Pulmonary sufactant. *N Engl J Med* 284:1185–1193, 1971.

8. Schechter CJ, O'Neill G, Schweppe HI Jr, et al: Asymptomatic cavitary pneumonitis due to amiodarone pulmonary toxicity. *Texas Heart Inst J* 12:371–375, 1985.

9. McGovern B, Garon H, Ruskin JM: Serious adverse effects of amiodarone. *Clin Cardiol* 7:131–137, 1984.

10. Pontopiddan H, Geffin B, Lowenstein E: Acaute respiratory failure in the adult. *N Engl J Med* 287:743–806, 1972.

11. Nalos PC, Kass RM, Gang ES, et al: Life-threatening postoperative pulmonary complications in patients with previous amiodarone pulmonary toxicity undergoing cardiothoracic operations. *J Thorac Cardiovasc Surg* 93:904–912, 1987.

12. Holland CL, Singh AK, McMaster PRB, et al: Adverse reactions to protamine sulfate following cardiac surgery. *Clin Cardiol* 7:157–162, 1984.

13. Rogers K, Milne B, Salerno TA: The hemodynamic effects of intra-aortic versus intravenous administration of protamine for reversal of heparin in pigs. *J Thorac Cardiovasc Surg* 85:851–855, 1983.

14. Sethna DH, Gray RJ, Chaux A, et al: *Postmyocardial Infarction Management and Rehabilitation*, New York, Marcel Dekker, 1983, pp 329–351.

15. Weedn RJ, Coalson JJ, Greenfield LJ: Effects of oxygen and ventilation on pulmonary mechanics and ultrastructure during cardiopulmonary bypass. *Am J Surg* 120:584–590, 1970.

16. Weeks KR, Chatterjee K, Block S: Bedside hemodynamic monitoring: its value in the diagnosis of tamponade complicating cardiac surgery. *J Thorac Cardiovasc Surg* 71:250–252, 1976.

17. Barash PG, Nardi D, Hammond G, et al: Catheter-induced pulmonary artery perforation. Mechanisms, management and modifications. *J Thorac Cardiovasc Surg* 82:5–12, 1981.

18. Lee ME, Matloff JM, Hackner E: Catheter-induced pulmonary artery hemorrhage (letter to the editor). *J Thorac Cardiovasc Surg* 83:796, 1982.

19. Dalen JE, Alpert JJ: *The Heart*, ed 6. New York, McGraw-Hill, 1985, pp 1105–1119.

20. Greenfield LJ, Zocco JJ: Intraluminal management of acute massive pulmonary thromboembolism. *J Thorac Cardiovasc Surg* 77:402–410, 1979.

21. Carlin GC, Howland WS, Ray C, et al: High frequency jet ventilation. A prospective randomized evaluation. *Chest* 84:551–559, 1983.

22. Haselton FR, Scherer PW: Bronchial bifurcations and respiratory mass transport. *Science* 208:69–71, 1980.

23. Borovetz HS, Hardesty RL, Griffith BP, et al: *Techniques in Extracorporeal Circulation*, ed 2. London, Butterworths, 1981, pp 642–681.

Chapter 24
RENAL FAILURE

CYNTHIA KRISTENSEN, M.D.

The incidence of acute renal impairment has fallen dramatically in the past 2 decades to 1.5 to 5% of open-heart operations (1–3). The proportion of acute renal failure (ARF) that is nonoliguric has risen, probably due to improved surgical and anesthetic techniques and better maintenance of tissue perfusion intra- and postoperatively. However, mortality of patients with oliguric ARF is still 65 to 90% in most series, primarily due to nonrenal complications (1, 2, 4, 5).

NORMAL RENAL FUNCTION

In normal humans, renal blood flow (RBF) and glomerular filtration rate (GFR) remain constant over a range of mean arterial pressures (MAP) from approximately 70 to 200 mm Hg (6). The preglomerular afferent arteriole constricts in concert with a rise of MAP and the postglomerular efferent arteriole constricts at lower MAP, such that large changes in glomerular perfusion pressure are prevented and glomerular filtration remains constant (6). In addition to this intrinsic system of autoregulation, extrinsic vasoconstrictor influences such as adrenergic nerve activity, norepinephrine and angiotension II act on pre- and postglomerular arterioles to diminish RBF under certain circumstances, whereas vasodilatory prostaglan-dins, bradykinin, and dopamine tend to augment RBF and GFR.

Effects of Anesthesia and Surgery on Renal Function

The effects of anesthetic agents on renal function are mediated by changes in cardiac output and vascular resistance, as well as neuroendocrine systems. With the exception of methoxyflurane, which has fallen out of use due to the nephrotoxicity of its metabolic products inorganic fluoride and oxalate, anesthetics are not a direct cause of renal injury (7, 8). On rare occasions, enflurane has been associated with toxic fluoride levels when used for long periods in patients with large fat stores.

More important than the specific anesthetic agents are the effects of surgery and cardiopulmonary bypass (CPB) on RBF, GFR, and endogenous vasoactive substances. MAP is lowered to 50 to 90 mm Hg, and mean blood flow rate is generally 2.2 to 2.4 liters/min/m² body surface area. Urine flow falls markedly during transition to bypass, remaining at 2 to 3 ml/min during CPB, and rises within the 1st hour following CPB termination. During CPB, circulating levels of vasopressin, vasoconstricting catecholamines, and angiotensin II rise (9–11). Investigations in the 1960s documented a fall in RBF by 30% or more early in CPB with rapid normalization following termination. Of note is that autoregulation of RBF appeared to be impaired within the 1st hour of CPB. Renal vasoconstriction occurred despite systemic blood flow rates comparable to normal cardiac output and correction of volume depletion and hypotension. GFR fell to approximately 50 to 60% of baseline during CPB and recovered less rapidly than RBF, but normalized by the 2nd postoperative day (12–15).

In general, it is safe to assume that even a MAP of 50 mm Hg during CPB does not adversely affect postoperative renal function as long as perfusion is maintained with fluid volume and vasodilators, and CPB time is not prolonged (5, 13). Fluid administration results in an increase in extracellular fluid volume from 20% of body weight preoperatively to 25% postoperatively, which may be reflected by a slight dilutional lowering of the serum creatinine concentration; creatinine measurement, however, is affected by other factors such as noncreatinine chromogens so that small changes in either direction may not accurately reflect changes in GFR (15). A diuresis typically ensues within the first 2 postoperative days, and the serum creatinine returns to the baseline level (13).

ACUTE RENAL FAILURE

ARF is a syndrome of acutely impaired renal function, characterized by progressive azotemia; that is, the inability to excrete creatinine and other products of daily metabolism. Blood urea nitrogen (BUN) concentration is an inaccurate indicator of renal function in the hypercatabolic postoperative patient. Oliguria is present if urine volume is less than 400 to 500 ml/24 hr; anuria is defined as less that 50 to 100 ml/24 hr. Nonoliguric ARF is generally a less severe form of ARF and is associated with fewer nonrenal complications and a better prognosis compared to oliguric ARF (4, 16). Nutritional, drug, and fluid and electrolyte management are greatly complicated in oliguric ARF.

The etiology of ARF is usually multifactorial in the surgical patient and involves both prerenal and renal causes (5). Reduced cardiac output, redistribution of blood flow away from the kidney as occurs during sepsis, and intense in-

trarenal vasoconstriction due to endogenous or exogenous vasopressors all cause glomerular hypoperfusion and ischemia even in the absence of diminished intravascular blood volume or lowered blood pressure. In turn, renal hypoperfusion, low urine flow, and acidemia sensitize the kidney to superimposed nephrotoxic insults.

The chronology of ARF can be divided into an initiation phase, an established, maintenance phase, and a recovery phase. The term acute tubular necrosis (ATN) is often used to describe established ARF regardless of etiology or urine volume.

Acute renal impairment following open-heart surgery is almost always initiated by renal ischemia (1–5). Low cardiac output postoperatively is the most critical and central factor; prolonged cardiopulmonary bypass (for more than 160 min) or aortic cross-clamp time (more than 40 min) are also associated with an increased incidence of postischemic ARF (1, 2). While MAP and mean systemic blood flow rates during CPB are not different in patients with or without ARF, patients with ARF more often received large doses of intraoperative pressors, probably reflecting hemodynamic instability (1, 2, 4). The complexity and number of surgical procedures performed and the extent of hemolysis correlate with an increased incidence of ARF due to their association with prolonged CPB (2, 5). Similarly, use of the intraaortic balloon pump does not of itself cause increased renal morbidity, but is used in unstable patients at greater risk of ARF (1). Susceptibility to postischemic renal failure varies markedly, and advanced age, hypertension, and preoperative renal insufficiency, cardiac dysfunction, or volume depletion increase risk due to an already compromised renal circulation (1–5).

The postischemic kidney loses its autoregulatory capacity and is very susceptible to repeated ischemic insults, even at systemic pressures that are well tolerated in normal kidneys (17). GFR may remain significantly depressed even when RBF is restored. In the early "functional" stage of postischemic renal impairment, prompt restoration of RBF by correction of volume deficits and normalization of cardiac output generally prevents deterioration to "fixed" renal failure. Obstruction of tubules by casts, swollen tubular cells, and cellular debris, as well as back-leak of filtrate across damaged tubular epithelium, appear to be responsible for the maintenance phase (18, 19). Renal vasoconstriction is present at this stage but its reversal does not improve glomerular function.

The severity of ARF also depends on superimposed complications, especially sustained hemodynamic instability, sepsis, treatment with nephrotoxic drugs (particularly aminoglycosides), and intravenous radiocontrast agent administration (5). Hemolysis while on CPB is often mentioned as a risk factor (4); in normal persons, free hemoglobin is not usually nephrotoxic unless hemolysis is massive, but under conditions of hypoperfusion and acidemia, tubular obstruction and epithelial damage may result. One must also consider less common complications such as drug-induced allergic interstitial nephritis, renal artery occulsion by large cholesterol plaques, cholesterol microvascular embolization, or glomerulonephritis associated with endocarditis.

Uncomplicated oliguric ARF generally lasts 1 to 4 weeks, and recovery of GFR is heralded by gradually increasing urine output even before the serum creatinine concentration declines.

Differential Diagnosis of Acute Renal Failure

Anuria is uncommon in ARF and, when present, should suggest urinary tract obstruction, overwhelming acute glomerulonephritis, severe untreated hypovolemia, bilateral renal vascular occulsion, or cortical necrosis. Alternating anuria and polyuria strongly suggest fluctuating postrenal obstruction.

Oliguria may be seen in any form of ARF. In prerenal azotemia, the GFR is relatively preserved despite a decline in RBF, so that glomerular solute excretion continues while tubular salt and water reabsorption is enhanced; urinary creatinine concentration, osmolality, and specific gravity are elevated and urinary sodium is low (20). In ATN, glomerular filtration is limited and the tubules do not adequately process the glomerular filtrate. Urinary solute concentrations and tonicity remain closer to that of plasma (isosthenuric). Nonoliguric patients tend

to have lower serum creatinine concentrations and shorter duration of ARF, consistent with less severe renal damage (16). It has been claimed that some patients with "pure" prerenal ARF may be nonoliguric, but most patients described had clinical courses suggestive of superimposed ATN (21).

A number of indices of glomerular and tubular function have been used to differentiate prerenal azotemia from oliguric ATN (Table 24.1) One must use caution in the interpretation of these tests, since overlap exists and exceptions are frequent (22). Patients with underlying sodium-avid conditions (congestive heart failure, cirrhotic liver disease, acute glomerulonephritis, nephrotic syndrome), intratubular (pigment nephropathy) or ureteral obstruction, radiocontrast-induced ARF, and acute interstitial nephritis have been described with oliguric ATN but a low fractional excretion of sodium (FE_{Na}). Patients who have recently (within 12 hr) received furosemide or mannitol, or those with marked hyperglycemia, may have elevated urinary sodium concentrations regardless of intravascular volume. Serial testing may be useful; the transition from functional to fixed ARF in the patient with hemodynamic instability may be reflected by a rise in the FE_{Na} from "prerenal" values immediately postoperatively to "ATN" values over ensuing days (23). Diagnostic indices are less helpful in the nonoliguric patient who tends to be less sodium retentive and have better-preserved overall function.

Urinary diagnostic indices should be used in conjunction with old-fashioned clinical acumen. The physician should look for signs of insufficient cardiac output or peripheral vasoconstriction; in addition, the following tests should be done: skin examination for evidence of cholesterol embolization or endocarditis; cardiac auscultation for a pericardial rub or a murmur suggesting endocarditis; urinalysis (Table 24.2); blood morphology for signs of hemolysis, etc. Measured and calculated values obtained from a Swan-Ganz catheter are valuable but should be used with the understanding that systemic and renal vascular resistance may be markedly different, and the pulmonary capillary wedge pressure

TABLE 24.1

URINARY DIAGNOSTIC INDICES IN ACUTE TUBULAR NECROSIS AND PRERENAL AZOTEMIA[a]

	Urine Sodium	Urine/ Plasma Creatinine	Urine/ Plasma Urea	RFI	FE_{Na}	Urine Osmolality	Urine Tonicity
	mEq/liter			%	%	*mosm/liter*	
Prerenal azotemia	<20	>40:1	>8:1	<1	<1	>500	>1.020
Acute tubular necrosis	>40	<20:1	<3:1	>3	>3	<350	1.010

[a]See comments in text regarding exceptions.
[b]RFI, Renal failure index = (urine Na)/(urine creatinine/plasma creatinine).
[c]FE_{Na} = [(urine Na/plasma Na)/(urine creatinine/plasma creatinine)] × 100

(PCWP) may not reflect left ventricular filling pressure under certain conditions, including sepsis and pulmonary hypertension.

Prevention and Treatment of Acute Renal Failure

The most important measures to prevent ARF are attention to adequate intravascular volume and maintenance of optimal cardiac output. Vasodilators, inotropic agents, and fluid volume should be chosen over vasopressors whenever possible to maintain blood pressure and cardiac output (1, 24). The intraaortic balloon pump should not be avoided if it is needed to maintain cardiac output. Careful surveillance for infection and prompt treatment are mandatory; a fall in urine output may be the first clue to sepsis, even before fever or leukocytosis. Broad-spectrum coverage may be initiated with aminoglycosides for 24 to 72 hr, but it is prudent to switch to less nephrotoxic antibiotics as soon as bacterial sensitivities are known. Administration of radiocontrast material immediately preoperatively has not been associated with increased risk of ARF in the hydrated, normal patient (1), but should be avoided postoperatively.

Oliguria (less than 30 ml/hr) or an acute fall in urine volume should prompt an immediate search for reversible causes, including an obstructed urinary catheter. Most importantly, the patient should be evaluated for signs of hypovolemia or inadequate cardiac output. Volume deficits should be corrected; if the cardiac index is low despite normal PCWP and ventilation is adequate, a volume challenge sufficient to increase the PCWP modestly (4 to 5 mm H_2O) should be considered.

A great deal has been written regarding the use of mannitol, loop diuretics, and dopamine for prevention of ARF and for conversion of oliguric to nonoliguric renal failure (17). Oliguric ARF is associated with great morbidity—including sepsis, pulmonary insufficiency, and gastrointestinal bleeding—and high mortality. Whether or not intervention that increases urine output can also improve renal function is controversial, and survival has not been shown to be better in nonoliguric ARF severe enough to require dialysis (1, 2, 4). If intervention is to be effective, it must be done early, prior to establishment of "fixed" ARF (25). While it is possible to augment urine volume in established ATN with high-dose diuretics or mannitol, their use in that setting does not improve survival and may provoke additional morbidity (ototoxicity, hyperosmolality, pulmonary edema). Also, these agents should not be used as "diagnostic" challenges, since such potent stimuli may increase urine output even in the volume-depleted patient.

Most retrospective studies report that the doses of mannitol and furosemide used during CPB were not different between patients with and without subsequent ARF (1–5). When mannitol is given during CPB, intraoperative GFR and urine volume increase, but postoperative renal function is not different than in patients without mannitol (26). Experimentally, mannitol increases blood flow in some models of ARF and increases urine flow more than does saline loading alone. Its protective effects may

TABLE 24.2

URINALYSIS IN ACUTE RENAL FAILURE IN THE POSTOPERATIVE PATIENT

Etiology	Urinary Microscopic Findings	Ancillary Findings
Prerenal	Bland or scant, with hyaline and finely granular casts	Signs of volume depletion or low cardiac output; signs of sepsis
ATN due to ischemia, aminoglycosides	Tubular epithelial cells, free or in casts; coarsely granular pigmented casts	
Allergic interstitial nephritis	Hematuria, pyuria, tubular epithelial cells; eosinophiluria early but inconsistent; RBC casts may be seen	Eosinophilia, fever, skin rash may be present but their absence is not useful diagnostically
Pigment nephropathy (hemoglobin, myoglobin)	Pigmented tubular cell and coarsely granular casts; positive dipstick for hemoglobin/myoglobin in absence of RBCs	Separated plasma is dark in massive hemolysis, clear in rhabdomyolysis; check haptoglobin, CPK, aldolase
Cholesterol embolization	Hematuria, pyuria, often eosinophiluria	Signs of peripheral embolization, livido reticularis, eosinophilia
Urinary infection	Pyuria; WBC casts may be seen in pyelonephritis; ± large bacteriuria	Fever, leukocytosis
Endocarditis	Hematuria, RBC casts, variable proteinuria	New cardiac murmur, fever, signs of peripheral embolism
Urinary tract obstruction	Dependent on etiology; crystals in acute or chronic calculus disease; scant or few histiocytes in hydronephrosis	Ultrasound high yield if hydronephrotic; KUB may show calcifications except in pure urate calculi; urine volume may fluctuate

be due to decreased swelling of tubular epithelium and prevention of tubular obstruction by solute diuresis (19). Loop diuretics, unlike thiazide diuretics, increase renal blood flow as well as solute diuresis and are postulated to decrease tubular obstruction. Prophylactic diuretics are not more effective in preventing postoperative ARF than is adequate volume repletion, however, and whether they have a role in reversing "incipient" ARF is unclear. Dopamine in low doses has been useful in maintaining urine flow in situations of low cardiac output and vasoconstriction (27); the combination of dopamine and furosemide has been purported to improve renal function. If these agents are effective, it appears to be due to the synergistic effects of improved perfusion and solute diuresis.

Recognizing the absence of good controlled studies, if oliguria persists, it seems prudent to carefully administer 12 to 25 gm of mannitol, with care to watch for intravascular volume overload that may result from the osmotically driven translocation of extravascular water into the plasma space. Furosemide (80 to 200 mg, no faster than 4 mg/min intravenously) may be given if vascular volume is replete; if successful, intermittent smaller doses may be used to maintain diuresis. Dopamine (1 to 3 µg/kg/min) may be useful, especially in the patient with low cardiac output. If urine volume remains depressed or if the serum creatinine continues to rise, these measures should be abandoned in favor of supportive treatment.

Supportive Therapy in Acute Renal Failure

The oliguric patient cannot handle large fluid volumes, and the nonoliguric patient may not appropriately conserve volume in the face of losses. Fluids must be adjusted to ensure adequate cardiac output, but pulmonary congestion must be avoided as well as extensive tissue edema, which may retard wound healing or contribute to skin breakdown; however, minor peripheral or sacral edema is usually of cosmetic importance only. Respiratory and GI fluid losses need to be considered, including their electrolyte contents. Intravenous medications are a large source of fluids, and often the sodium or free water content of those fluids is forgotten.

Hyponatremia may be associated with normal, low, or increased extracellular fluid volume, and indicates free water excess relative to sodium; it is often the result of excessive hypotonic fluid administration, with or without diuretic use. A serum sodium below 125 mEq/liter requires treatment. If the patient is asymptomatic, fluid restriction or normal saline is generally adequate. If symptomatic, and the hyponatremia is acute (less than 2 days), saline plus furosemide or dialysis should be employed, with care to acutely correct to a serum sodium no higher than 125 to 130 mEq/liter. Chronic (for more than 3 days) hyponatremis should probably be corrected slowly (less than 0.5 mEq/liter/hr) (28). If the patient received mannitol without diuresis or is hyperglycemic, serum sodium is diluted by translocated water (-1.6 mEq/liter sodium for every 100 mg/dl glucose over 100 ml/dl). Hypernatremia in outpatients is usually associated with intravascular volume depletion, but postoperatively can also result from hypertonic fluids used in resuscitation or treatment of acidosis, or diuretics without adequate free water replacement.

Potassium should be eliminated from intravenous fluids in the oliguric patient; hyperkalemia is less of a problem in the nonoliguric patient, but serum potassium should be monitored frequently (29). Potassium-sparing diuretics should be avoided, and the potassium content of medications should be considered. ECG manifestations of hyperkalemia include peaked T waves (K+ more than 5.5 mEq/liter, approximately), lengthened P-R interval (more than 6.0 mEq/liter), widened QRS complex and flattened P wave (more than 6.5 mEq/liter), deep S wave (more than 7.0 mEq/liter), and finally, a sine wave (more than 8.0 mEq/liter). Emergency treatment for hyperkalemia is outlined in Table 24.3. It should be emphasized that glucose, insulin, bicarbonate, albuterol, and calcium do not eliminate potassium from the

body, and are only temporizing measures.

Hyperchloremic metabolic acidosis associated with renal dysfunction is due to impaired excretion of the daily acid load; an anion gap due to retained anions may occur when ARF is severe. A serum bicarbonate of 18 to 20 is usually well tolerated; adding bicarbonate to daily fluids obligates a sodium load which is often contraindicated in the oliguric patient. Increased acid production (lactic acid, ketoacids) causes a precipitous decline in serum bicarbonate, and correction of the underlying disorder is essential. Acute bicarbonate therapy is unnecessary unless pH is 7.1 or less or serum bicarbonate is 10 mEq/liter or less. Alkalemia is generally the result of vomiting or nasogastric suction and chronic diuretic use. Repletion with chloride-containing fluids is corrective.

Medications in the Patient with Acute Renal Failure

Close attention to drug dosing is mandatory. Drugs that are excreted or metabolized by the kidneys usually require dose or interval adjustment (30). Whenever possible, drug levels should be obtained, especially in the patient whose renal function is changing. For initial dosing, an approximation of creatinine clearance can be made with the formula:

$$C_{cr} = \frac{(140 - age) \times (wt\ kg)}{72 \times S_{cr}\ mg/dl}\ (\times .85\ for\ women)$$

Aminoglycosides should be dosed so that adequate therapeutic peaks are obtained, as well as low troughs, to minimize nephrotoxicity. To achieve this, the interdose level will require lengthening. For other drugs such as digoxin, in which a steady-state blood level is desired, both dose and dosing interval must be changed. Some, but not all, penicillins and cephalosporins require dose adjustments. Insulin is metabolized by the kidney and requirements fall in renal failure; glycemia is also complicated by catabolic stress, so that blood sugar should be carefully monitored. Consult any of the recently available reviews of drug therapy in renal failure for dosing guidelines.

Heart failure and liver disease also alter phar-

TABLE 24.3

ACUTE TREATMENT OF HYPERKALEMIA

Indication	Treatment	Mechanism	Onset of Action
Any ECG findings other than peaked T waves	Calcium gluconate 10–30 ml of 10% solution	Antagonizes membrane effects	Few minutes
K > 6.5 mEq/liter	$NaHCO_3$ 50–100 mEq, glucose 50 gm plus regular insulin 10 units i.v.	Redistributes K	15–30 min
	Albuterol 10–20 mg by nebulizer	Redistributes K^+	15–30 min
	Sodium polystyrene sulfonate (Kayexalate) (cation exchange resin)	Removes K	1–2 hr
	Enema 50–100 gm in 50–100 ml 70% sorbitol	Removes approximately 0.5 mEq/gm	
	Oral 20–50 gm in 100 ml 20% sorbitol	Removes approximately 1 mEq/gm	
	Hemodialysis	Removes up to 25–30 mEq/hr	Few minutes after starting
	Peritoneal dialysis	Removes 10–15 mEq/hr	

macodynamics, and many drugs that are not excreted by the kidneys have effects that are synergistic with uremic complications, such as anticoagulants, sedative-hypnotics, analgesics, etc. For instance, repeated parenteral doses of meperidine cause significant neurotoxicity due to its metabolite normeperidine, especially if hepatic insufficiency coexists.

Many drugs have predictable, often non-dose-related, side effects that are deleterious in the patient with renal insufficiency. Nonsteroidal anti-inflammatory drugs cause functional renal impairment in the postischemic kidney and may result in serious hyperkalemia. Converting enzyme inhibitors decrease kaliuresis and should be used with great caution. Haloperidol blocks dopaminergic receptors and inhibits the vasodilatory effects of dopamine. Tetracycline hydrochloride should be avoided because of its catabolic effects; other tetracyclines can be used.

Radiocontrast agents are especially hazardous to renal function in the postischemic kidney. At greatest risk are patients with diabetic nephropathy (creatinine 2 ml/dl or higher), multiple myeloma, advanced age (more than 60 years), preexisting renal insufficiency, and vol-

ume depletion. If contrast agents must be used, adequate intravascular volume must be maintained; mannitol or furosemide or both given during and immediately after the study may be effective in reducing nephrotoxicity.

Dialysis for Postoperative Acute Renal Failure

The goals of dialysis in postoperative ARF are control of fluid volume, correction of serious electrolyte and acid-base disturbances, and prevention of uremic symptoms. Dialytic fluid removal allows "space" for hyperalimentation and parenteral medications and may improve platelet function. Most deaths in patients with postoperative ARF are not due to uremia, and dialysis is not indicated in the patient with irreversible, lethal nonrenal complications (1).

Rather than await uremic complications, most nephrologists choose to begin dialysis when the creatinine is 6 to 8 ml/dl, especially if the patient is oliguric. While hemodialysis is more frequently used, either hemodialysis or peritoneal dialysis is effective. Hemodialysis is approximately 5 times as efficient as peritoneal dialysis in solute fluid removal. Hypotension can be avoided by the use of small, noncompliant dialyzers, bicarbonate dialysate, hypertonic dialysate, and careful management of fluid removal. Anticoagulation can be minimized or eliminated altogether by using fast blood flow rates and nonthrombogenic dialyzers, or regional citrate anticoagulation may be used. Vascular access may be obtained by a femoral or subclavian catheter. Peritoneal dialysis has the advantage of requiring minimal equipment and no specialized personnel. It is less efficient at potassium removal than are exchange resins, but its slow, continuous nature makes it preferable for patients with marked hemodynamic instability. Poor drainage with overfilling of the peritoneal cavity and subsequent diaphragmatic elevation and reduced venous return may compromise ventilatory and cardiac function. Peritonitis or exit site infections, especially if "acute" straight catheters are used, are common. Hemodialysis should be used in the patient with a very high BUN or who otherwise requires rapid, efficient solute or fluid removal, or the patient with prior abdominal surgery.

Recently, continuous arteriovenous hemofiltration (CAVH) and continuous arteriovenous hemodialysis (CAVHD) have been successfully used to treat ARF (31). Vascular access is gained via large-bore arterial and venous catheters (femoral or a Scribner shunt), and arterial blood is heparinized and circulated through a highly permeable dialyzer. An ultrafiltrate of plasma is formed across the dialyzer membrane and drains from the dialyzer into a Foley bag. Ultrafiltrate volume is dependent on the hydrostatic pressure of the blood within the dialyzer, so that fluid loss decreases when blood pressure falls. Intravenous fluid replacement may be given either before or after the dialyzer. IN CAVH, 8 to 15 liters of ultrafiltrate may be lost per day; this may represent adequate solute removal (5 to 10 ml/min urea clearance), especially if the patient is not hypercatabolic or has residual renal function. CAVHD is similar except that peritoneal dialysate (1.5% Dianeal) flows countercurrent to blood through the dialyzer at 900 ml/hr, and out to the Foley bag; urea clearances of 15 to 25 ml/min are obtained by a combination of plasma ultrafiltration and diffusion across the dialyzer membrane. These two methods offer

significant, continuous fluid removal while minimizing the risk of hypotension, and can be used with MAP as low as 60 to 70 mm Hg. Unfortunately, both methods require anticoagulation except in the thrombocytopenic patient. CAVHD has the advantage of additional solute clearance and lesser heparin requirements (300 to 500 units/hr). Both can be done by intensive care unit personnel.

Cardiac Surgery in the Patient with Chronic Renal Disease

The nondialyzing patient with chronic renal insufficiency requires the same care in management of fluids and cardiac output that the normal patient does (32). The risk of ARF is greater, and lesser insults will result in greater loss of renal function. No medication should be used without careful consideration of its metabolism, interactions, etc. If the patient is very close to requiring dialysis, consideration should be given to preoperative dialysis or to intraoperative temporary access placement. A single intraoperative dialysis can be very useful in such patients and should be considered in view of the ready vascular access provided during cardiopulmonary bypass.

Chronic dialysis should no longer be considered a major contraindication to open-heart surgery, and several centers have reported excellent patient survival following coronary artery bypass or valve replacement (33, 34). Peritoneal dialysis may be performed up until surgery; hemodialysis is usually performed the day prior to surgery. The aim is to completely correct volume excess, but postdialysis hypovolemia should be avoided since it leads to hypotension at the induction of anesthesia. A postdialysis potassium of 3 mEq/liter is desirable, so that the potassium at surgery is approximately 4 mEq/liter. Alkalosis should be avoided; combined with hyperventilation during anesthesia it may cause a hazardous alkalemia. Phosphorus should ideally be 4 to 6 mg/dl. The optimal BUN level for platelet function is unknown, but should probably be 50 ml/dl or less preoperatively. Heparin effects will be gone within 2 to 3 hr following hemodialysis. Prolonged bleeding time may also be shortened, though inconsistently, by conjugated estrogen treatment (0.6 mg/kg/

day intravenously for 5 days, peak action days 5 to 7), desmopressin acetate (DDAVP) (0.3 mg/kg intravenously over 1 hr or 3 μg/kg intranasally; subsequent doses are less effective), cryoprecipitate (10 units), and by maintaining hematocrit at 30% or higher. The optimal hematocrit for surgery is unclear, and will depend on anticipated blood losses and the severity of ischemic heart disease.

Intraoperatively, the hemodialysis vascular access must be protected. Pressure should not be exerted on that extremity by either a blood pressure cuff or patient positioning. Intravenous infusions should not be given through the access or any vessel above the access, including the ipsilateral subclavian vein. Hypotension also increases the risk of a thrombosed access.

Potassium should be monitored frequently. Hyperkalemia may result from release of intracellular potassium by depolarized muscle following administration of muscle relaxants such as succinylcholine, or from tissue trauma, hypercatabolism, acidosis, or resorption of internal bleeding; high-potassium cardioplegic solutions, transfusions, and some medications introduce exogenous potassium. Insulin and catecholamines are important in acutely redistributing potassium from plasma to the intracellular space; diabetics and possibly patients on β-adrenergic blocking agents are at particular risk of hyperkalemia (29).

Hemodynamic monitoring is essential to guide postoperative fluid management; dialysis will be necessary to treat hypertension due to volume overload, while antihypertensives (intravenous labetalol, nitroprusside) will be required if volume is low. Hypotension may be the result of cardiac failure, volume depletion, or pericardial effusion, even in the absence of a friction rub.

Peritoneal dialysis may be resumed immediately postoperatively. The decision to hemodialyze should be made on a day-by-day basis and should not be delayed if indications such as volume overload, hyperkalemia, or hyponatremia are present. Underdialysis should be avoided since the postoperative patient is catabolic and prone to uremic complications. Heparin-free dialysis for 1 to 2 weeks is preferable; regional citrate anticoagulation may be used. CAVH or CAVHD may also be useful,

especially if the patient is unstable or receiving hyperalimentation; if arterial flow from the vascular access is inadequate, a femoral artery may be cannulated. The heparin dose should be minimized, guided by the activated clotting time.

As with the ARF patient, careful attention must be paid to medications, including their sodium and potassium contents, and to drug levels. Fever may be blunted in the azotemic patient, so slight temperature elevations should be considered significant.

References

1. Abel RM, Buckley MJ, Austen WG, et al: Etiology, incidence, and prognosis of renal failure following operations. *J Thorac Cardiovasc Surg* 71:323–333, 1976.
2. Yeboah ED, Petrie A, Pead JL: Acute renal failure and open heart surgery. *Br Med J* 1:415–418, 1972.
3. Gailiunas P, Chawla R, Lazarus JM, et al: Acute renal failure following cardiac operations. *J Thorac Cardiovasc Surg* 79:241–243, 1980.
4. Bhat JG, Gluck MC, Lowenstein J, et al: Renal failure after open heart surgery. *Ann Intern Med* 84:677–682, 1976.
5. Hilberman M, Myers BD, Carrie BJ, et al: Acute renal failure following cardiac surgery. *J Thorac Cardiovasc Surg* 77:880–888, 1979.
6. Margolis BL, Stein JH: The renal circulation. *Int Anesthesiol Clin* 22:35–63, 1984.
7. Mazze R: Nephropathies associated with the use of anesthetics. *Monographs in Applied Toxicology* 1:422–436, 1982.
8. Wickstrom I, Sefansson T: Effects of prolonged anesthesia with enflurane or helothane on renal function in dogs. *Acta Anesthesiol Scand* 25:228–234, 1981.
9. Taylor KM, Morton IJ, Brown JJ, et al: Hypertension and the renin-angiotensin system following open-heart surgery. *J Thorac Cardiovasc Surg* 74:840–845, 1977.
10. Wu W, Zbuzed VK, Bellevue C: Vasopressin release during cardiac operation. *J Thorac Cardiovasc Surg* 79:83–90, 1980.
11. Fedderson K, Aurell M, Delin K, et al: Effects of cardiopulmonary bypass and prostacyclin on plasma catecholamines, angiotension II and arginine-vasopressin. *Acta Anaesthesiol Scand* 29:224–230, 1985.
12. Lundberg S: Renal function during anaesthesia

and open-heart surgery in man. *Acta Anaesthesiol Scand* 27:9–81, 1967.

13. Porter GA, Kloster FE, Herr RJ, et al: Relationship between alterations in renal hemodynamics during cardiopulmonary bypass and postoperative renal function. *Circulation* 34:1005–1021, 1966.

14. Mielke JE, Maher FT, Hunt JC, et al: Renal performance in patients undergoing replacement of the aortic valve. *Circulation* 32:394–405, 1965.

15. Bourgeois BF, Donath A, Paunier L, et al: Effects of cardiac surgery on renal function in children. *J Thorac Cardiovasc Surg* 77:283–286, 1979.

16. Anderson RJ, Linas SL, Berns AS, et al: Nonoliguric acute renal failure. *N Engl J Med* 296:1134–1138, 1977.

17. Madias NE, Harrington JT: Postischemic acute renal failure. In Brenner BM, Lazarus JM (eds): *Acute Renal Failure.* Philadelphia, WB Saunders, 1983.

18. Myers BD, Moran SM: Hemodynamically mediated acute renal failure. *N Engl J Med* 314:97–105, 1986.

19. Zager RA, Mahan J, Merola AJ: Effects of mannitol on the postischemic kidney. *Lab Invest* 53:433–442, 1985.

20. Miller TR, Anderson RJ, Linas SL, et al: Urinary diagnostic indices in acute renal failure. *Ann Intern Med* 89:47–50, 1978.

21. Miller PO, Krebs RA, Neal BJ, et al: Polyuric prerenal failure. *Arch Intern Med* 140:907–909, 1980.

22. Zarich S, Fant LST, Diamond JR: Fractional excretion of sodium. *Arch Intern Med* 145:108–112, 1985.

23. Hilberman M, Derby GC, Spencer RJ, et al: Sequential pathophysiological changes characterizing the progression from renal dysfunction to acute renal failure following cardiac operation. *J Thorac Cardiovasc Surg* 79:838–844, 1980.

24. Maseda J, Hilberman M, Dereby GC, et al: The renal effects of sodium nitroprusside in postoperative cardiac surgical patients. *Anesthesiology* 54:284–288, 1981.

25. Dixon BS, Anderson RJ: Nonoliguric acute renal failure. *Am J Kidney Dis* 2:71–80, 1985.

26. Berman LB, Smith LL, Chisholm GD, et al: Mannitol and renal function in cardiovascular surgery. *Arch Surg* 88:239–243, 1964.

27. Davis RF, Lappas DG, Kirklin JK: Acute oliguria after cardiopulmonary bypass: renal functional improvement with low-dose dopamine infusion. *Crit Care Med* 10:852–856, 1982.

28. Sterns RH: Severe symptomatic hyponatremia: treatment and outcome. *Ann Intern Med* 107:656–664, 1987.

29. Weber DO, Yarnoz MD: Hyperkalamia complicating cardiopulmonary bypass: analysis of risk factors. *Ann Thorac Surg* 34:439–445, 1982.

30. Benner WM, Aronoff GR, Morrison G, et al: Drug prescribing in renal failure: dosing guidelines for adults. *Am J Kidney Dis* 3:155–193, 1983.

31. Sigler MH, Teehan BP: Solute transport in continuous hemodialysis: a new treatment for acute renal failure. *Kidney Int* 32:562–571, 1987.

32. Burke GR, Gulyassy PF: Surgery in the patient with renal disease and related electrolyte disorders. *Med Clin North Am* 63:1191–1230, 1979.

33. Francis GS, Sharma B, Collins AJ, et al: Coronary-artery surgery in patients with end-stage renal disease. *Ann Intern Med* 92:499–503, 1980.

34. Opsahl JA, Husebye DG, Helseth HK, et al: Coronary artery bypass surgery in patients on maintenance dialysis: long-term survival. *Am J Kidney Dis* 12:271–274, 1988.

Chapter 25
GENERAL SURGICAL COMPLICATIONS FOLLOWING CARDIAC SURGERY

STEPHEN J. SHAPIRO, M.D., F.A.C.S.
LEO A. GORDON, M.D., F.A.C.S.

The postoperative cardiac surgical patient offers a challenging and complex scenario for the diagnosis of acute intraabdominal conditions. The age of the patient, the changes induced by cardiac bypass, sedation, and metabolic alterations of the postoperative period all combine to cloud the basic patterns of these disease entities.

Although they occur in only 1% of postoperative cardiac surgical patients, the mortality of these entities is approximately 20 to 50%. For this reason, a rapid, well-thought-out workup is essential to the patient's survival. There is a natural reluctance to transport the intubated, early postoperative patient to a variety of diagnostic tests. Today, given the availability of many portable units (nuclear scans, ultrasonography, etc.) bedside diagnosis is more feasible.

Potential mechanisms to explain the occurrence of intraabdominal problems following open-heart surgery include, among others, preexisting conditions aggravated by the trauma of surgery, hypoperfusion caused by extracorporeal bypass, and intraaortic balloon pumping. Rather than elaborate these theoretical considerations, this chapter will stress the practical approach to the diagnosis of acute intraabdominal disease.

The suspicion of intraabdominal disease in the postoperative cardiac surgical patient may be heightened in a variety of clinical situations. These situations are described in the paragraphs that follow.

CLUES TO THE PROBLEM

Abdominal Signs and Symptoms

Abdominal Pain. Though the patient is sedated and intubated, many intraabdominal problems may present in the usual fashion, for example, right upper quadrant pain in biliary tract disease, diffuse upper abdominal pain in pancreatitis, diffuse pain in bowel ischemia. If the pattern is typical, even given the presence of a recent sternotomy and chest tubes, it should be pursued.

Abdominal Distension. Although ileus is frequent, progressive distension and persistently absent bowel sounds may herald a developing acute intraabdominal condition.

Guarding and Rigidity. Generalized board-like rigidity is almost never present in normal convalescence and may suggest an acute perforation. Localized guarding and rigidity should heighten the suspicion for an acute problem such as cholecystitis or appendicitis.

Abnormal Blood Tests

Routine postoperative blood tests provide a wealth of laboratory data. Often, a markedly abnormal value may herald a developing problem—a very high amylase or lipase, a persistently elevated WBC with left shift, etc. Although certain routine values will be transiently elevated due to recent surgery, a persistently abnormal value may lead to early workup. Transient hyperbilirubinemia, hyperamylasemia, and leukocytosis are frequently seen after cardiac bypass.

UNEXPLAINED SEPSIS

As in any other clinical situation, unexplained sepsis may suggest significant intraabdominal pathology and should be vigorously pursued.

PROCEEDING WITH THE WORKUP (TABLE 25.1)

History and Physical.   A careful review of the patient's prior GI history and an even more careful repeat physical examination are essential. Frequently, such problems have their roots in a preexisting condition. Many times the fixation on the cardiac problem and surgery can obscure some key points in the patient's history. Among the advantages of engaging a new consultant in this situation is to have him or her perform a careful review of the record or conduct an interview with the family to get a hint of any preexisting conditions. A review of the hospital course and a careful physical examination with special attention to the chest, ab-

TABLE 25.1

EVALUATION OF SUSPECTED POSTSURGICAL ABDOMINAL PATHOLOGY

1. Careful review of history, preoperative and intraoperative
2. New physical examination
3. Review of recent blood work
4. Plain films of abdomen and chest

domen, and perineum by an experienced general surgeon is invaluable. This can be made difficult by the technology of the intensive care unit and the intubated, sedated, and monitored patient. Perirectal abscesses, orchitis, fasciitis and other extraabdominal conditions have all been "discovered" by a new examiner doing a thorough examination.

Laboratory.   Specific blood work important in the differential diagnosis of an acute intraabdominal condition include a CBC; serum amylase, lipase, calcium, and liver function studies (including TD bilirubin, alkaline phosphatase, SGOT, SGPT, and prothrombintime); as well as blood and urine cultures and stool examination.

Plain Films of the Abdomen.   Plain films of the abdomen are the general surgeon's electrocardiogram. Simultaneous with the thought of surgical consultation should be the ordering of a flat and either erect or lateral decubitis film of the abdomen. The bowel pattern, extraluminal gas, stippled gas, or pneumobilia may be of help in defining the problem. A chest film is extremely important in evaluating a suspected intraabdominal condition. As Hamilton Bailey said, "The abdomen extends from the chin to the knees."

Ultrasonography.   In suspected cases of biliary tract disease or pancreatitis, the ultrasound scan can be helpful if a definite abnormality is detected. The bedside availability of this test has proved to be a useful adjunct to the diagnosis of acute intraabdominal disease.

Nuclear Scans.   The hepato-iminodiacetic acid (HIDA) scan has been helpful in cases of acute cholecystitis. Also, the indium-tagged white blood cell study can be helpful in the diagnosis of intraabdominal abscess. Occult gastrointestinal bleeding may be defined by the technetium pyrophosphate–tagged red blood cell study. Bedside availability has enhanced the use of these nuclear studies.

Contrast Studies.   Contrast studies of the bowel using water-soluble agents such as Gastrografin have a select usefulness in the critically ill patient.

Endoscopy.   Bedside flexible sigmoidoscopy can assist in the diagnosis of colonic bleeding or ischemia or recognition of pseudomembranous colitis. Upper-GI endoscopy can pinpoint the cause and sometimes treat gastroduodenal hemorrhage.

Bedside laparoscopy using a small instrument has a limited role in detecting intraabdominal hemorrhage, ischemia, or traumatic lesions (ruptured spleen or liver).

Exploratory Laparotomy. This is included in a list of investigative studies and has been labeled the "ultimate diagnositc test." The ideal approach is to begin with a definitive diagnosis, especially in more seriously ill patients. Unfortunately, as the managing team continues their diagnositc search, the patient's condition may deteriorate. Most stable postoperative cardiac patients will tolerate a laparotomy far better than persistent sepsis from an intraabdominal cause. Many older patients, sedated and medicated, will not display the usual patterns of abdominal pain, fever, or leukocytosis, and can easily mask ongoing pathology. Persistent sepsis, even with negative studies, may properly lead to diagnostic exploratory laparotomy.

MAJOR CAUSES OF GASTROINTESTINAL COMPLICATIONS AND THEIR MANAGEMENT

Acute intraabdominal conditions requiring urgent surgery will occur in approximately 1% of all cardiac surgical patients (Table 25.2). The conditions described below will account for the majority of these cases.

Ileus. The occurrence of painless abdominal distension following cardiac surgery is a frequent event. The ileus may be generalized or specifically localized to the colon. This usually re-

TABLE 25.2

GENERAL SURGICAL COMPLICATIONS IN POSTOPERATIVE CARDIAC SURGICAL PATIENTS

1. Ileus
2. Acute cholecystitis
3. Gastroduodenal disease
4. Mesenteric ischemia
5. Acute pancreatitis
6. Other vascular disease
7. Intraabdominal bleeding, liver, or splenic injury
8. Lower thoracic pathology
9. Miscellaneous conditions

sponds to nasogastric decompression and nutritional support, should the problem continue. The pattern of ileus is important. If generalized, the suspicion of concurrent general surgical pathology (adhesive obstruction of colonic lesion) is low. If localized to the colon, Ogilvie's syndrome (nonobstructive colon dilation) may be present. Although usually benign, a colon ileus may be of concern due to increasing cecal size or the presence of localized findings. If colonic distension is present with a cutoff on plain abdominal film, a Gastrografin study to delineate a mass lesion is necessary.

Most small bowel or colonic ileuses will resolve as the acuity of the patient's postcardiac surgical condition improves.

Biliary Tract Disease. This accounts for approximately one-third of urgent intraabdominal conditions in the postoperative cardiac surgical patient. A history of gallstones may be identified in many cases. The onset of upper abdominal pain, fever and right upper quadrant tenderness, or the presence of a tender right upper quadrant mass should suggest acute obstructive cholecystitis. The older patient presents a more difficult clinical challenge, because disordered liver function tests and fever may be the only presenting signs. The diagnosis can be confirmed by ultrasonography and the HIDA scan.

Acalculous cholecystitis is more frequently seen in the postoperative cardiac surgical patient. Its clinical identification can be more difficult and the signs more subtle; for example, the ultrasound scan may show only wall thickening or pericholecystic fluid, sludge without stones, and only modest intraluminal distension (Fig. 25.1) The HIDA scan can be particularly helpful in these patients and may lead to early operative intervention.

Fever, jaundice, and upper abdominal pain do not always mean biliary tract disease. In the postoperative cardiac patient, many entities may mimic biliary tract disease. Jaundice and fever are frequently seen in the postoperative cardiac bypass patient. Red blood cell breakdown, liver hypoperfusion, and numerous drugs may all contribute to hyperbilirubinemia.

Additional diagnostic studies such as transhepatic cholangiography (THC), endoscopic

FIGURE 25.1

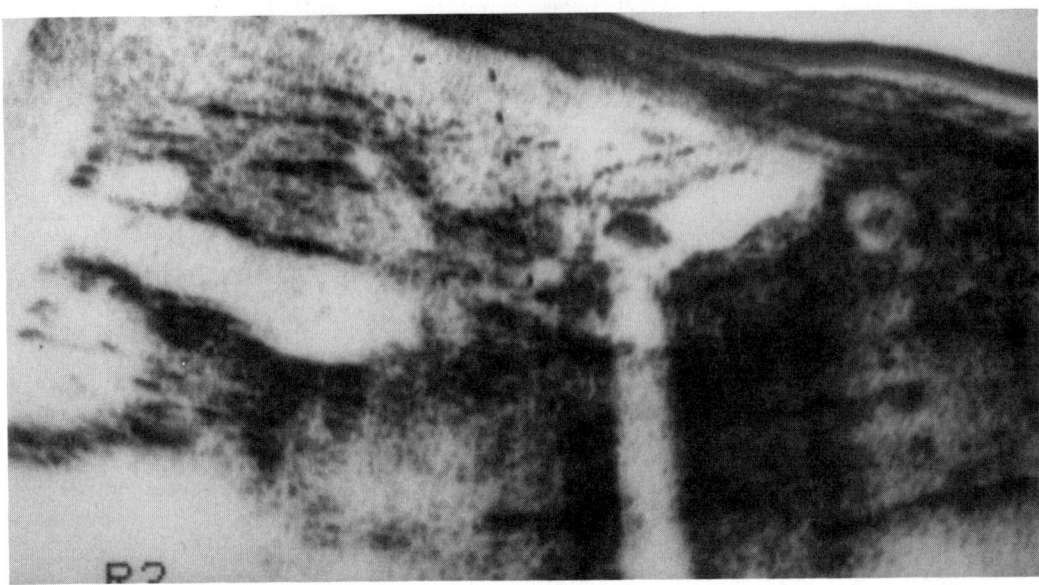

Ultrasound scan of gallbladder showing a stone and thickened gallbladder wall.

retrograde cannulation of the pancreatic duct (ERCP), as well as the studies mentioned above may be important in further defining the clinical problem. Confusing clinical presentations in poor-risk patients may require the anatomic detail that only these additional procedures can give.

The following case is a typical example.

J.W. is a 72-year-old white male who underwent coronary artery bypass grafting 5 days ago. On the 4th postoperative day he was noted to be deeply jaundiced, mildly febrile, and minimally tender in the right upper quadrant. Ultrasound was equivocal. Liver function tests were mildly abnormal except for a bilirubin of 10. There was no evidence of hemolysis. Because of the concern over extrahepatic biliary obstruction, a skinny-needle THC was performed. No evidence of obstruction was found (Fig. 25.2). The patient's jaundice resolved.

The use of ERCP and urgent sphincterotomy should be considered in the patient with obstructive jaundice whose operative mortality is felt to be prohibitive. As the expertise of interventional gastroenterologists improves, this technique may be more frequently employed.

Acute obstructive cholecystitis secondary to

an impacted stone or acute acalculous cholecystitis is best treated by cholecystectomy with operative cholangiography. In the diabetic patient, operative intervention should be early, given the high risk of gangrene and perforation. In the patient who is hemodynamically unstable, cholecystostomy under local anesthesia to decompress the gallbladder may be life saving.

Ascending cholangitis should be rapidly diagnosed, especially in the patient with a prosthetic cardiac valve or graft. The frequent septicemia seen with this entity can be lethal. Intraoperative cholangiography is essential in defining ductal anatomy and identifying common duct stones. The addition of common duct exploration and removal of common duct stones with T-tube drainage is effective. The use of biliary bypass or sphincteroplasty is governed by the operative findings.

Acute obstructive cholangitis, characterized by right upper quadrant pain, jaundice, fever, Gram-negative shock, and confusion, is a true surgical emergency. Immediate decompression of the common duct is essential. In the hemodynamically unstable, high-risk, cardiac surgical patient, ERCP with sphincteroplasty (Fig. 25.3) or transhepatic decompression should be

FIGURE 25.2

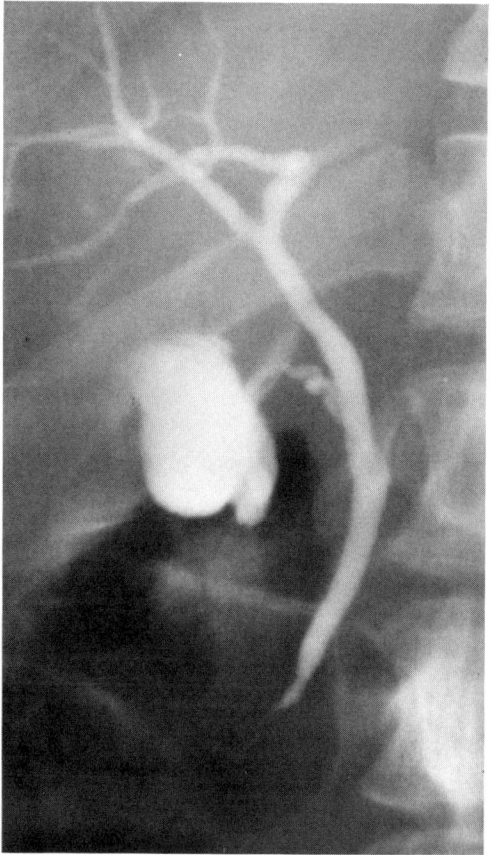

"Skinny needle" cholangiogram showing a normal extrahepatic biliary tree.

FIGURE 25.3

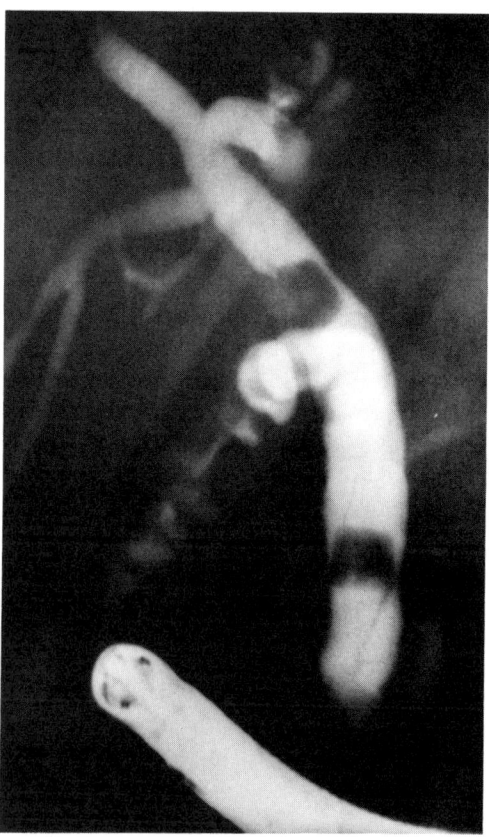

ERCP prior to sphincterotomy showing common duct stones.

considered. The use of these modalities is limited since many of these patients are on anticoagulants. Further availability is limited by the specific expertise that is needed. The availability of an interventional radiologist and gastroenterologist is essential to this diagnositc and therapeutic approach.

Gastroduodenal Disease.   Upper gastrointestinal hemorrhage is the most common gastroduodenal disease seen in this setting. Stress gastritis and peptic ulcer disease are most common and may be aggravated or caused by cardiac surgery. Upper gastrointestinal bleeding has become less frequent with the judicious use of gastric alkalinization and intravenous histamine blockers. Nevertheless, bleeding and even perforation still occur.

Other causes of upper tract bleeding may oc-

cur as well. Mallory-Weiss tears and erosive processes from adjacent organs and undetected bleeding tumors also have been seen in these situations.

Indications and timing of surgery in these patients do not lend themselves to a formula approach. When the supportive treatment is ineffective, surgical treatment should be considered. Coagulopathy, hypotension, and even a depleted blood bank may all result if surgical intervention is unduly delayed.

GI bleeding should lead to early endoscopy to define both the site of bleeding and the underlying pathology. This information can influence the immediate medical therapy and its prognosis and provide invaluable information for the surgeon.

Several management points should be stressed when dealing with the upper-GI bleeder. A large-bore nasogastric tube is help-ful for the administration of antacids. These antacids should be given in amounts sufficient to affect the gastric pH rather than in amounts given by a set protocol. It is helpful to measure the gastric pH to check the gastric acidity, and to double the previous amount of antacid if the alkalinization is ineffective. Too often, a patient is said to have failed medical treat-ment when in fact the treatment was inade-quately administered.

While iced-saline lavage may be helpful in gauging the vigor of a bleed, one of the main drawbacks is trauma to the gastric wall from overzealous suction. Gentle aspiration is the goal. Many upper GI tract bleeders would have been successfully treated were it not for the trauma induced in the gastric wall from mucosal trauma.

Mesenteric Ischemia.   Of all the intraabdom-inal entities that can trouble the postoperative patient, none is more elusive or lethal than intestinal ischemia. Poor cardiac output, debris embolized through the mesenteric blood supply, vessel dissection from an intraaortic balloon, as well as the effect of cardiopulmonary and va-soconstrictive drugs can all contribute to intes-tinal ischemia.

Frequently, an intraoperative event may her-ald suspicion of postoperative intestinal is-chemia. A lengthy pump run with prolonged hypoperfusion, or a suspicion of embolization during balloon placement may lead to a higher clinical suspicion of ischemic intestinal disor-ders.

Diffuse pain out of proportion to the physical examination findings, blood in the stool, unex-plained sepsis due to enteric organisms, as well as subtle, nearly hidden stippled gas on a plain abdominal x-ray film may all herald a mesen-teric vascular catastrophy (Fig. 25.4).

There is no easy answer. Mesenteric angiog-raphy, in most centers, has not proved helpful in either the diagnosis or treatment of clinically suspected mesenteric ischemia. Laparoscopy for preoperative diagnosis cannot adequately visu-alize the entire small bowel. The often focal nature of small bowel ischemia makes this tech-nique unreliable for full visualization of the small intestine. Contrast bowel studies may give a clue as to the diagnosis, but cannot distinguish

FIGURE 25.4

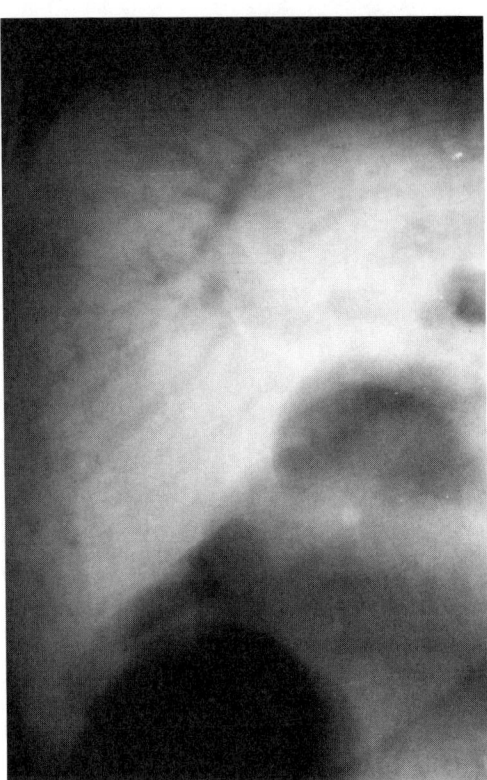

Hepatic portal venous gas in a patient with mesenteric ischemia.

ischemia from infarction. Sigmoidoscopy can help should colonic ischemia be suspected.

In cases of suspected ischemia, more testing and consequently longer waiting results in higher mortality. Early laparotomy with appropriate re-section, reconstruction, or embolectomy ap-pears to be the safest course.

The surgical approach consists mainly of re-section of infarcted intestine. The main oper-ative problem is one of assessing intestinal viability. Doppler assessment and fluorescein dye testing have been advocated. The most reliable index appears to be the presence of freely bleed-ing mucosal vessels at the resection margins. Normal-locking mucosa, free of ulcerations, is also a sign of viability.

We do not favor a routine "second-look" procedure in all cases. If the patient is doing clinically well, he or she is observed. Obvious deterioration or sepsis mandates a reexploration.

The advent of the Hickman catheter and refined methods of long-term or home hyperalimentation have aided greatly in the postoperative management of bowel ischemia.

Acute Pancreatitis. Pancreatitis may be seen in a variety of postoperative settings. Postoperative pancreatitis amounts for about 10% of all types of pancreatitis. Most frequently, it follows surgery of the upper abdomen where local trauma is believed to play a role.

Hyperamylasemia is not rare during normal convalescence in the cardiac surgical patient. Fortunately, very few patients will develop clinically significant pancreatitis. The etiologic factors in postoperative cardiac surgical pancreatitis include hypotension, splanchnic vasoconstriction, and thromboembolic phenomena.

When clinical signs of acute pancreatitis develop, treatment should consist of gastric decompression and judicious fluid replacement. Serial ultrasonography of the upper abdomen has been helpful in detecting early pseudocyst or abscess formation. The development of hemorrhagic pancreatitis is usually a lethal event that should be treated with the same vigor as in the patient who has not had recent surgery.

If the pancreatitis is biliary in nature, timing of operative intervention is crucial, and intervention should be early in any worsening clinical situation.

The use of transhepatic percutaneous techniques for common bile duct visualization and biliary decompression has been gaining acceptance. This can be most helpful in defining ductal anatomy and visualization of common duct pathology.

In critically ill patients with clinical pancreatitis and demonstrated common duct pathology, there is some recent interest in the use of ERCP for both diagnosis and relief of common duct obstruction (vide supra).

Fortunately, most cases of pancreatitis in postoperative cardiac surgical patients are self limited and will respond to fluid support and nasogastric suction.

Other Vascular Causes. The patient with coronary artery disease or valvular heart disease may have concurrent vascular pathology that may present in the postoperative state. Dissecting aneurysm and pseudoaneurysm, distal embolic phenomena, as well as extracranial carotid occlusive disease are not infrequent. Adequate preoperative assessment and the increasing use of combined or staged procedures have lessened the complications from these entities somewhat. Nevertheless, the mechanics by bypass and balloon pumping must lead to consideration of these factors.

Back pain, exquisite limb pain from ischemia, and neurologic disturbances should be viewed in the context of vascular problems rather than metabolic problems in the postoperative patient. Angiography or noninvasive vascular testing may be helpful.

Intraabdominal Bleeding and Liver or Splenic Injury. Intraabdominal hemorrhage may present during or following cardiac surgery. Although rarely seen, intraabdominal bleeding can occur during abdominal extensions of thoracic incisions. Misplaced chest tubes have resulted in hepatic or splenic injuries. Trauma to other upper abdominal organs can also result in massive intraabdominal hemorrhage. Preexisting hepatic lesions, such as hamartomas, angiomas, or hepatomas can spontaneously rupture in the patient on anticoagulants and extracorporeal bypass.

In the absence of excessive thoracic bleeding, one should consider an abdominal cause for a decreasing hematocrit, especially with a dull, "doughy," tender abdomen.

The diagnostic workup for suspected intraabdominal bleeding should include abdominal lavage. We favor the open technique, using a direct cutdown and direct visualization of the peritoneum. This has been helpful in eliminating false-positive lavages and intraabdominal injury.

Bedside laparoscopy, using the 1.5-mm laparoscope, is well tolerated even without sedation and can enable directly visualizing the major organs. Significant intraperitoneal hemorrhage and disruption of the major organs can be detected. Computerized tomography can also detect free fluid and disruption of the major organs. Ultrasonography and angiography have little role in the diagnositc evaluation of intraabdominal bleeding.

Lower Thoracic Pathology. Just as in the unoperated patient, the postoperative cardiac sur-

FIGURE 25.5

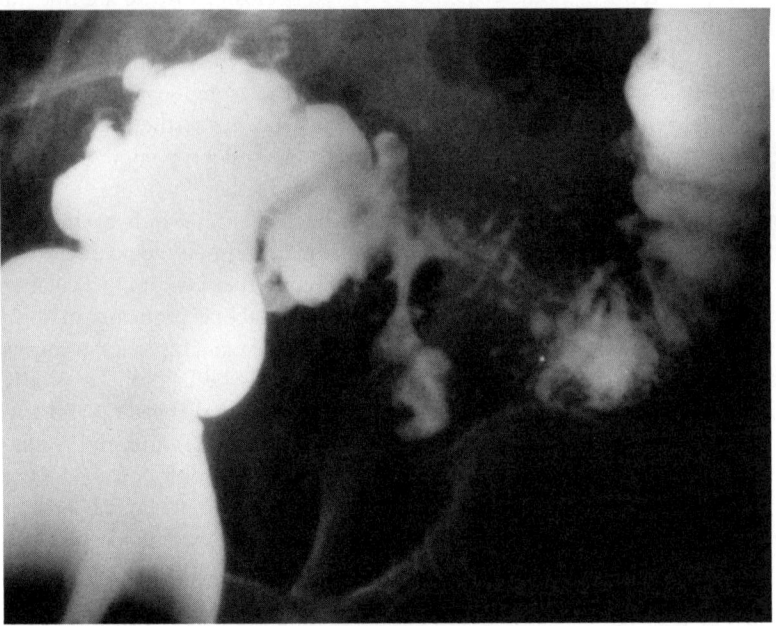

Acute diverticulitis in a postoperative cardiac surgical patient.

gical patient may present with upper abdominal pain due to lower thoracic pathology. Lower lobe pulmonary emboli with infarction, inferior wall myocardial infarction, mediastinitis, and muscular pain from chest tube exit sites may all be confused with upper abdominal surgical conditions.

Miscellaneous Conditions. The postoperative cardiac surgical patient can have any disease any other patient can have, which many times will present in the postoperative period. Acute diverticulitis, appendicitis, and lower gastrointestinal bleeding from any colonic source can occur (Fig. 25.5).

Incarcerated inguinal hernias, perirectal abscess, and orchitis must also be considered in the differential approach to abdominal pain.

Retroperitoneal pathology such as acute pyelonephritis, perinephric abscess and renal stones, as well as retroperitoneal tumors may present as acute abdominal conditions.

The physician should approach these problems independent of the postoperative state of the patient, because delay contributes to mortality from these conditions.

SUMMARY

Gastrointestinal problems following cardiac surgery are rare but, when they occur, carry a high morbidity and mortality. The workup of these problems has its foundation on a careful review of the patient's preoperative and intraoperative history, as well as a complete physical examination. The diagnosis of the more common entities can be facilitated by plain radiography and the limited use of ultrasound and contrast studies. Prolonged workups to obtain a definitive diagnosis may delay needed surgical intervention, such as in unexplained sepsis in a deteriorating patient which should lead to early laparotomy.

Suggested Readings

1. Aranha GV: The reasons for gastrointestinal consultation after cardiac surgery. *Am Surg* 50:301–304, 1984.
2. Feiner H: Pancreatitis after cardiac surgery. *Am J Surg* 131:684–688, 1976.
3. Hanks JB: Gastrointestinal complications after

cardiopulmonary bypass. *Surgery* 92:394–400, 1982.

4. Howard RJ: Acute acalculous cholecystitis. *Am J Surg* 141:194–198, 1981.

5. Moneta G: Hypoperfusion as a possible factor in the development of gastrointestinal complications after cardiac surgery. *Am J Surg* 149:648–650, 1985.

6. Pinson CW: General surgical complications after cardiopulmonary bypass surgery. *Am J Surg* 148:133–137, 1983.

7. Reath DB: General surgical complications following cardiac surgery. *Am Surg* 49:11–14, 1983.

8. Roise DM: Patterns of severe pancreatic injury following cardiopulmonary bypass. *Ann Surg* 199:168–172, 1984.

9. Savina JA: Factors encouraging laparotomy in acalculous cholecystitis. *Crit Care Med* 13:377–380, 1985.

10. Steed D: General surgical complications in heart and heart-lung transplantation. *Surgery* 98:739–745, 1985.

11. Svensson LG: A prospective study of hyperamylasemia and pancreatitis after cardiopulmonary bypass. *Ann Thorac Surg* 39:409–411, 1985.

12. Wallwork J: The acute abdomen following cardiopulmonary bypass surgery. *Br J Surg* 67:410–412, 1980.

Chapter 26
COGNITIVE AND PSYCHOLOGICAL CHANGES

RICHARD J. GRAY, M.D.

There is perhaps no medical intervention with so great a psychological as well as physical impact as cardiac surgery. This is to be expected, considering the central theme played by the heart in religion, literature, and the visual arts. Widely attributed as the seat of the soul, the heart was believed to have great powers before its true function was even known. This is exemplified in the following quotation, attributed to Huang Ti (2697 to 2597 BC), taken from *The Yellow Emperor's Classic of Internal Medicine*: "The heart is the root of life and causes the versatility of the spiritual faculties. The heart influences the face and fills the pulse with blood" (1). Leonardo da Vinci writes, "The heart . . . moves of itself and does not stop unless forever" (2); and William Boyd, in *Pathology for the Surgeon*, states, "Of all the ailments which may blow out life's little candle, heart disease is the chief" (3). These quotations demonstrate the great respect with which the heart is regarded, but also highlight the mystery and pehaps the fear surrounding diseases of the heart as expressed by these eminent men of science in medicine from totally different eras. Numerous daily expressions such as "heartsick," "heart-rending," "lighthearted," "coldhearted," and "heavyhearted" all have implications regarding our beliefs of the importance of the heart. Perhaps it should not be surprising that special significance is placed on surgery in which the heart is actually exposed, handled, incised, and even, in some cases, removed.

SENSATIONS BEFORE AND EARLY AFTER SURGERY

Preoperatively, anxiety is one of the principal symptoms and can be disabling, especially if the patient is unfortunate enough to be on a long waiting list for surgery (4). After hospitalization, even more anxiety provoking is the sudden cancellation and postponement of surgery due to change in the surgical schedule. Styles of coping with preoperative anxiety are a function of personality characteristics and appear to fit two general patterns: those who tend to avoid or deny the threatening aspects of an impending operation, characterized as *repressors*; and those who approach their anxiety by intellectualizing and striving to know as much as possible about their upcoming surgery, called *sensitizers* (5). It is apparent that patients become more polarized in their adoption of either of these coping styles as the risk of impending surgery increases. Furthermore, it appears that patients having a longer duration of preoperative complaints and, even more specifically, those who have valvular heart disease (rather than coronary artery disease) tend to use sensitization (the desire to know more) rather than repression as a coping style (6).

The practical application of these concepts

can be seen in observing the experienced clinician discuss the risks of upcoming surgery who, responding to seemingly the slightest verbal or nonverbal clues, knows just what to tell his or her patient. Certain patients, after a brief and honest appraisal of the risks of surgery, simply want to know that they will survive and benefit from the operation; others would be offended by the simplicity of this discussion and may wish a lengthy scientific or technical explanation of the surgical procedure and its outcome. The most successful physician must learn which of these two different approaches will be most successful with each individual patient. For those patients wishing a more detailed explanation, it should be kept in mind that the concepts of cardiopulmonary bypass might be quite foreign and may require additional explanation (some patients even assume the heart and lungs are removed during surgery).

On the day immediately following surgery most patients are quite convivial, expressing great optimism about their recovery and surprise over the lack of significant discomfort. Within 1 to 2 days this enthusiasm is exchanged for a more realistic approach as they realize that they are more severely afflicted by the trauma of the operation than they had thought. Realization that even slight position changes in bed, coughing, and deep breathing all produce incisional discomfort; confrontation with their own physical weakness; lack of appetite and perhaps inability to sleep; viewing the convalescence as a long and dreary period—all contribute to a much changed attitude and the first traces of hospital depression.

EARLY POSTOPERATIVE CHANGES IN MOOD

The depression that begins a few days after surgery is so common that it does not constitute a complication in the majority of patients. It will often be commented on by family and friends and makes the medical and nursing care of such patients a good deal more time-consuming. It is occasionally severe enough to affect eating and sleeping habits and retard physical activities and convalescence. Preoperative mood tendencies (such as depression) may serve as a helpful

predictor of more severe postoperative involvement (7), and lengthy postoperative complications often lead to depression, but few other preoperative factors are useful. On the contrary, younger and previously more healthy patients are often the most frustrated with slow postoperative recovery and, hence, more prone to depression and anger.

Any patient undergoing major surgery is in a unique situation, totally dependent on others and devoid of his or her usual rights as an adult with respect to such important factors as what and when he or she will eat, timing of bedtime, use of toilet facilities, and complete lack of privacy. This is often expressed as anger and hostility or, under certain circumstances, paranoid ideation. Anger is most often expressed toward the patient's spouse, significant other, or the nursing staff. Occasionally attempts to regain control are seen in refusal to cooperate with treatments, regimens, or medical recommendations. The ability to tolerate this loss of control is often predictable, based on certain personality traits or life-style expectations preoperatively. These understandable but often profound changes in mood must be dealt with supportively, but should be differentiated from true disordered thought processes often not amenable to rational measures and with potentially different medical implications. Depression occurring during this early period is self-limited in almost all cases, and requires only supportive therapy. Hostility and paranoid ideation require a tactful and understanding approach, a full explanation of the rationale behind the treatment plan, and assurance that the patient can control certain aspects of his or her therapy.

CHANGES IN THOUGHT PROCESS

More profound alterations in mood and sensorium, such as delirium (either quiet or agitated) and other forms of psychoses, are less common. However, when more actively sought by interview techniques, delirium may be present in as many as 40% of patients undergoing valvular surgery (4, 8). Delirium usually begins 3 to 5 days after surgery and is first noted as an inappropriate remark or a more dramatic agitated outburst. The quiet or nonagitated version will often go undetected by the physician as the patient answers seemingly appropriate "Yes" or "No" to simple questions at the time of the daily hospital visit. Nursing staff or family will soon discover that the patient may be completely disoriented in all spheres, unable to recognize family and friends, and totally ignorant of the reasons for his or her hospitalization. In retrospect, patients may describe an illusion beginning with the hissing noise from an air conditioning vent or oxygen mask or other noises outside the room, which then develops into hallucinatory phenomena. On occasion, periods of lucidity alternate with disorientation, often at night or in the early morning hours. This condition may persist for 3 to 4 days. The occurrence of quiet delirium should occasion a brief neurologic examination but the extremely low yield of more costly and risky testing such as computed tomographic imaging, EEG, and lumbar puncture is of questionable value in this situation. Aside from the possibility of sedative, narcotic, or sleeping pill–induced drug reaction, the specific medical or psychiatric mechanism remains unknown and supportive therapy is indicated.

Agitated delirium is the variety that has been referred to in other situations as "CCU psychosis" or "postoperative psychosis." In agitated delirium, patients may exhibit emotional outbursts such as shouting or may attempt quitely but persistently to get out of bed and disconnect all tubes, catheters, etc. These patients have substantial risk of self-harm, and initial therapy should entail the use of soft restraints and antipsychotic sedation. Haloperidol 1 to 2 mg given intramuscularly every 4 hr has been extremely successful in initial control of this behavior. Many such patients spend 1 to 2 sleepless nights, but when sleep is finally achieved will awaken refreshed and recovered. As with quiet delirium, brief physical examination is indicated and review of all medications should be conducted; however, in contrast to quiet delirium in which sedatives are usually discontinued, this type of disorientation often requires sedative therapy. As with quiet delirium, recovery usually takes place in approximately 3 days, and no unusual consequences ensue. Patients may also manifest perceptual distortions, visual and auditory hallucinations, as well as paranoia and even acute paranoid schizophrenia, during certain periods of time (8). The occurrence of this syndrome has been linked to the performance of valvular surgery more than with coronary bypass, with which the incidence is reported to be much lower (16%) (9). Sleep deprivation, a protracted stay in the intensive care unit, excessive

FIGURE 26.1

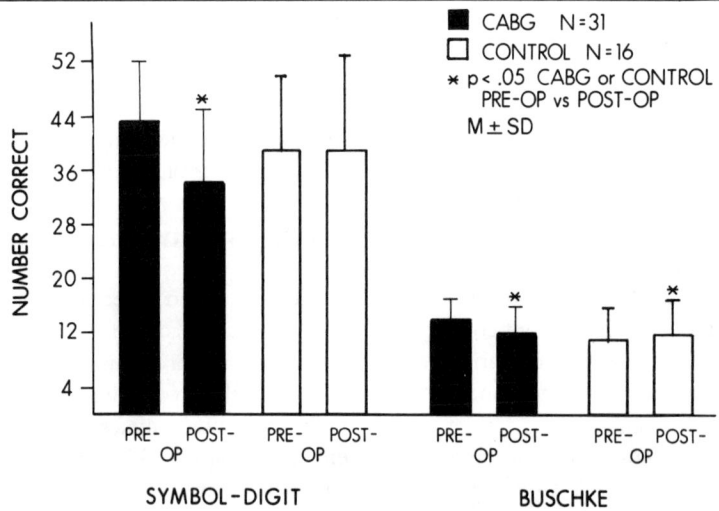

Symbol digit modalities—Buschke Word List test scores before and after surgery in 31 coronary bypass surgery patients and 16 general surgery control patients. (From Raymond M, Conklin C, Schaeffer J, et al: Coping with transient intellectual dysfunction after coronary bypass surgery. *Heart Lung* 13:531–539, 1984. Used with permission.)

FIGURE 26.2

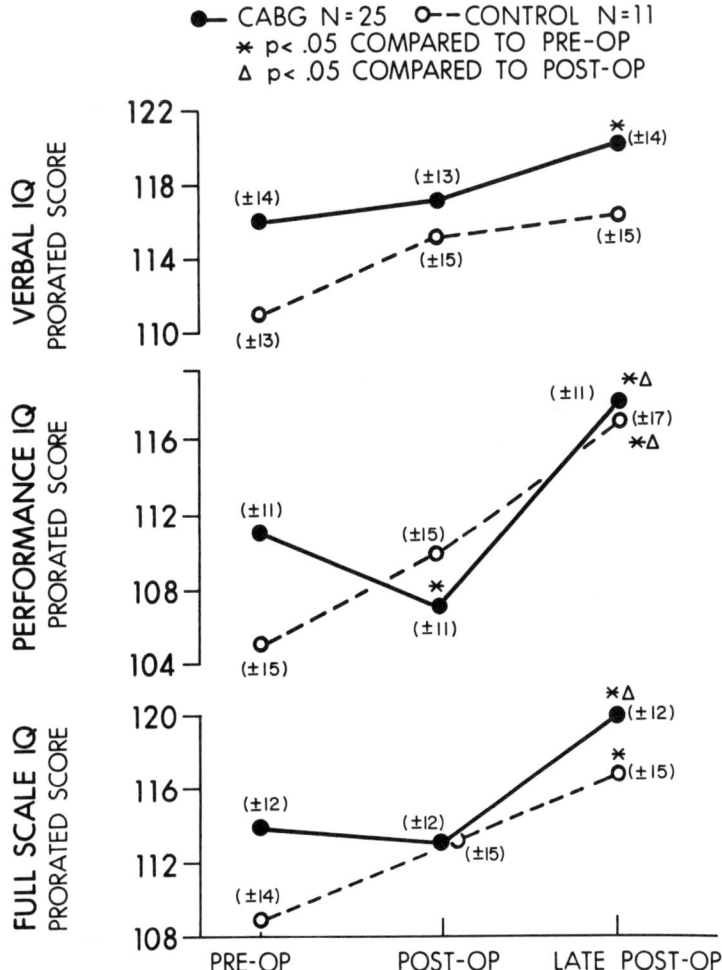

● — CABG N=25   ○ — — CONTROL N=11
* p< .05 COMPARED TO PRE-OP
Δ p< .05 COMPARED TO POST-OP

WAIS IQ scores 6 weeks after surgery in 25 coronary surgery and 11 general surgery patients. (From Raymond M, Conklin C, Schaeffer J, et al: Coping with transient intellectual dysfunction after coronary bypass surgery. *Heart Lung* 13:531–539, 1984. Used with permission.)

sensory input or lack thereof, and absence of orienting day and nighttime clues have also been blamed. Although advanced age may be a factor, neither the duration of anesthesia or cardiopulmonary bypass nor the presence of hypothermia is an important predisposing factor.

COGNITIVE DISTURBANCES

Abnormalities of intellect may be quite mild and consist of a brief retrograde amnesia for the days just preceding surgery, but more often patients will report substantial recent memory loss such as forgetting a friend's name or telephone number. Difficulty performing simple tasks of arithmetic such as balancing one's checkbook, and poor concentration span, resulting in frustration in reading a novel or watching television, are common. Poor coordination and judgment of distances and slow reaction time all make automobile driving dangerous. Formal testing has revealed transient abnormalities of performance-related IQ scores as measured by testing using the Wexler memory scale (10) or the Wexler adult intelligence scale (WAIS) (11). These changes are summarized in Figures 26.1 and 26.2.

Whether symptomatic or not, many patients are afflicted by a measurable decrease in cognitive skills, which usually affects memory and other nonlanguage visual-spatial relationships. Fortunately, follow-up testing indicates restitution of faculties, generally by 6 weeks, consistent with symptomatic reporting. The impact of these changes on hospital convalescence can be quite great, however, because a large amount of new information must be learned by the patient and his or her family. A comprehensive understanding of the surgical findings and possible implications for future prognosis, understanding of changes in diet, wound care, various medication regimens and their possible side effects, and other postoperative dos and don'ts all require extensive teaching. Unfortunately, limitations of memory and attention span often interfere with this process and necessitate inclusion of family and friends in teaching sessions and presentation of postoperative information repeatedly using a variety of audiovisual aids. It is most important to reassure the patient and family that intellectual shortcomings are common and fortunately temporary. Returning to work, especially work with heavy intellectual demands, should take these factors into consideration.

Discussion of mood changes after hospital discharge is included in Chapter 30.

References

1. Huang Ti: *Nei Ching Su Wen*, book 3, section 9. In Veith I (trans): *The Yellow Emperor's Classic of Internal Medicine.*

2. da Vinci L: *Dell' Anatomia*, foglia B. In MacCurdy E (trans): *The Notebooks of Leonardo da Vinci*, vol 1, chapter 3.

3. Boyd W: *Boyd's Pathology for the Surgeon*, ed 8 Anderson WA (ed). Philadelphia, WB Saunders, 1967.

4. Egerton N, Kay JH: Psychological disturbances associated with open-heart surgery. *Br J Psychiatry* 110:433–439, 1964.

5. Bryne D: The repression-sensitization scale: rationale, reliability and validity. *J Pers* 29:334–349, 1961.

6. Trager H, Flemming B, Nordmeyer J, et al: Psychological effects of preoperative doctor-patient communications. In Becker R (ed): *Psychopathological and Neurological Dysfunction Following Open-Heart Surgery.* New York, Springer-Verlag, 1982, pp 129–136.

7. Kimball CP, Quinlan D, Osborne F, et al: The experience of cardiac surgery. V. Psychological patterns and prediction of outcome. *Psychother Psychosom* 22:310–319, 1973.

8. Kornfeld DS: Psychiatric complications of open-heart surgery. *N Engl J Med* 273:287–292, 1965.

9. Rabiner CJ, Willner AE, Fishman J: Psychiatric complications following coronary bypass surgery. *J Nerv Ment Dis* 160:342–348, 1975.

10. Savageau JA, Stanton BA, Jenkins CD, et al: Neuropsychological dysfunction following elective cardiac operation. *J Thorac Cardiovasc Surg* 84:585–594, 1982.

11. Raymond M, Conklin C, Schaeffer J, et al: Coping with transient intellectual dysfunction after coronary bypass surgery. *Heart Lung* 13:531–539, 1984.

Chapter 27
NURSING CARE OF THE CARDIAC SURGICAL PATIENT

ROBERT E. LEE, R.N., M.S.N., C.C.R.N., C.N.A.
RACHEL RAMOS, R.N., M.S.N., C.C.R.N.

Nursing care of any particular group of patients varies from nurse to nurse, from patient to patient, and from one medical facility to another. Care of the cardiac surgery patient is no different. Institutional policy, type of patient, equipment, and available technology all play major roles in this variance.

This chapter includes discussions of planning for the patient, immediate admission of the patient from surgery to the intensive care unit (ICU), assessment, care planning using nursing diagnoses, and patient education and transfer planning prior to leaving the ICU.

PLANNING FOR THE PATIENT

Nursing care of the cardiac surgery patient starts several hours prior to the patient's arrival in the ICU. This includes preparing the environment for the patient and ensuring that all necessary supplies are available and that the equipment to be used is functioning properly.

The bed must have side rails with appropriate locks, a grounding plug that is secured, and properly functioning head, foot, height, Trendelenburg, and reverse Trendelenburg positions. The mattress is covered with material to prevent skin irritation and discomfort. An eggcrate mattress is commonly used for this purpose. To warm the patient after surgery, a hyperthermia blanket is placed on the bed. Attention must be given to protecting the patient from burns; therefore, it is recommended that a bath blanket and sheet cover the hyperthermia blanket. The bed is equipped with an intravenous pole, a cardiac monitor with cable and new lead wires (to prevent cross-contamination from previous patient use), an Ambu bag with reservoir and connecting tubing, and an oxygen tank.

The numerous supplies that will be needed during the postoperative course are placed in the room to allow the nurse to function most efficiently and stay in attendance with the patient. Essential items include lidocaine for both bolus and drip, syringes, needles, tape, nasogastric irrigation, antacid, potassium, sterile distilled water and saline, heparin, blood tubes, chest tube strippers, and chest tube clamps. Other supplies necessary will be dependent on the operative procedure performed and specific institutional practices.

The ICU is a highly technical area requiring the use of numerous pieces of equipment to meet the patient's various needs. The nurse must be trained in the use of all equipment. Periodic checks by the biomedical engineers are essential to ensure proper working condition. Equipment most commonly used in caring for the cardiac surgery patient includes a ventilator; hypo/hyperthermia machine; cardiac monitor with hemodynamic monitoring capabilities; transducers; nasogastric, chest, and tracheal suction; intravenous infusion pumps; and atrial and ventricular pacemakers. It is also necessary to have atrio-ventricular sequential pacemakers, overdrive pacemakers, and the equipment necessary to determine clotting times, hematocrit, and sodium and potassium levels. A defibrillator, crash cart, and sterile instruments and supplies needed to open the chest incision must be close at hand. Finally, a flow sheet that is both systematic and comprehensive is placed in the room for accurate and timely documentation by the nurse. The flow sheet is accessible to other health team members.

The decision as to which nurse will care for the patient is made by the nurse manager or charge nurse. This decision should be based on the experience and expertise of the nurse as well as the operative procedure and complications associated with it. The nurse who will care for the patient should be informed promptly in order to ready the room and prepare for the admission. Other nurses must also be informed so that they may provide assistance as necessary.

ADMISSION OF THE PATIENT TO THE ICU

After surgery the patient is admitted to the ICU or other recovery area. This is a systematic process requiring the nurse to be alert, prepared, and in control of the admission. The nursing focus is on patient safety and stability.

The patient arrives in the unit and is immediately placed on assisted ventilation. The nurse assesses for bilateral breath sounds and adequate aeration. Cardiac rhythm from the portable monitor and an initial blood pressure are determined. Connecting the arterial and other hemodynamic lines to transducers is essential but may be delegated to another nurse, an anesthesia technician, or other appropriately trained personnel. The bed is grounded, and

cardiac monitoring is changed from the portable battery-operated monitor to the room or wall-mounted monitor. Chest tubes, which are attached and secured to a drainage device, are checked and suction is applied as ordered.

Intravenous lines are checked for patency, and all infusions of medications (antiarrhythmics, vasopressors, etc.) should be quickly checked for accuracy of concentration and regulated on the infusion devices. The hyperthermia blanket is then connected. The Foley catheter is checked for patency, and accumulated volume and color of urine are noted. The next step is to obtain admission laboratory work, which usually includes complete blood count, electrolytes, blood urea nitrogen, creatinine, glucose, prothrombin time, and partial thromboplastin time. Cardiac enzymes may also be included.

Throughout this process, which routinely takes less than 15 min, the surgeon or anesthesiologist will give the nurse a brief patient history, discuss any problems encountered during the operative procedure that may affect postoperative care, and state any patient allergies.

Following the initial admission, a general assessment is performed. Heart rate and rhythm are determined. If premature ventricular contractions are noted secondary to bradycardia, atrial pacing is generally instituted. The type, rate, mode, milliamperes, and adjusted threshold are documented. The patient's general condition, status of dressings, placement and number of pacer wires (atrial and ventricular), peripheral pulses, heart sounds, verification of nasogastric tube placement, and regulation of intermittent suction are also checked. Restraints may also be applied to both wrists to prevent the patient from disturbing the various lines and tubes, which could potentially result in self-injury.

Hemodynamic lines, and the valuable parameters they measure, are frequently used in the cardiac surgery patient. Due to their importance, the authors have chosen to address the basic management of hemodynamic lines and transducers.

Hemodynamic Lines

Many patients will have a flow-directed catheter in place after open-heart surgery. These catheters, as well as intraarterial line catheters, are connected to electronic systems through transducers that will change the varying pressures sensed to varying electronic signals (1). To ensure accurate hemodynamic parameters, calibration of both the transducer and the amplifier is necessary. Various methods for calibration can be used; however, the simplest method is to use a mercury manometer. This procedure is explained in most critical care nursing texts. It is recommended that equipment be calibrated on a frequent, routine basis to ensure that accurate pressure measurements are being determined (2).

There are other important considerations when using hemodynamic lines: (a) the tubing used should be stiff and noncompliant, (b) tubing length should be 100 cm or less, and (c) a continuous flush device should be employed with a heparinized solution to prevent catheter occlusion (1). The heparinized solution should be placed in a pressurized device to maintain approximately 300 mm Hg pressure. This, along with the continuous flush device, will deliver 3 to 5 ml/hr of solution through the catheters.

The nurse must be aware of possible monitoring problems and complications when using hemodynamic monitoring. These include the following: (a) dampened pressure waveforms caused by clots, air bubbles, kinked catheters, and loose connections; (b) dislodgment or malposition of the catheter; (c) sepsis; (d) embolism; (e) arteriospasm; and (f) hemorrhage. If any of these problems or complications are noted, appropriate intervention should be initiated.

After ensuring proper calibration of transducers and amplifiers, complete hemodynamic parameters should be obtained. These include the pulmonary artery systolic, diastolic, and mean pressures; the right atrial pressure; and the pulmonary capillary wedge pressure. Cardiac output is then determined. Once again, depending on institutional practice, unit standards, or physician orders, the cardiac index, systemic vascular resistance, and stroke volume index will be calculated.

The cardiac index (CI) is the patient's cardiac output (CO) per square meter of body surface area (BSA) (3). To determine cardiac index, the cardiac output is divided by the BSA, which can be obtained using the Dubois Body Surface Chart. Normal range for CI is 2.5 to 3.5 liters/

min. Systemic vascular resistance (SVR) is the resistance against which the left ventricle must eject to force out its stroke volume with each beat (4). Also known as afterload, this can be determined by using the following formula: SVR = (MAP − RAP)/CO × 80, with MAP being the mean arterial pressure and RAP the right atrial pressure. Normal range is 800 to 1200 dynes/second/cm^{-5}. Stroke volume index (SVI) is the stroke volume (SV) adjusted for BSA. The formula is SVI = (CI)/HR × 1000, or SVI = SV/BSA, with HR being the patient's heart rate. Normal range for stroke volume index is 35 to 45 ml/beat/m^2.

After obtaining hemodynamic parameters and determining cardiac output, as well as other cardiac calculations, further general assessment can then take place. This should include determining actual urinary and chest tube drainage. The drainage is assessed for amount, color, and consistency. Ventilator settings are checked against the physician orders and documented. All medication infusions require review of the drug, fluid concentration, rate of infusion, and the location and integrity of the site. The hyperthermia device is regulated based on the patient's core temperature. Pupils are checked, and any responses of the patient to verbal or tactile stimuli are noted.

After completion of the general assessment, all findings must be documented. Documentation is essential, and a comprehensive flow sheet is needed for this purpose. A copy of the 24-hr intensive care flow sheet used at Cedars-Sinai Medical Center, Los Angeles, is shown in Figure 27.1.

Once the patient is stabilized, an electrocardiogram and upright portable chest x-ray are routinely performed. The family is then allowed to visit the patient. This provides the nurse the opportunity to meet the family, explain the various tubes and devices, discuss the patient's condition, and summarize the plan of care. This simple but often overlooked process is essential to allay the fears and anxiety of the family (5).

ASSESSMENT

General assessment criteria, as previously described, are necessary to obtain baseline information and ensure patient safety and stability. A

FIGURE 27.1

DATE: _____   RM. # _____

ALLERGIES		TIME →	0800 ↘	0900	1000		0700
ABBREVIATIONS:		240					
	A - Arterial Line	230					
		220					
	D - Dinamap	210					
		200					
	PA - Pulmonary Artery	190					
	Pressure	180					
		170					
	PCW - Pulmonary Capillary	160					
	Wedge Pressure	150					
		140					
H	RA - Right Atrial	130				→	
E	Pressure	120					
M		110					
O	CO - Cardiac Output	100					
D		90					
Y	ICP - Intra-Cranial	80					
N	Pressure	70					
A		60					
M	PVR - Pulmonary Vasc. Res.	50					
I		40					
C	CI - Cardiac Index	30					
		TEMP					
S	SVR - Systemic Vascular	EKG					
T	Resistance	HEART RATE					
A							
T	SVI - Stroke Volume	B/P S/D					
U	Index	B/P MEAN				→	
S							
	SVRI - Systemic Vascular	RA					
	Resistance Index	PA S/D					
	CVP - Central Venous	PCW					
	Pressure						
	ABP - Augmented B/P						
I							
V							
D						→	
R							
I							
P							
S							
M							
E							
D						→	
S							

24-hr ICU flow sheet. Also included in this chart are patient name, ID no., physician name, hospital admission date, hospital day no., diagnosis, operation, operation date, postoperation day no., age, BSA, weight, and blood type. Chart continues through 24 hr (*arrows*).

FIGURE 27.1   (Continued)

V		AIRWAY					
E		SOURCE/MODE					
N		F_1O_2 OR LPM					
T		R SET R RATE					
I		PEEP/PIP					
L		TIDAL VOL.					
A							
T							
O							
R							
B		TIME DRAWN				→	
L		SAMPLING SITE(S)					
O		pH					
O		PCO_2					
D		PO_2					
G		HCO_3					
A		O_2 SAT/O_2 CONT					
S							
I	BLOOD						
	PLASMA						
N	ORAL - PO						
T	NGT						
A	FLUSH						
K	CO - Cardiac					→	
E	Output						
	IV's						
		URINE					
	NGT - Nasogastric Tube	STOOL					
O	ICP - Drain						
U	SUMPS						
T	EMESIS						
P	CT - Chest Tubes					→	
U	PL - Pleural						
T	M - Mediastinal						
	P - Pericardial						
L		TIME DRAWN →					
A							
B							
R						→	
E							
S							
U							
L							
T							
S							
NURSE'S INITIALS ————————→							
SIGNATURE		SIGNATURE					

comprehensive, systematic assessment is now indicated. It should be conducted and documented within 2 hr of admission. The authors recommend a systems format using the American Association of Critical Care Nurses Process Standards (6). The cardiovascular, respiratory, neurologic, renal, gastrointestinal, and integumentary systems are included. Other important data can be obtained by reviewing the patient's previous medical history and medications, preoperative anxiety level, social support system, preoperative instructions, etc. The details of the assessment will vary among nurses and standards of practice adopted at various institutions. Therefore, the authors feel that listing comprehensive physical assessment criteria is beyond the scope of this chapter. However, it is important to remember that the data collected form the basis of the nursing process and allow for specific and individualized care planning.

CARE PLANNING

Critical care nursing incorporates independent, dependent, and interdependent functions in providing patient care and care planning. The authors advocate using a patient care plan that focuses on achieving established patient outcomes, *not* a nursing care plan that focuses on the nurse and nursing outcomes. The authors have found that the patient focus results in more comprehensive and less fragmented care, promotes multidisciplinary involvement, and limits the various documentation forms required to plan for the holistic needs of the patient. A copy of the patient plan of care used at Cedars-Sinai Medical Center is shown in Figure 27.2.

The nursing process is a problem-solving approach that consists of assessment, planning, implementation, and evaluation. Numerous problems or needs that are specific to the postoperative cardiac surgery patient can be identified. Once identified, all causative and contributing factors need to be examined. These factors verify whether the problem or need actually or potentially exists. An actual problem is clinically validated by identifiable defining characteristics, whereas a potential problem may

exist if certain nursing interventions are not determined and implemented (7).

To add to the body of nursing knowledge, promote clinical nursing research, and evaluate nursing interventions related to positive patient outcomes, the authors advocate the use of nursing diagnoses in care plan development. Nursing diagnoses, as defined by Gordon, are the actual or potential health problems that nurses, by virtue of their education and experience, are capable and licensed to treat (8).

The following is a brief case study of a cardiac surgery patient. Many nursing diagnoses are applicable to the cardiac surgery patient. Using the nursing process–patient plan of care format, several of the most frequently used nursing diagnoses are presented. The nursing diagnoses are taken from the accepted list by the North American Nursing Diagnosis Association (NANDA).

Mr. R.S., a 55-year-old Caucasian male, was admitted to the hospital because of increasing substernal chest pain. He was in a normal state of health until 3 weeks ago, when he noticed dull, substernal pain radiating to the left arm, accompanied by diaphoresis and shortness of breath. The pain was relieved by rest; however, he noticed the same incidence induced by low levels of exercise, extreme emotions, or heavy meals. Mr. R.S. was diagnosed as having unstable angina and underwent cardiac catheterization which showed triple vessel disease. He therefore underwent coronary artery bypass graft surgery.

Initial assessment on the patient's arrival in the intensive care unit showed that Mr. R.S. was in sinus bradycardia with a heart rate of 50 beats/min; blood pressure of 90/50; temperature 91°F; hemodynamic pressures of PA = 20/7, RA = 4, PCW = 7, CO = 3.01, CI = 1.87, SVR = 2500, SVI = 25. Heart sounds were regular S_1, S_2, without S_3, S_4, or murmurs. He had two atrial and two ventricular wires, as well as two mediastinal chest tubes that were connected to two underwater-seal drainage bottles with minimal drainage. He also had a radial arterial

FIGURE 27.2

PATIENT I.D.		CEDARS-SINAI MEDICAL CENTER

CEDARS-SINAI MEDICAL CENTER
PATIENT PLAN OF CARE

MEDICAL DIAGNOSIS

LONG TERM GOALS

NUTRITION CARE GOALS: "The Standard Nutrition Care Plan (No. 1) is automatically implemented for all patients given an enteral diet.
Refer to additional Nutritional Care Plan(s) No.(s) -

Discharge Planning Conference: OUTCOME

DATE:	NURSE'S INITIALS:

Date/Initials			Nursing Diagnosis/	Expected Outcomes	Interventions	Date/Initials	
Entry	Resolved	#	Etiological Factors			Update	DC'D

NAME	TITLE	INIT.	NAME	TITLE	INIT.	NAME	TITLE	INIT.	NAME	TITLE	INIT.	NAME	TITLE	INIT.

Form No. 3701-11 Rev. 5/87

Patient care plan. (Courtesy of Cedars-Sinai Medical Center, Los Angeles).

line and a five-lumen flow-directed catheter via the right internal jugular vein. All peripheral pulses were present but faint.

Mr. R.S. had an endotracheal tube that was connected to a ventilator. Breath sounds were equal, diminished in the bases, with scattered rhonchi. Arterial blood gas on 50% FiO_2 revealed pH = 7.30, PO_2 = 85, with 94% saturation, PCO_2 = 38, and $pHCO_3$ = 18.

His skin was cool, pale, and dry. He had a sternal dressing with minimal drainage and a right leg dressing with Act bandage. His abdomen was soft and nondistended, and bowel sounds were absent. A nasogastric tube was connected to low-intermittent suction. The Foley catheter was connected to gravity drainage, and urine output was 20 to 30 ml/hr.

Mr. R.S. was unresponsive to verbal and tactile stimuli. His pupils were equal, approximately 2 cm, and reacted sluggishly to light.

His wife and two sons were very anxious about his hospitalization, the outcome of surgery, and possible limitations imposed by his heart disease.

The following care plan was established.

Etiologic Factors, Nursing Diagnosis	Expected Outcomes	Interventions
1. Decreased cardiac output related to hypothermia, hypovolemia, arrhythmias.	Patient will maintain hemodynamic stability as demonstrated by CI ≥ 2.0, SVR = 800–1200, Temp = 97°F, Sinus rhythm = 60–100/min, SBP = 110–140.	1. Apply warming blankets until temperature is 96°F. 2. Place patient in Trendelenburg position, in case of severe hypotension. 3. Start atrial pacing for sinus bradycardia. 4. Administer volume (albumisol, blood or blood products) as ordered. 5. Correlate pharmacologic therapy with hemodynamic parameters. 6. Monitor chest tube drainage and note color, amount, fluctuation, and presence of clots. 7. Monitor hemodynamic parameters constantly. 8. Perform intraaortic balloon therapy as indicated.[a]
2. Impaired gas exchange related to tracheobronchial secretions, hypoventilation, atelectasis.	Patient will demonstrate adequate oxygenation and ventilation as evidenced by arterial blood gases: PO_2 ≥90, PCO_2 35 to 45. Lungs will be clear by auscultation and chest x-ray.	1. Establish and maintain patient airway by suctioning endotracheal tube as needed; bagging the patient with 100% oxygen before and after suctioning; turning every 1 to 2 hr as condition permits. 2. Monitor arterial blood gases[b]: a. 30 min after a change in ventilator settings;

[a]Intraaortic balloon pump (IABP) therapy is often required when the various interventions mentioned in the foregoing are not effective. The IABP is a circulatory assist device that utilizes the principle of counterpulsation by diastolic augmentation. The IABP catheter is a long, thin, multichambered or single-chambered catheter inserted through an artery (usually femoral) via a cutdown procedure or percutaneously. The catheter is inserted retrograde through the aorta until it lies in the descending thoracic aorta distal to the left subclavian artery.

The balloon catheter inflates during diastole by the rapid infusion of a gas (usually helium), raising the intraaortic pressure. The balloon is then rapidly deflated immediately prior to the next systole. During diastole, when the balloon is inflated, the diastolic pressure is augmented (increased), thus coronary artery perfusion is enhanced. During systole, when the balloon is deflated, cardiac output is increased by decreasing systemic vascular resistance or afterload, thus reducing myocardial oxygen consumption through decreased left ventricular workload (4).

The catheter is connected to an external pump device that triggers inflation and deflation of the balloon. This triggering device is in synchrony with the mechanical events of the heart—systole and diastole—which are determined from the patient's ECG.

The nurses' responsibilities in IABP management include the following interventions: (a) Maintain a stable ECG signal and intraarterial pressure tracing on the oscilloscope. (b) Keep the extremity with the balloon in straight alignment. (c) Maintain the head of the bed between 0 and 30° at all times. (d) Perform nerve and circulation checks of the extremity distal to the insertion site and compare to the other extremity. (e) Check balloon insertion site for bleeding, swelling, tenderness, and hematoma. (f) Keep IABP catheter visible at all times. (g) Assess pump device settings, e.g., mode, ratio, balloon volume, and inflation-deflation timing. (h) Assess catheter for moisture, kinks, and cracks. (i) Check arterial pressure tracing for appropriate diastolic augmentation. (j) Turn patient every 2 hr, side to side, to prevent respiratory or integumentary complications. (k) Obtain platelet, hematocrit, partial thromboplastin time (PTT), and prothrombin time (PT) as ordered. (l) Educate patient and family regarding the use of IABP therapy and the plan of care.

[b]Arterial blood gas protocol used in the cardiac surgery ICU at Cedars-Sinai Medical Center, Los Angeles.

Etiologic Factors, Nursing Diagnosis	Expected Outcomes	Interventions
		b. after an increase in respiratory rate of eight breaths or more from previous rate unrelated to activity;
		c. in the presence of extreme restlessness, confusion, or lethargy;
		d. if nasal flaring is noted;
		e. in the presence of adventitious breath sounds not previously noted;
		f. if cyanosis of skin, mucous membranes, or nail beds unrelated to previous assessment is noted;
		g. when there are no audible breath sounds in either right or left lung fields.
		3. Perform portable upright chest x-ray every morning and as ordered.
3. Ineffective family coping related to knowledge deficit— outcome of surgery, heart disease.	Family will verbalize fears and anxieties. Family will participate in care measures as determined with the nurse and will work independently with the health team.	1. Encourage family to verbalize fears, anxieties, previous experiences with illness, coping mechanisms used and their effectiveness.
		2. Orient family to the ICU environment and routine procedures.
		3. Keep family informed of patient's status and progress.
		4. Include the family in care measures when appropriate.
		5. Refer to available support services.
4. Impaired verbal communication related to intubation.	Patient will use nonverbal techniques of communication to express his or her needs. Patient will cooperate with the plan of care.	1. Assess patient's orientation and ability to hear, read, write, and use primary language.
		2. Use nonverbal communication techniques, such as hand signals, head nods, paper and pencil, etc.
		3. Anticipate common needs, such as pain relief, need to urinate, drink, change position, etc.

Etiologic Factors, Nursing Diagnosis	Expected Outcomes	Interventions
		4. If language barrier exists, use family members or translator to provide phonetically spelled words in native language.
		5. Inform patient of his or her condition and progress, procedures, and plan of care.
		6. Explain that the inability to talk is temporary.
5. Alteration in comfort: pain related to surgical incision, knowledge deficit regarding proper coughing and deep breathing.	Patient will acknowledge absence or decrease of pain. Patient will demonstrate effective use of noninvasive relief measures.	1. Assess the location, intensity, duration, and activity associated with pain.
		2. Determine patient's beliefs and implications of pain psychologically and culturally.
		3. Explain all procedures and possible associated discomfort prior to implementation.
		4. Encourage patient input into care measures.
		5. Provide pain medication as ordered.
		6. Educate patient and family regarding: a. proper coughing, deep breathing, use of pillow to support the chest when coughing or turning; b. noninvasive relief measures such as relaxation techniques, massage, guided imagery; c. expected course of pain from the surgery.
		7. Evaluate patient's response to pain relief measures.
6. Ineffective airway clearance related to intubation, weakness, presence of tracheo-bronchial secretions, improper coughing and deep breathing technique, pain.	Patient will demonstrate effective coughing, deep breathing, and use of incentive devices. Patient's lungs will be clear on auscultation and chest x-ray.	1. If intubated, ensure patient readiness for extubation: hematocrit >26%, O_2 saturation >95% on FiO_2 of 0.4 positive end-expiratory pressure (PEEP) no greater than 5 cm, pH and PCO_2 within normal limits; patient is awake, alert, follows commands, can lift head off the pillow and take deep breaths independent of ventilatory support.

Etiologic Factors, Nursing Diagnosis	Expected Outcomes	Interventions
		2. Maintain patent airway by suctioning, proper positioning, providing adequate hydration.
		3. Demonstrate proper coughing, deep breathing, and use of support devices (e.g., cough pillow).
		4. Provide adequate rest periods between various nursing care measures.
		5. Medicate for pain prior to pulmonary toilet.
		6. Encourage movement and ambulation as conditions permits.
7. Potential for infection related to surgical incision, presence of indwelling lines: intravenous, intraarterial and flow-directed catheters, chest tubes, Foley catheter.	Patient will demonstrate no signs and symptoms of infection as evidenced by the surgical incisions, temperature 99°F or less, white blood count, 14,000 or less.	1. Use aseptic technique in changing dressings and handling invasive lines.
		2. Observe incisions for signs of infection: redness, swelling, tenderness, presence of abnormal drainage.
		3. Monitor temperature every 4 hr and as necessary.
		4. Monitor for elevated white blood count.
		5. Obtain cultures of the wound as ordered.
		6. Administer antibiotics as ordered.
		7. Educate patient and family regarding:
		a. proper care of the surgical incisions;
		b. proper hand-washing technique;
		c. signs and symptoms of infection.
8. Potential for fluid volume deficit: bleeding related to altered clotting factors (inadequate reversal of heparin effect postpump), rupture of graft anastomosing sites.	Patient will demonstrate no signs of bleeding as evidenced by normal clotting factors, hematocrit levels within acceptable limits, and minimal chest tube drainage.	1. Monitor clotting parameters (PT, PTT, platelet count, etc.) and hematocrit.
		2. Monitor chest drainage every hour and as necessary.
		a. Note color, consistency, and amount of drainage.
		b. Maintain patency by milking or stripping chest tubes as necessary.

Etiologic Factors, Nursing Diagnosis	Expected Outcomes	Interventions
		c. Apply thoracic suction to chest tubes as ordered.
		d. Turn patient from side to side every 1 to 2 hr to promote drainage as condition permits.
		e. Tape chest tubes and drainage tubing connection sites.
		3. Monitor and record intake and output.
		4. Administer blood or blood products or heparin antidote (protamine sulfate) as ordered.
		5. Apply pressure dressings over bleeding areas.
		6. Prevent elevation of blood pressure that may rupture graft anastomosis by sedating patient and titrating vasopressor agents.
		7. Implement autotransfusion device as ordered.
9. Potential for injury related to altered sensorimotor function secondary to anesthesia or sedation; postoperative cardiovascular accident.	Patient will show no evidence of physical injury.	1. Assess neuromuscular function every hour until stable.
		2. Apply body or wrist restraints for safety.
		3. Keep indwelling lines secured and away from patient's reach.
		4. Maintain bed at its lowest position with side rails up at all times.
		5. Maintain soft, indirect lighting in room.
10. Anxiety related to the ICU environment, hospitalization, and the outcome of surgery.	Patient will verbalize anxieties and fears. Patient will participate in the plan of care.	1. Encourage patient to verbalize fears and anxieties.
		2. Give clear, concise explanations of care and procedures. Repeat explanations as necessary.
		3. Inform patient regarding status and progress of his or her condition.
		4. Allow family members to assist in supporting the patient.
		5. Encourage patient to participate in decision making and care measures as condition permits.

IMPLEMENTATION

When caring for the cardiac surgery patient, the nurse prioritizes the patients' problems. Those related to the circulatory and respiratory systems—such as decreased cardiac output, impaired gas exchange, and ineffective airway clearance—are most important, and interventions are initiated immediately. As the patient wakes up from anesthesia, interventions related to psychological needs, such as anxiety and coping, are implemented. Problems that are not present but may occur, such as potential for infection or injury, are also considered. With potential problems, nursing activities are preventive in nature (7).

The interventions or plan of actions identified by the nurse during the planning phase of the nursing process are organized to accomplish the expected patient outcomes. These activities are aimed at reducing, preventing, or eliminating the causative or contributing factors that affect the altered state of the patient. Input, as available, from the patient and significant others is incorporated in the plan. This encourages the patient and significant others to participate in the process. It also places responsibility on the patient to perform some self-care activities as his or her condition permits.

EVALUATION

The effectiveness of both nursing and patient activities is evaluated using the expected outcomes previously determined during the planning phase. Evaluation is an ongoing process. It indicates whether the established nursing diagnoses were correct and whether the plan of actions was effective and efficient in meeting the desired patient outcomes. Interventions may then be modified based on the evaluation and as the patient's condition changes. The patient is encouraged and educated to perform more activities—from further decision making to actual physical care measures within the physiologic limits of the condition. Once the expected outcomes are achieved and no instruction or health promotion is required from the nurse, the problem is resolved.

For example, the problem of impaired verbal communication related to intubation is resolved once the patient is extubated. Interventions associated with ineffective airway clearance, such as suctioning the endotracheal tube, no longer apply. However, the problem of ineffective airway clearance may still exist. It now becomes the nurse's responsibility to teach, assist, and encourage the patient in proper coughing and deep breathing techniques.

PATIENT EDUCATION AND TRANSFER PLANNING

Patient education is an ongoing process that begins once the patient is alert and continues throughout the hospitalization. Each encounter with the patient is a teaching-learning process, whether it be a defined strategy or offering information on his or her current status (9). Using Guzzetta's model for integrating education and the nursing process, patient education may occur in relation to one or all of the nursing diagnoses (9). Once the patient's condition is stable, the nursing care emphasis moves from meeting the physiologic needs of the patient to teaching information and skills the patient requires to participate in, achieve, and maintain self-care. This occurs most frequently during a "weaning" process in the intensive care unit when tubes, lines, and equipment are removed from the patient and the patient is informed of his or her ongoing progress (9). Following this, patients are prepared for what to expect when transferring from the intensive care unit to the step-down unit.

At this point in the intensive care stay, the patient is instructed to continue the various skills he or she has been performing. These skills may include coughing, deep breathing exercises, use of any incentive respiratory devices, range-of-motion exercises, and ambulation within the limits of the condition. Signs and symptoms the patient should report to the nurse are stressed to both the patient and the family so as to detect and prevent possible complications. To ensure continuity of care, the importance of documenting the educational process and the patient-family responses cannot be overemphasized.

When the patient transfers to new surroundings, it is necessary that the nurse ensure patient comfort and instruct the patient as to the bed operations, telemetry monitoring, nurse call system, etc. There is a trusting relationship between patient, family, and nurse, and the intensive care nurse may make the patient and family aware that he or she is available if they have questions or concerns. Finally, the nurse must update the plan of care and provide a comprehensive report to the nurse accepting responsibility for the patient. This should include a brief history, current patient problems and needs, progress toward achieving the desired expected outcomes, and further support and education the patient and family may require.

SUMMARY

Nursing care of the cardiac surgery patient is a difficult and challenging process. For patients to achieve positive outcomes, the nurse must be well aware of the dynamic nature of the intensive care environment, the patient as a holistic entity, and his or her own intellectual and cognitive abilities. This chapter has pro-

vided an overview of the nursing management of the cardiac surgery patient.

References

1. *Guide to Physiological Pressure Monitoring.* Waltham, MA, Hewlett-Packard Co., 1977, pp 5–12.
2. Schroeder J, Daily E: *Techniques in Bedside Hemodynamic Monitoring.* St Louis, CV Mosby, 1976, pp 54, 55.
3. Millar S, Sampson L, Soukup M (eds): *AACN Procedure Manual for Critical Care.* Philadelphia, WB Saunders, 1985, p 68.
4. Quall S: *Comprehensive Intra-aortic Balloon Pumping.* St. Louis, CV Mosby, 1984, pp 85, 202–204.
5. Rodgers C: Needs of relatives of cardiac surgery patients during the critical care phase. *Focus on Critical Care* 10:50–55, 1983.
6. Thierer J, Perhus S, McCracken ML, et al (eds): *AACN Standards for Nursing Care of the Critically Ill.* Reston, VA, Reston Publishing, 1981, pp 55–104.
7. Carpenito LJ: *Nursing Diagnosis Application to Clinical Practice.* Philadelphia, JB Lippincott, 1983, p 20.
8. Gordon M: Nursing diagnosis and the diagnostic process. *Am J Nursing* 76:1299, 1976.
9. Guzzetta CE: Can critically ill patients be taught? In Billie DA (ed): *Practical Approaches to Patient Teaching.* Boston, Little, Brown, 1981, pp 258–267.

Section 5
THE INTERMEDIATE PHASE:
LEAVING THE HOSPITAL

Chapter 28
PATIENT EDUCATION PROGRAMS

VIRGINIA RURYCZ, R.N.

The primary goals of postoperative teaching are (a) to increase knowledge of and compliance with health-promoting behavior and (b) to provide opportunities for patients and their families to ask specific questions about matters pertaining to the recovery period as an important basis for anxiety reduction. Additionally, those aspects of preoperative teaching that remain relevant during the postoperative period should be continued.

To accommodate the postoperative cognitive and psychological changes, multiple teaching methods are needed. Lectures, slide and sound presentations, handouts, and both individual and group teaching for patients and their families are supplemented with demonstrations of how the heart works. What was done during surgery is explained using heart models and examples of prosthetic valves, Dacron grafts, pacemakers, and implantable defibrillation patches as appropriate, and other items that may have been used in surgery or may have been placed in the patient.

At our institution, classes are divided into the following five major categories, a different one of which is taught each day of the week. These topics form the basis for the organization of this chapter.

1. Nutrition
2. Stress Management
3. Discharge Instructions
4. Coping after Heart Surgery
5. Topics of Special Interest

Liaison nurses conduct the classes in groups and individually, with the aid of dieticians, social workers, and psychologists.

As part of his or her postoperative teaching, each patient is given a copy of a locally prepared booklet entitled "Heart to Heart" (1). In this chapter we have reproduced sections of that booklet. This chapter focuses on highlights and guidelines that we follow or present in our postoperative teaching.

Since knowledge retention is limited during the acute phase (2), the patient is encouraged to return following hospital discharge to repeat some if not all of the classes. When the patient returns for his or her 6-week postoperative visit, the liaison nurse uses this opportunity to review risk factor modification and determine compliance with the diet, physical exercise, weight control, stress management, and medication recommendations.

NUTRITION

Because of the relationship between diet and coronary artery disease, proper eating habits are discussed before admission to the hospital. While in the hospital the diet is controlled, and it is at this time that we place great emphasis on making diet and eating habits compatible with the patient's life-style and the needs of a healthy heart. We use American Heart Association guidelines emphasizing calorie-controlled, nutritionally balanced menus that are low in fat, cholesterol, and sodium.

Patients (and family members) are taught about the nutritional content of foods, which to avoid, which to emphasize, and how to plan menus and eat appropriately but well. As needed, we recommend behavioral training programs on eating. The level of detail should not only deal with what foods to eat, but also instruct in such matters as food preparation and cooking.

Thus, fatty meats (salami, sausage, etc.) as well as marbled red meats (prime rib, brisket, short ribs, etc.) are to be avoided, as well as whole milk, cheeses made from whole milk, and organ meats. Butter and animal fats are strictly forbidden, and eggs are to be minimized, if not eliminated. The relationship of dietary fats and cholesterol and the risk associated with elevated serum cholesterol, and the difference between high- and low-density lipoproteins (HDL and LDL) should be explained.

Patients are also taught that certain fats do not lead to higher cholesterol. Polyunsaturated fats, as are found in safflower or corn oil and fish oils, have this property. Also, monosaturated fats are helpful in lowering cholesterol or LDL. Olive and peanut oils are major sources of this type of fat.

The importance of complex carbohydrates such as in cereals, rice, grains, and pasta is taught. We emphasize the merit of eating fresh fruits and vegetables and how to look out for the unexpected, such as excessive salt or sodium concentration in packaged foods.

The nutritional guidelines we suggest are those of the original American Heart Association prudent diet (3). They include:

1. Reduce fat to approximately 30% of total caloric intake. Less than one-third of this is to be from saturated fats, up to one-third from polyunsaturated fats, and the remainder from monosaturated fats. Patients also need to understand that fatty foods have a much higher concentration of calories than do other foods.

2. Reduce cholesterol intake to no more than 300 mg per day.

3. Increase the total amount of complex carbohydrates in the diet to approximately 55% of the total calories.

4. Reduce sodium intake preferably to 2 gm per day, but not more than 3 gm per day.

5. Achieve or maintain appropriate body weight through proper calorie intake.

To ensure that patients and their families understand the nutritional guidelines, a dietician should meet with the patients and *all* available family members. All family members are encouraged not only to participate insofar as the patient's diet is concerned, but, to the extent feasible, to adopt similar eating habits.

Special Nutritional Problems

Patients and their families are often concerned with special nutritional problems such as eating out, buying packaged foods, and problems associated with following recipes while cooking at home.

Eating in restaurants presents no special problems as long as the patient uses reasonable judgment. Many restaurants will honor requests for low sodium (or no MSG), margarine instead of butter, and similar requests. Other useful hints include having fruit for desert, eating potatoes without sour cream or butter, ordering salad dressing on the side, and avoiding fried foods. One economical hint is to order an appetizer in lieu of an entree. Many restaurants have fat and cholesterol controlled menu items such as those included in the American Heart Association Dine to Your Heart's Content program.

Packaged foods are less problematic now that labels must list all ingredients. Patients should be urged to read and understand labels based on the fact that ingredients are listed in order of prevalence. They also must learn that labeling may indicate the presence of three or four different forms of sodium.

Since most patients eat the majority of their meals at home, educational effects should focus on proper menu planning, cooking methods, and ingredient substitution or recipe modification. Patients (and others in the family who may do the cooking) can be taught ways to substitute ingredients and still provide tasty and nutritious dishes. Some examples are the use of the lowfat yogurt instead of sour cream, margarine instead of butter, ricotta instead of cream cheese, nonstick sprays for frying, egg substitutes, etc. We also advise patients to be on the lookout for such items as lard, hydrogenated vegetable shortening, coconut or palm oils, and other disguises for unwanted saturated fats. The use of a prepared shopping list is recommended to minimize unwise impulse buying.

Sample menus are provided to encourage patients and their families to plan properly and to indicate the wide variety of foods still available to them. Figure 28.1 is an example of a daily menu used at Cedars-Sinai Medical Center and indicates the variety of foods that may be selected for the meals in one day.

STRESS MANAGEMENT

Stress is a part of our everyday lives and is considered by some to be a leading factor in coronary artery disease. Chronic stress has been implicated in adrenergic effects which are cumulative in nature (4). The potential long-term effect is to vitiate the body's immune reaction and thus increase susceptibility to disease processes.

In the stress management class, patients should be taught to understand the signs of stress and ways to manage it. They should also be taught to differentiate between mild stress that does not produce substantial anxiety or adrenergic effect (and which may in fact be productive) and the more devastating and destructive stress.

Stress reactions manifest themselves in different ways. A given individual may display any one or more of the following signs: tachycardia, hypertension, headache, shallow breathing, perspiration, and emotional reactions such as anxiety, fright, anger, and inappropriate frustration, to mention but a few of the more common reactions. The important thing to learn is how to recognize the stress reactions in oneself and what to do to reduce or control the stress, if not eliminate it altogether.

Patients can be taught to ascertain if their

reactions to stress are beneficial or detrimental. The goal is to teach the patient how to eliminate the detrimental reactions and substitute for them reactions that tend to reduce stress but are health-promoting and beneficial. For example, if the reaction to stress is to eat or to smoke (two common detrimental reactions), a healthier response would be to substitute exercise for the detrimental response.

Many patients will have "type A" personalities (5) and may tend to take on too much within a limited time frame. They are taught to schedule better, to ask for help, and, perhaps most important, to learn how to say no. Patients are taught to balance work and play or leisure activities and to emphasize the importance of hobbies and recreation, but predominantly those that are relaxing and enjoyable. Our patients are told that not only do they deserve free time each day, they need it.

Stress management teaching should include the role of rest, sleep, and relaxation in managing stress; how to use leisure time activities to reduce stress; the interrelationship between exercise or physical activity and heart and lung capacity; learning to accept things you cannot change or over which you have no control; and the value of talking about problems and not holding them in. One can increase frustration tolerance by learning to "let go" of anger, hostility, and similar feelings.

A psychologist is available as a consultant in connection with stress management or will make recommendations for further follow-up when it seems warranted.

At the completion of the stress management class relaxation exercises are presented, using various techniques such as breathing control, focusing, and imagery. Patients sit erect with their feet flat on the floor, hands in their laps, and eyes closed. They then inhale deeply through the nose counting slowly to four, and then exhale through the nose. This is repeated for 10 min, during which patients are asked to focus on their breathing and counting. As they continue to breathe slowly they are asked to imagine the air flowing through their bodies bringing warmth, energy, and releasing muscle tightness. At the completion of the 10 min patients slowly open their eyes and remain seated and relaxed

FIGURE 28.1

Breakfast

Name _____ Room _____

SU	MO	TU	WE	TH	FR	SA

PLEASE CIRCLE SELECTIONS

CHOLESTEROL/FAT CONTROLLED MENU
THE LOW CHOLESTEROL DIET ALLOWS 1 EGG ON TUESDAY AND THURSDAY

Fruits & Juices
_Orange Juice
_Grapefruit Juice
_Apple Juice
_Cranberry Juice
_Prune Juice
_LS Vegetable Juice
_Grapefruit Sections
_Stewed Prunes
_Seasonal Fresh Fruit
_Applesauce
_Ripe Banana

Cereals
_Creamed Wheat
_Oatmeal
_Whole Grain Cereal
_Cheerios
_Rice Krispies
_Puffed Wheat
_Cornflakes
_Bran Flakes
_Shredded Wheat
_All Bran*
_2 TB Bran

Beverages
_4 oz Nonfat Milk
_4 oz Lowfat Milk
_8 oz Lowfat Milk
_Nonfat Choc. Milk
_Hot Chocolate(nonfat)
_4 oz NonDairy Creamer
_Decaf Coffee
_Coffee Creamer
_Coffee
_Herb Tea/Lemon
_Tea/Lemon

Entrees
_Low Chol Omelette
_Scrambled Egg
_Soft Cooked Egg
_Hard Cooked Egg
_Mozzarella Cheese
_LF Cottage Cheese

Breakfast Breads
_Bagel
_Sourdough Roll
_Wheat Bread
_White Bread
_Rye Bread
_Reg Crackers
_LS Wheat Crackers
_Melba Toast
_Matzo

Condiments
_Sweet Margarine
_Jelly
_Jam
_Honey
_Pepper
_Sugar Sub

LS = LOW SODIUM
LF = LOW FAT
* = HIGHER IN SODIUM (more than 500 mg/serving)

Moist Towelette

If you have not received what you circled or have any other food service concerns, please call the Food & Nutrition Hot Line, x4444.
REV. 1/88

F

Lunch

Name _____ Room _____

SU	MO	TU	WE	TH	FR	SA

PLEASE CIRCLE SELECTIONS

CHOLESTEROL/FAT CONTROLLED MENU

Appetizers
_Cranberry Juice
_Orange Juice
_Grapefruit Juice
_Apple Juice
_Apricot Nectar
_LS Vegetable Juice
_LS Tomato Soup
_LS Vegetable Soup
_LS Chicken Broth

Salads/Side Dishes
_Tossed Salad
_Lettuce & Sl Tomato
_Cole Slaw
_Sliced Turkey
_LF Cottage Cheese
_Mozzarella Cheese
_LS Tuna Salad Cup

Dressings/Spreads
_Diet Italian Dressing
_Diet French Dressing
_Italian Dressing
_French Dressing
_1000 Isle Dressing
_Catsup
_Mustard
_Lite Mayonnaise

Breads
_Sourdough Roll
_Dinner Roll
_Wheat Bread
_White Bread
_Rye Bread
_Reg Crackers
_LS Wheat Crackers
_Melba Toast
_Matzo

Condiments
_Sweet Margarine
_Jelly
_Cranberry Sauce
_Lemon
_Vinegar
_Pepper
_Sugar Sub

Beverages
_4 oz Nonfat Milk
_4 oz Lowfat Milk
_8 oz Lowfat Milk
_Nonfat Chocolate Milk
_Lemonade
_Decaf Coffee
_Coffee Creamer
_Coffee
_Herb Tea/Lemon
_Tea/Lemon
_Iced Tea/Lemon
_Reg / _Diet Lemon-Lime
_Reg / _Diet Cola

Entrees (Choose 1)
_Baked Dark Meat Chicken
_Baked Orange Roughy
_Lean Roast Beef & Gravy
_Cornish Hen
_Broiled Chicken Breast
_Broiled Halibut/Lemon
_Baked Turkey
_Chicken Stew
_LS Turkey Sandwich with Lettuce & Tomato
_Seafood Pasta Salad*
_Cottage Cheese & Fresh Fruit Platter

_Brown Gravy*
_LS Brown Gravy

Vegetables
_Rice
_Baked Potato
_Duchess Potatoes
_Pilaf
_Green Peas
_Mashed Winter Squash
_Corn
_LS Stewed Tomatoes
_Green Beans
_Carrots
_Chopped Spinach

Desserts
_Applesauce
_Pears
_Grapefruit Sections
_Fruit Cup
_Seasonal Fresh Fruit
_Orange Wedges
_Fresh Apple
_Fruited Yogurt
_Flavored Gelatin
_Fruited Gelatin
_Angel Food Cake
_Fruit Ice
_Vanilla Wafers
_Graham Crackers
_Baked Apple Dessert

LS = LOW SODIUM
LF = LOW FAT
* = HIGHER IN SODIUM (more than 500 mg per serving)

Moist Towelette

If you have not received what you circled or have any other food service concerns, please call the Food & Nutrition Hot Line, x4444.

F

Sample daily menus for cholesterol and fat controlled diet. (Courtesy of Food and Nutrition Services, Cedars-Sinai Medical Center, Los Angeles, CA.)

FIGURE 28.1 (Continued)

Dinner

Name _____ Room _____

| SU | MO | TU | WE | TH | FR | SA |

PLEASE CIRCLE SELECTIONS

CHOLESTEROL/FAT CONTROLLED MENU

Appetizers
_Cranberry Juice
_Orange Juice
_Grapefruit Juice
_Apricot Nectar
_LS Vegetable Juice
_LS Tomato Soup
_LS Vegetable Soup
_LS Chicken Broth

Salads/Side Dishes
_Tossed Salad
_Lettuce & Sl Tomato
_Cole Slaw
_Small Vegetable Salad
_Sliced Turkey
_LF Cottage Cheese
_Mozzarella Cheese
_LS Tuna Salad Cup

Dressings/Spreads
_Diet Italian Dressing
_Diet French Dressing
_Italian Dressing
_French Dressing
_1000 Isle Dressing
_Catsup
_Mustard
_Lite Mayonnaise

Breads
_Sourdough Roll
_Dinner Roll
_Wheat Bread
_White Bread
_Rye Bread
_Reg Crackers
_LS Wheat Crackers
_Melba Toast
_Matzo

Condiments
_Sweet Margarine
_Jelly
_Cranberry Sauce
_Lemon
_Vinegar
_Pepper
_Sugar Sub

Beverages
_4 oz Nonfat Milk
_4 oz Lowfat Milk
_8 oz Lowfat Milk
_Nonfat Chocolate Milk
_Lemonade
_Decaf Coffee
_Coffee Creamer
_Coffee
_Herb Tea/Lemon
_Tea/Lemon
_Iced Tea/Lemon
_Reg / _Diet Lemon-Lime
_Reg / _Diet Cola

Entrees (Choose 1)
_Baked Orange Roughy
_Broiled Chicken Breast
_Lean Roast Beef & Gravy
_Baked Dark Meat Chicken
_Cornish Hen
_Broiled Halibut/Lemon
_Baked Turkey
_Chicken Stew
_LS Turkey Sandwich with
  Lettuce & Tomato
_Seafood Pasta Salad*
_Cottage Cheese & Fresh
  Fruit Platter

_Brown Gravy*
_LS Brown Gravy

Vegetables
_Rice
_Baked Potato
_Duchess Potatoes
_Pilaf
_Green Peas
_Mashed Winter Squash
_Corn
_LS Stewed Tomatoes
_Green Beans
_Carrots
_Chopped Spinach

Desserts
_Applesauce
_Pears
_Grapefruit Sections
_Fruit Cup
_Seasonal Fresh Fruit
_Orange Wedges
_Fruit Cup
_Seasonal Fresh Fruit
_Orange Wedges
_Fresh Apple
_Fruited Yogurt
_Flavored Gelatin
_Fruited Gelatin
_Angel Food Cake
_Fruit Ice
_Vanilla Wafers
_Graham Crackers
_Baked Apple Dessert

LS = LOW SODIUM
LF = LOW FAT
* = HIGHER IN SODIUM (more
      than 500 mg per serving)

Moist Towelette

If you have not received what you circled or have any other food service concerns, please call the Food & Nutrition Hot Line, x4444.

F

Night Snack

Name _____ Room _____

| SU | MO | TU | WE | TH | FR | SA |

PLEASE CIRCLE SELECTIONS

CHOLESTEROL/FAT CONTROLLED MENU

Providing your diet allows, night food service
will be delivered to you by 8:30 PM.

Kitchen closes at 8:45 PM

Please check selections below.
Limit choices to two (2) items.

_Mozzarella Cheese
_Melba Toast
_Cornflakes (order milk)
_LS Cornflakes (order milk)
_Diet Flavored Gelatin
_Applesauce
_Fresh Apple
_Fruit Ice
_Graham Crackers

_Orange Juice
_Grapefruit Juice
_Prune Juice
_4 oz Nonfat Milk
_4 oz Lowfat Milk

LS = LOW SODIUM
LF = LOW FAT
* = HIGHER IN SODIUM (more
      than 500 mg per serving)

Moist Towelette

If you have not received what you circled or have any other food service concerns, please call the Food & Nutrition Hot Line, x4444.

F

for a few more minutes. As described by Lazarus and Folkman, this helps to teach that "as we learn to relax and take time to improve our health, we begin to feel better about ourselves in ways that help us deal with stress" (6).

DISCHARGE INSTRUCTIONS

In one sense, almost all postoperative teaching may be viewed as part of discharge instructions. As used here, however, this class refers to those aspects of instruction given to cover the period directly after the patient leaves the hospital. Included here are scheduling follow-up visits, medications, prevention of incision infection, as well as activities in which the patient should or should not engage. Since exercise and activities are so intimately related, exercise instructions are also discussed at this time, noting that it is also discussed as a part of stress management. Figure 28.2 illustrates the Discharge Instructions checklist that is used at Cedars-Sinai Medical Center.

Surgical Healing

The following information is discussed in class and is given as part of the Heart to Heart booklet. Not all aspects of the booklet apply to all patients; that is, unless the patient has had a valve replacement, those pages that deal with infection in the valve replacement patient are not applicable (and in fact are removed from the patient's copy of the booklet). Patients are informed that the chest incision goes through the skin, muscle, and bone, and that the skin and muscle are the first to heal, often by the time the patient is discharged from the hospital. The sternum takes much longer to heal (12 weeks) and pain or discomfort is common when coughing, sneezing, burping, or turning in bed. Patients are told that any Steri-Strips used after suture removal will likely fall off in the shower, but if this has not happened by the 3rd day they should simply be removed. The fact that, for bypass surgery, the saphenous vein was removed and used to make the bypasses is discussed. This may result in swelling of the leg and often a burning or tingling sensation. Patients are taught to elevate the leg when not walking,

and not to sit with the legs crossed at the knee or ankle. The special chest discomfort associated with use of the internal mammary artery is also discussed.

Activities and Exercise

Table 28.1, adapted from our Heart to Heart booklet, presents a summary of the information given to our patients concerning the activities they may or may not engage in directly after discharge from the hospital and when they may start a given activity.

Depending on such factors as the patient's age and general health, the need for appropriate physical activity is emphasized. Thus, exercise regimes vary considerably from one patient to another and, therefore, each patient should develop his or her own regimen with his or her own physician and liaison nurse. Practically everybody can enjoy and benefit from walking, an activity that requires no special skills, equipment, or facility. as soon as the patient is out of intensive care, we begin the walking program while monitoring for any abnormal response.

Upon discharge, patients are instructed to continue a similar amount of walking for a period of 7 to 10 days and thereafter to increase the amount of walking daily in accordance with guidelines provided. The amount of walking or exercise varies considerably from one person to another depending on age, sex, previous physical fitness, health status, and type of surgery. We establish individualized goals for each patient to attain at the time of his or her 6-week visit and prepare new goals as appropriate, again on an individualized basis, realizing the importance of setting realistic, achievable goals. The goal in the walking program is to have patients first achieve 2 miles in 40 min, and then 3 miles in 60 min, provided there are no contraindications or other limitations. This can be adjusted downward for those who cannot achieve the goal.

Patients are taught that not only do walking and exercise benefit them physically, but they also are of great psychological benefit in reducing anxiety and depression and enhancing their self-esteem and emotional stability. We instruct our patients to follow the guidelines listed here in planning their walking or exercise programs:

FIGURE 28.2

PATIENT EDUCATION RECORD
Cardiac Surgery

DISCHARGE INSTRUCTIONS

PURPOSE:

1.) To facilitate patient's compliance after discharge.
2.) To facilitate easier transitions from hospital setting to home.
3.) To provide educational material as a resource.
4.) To assist patient in identifying the need for modification in lifestyle.

RESOURCE MATERIALS:
Discharge Booklet
Medication List

EDUCATIONAL MEETINGS ATTENDED: _____

CONTENT REVIEWED:

	YES	NO		YES	NO
Coronary Artery Disease			Activities / Restrictions		
Valvular Disease			Walking Goals		
Coronary Artery Bypass Graft			Driving		
Valve Replacement			Stairs		
Risk Factors			Lifting		
Infection Prevention			Flying		
Pacemaker Implantation			Housework		
Pulse-Taking			Swimming / Jacuzzi / Sauna		
Bathing / Showering			Golf / Tennis / Jogging		
Incisional Care			Other:		
Sensations			Return to Work		
Weighing			Sexuality		

PATIENT / FAMILY OBJECTIVES   COMPLETED: YES   NO

1.) Verbalized definition of the disease process;
2.) Verbalized understnding of surgical procedure in general terms;
3.) Verbalized the need for and ways to modify lifestyle;
4.) Stated intent to comply with activity regime and restrictions.

FOLLOW-UP APPOINTMENTS:
_____
_____

ADDITIONAL COMMENTS:
_____
_____
_____
_____
_____

DATE_____   R.N.
                        Cardiac Surgical Liaison Nurse

Hospital discharge instruction checklist used in discharge teaching at Cedars-Sinai Medical Center, Los Angeles, CA.

1. Do not walk or exercise immediately after eating. Food digestion requires significant blood flow, thus competing with needs of the muscles, and places additional demands on the heart.

2. Be sure to warm up and cool down properly.

3. Do not exercise outdoors during the hot part of a day or when it is especially humid or smoggy. These factors also result in extra demands on heart function.

TABLE 28.1

RECOMMENDED ACTIVITIES AND THEIR INTRODUCTION DURING CONVALESCENCE[a]

Activity	Guidelines	Activity	Guidelines
Shower	Begin in hospital as soon as temporary pacing wires and staples removed. Shower stools are provided. Use warm (not hot or cold) water. Back to shower spray.	Stairs	You may climb stairs BUT, for the first 6 to 8 weeks go slowly, one at a time, and rest if you feel yourself getting winded or tired. As you progress you may increase the number of steps or the frequency of climbing. If you feel dizzy or fatigued or short of breath STOP, SIT DOWN, AND REST. The feeling should pass and you may resume. If the feeling persists, do not climb any more and contact your physician.
Tub bath	Wait at least six weeks after surgery before taking a tub bath. Getting in and out stresses muscles of chest, arms, and back and places stress on incision.		
Sauna or steam bath	NEVER! Places too much demand on circulatory system which may result in a rapid fall of blood pressure and an inadequate return of blood flow to the heart and brain.	Dining out	This is permissible as long as you feel comfortable and follow the nutritional guidelines.
Hot tub	Avoid for 6 to 8 weeks after surgery. Then, for patients who DO NOT HAVE arrythmias, hot tubs are permissible but keep the water temperature UNDER 95 degrees.	Travel	Delay vacations or extended trips away from home for at least 8 weeks.
		Housework	You may begin light housekeeping tasks when you feel physically comfortable but avoid lifting as described above. You should not expect to assume total responsibility for housework for at least 8 weeks and longer.
Driving a car	Do not drive for approximately 6 to 8 weeks following surgery. During this period your reactions and alertness may decrease. Wait until the sternum is sufficiently well healed before driving. When you do start to drive, limit yourself at first. Also, avoid rapid acceleration, braking, and sharp turns. Note, if you have an accident after surgery you may incur special legal liabilities not otherwise there. Check with your insurance carrier, attorney, etc.	Returning to work	Returning to work depends upon the type of work you do, the level of stress or tension on the job, and your physical stamina. This decision needs to be made jointly by you and your physician together. You may do paper work and make work related phone calls while recuperating at home but remember stop and rest if you get tired. When you do return to work, plan on working no more than half days at first, gradually increasing to full days.
Passenger in a car	Wear your seat belt but, while your chest incision is healing, cushion the belt with a pillow against your chest for added comfort and to prevent irritation to the incision.	Resting	Take frequent rest periods, especially when first returning home. At least two of the rest periods each day should be a minimum of 30 minutes although as much as an hour is preferred. Plan your activities and your day each day so that you don't feel rushed or tense (a good practice to continue beyond your recuperation). If you get tired or fatigued, no matter what you are doing, stop and rest for at least fifteen and as much as thirty minutes.
Golf, swimming, hiking	Avoid these activities until the sternum has healed sufficiently (about 3 months) although putting and chipping is permissible after 6 to 8 weeks.		
Lifting	DO NOT LIFT MORE THAN 10 POUNDS during the first 8 weeks after surgery. Note that grocery bags when full often weigh in excess of 10 pounds. Think about this weight limitation especially with respect to children and pets as well as groceries and other commonly lifted objects. Once the sternum heals, there is no restriction; lift as you did before surgery.		

[a]From the discharge booklet "Heart to Heart." Courtesy Cedars-Sinai Medical Center, Los Angeles, CA.

4. Walk at a comfortable pace. Fatigue without exhaustion should be your guide. "All-out" efforts are especially demanding on the heart and are to be avoided. The walk or exercise should be enjoyable and not stressful.

5. Dress appropriately and comfortably. Use good lightweight walking shoes with slightly elevated heals, a well-supported arch, and flexible soles.

6. Be alert to warning signs. If you feel dizzy, are short of breath, faint, have chest pain (other than the incision), feel a pounding or fluttering sensation in the chest, are are unusually weak, STOP, AND DO NOT CONTINUE your program until you check with your physician.

In addition to the above program, we encourage patients to take advantage of the outpatient Cardiac Rehabilitation Program. This is a supervised, monitored exercise program, described in detail in Chapter 29.

COPING WITH THE OPEN-HEART PATIENT

This class is particularly oriented for family members and others who have to deal with the recuperating open-heart surgical patient. Necessarily, much of the material presented in this class is a repetition of that presented in other classes. The difference is the focus—what the family member can expect and how he or she can help. The following is the outline of the class given to the family members. It illustrates the topics presented and the emphasis placed on those topics.

Someone close to you is in the hospital, either having or recovering from heart surgery. So far, all of the attention has been focused on the patient, but what about you? You, too, are in a crisis situation, experiencing much pain and anxiety. We are here for you!

For your own survival certain measures are encouraged:

1) Recognize and take care of your own basic needs . . .
   eating, sleeping, resting.

2) Avoid unnecessary stress. For example:
   • Avoid people who are demanding.
   • Avoid waiting in lines.
   • Give up smoking later.
   • Go on a diet later.
   • Put off as much as possible the things you don't want to deal with and are not relevant to the present

3) Recognize and respect your own feelings . . .
   fear, anger toward the patient, anger toward the doctor, or that ever-present sense of guilt.

4) Talk with someone about your feelings.

5) Pamper yourself. Find ways of soothing yourself.

6) Use stress management techniques. For example:
   • Deep breathing.
   • Close your eyes and think of a pleasant place.
   • Attend our stress management class.

The ultimate stress reliever would be for the patient to recover but, in the meantime, what would help you most in coping during this critical period? Remember that you can best help your family member by being available in an unstressed way. If you are overburdened, anxiety-ridden, depressed, etc., you are likely to convey those feelings to the patient. Take care of yourself and you will be better able to provide the support and comfort the patient needs.

Finally, we stress that we expect the patient to return to a full and useful life and to return to the activities that were usual before the illness. Therefore, we encourage family members to try to get patients to do things for themselves as soon as practical and not to treat the patient as an invalid.

TOPICS OF SPECIAL INTEREST

We conduct a class in what is known as Topics of Special Interest. These are selected because we feel they need to be emphasized or because patients and families ask may questions or seem especially concerned about these topics.

They include (a) sex after open-heart surgery, (b) arrhythmias, (c) physical fitness, (d) current treatment for coronary artery disease, (e) coronary risk factors, (f) smoking cessation, and (g) cardiopulmonary resuscitation.

We have selected two of these topics to illustrate the type of material we cover and the coverage that we provide. The topics selected, sex and coronary risk factors, are ones about which we receive many questions, and about which there are many misconceptions.

Sex and the Open-Heart Patient

Sex information is provided in a group setting. Additionally, we counsel patients and their sex partners in a private setting as they may require.

The basic fear is that sexual intercourse will place a heavy strain on the heart and possibly lead to a "heart attack" or other dire consequence.

Hellerstein and Friedman have described the physiologic demands of coitus in a group of post–myocardial infarction patients having intercourse in the usual setting and with the usual sex partner. They found the average peak coital heart rate was only 117 beats/min, and the duration of the elevated heart rate was less than 10 min (7). In several of their patients, the work situations often resulted in higher heart rates for more extended periods on a regular and daily basis than did coital activities for the same patients. Studies by Siewicki in which heart rate and blood pressure were measured while climbing stairs and during coitus in the same type of home setting confirm that the effect on the heart is about the same for coitus as it is for climbing two flights of stairs (8).

Depending on patient interest and sophistication we may go into the studies such as the ones just cited. We believe that factual information will help allay fears and dispel the many misconceptions that we encounter. The following, quoted from our manual on discharge instructions, is an example of the information given all patients and their sex partners.

Most patients will demonstrate sexual interest in three to four weeks after surgery. However, sexual activity should be resumed gradually; the ability to exercise without discomfort (such as walking two miles) is a prerequisite for resuming lovemaking. Prior to this, however, touching, caressing, holding and closeness can be satisfying not only as part of sexual activity, but as a source of comfort and renewal.

All sexual positions are acceptable, but initially you should assume a position of comfort. Oral sex, if desired, places no additional demand on the heart. If you find it acceptable, masturbation might be the first step towards sexual satisfaction. This allows you to control the amount of stimulation and lessens the pressure of pleasing your partner. Manual stimulation may be enough to satisfy your partner until you are ready to resume full sexual relations.

Amphetamines, amyl nitrate, cocaine, mood altering drugs, and other stimulants are unsafe for the heart and should not be used. Marijuana has been shown to increase the heart rate as well as the oxygen demand of the heart muscle, and therefore should not be used.

Pregnancy should be avoided until recovery is completed. In certain congenital heart conditions even after corrective surgery, pregnancy may not be advisable. Be sure to speak with your physician or cardiac surgeon about the best method of birth control for you.

Remember, although you may not be able to return to having sexual intercourse immediately upon discharge, you are able to share in tender loving and care. These activities convey a positive sense of closeness between you and your partner.

Coronary Risk Factors

During this class each patient is asked to identify those risk factors that exist for all persons generally, and those particularly related to the patient. Only by this awareness can the patient begin to modify his or her life-style or behavior to minimize the effect of those factors under the patient's control. The potential impact of common risk factors is illustrated in Figure 28.3 and is discussed more fully in Chapter 31. We concentrate on being sure that the pa-

FIGURE 28.3

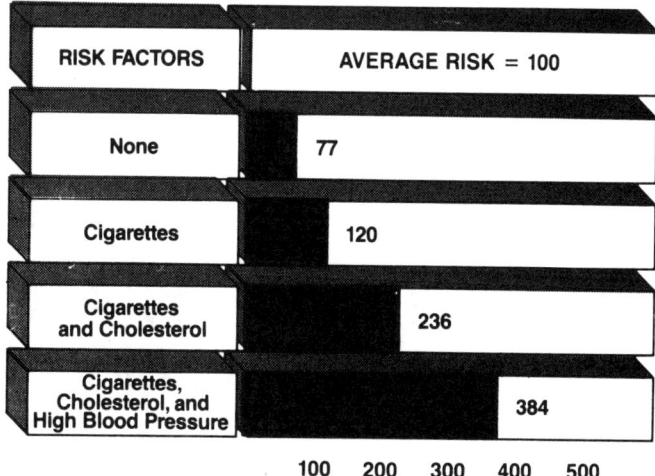

RISK FACTORS	AVERAGE RISK = 100
None	77
Cigarettes	120
Cigarettes and Cholesterol	236
Cigarettes, Cholesterol, and High Blood Pressure	384

100   200   300   400   500

Impact of common risk factors. The dangers of heart attack increase with the number of risk factors present. This chart shows how a combination of three major risk factors can increase the likelihood of heart attack. For purposes of illustration, this chart uses an abnormal blood pressure level of 310 in a 45-year-old man. (Adapted from *Heart Facts 1985*. Dallas, TX, American Heart Association, 1985, p 4.)

tient understands the risk factors that apply to him or to her, and understands what can be done about them. Each patient is urged to verbalize positive actions that he or she will take upon leaving the hospital with respect to modifying his or her risk factors.

CONCLUSION

In this chapter we provided an overview of postoperative teaching as presented to our cardiac surgical patients and their families. The focus of that training is to prepare the patient to return as rapidly as possible to normal life, consistent with his or her medical condition. We also focused on reducing the anxiety and fear that frequently accompany the recuperation period.

We emphasized adaptive behavior that promotes good health and that reduces the probability of exacerbating the original condition. To do this we use techniques of learning theory designed to maximize understanding and compliance, and present a variety of topics in such

areas as stress management, nutrition, exercise and activities, surgical healing, and sex.

References

1. Rogoz B: Nursing care of the cardiac surgery patient. *Nurs Clin North Am* 4:631, 1969.
2. Pitorak E: Open-ended care for open-heart patient. In Lewis EP (ed): *Nursing in Cardiovascular Disease*. New York, AJN Company, 1974.
3. Cassaday J, Altrocchi J: Patient concerns about surgery. *Nurs Res* 9:220, 1960.
4. Lazarus RS: *Psychological Stress and the Coping Process*. New York, McGraw-Hill, 1966.
5. Lazarus RS, Averill JR, Opton EM Jr: The psychology of coping, issues of reseach and assessment. In Godho GV, Hamburg DA, Adorus JE (eds): *Coping and Adaptation*. New York, Basic Books, 1974, p 249.
6. Lazarus RS, Folkman S: *Stress, Appraisal, and Coping*, New York, Springer Verlag, 1984.
7. King KB: Measurement of coping strategies, concerns and emotional response in patients undergoing coronary artery bypass grafting. *Heart Lung* 14:579, 1985.
8. Fuerst EV, Wolff LV, Weitzel MH: The nurse or a health teacher. In *Fundamentals of Nursing*. Philadelphia, JB Lippincott, 1974, p 148.

Chapter 29
EXERCISE REHABILITATION AFTER CORONARY BYPASS GRAFT SURGERY

DHUN H. SETHNA, M.D.
JACK M. MATLOFF, M.D.
RICHARD J. GRAY, M.D.

Cardiac rehabilitation is a multidisciplinary intervention designed to restore cardiac patients to optimal levels of physical, psychologic, social, and vocational function (1). For patients convalescing from open-heart surgery, an individualized exercise prescription is an essential component of their recovery. A deconditioned state is virtually unavoidable after any major surgery, and this is particularly true after cardiovascular operations. Debilitating effects of the actual procedure, along with bed rest and the metabolic demands of recuperation, can significantly and rapidly depress levels of physical fitness. Decreased skeletal muscle mass, contractile strength, and efficiency have all been associated with postoperative deconditioning (2).

Definite hemodynamic alterations occur after deconditioning and bed rest. In one study, young men confined to bed rest for 3 weeks showed a 20 to 25% decrease in maximum volume of oxygen use (VO_2 max) (3). Besides decreasing functional capacity, prolonged bed rest results in orthostatic hypotension and can lead to venous thrombosis from loss of blood volume, because plasma loss may exceed loss of red blood cell mass. Pulmonary function is also compromised, and negative nitrogen and calcium balance can result (4). Instituting physical training very early after coronary artery bypass surgery is not associated with a higher morbidity or mortality. On the contrary, duration of hospitalization may be shortened, and improved functional capacity at the time of discharge results in earlier and more complete resumption of normal activities.

INITIATION OF EXERCISE THERAPY

Patients who have undergone coronary bypass surgery with an uncomplicated perioperative clinical course should begin activity 24 to 48 hr after surgery, and occasionally while still in the cardiac surgical intensive care unit. An uncomplicated perioperative course is one in which there is no significant arrhythmia, hemodynamic instability, active bleeding, or serious postoperative neurologic or pulmonary complications. The occurrence of an uncomplicated perioperative myocardial infarction need not alter plans for early exercise therapy.

Most patients are extubated on the evening of surgery or the following morning. On the 1st postoperative day, activity should approximate 1 to 2 metabolic equivalents (MET); that is, 1 to 2 times the resting metabolic rate (1 MET is equivalent to an oxygen consumption of 3.5 ml/kg/min). Recommended activities include partial self-care (washing hands and face, brushing teeth), simple active and passive arm and leg movements, and active plantar and dorsiflexion of ankles several times a day. If mediastinal chest tubes have been removed, the patient is encouraged to sit with the head of the bed raised to a 45° angle and with the trunk and arms supported by an over-bed table. The patient should also dangle his or her legs on the side of the bed at least once on this day. Young and middle-aged, otherwise healthy patients may be assisted to a bedside chair in the afternoon of the 1st postoperative day, or may even be transferred from the intensive care unit by wheelchair to a monitored ward bed.

By the 2nd postoperative morning, the patient is usually eating a soft diet by himself or herself and is assisted to a bedside chair. A bedside commode can be used at this time; indeed, the commode involves less energy expenditure and myocardial work than does the use of a bedpan (5). On transfer from the intensive care unit (usually 24 to 48 hr after surgery), some patients may walk around the room with the help of a nurse. They should be monitored clinically and electrocardiographically at all times, and the extent of ambulation is decreased if any of the following criteria are observed: (*a*) a heart rate greater than 20 beats/min above the resting heart rate (9); (*b*) occurrence of an arrhythmia or S-T segment displacement; (*c*) decrease in systolic blood pressure; or (*d*) development of chest pain, fatigue, or dyspnea. The usual blood pressure response to exercise is an elevation of systolic pressure; the absence of which is evidence that cardiac output is not meeting the demands of exercise. Isometric maneuvers, which may elevate blood pressure and

precipitate arrhythmias, contribute little to cardiovascular conditioning and are avoided.

PROGRESSIVE IN-HOSPITAL EXERCISE

The objectives of rehabilitation after release from the intensive care unit are to help alleviate problems associated with bed rest, reduce anxiety and depression, develop the patient's confidence, provide education regarding modification of risk factors, increase the chance of earlier hospital discharge, and provide surveillance for optimal patient management (6). In general, low-intensity (2 to 3 MET) isotonic calisthenics and exercises designated to maintain muscle tone, coordination, and joint mobility are initiated (7). Range-of-motion exercises are particularly useful for restoring flexibility and maintaining muscle tone. Exercises used at the author's institution are shown in Figures 29.1 to 29.8. Soft tissue and bone damage of the chest wall may occur during the surgical procedure. If this area does not receive range-of-motion exercise, adhesions may develop and the musculature can weaken. Patients may tend to favor the arm, shoulder, and chest areas, and this can accentuate later problems of poor posture and strength. About 95% of patients after coronary artery bypass surgery can perform upper extremity range-of-motion exercise without overt problems (8).

At each stage of recovery, the level of activity chosen is one that can be performed without

FIGURE 29.1

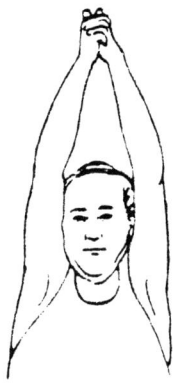

Shoulder flexion: Clasp both hands together, keeping elbows straight. Lift arms over head. (Five times.)

FIGURE 29.2

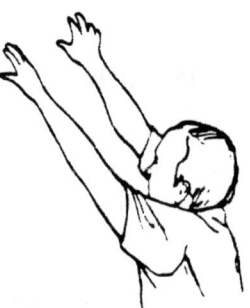

Wall climbing: Stand facing the wall and "walk" the fingers of both hands up the wall as high as possible. (Five times.)

hazardous, abnormal responses. A distinction between discomfort and pain must be appreciated by the patient, because incisional discomfort is unavoidable. Administration of analgesics timed to coincide with planned activity periods may enhance exercise tolerance. Thoracic skeletal pain during normal postoperative convalescence can be quite remote from the sternum, and may involve the axilla, lateral chest, dorsal and cervical spine, and shoulder. Rehabilitation should be decreased or even discontinued temporarily if any untoward reaction or discomfort other than the above is experienced. Sternal instability, as evidenced by clicking, grating, or movement on careful palpation occurs in about 5% of patients, and should be promptly reported to the surgeon. When this occurs, upper ex-

FIGURE 29.3

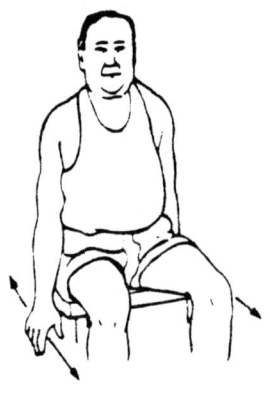

Arm swinging: Sit in a chair, allowing arms to hand loosly at sides. Swing arms forward and backward. (Ten times.)

FIGURE 29.4

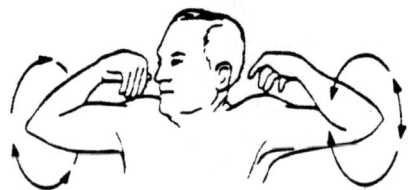

Elbow circling: Place fingertips on shoulders. Move elbows in a circle, going up and back. Repeat in opposite direction. (Five times each.)

tremity and trunk range-of-motion exercise should be temporarily curtailed.

The patient should sit in a chair for all meals, frequently getting in and out of bed and standing up; walking (with assistance initially, as for all activity) is encouraged. Ambulation is the primary mode of aerobic activity in the inpatient program, since this is also the patient's means of transportation. Casual but routine walks with a nurse gradually supplement the calisthenics, and a walking program is initiated in the hospital corridors, wherein distance walked and pace are progressively increased. Frequent observations of vital signs determine when the pace may be increased and the distance extended. Assistance during walking is usually required for 48 hr (3rd to 5th postoperative days). Thereafter, the average patient should feel stable enough to walk alone or with a family member. By the 6th or 7th postoperative day, he or she should walk comfortably alone. At this time, most patients are able to ambulate about 400 feet. When such a level of activity has been reached, the patient is often ready for discharge from the hospital.

The recommended frequency of inpatient exercise training is 2 or 3 times per day. Because of fatigue, frequent shorter sessions are often

FIGURE 29.5

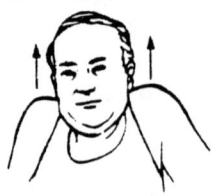

Shoulder shrugging: Hunch shoulders up and down. (Five times.)

FIGURE 29.6

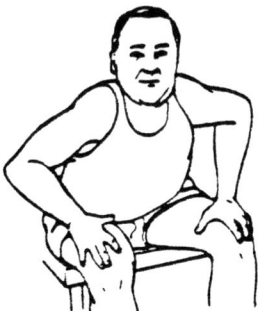

Trunk flexion: Sit in a chair with hands resting on knees. Bend forward from the waist and then straighten up. (Five times.)

better tolerated, at least one of which should be conducted by the rehabilitation staff and should include range-of-motion exercises. Most early inpatient activities can be performed at the patient's bedside, with ambulation around the room or the ward. In a prospective study of 521 consecutive postoperative coronary bypass patients who were referred for rehabilitation from 1978 to 1980, the program was initiated as early as 12 hr after operation (9). Heart rate and systolic pressure were only moderately elevated at 2 MET. New ventricular arrhythmias occurred in 22% of patients during exercise, but few required treatment. Ten percent of patients showed a fall in systolic blood pressure during exercise, but this was rarely symptomatic. Blood

FIGURE 29.7

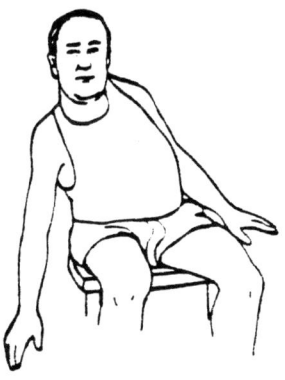

Lateral trunk flexion: Sit in a chair with arms hanging loosly at sides. Bend sideways as if to touch floor with right hand. Repeat to the other side. (Five times.)

FIGURE 29.8

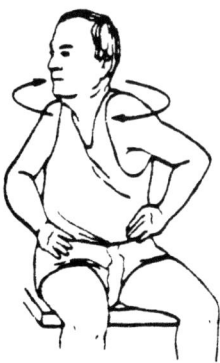

Trunk rotation: Sit in a chair and place hands on sides and waist. Looking over right shoulder, turn shoulders to the right. Repeat, moving shoulders and looking to the left. (Five times.)

pressure decreased in some patients during stair climbing.

PREDISCHARGE LOW-INTENSITY CARDIAC FUNCTION TESTING

A low-intensity treadmill test may be performed the day before hospital discharge. The test is explained in detail and an informed consent is signed. For morning tests breakfast is withheld, and for afternoon tests breakfast but not lunch is allowed, because S-T segment or T wave changes may be associated with the postprandial state. A standard 12-lead ECG is recorded, and blood pressure, S-T segments, T waves, and cardiac rhythm are evaluated in the supine and standing positions and during hyperventilation and the Valsalva maneuver. Treadmill exercise is then started at a low speed (2.7 km/hr) and 0° elevation (1.7 MET). The speed or the elevation or both are increased every 3 min, so that at successive stages the work rates are 2.5, 3.4, 4.2, 5.4, and 6 to 7 MET. The speed may be held at 2.7 km/hr and the elevation increased by 2 to 3° per stage up to a maximum of 14° grade (6 to 7 MET). Alternatively, the speed may be increased at the first two stages to 4.0 and 5.4 km/hr respectively at zero grade; thereafter, speed is held at 5.4 km/hr, and the grade is increased by 2° per stage up to a maximum of 6° grade (6 to 7 MET).

The test is stopped if the patient develops (*a*) symptoms of angina, excessive fatigue, dyspnea, or claudication; (*b*) a decrease in systolic blood pressure of more than 10 mm Hg relative to the preceding pressure; (*c*) cardiac arrhythmias (significant supraventricular ectopics, salvos of three or more ectopic beats, Mobitz type 2 or third-degree heart block); (*d*) a target heart rate of 130 beats/min; or (*e*) the intended maximal exercise level (7 MET). S-T segment depression would be a relative indication for stopping the test. If a patient is receiving β-adrenergic blocking medication, a target heart rate of 100 beats/min may be used. In a large prospective study of patients after coronary artery bypass, heart rate increased an average of 33 beats/min over resting levels during a symptom-limited treadmill test (9). However, this exertion was perceived as "very difficult" by 16.5% of patients, and "somewhat difficult" by another 13%. Because of this, it has been recommended that the upper limit for the increase in heart rate from rest during inpatient exercise programs be set at 20 beats/min (9).

A patient taking a cardioactive drug should continue medication during the test exactly as if he or she were at home. This is important, since one of the purposes of functional testing is to detect symptoms of cardiac decompensation or cardiac arrhythmia that might be dangerous if the same work rate were developed at home.

Low-intensity treadmill testing assesses postoperative functional capacity and allows a safe target heart rate to be determined. Each patient is instructed to measure his or her pulse before and after exercise. Should the measured pulse rate exceed the target figure, the patient is advised to decrease activity. Finally, the occurrence of exercise-induced arrhythmias or ischemia must be evaluated when making recommendations for continuing rehabilitation at home (Table 29.1).

POSTDISCHARGE PROGRAM

The goal of an outpatient program is to enable the cardiac patient to safely regain and maintain optimal levels of physical, psychosocial, and vocational functions. Focus shifts from

TABLE 29.1

ENERGY COST OF COMMON ACTIVITIES[a]

1–2 MET level

Reading	Dressing
Letter writing	Shaving while sitting
Playing cards and table games	Relaxing with immediate family
Sedentary hobbies at table level	Slow walking on level at 1.6 km/hr (fewer than 80 steps/min)
Hand sewing	Exercises as prescribed by the therapists
Light desk work	
Typing (electric)	
Light dusting	

2–3 MET level

Typing	Work involving use of hands, standing and walking
Showering	
Shampooing hair with assistance	Ironing
Small home repairs	Use of washer and dryer with light loads
Playing piano	Making beds
Peeling vegetables	Meal preparation
Snack preparation	Auto driving (low-stress area)
Washing small clothes by hand	Walking at 4.8 km/hr (120 steps/min)
Light polishing	Exercise as prescribed by the therapists
Folding clothes	In moderation:
Having a few visitors in	Dining out
Walking at 3.2 km/hr (fewer than 100 steps/min)	Religious services
Exercises as prescribed by the therapists	Movies
All self-care	Concerts
	Plays

4–5 MET level

Mopping, cleaning windows	Normal social activities (e.g., entertaining, attending meetings)
Vacuuming carpets	Grocery shopping (avoid standing in lines and carrying)
Light gardening	
Carrying out garbage, using a dolly	
Golf, using a cart	Walking at 5.6 km/hr (more than 120 steps/min)
Bowling	
Ballroom dancing	
Swimming at 20 m/min	Walking up stairs slowly, pausing at each level

[a]These are recommended activities at various MET levels. One MET is the resting energy expenditure (equivalent to an oxygen consumption of 3.5 ml/kg/min). Remember to incorporate good body mechanics and apply energy conservation techniques with all activities. Always follow the guidelines for the home exercise program.

performing activities of daily living and ambulation to improving the level of cardiorespiratory conditioning and overall fitness. In general, the calisthenics initiated in the hospital are continued, with a progressive increase in the number of repetitions, the maximum number being attained by 4 to 6 weeks. Routine casual walking, both around the house and outside, is continued and progressively increased. Stationary cycling may be restricted until the leg incision has sufficiently healed.

The patient is warned that swelling of the venous donor ankle may occur initially, and that this is not an indication for decreasing the level of activity. Leg elevation and occasionally elastic stockings are required to decrease ankle swelling. Muscle soreness and thoracic skeletal pain should have decreased appreciably at this stage of rehabilitation, and the patient should be able to undertake increasing amounts of exercise with better overall tolerance and less discomfort and fatigue.

If the patient encounters no shortness of breath, chest discomfort, or palpitations with this regimen, then approximately 2 weeks after surgery a program of sustained daily walking is initiated (10). Initially, ½ mile is covered in 15 min. The distance is increased, if well tolerated, to 1 mile in 20 min, and then more gradually to 2 miles in 45 min. By the end of 8 weeks the average, uncomplicated patient should be walking 3 miles in 1 hr. When patients can walk at 3.5 miles/hr, 5% grade, during training, they are capable of jogging. This would be equivalent to 6 MET. Loose-fitting clothing and comfortable shoes are advised. Exercise should be avoided during extreme weather conditions (heat, cold, humidity, ozone alerts) and after meals. Fatigue is a desirable result of exercise, but exhaustion is to be avoided. The patient is instructed to stop the exercise program and consult a cardiologist if unusual discomfort or stress occurs. Exercise is also to be avoided if the patient is ill or overly tired.

Considerable variation in exercise tolerance is seen, depending on preoperative status, sex, age, motivation, and the presence of associated disease. The exercise prescription must be individually tailored to clinical condition and response; in general, if the duration of activity can be doubled or tripled at a given intensity without symptoms, progression to the next higher level of intensity is indicated (11). The response to a higher duration and frequency of activity may be monitored by the patient, based on the presence or absence of symptoms and the heart rate attained.

The eventual optimal exercise session consists of a warm-up period (10 min), a dynamic period during which the treal training exercise is done (40 min), and a cooling down period (10 min) (11). The warm-up period usually consists of calisthenics designed to stretch the major muscles and joints; this should always precede the dynamic interval. The dynamic interval comprises sustained walking, programmed to increase the heart rate to 70 to 85% of the measured maximum as determined by treadmill testing. The cool-down period involves low-intensity exercise, allowing the heart rate to decrease slowly and preventing pooling of blood in the legs; it avoids undesirable complications of abrupt stopping, such as syncope, lightheadedness, or nausea.

RETURNING TO WORK AND LIFETIME EXERCISE

Approximately 8 to 10 weeks after surgery, a submaximal (85% of predicted maximal heart rate) treadmill exercise should be performed. The results of this evaluation are used to further advise the patient regarding return to work and continuing exercise prescription. At this stage, physical function can be further enhanced by participation in individual or supervised community physical conditioning programs.

To maintain training, the exercise prescription should require (a) an intensity of 70 to 80% of the maximum heart rate safely achieved at prior exercise stress testing; (b) a duration of 30 to 60 min per session, including warm-up and cooling-down periods; and (c) a frequency of 3 to 4 times per week, preferably not on successive days. It is not known whether similar benefit could be obtained with a less-prolonged or a less-intense exercise training program. The patient is encouraged to work out at the same time and on the same days of the week to establish a routine. The level of exertion is increased only after appropriate testing, and if exercise is discontinued for 2 or more weeks, reevaluation may be required.

Driving a car is acceptable after 6 weeks; the patient should drive on side streets for 2 weeks and progress gradually to main highways. A person who can walk at a speed of 3 miles/hr without difficulty or symptoms can return readily to most semisedentary occupations that require an energy expenditure of 3 to 4 MET. Occupations demanding a higher energy expenditure call for more intense and prolonged training before returning to work. Nevertheless, most patients can return to physically demanding work 2 months following bypass surgery, and work that requires less physical activity can be initiated whenever the patient is ready, as determined by a physician who knows the individual well.

Studies on the resumption of gainful employment after bypass surgery indicate that the determinants of return to work are largely present before operation and are predominantly nonmedical: patient expectations and attitudes play an important role. Preoperative employment consistently favors return to work after operation, as do higher educational levels and family incomes. Participation in an inexpensive rehabilitation program involving simple calisthenics and graduated walking has been shown to significantly increase employment rates after operation (12).

References

1. Hellerstein HK, Ford AB: Rehabilitation of the cardiac patient. *JAMA* 164:225–231, 1957.
2. Taylor HL, Henschel A, Brozek J, et al: Effects of bed rest on cardiovascular function and work performance. *J Appl Physiol* 2:223, 1949.
3. Saltin B, Blomquist G, Mitchell JH, et al: Response to exercise after bedrest and after training. *Circulation* 38(Suppl 7):1–78, 1968.
4. Robinson G, Froelicher VF, Utley JR: Rehabilitation of the coronary artery bypass graft surgery patient. *J Cardiopulmonary Rehab* 4:74–86, 1984.
5. Wenger NK, Gilbert CA: Rehabilitation of the myocardial infarction patient. IN Hurst JW, Logue RB (eds): *The Heart*, ed 4. New York, McGraw-Hill, 1978.
6. Pollock ML, Pels AE III, Foster C, et al: Exercise prescription for rehabilitation of the cardiac patient. In Pollock ML, Schmidt DH (eds): *Heart Disease and Rehabilitation*, ed 2. New York, John Wiley & Sons, 1986.
7. Oberman A, Kouchoukos NT: Role of exercise after coronary artery bypass surgery. In Wenger NK (ed): *Exercise and the Heart*. Philadelphia, FA DAvis, 1978, pp 155–172.
8. Metier CP, Pollock ML, Grave SJE: Exercise prescription for the coronary artery bypass surgery patient. *J Cardiopulmonary Rehab* 6:85–103, 1986.
9. Dion FW, Grovenow P, Pollock ML, et al: Medical problems and physiologic responses during supervised inpatient cardiac rehabilitation. *J Cardiopulmonary Rehab* 2:248–254, 1982.
10. Sethna DH, Gray RJ, Chaux A, et al: Rehabilitation after coronary bypass surgery. In Vyden JK (ed): *Post-Myocardial Infarction Management and Rehabilitation*. New York, Marcel Dekker, 1983, pp 329–351.
11. The Committee on Exercise: *Exercise Testing and Training of Individuals with Heart Disease or at High Risk for Its Development: A Handbook for Physicians*. Dallas, TX, American Heart Association, 1975.
12. Crosby IK, Wellons HA Jr, Martin RP, et al: Employability—a new indication for aneurysmectomy and coronary revascularization. *Circulation* 62(Suppl 2):79–83, 1980.

Chapter 30
PSYCHOSOCIAL ADJUSTMENT

RICHARD J. GRAY, M.D.

Alterations in mood and difficulty in adjusting to postoperative life can discolor all aspects of the results from well-conceived, uncomplicated cardiovascular surgery. Although often self-limited, an understanding of the situation is essential in helping the patient and his or her family through these often very dark-appearing times and will aid in understanding the patient's assessment of his or her physical recovery as well.

CHANGES IN MOOD

Depression usually begins in the hospital and often continues for a few weeks after discharge. Other patients will first become depressed shortly after leaving the hospital. Most patients report the worst symptoms 1 to 2 weeks after leaving the hospital, with resolution in 6 weeks. Persistence much beyond 2 months, especially of symptoms that interfere with the patient's lifestyle, should trigger reappraisal of both medical and social factors that may be worsening the situation. Possibly offending medications should be evaluated and discontinued or replaced with others. These would include virtually all β-blockers, many sedatives and tranquilizers, and certain antihypertensives such as α-methyldopa and clonidine. Rare examples of such reaction to even calcium channel blockers have also been reported. Important contributors to exogenous depression include such common factors as medical expenses, uncertain work status, and disrupted home and family life resulting from hospitalization and surgery. While these obstacles to recovery are rarely easily removed, every possible support should be given in an effort to help the patient cope with the situation. Medical therapy of depression is rarely used or needed. This is because of the delayed onset of usual antidepressant medications often competing with the self-limited natural history of postoperative depression, the fear of cardiac side effects from antidepressant medications, and disappointing response in the presence of exogenous factors.

Thus, while postoperative depression is extremely common, virtually all symptoms are resolved by 6 to 8 weeks in most patients. Disabling symptoms beyond this are occasionally the result of exogenous factors, but usually imply the existence of a more profound underlying condition possibly triggered by the surgery. Professional (i.e., psychiatric or psychological) help should definitely be considered for disabling symptoms not responsive to the usual supportive measures by 4 and certainly 6 months after surgery. It should be kept in mind that in surveys, 10 to 15% of patients may report elevated levels of either anxiety or depression more than 1 year after surgery (1, 2).

Sharp swings in mood also characterize the patient for several weeks after surgery. Moments of elation are often followed within hours, or sometimes minutes, by periods of gloom or even crying spells. Interestingly, the crying is often triggered by words of kindness or reassurance from a family member or visiting friend. Other patients report free-flowing tears in response to an emotionally laden television drama. Such events are disturbing and puzzling to patients, especially men who are unaccustomed to such emotional fullness. The physiologic explanation (if indeed there is one) is unknown. This type of behavior is often seen even in the absence of postoperative depression and seems to be unrelated to preoperative personality traits, but fortunately disappears without consequences in 4 to 6 weeks. Reassurance is obviously in order.

PSYCHOSOCIAL ADJUSTMENT

The "quality of life" resulting from heart surgery has been the subject of much scientific interest. While improvement in quality of life is meant to imply benefit in the area of certain physical factors such as absence of angina, improvement in congestive heart failure symptoms, removal of activity limitations, improved work and recreational status, and freedom from hospitalization, other less concrete aspects have also been examined, especially after coronary bypass. An interesting follow-up was conducted for up to 4½ years after bypass to determine overall satisfaction with life (pleasure, nervousness, mood), return to work status, return to sexual activity, and status with regard to certain behavioral coronary risk factors such as smoking, weight loss, and exercise (3). Pleasure in life had improved substantially after surgery; 60% were extremely pleased that they had undergone surgery, and only 4% were displeased. Overall ratings of nervousness and mood status were rated by patients as being either much better or slightly better in a majority of patients. Seventy-seven percent of patients were working at the time of surgery, and 76% were working 9 months after surgery. Patients who returned to work were significantly younger, showed more improvement in angina, and were more likely to have type A behavior pattern preoperatively and postoperatively. At 9 months, only 38% of

patients reported being sexually active at least once a week and 31% reported no sexual activity, whereas preoperatively 67% had been sexually active at least once a week and only 11% reported no sexual activity. As with working, postoperative increase in sexual activity correlated with preoperative cardiac impairment (New York Heart Association functional class), return to work, and pre- and postoperative type A rating. Overall, however, sexual satisfaction declined early after surgery. Compliance with recommendation to change behavioral coronary risk factors such as smoking was successful in that only one-third of those smoking preoperatively were doing so after surgery, and the majority of those advised to change their exercise pattern did so. Unfortunately, weight loss was not satisfactorily achieved, and despite recommendations to "slow down" after surgery, type A behavior pattern activity was unchanged in 75%, and only 5% changed from type A to type B despite the fact that 30% thought that they had slowed down greatly. A more pessimistic view is reported in another study from a different geographic location within the United States, which found a high incidence of psychological and social disablement despite a good physical outcome from bypass surgery. Unemployment and sexual dysfunction were reported by 83 and 57%, respectively. Other evidence of maladjustment included a "constricted social life," low self-esteem, and lack of pleasure from close relationships. All of the latter, however, might be expected in a population, as this one was, of largely unemployed individuals (4). In another study of functional benefits following coronary bypass graft surgery, sexual functioning was essentially unchanged in approximately one-half of the patients, and the remainder was divided into those in whom it was improved and those in whom it was worsened after surgery (5).

A very relevant but often neglected aspect is the effect of surgery on family life, especially a patient's spouse. As might be expected, living with a depressed, convalescing surgical patient with wide and unpredictable mood swings can be difficult, to say the least. Additional discord often arises over a spouse's well-meant insistence on compliance with behavior modification such as exercises, changes in diet, and smoking. During postoperative office visits, the physician often finds himself or herself caught in the midst of some type of recurrent family debate once these subjects are brought up. The approach that no one is "to blame" should be used, and both parties are always reassured to hear that such discord is common, even expected, and fortunately transient. This family strife has been confirmed in an interesting study, which reported that 40 to 50% of spouses reported levels of depression severe enough to warrant treatment (6).

In an interesting review of 142 survivors of open-heart surgery, over 90% of patients showed improvement in physical condition compared with preoperative evaluation, but general psychological adjustment declined after surgery with significant psychological hindrances to recovery in approximately one-third (7). At 1 year postoperatively, on average, patients tended to become more passive, others exhibiting anxiety, depression, poor self-esteem, passive dependency, somatic preoccupation, paranoid tendency, and withdrawal. Other patients also exhibited impaired sexual and marital functioning. A high psychological risk group was characterized preoperatively by disorganization, anxiety, paranoid tendencies, hedonism, and high levels of psychologic activity. Whether because this study was confined to patients with chronic rheumatic valve disease or for other reasons, the results do not reflect the expected outcome from contemporary surgery, yet the preoperative description of a high-risk psychological profile remains an apt one.

RETURN TO WORK

Timing of return to work must be guided by cardiovascular status, musculoskeletal healing, incisional pain, and satisfactory progress in the area of emotional and intellectual well-being, the tempo for all of which will be modified by the patient's own motivation toward convalescence and return to normal activities. This is one area where type A behavior will promote more rapid return of normal behavior (3). Chapter 29 more fully discusses assessment of cardiovascular and other physical factors with

regard to work. By 6 to 8 weeks most patients are psychologically and intellectually able to return to work. Return to work as late as 10 weeks would still be considered normal convalescence, especially in more physically demanding or highly stressful occupations.

Much has been written about the success or failure of cardiac surgery, especially coronary bypass, to promote return to work. In an often-quoted early paper examining vocational and emotional status of a large group of surgical patients, the likelihood of returning to work was most clearly related to the duration of preoperative unemployment. A "law of the year" was proposed, which stated that if a person was unemployed for more than a year for any reason, the chance of postoperative reemployment is poor (8). Surgery in these patients predominantly consisted of valvular procedures and repair of certain adult congenital defects. In this analysis, 41% of patients felt unable to work, mostly for health reasons. Similar results in coronary bypass patients, despite differences in disease process and possibly chronicity of symptoms, have been confirmed in numerous more recent studies. Reported rates of return to work vary tremendously, but generally are between 60 and 90% (9–12). The incidence of employment also tends to decline with time after surgery due to advancing age and possibly recurrence of symptoms. In the quality-of-life analysis of patients randomized to surgical therapy in the Coronary Artery Surgery Study (CASS), approximately 70% of patients were working at 1 year, and approximately 55% were working 5 years after surgery (13). Unquestionably, the most important factor in return to work is preoperative unemployment for 3 months or more (15, 16). Other factors such as age over 55, preoperative work as a laborer, and educational level are also important (9–12). It is apparent that surgical therapy for coronary atherosclerosis (in contrast to medical therapy) does not overtly enhance return-to-work rates (13–15). This is true in large groups of patients because chronic disabling angina is less often an acceptable way of life, and therefore a singular cause of unemployment. In broad terms, rates of employment tend to decline slightly after surgery (10, 13, 16). The reasons for this 5 to 10% decline include acceptance of an early retirement of patients in their early 60s, disinclination to return to the physical or stressful demands of certain jobs on doctor's advice, and, most important, recurrence of angina. A specialized vocational rehabilitation program has been successful in enhancing return-to-work rates for coronary bypass patients (14). Based on personal knowledge of the individual patient, prediction of postoperative work is much easier, based quite simply on the three factors of preoperative employment, postoperative physiologic outcome, and, most important, motivation of the patient.

References

1. Rabiner CJ, Willner AE: Psychopathology observed on follow-up after coronary bypass surgery. *J Nerv Ment Dis* 163:295–301, 1976.
2. Wilson-Barnett J: Assessment of recovery: with special reference to a study with post-operative cardiac patients. *J Adv Nurs* 6:435–445, 1981.
3. Kornfeld DS, Heller SS, Frank KA, et al: Psychological and behavioral responses after coronary artery bypass surgery. *Circulation* 66(Suppl III):24–28, 1982.
4. Gundle MJ, Reeves BR, Tate S, et al: Psychosocial outcome after coronary artery surgery. *Am J Psychiatry* 137:1591–1594, 1980.
5. Stanton BA: Functional benefits following coronary artery bypass graft surgery. *Ann Thorac Surg* 37:286–290, 1984.
6. Goldschmidt T, Brooks N, Sethia B, et al: Coronary artery bypass surgery—impact upon a patient's wife—a pilot study. *Thorac Cardiovasc Surg* 32:337–340, 1984.
7. Heller SS, Frank KA, Kornfeld DS, et al: Psychological outcome following open-heart surgery. *Arch Intern Med* 134:908–914, 1974.
8. Blachly PH, Blachly BJ: Vocational and emotional status of 263 patients after heart surgery. *Circulation* 38:524–532, 1968.
9. Smith HC, Hammes LVH, Gupta S, et al: Employment status after coronary artery bypass surgery. *Circulation* 65(Suppl II):120–125, 1982.
10. Gutmann MC, Knapp DN, Pollock ML, et al: Coronary artery bypass patients and work status. *Circulation* 66(Suppl III):33–42, 1982.
11. Oberman A, Wayne JB, Kouchoukos NT, et al: Employment status after coronary artery bypass surgery. *Circulation* 65(Suppl II):115–119, 1982.
12. Danchin N, David P, Robert P, et al: Employment following aortocoronary bypass surgery in young patients. *Cardiology* 69:52–59, 1982.
13. CASS Principal Investigators and their associates. Coronary Artery Surgery Study (CASS): a randomized trial of coronary artery bypass surgery. Quality of life in patients randomly assigned to treatment group. *Circulation* 68:951–960, 1983.
14. Boulay FM, David PP, Bourassa MG: Strategies for improving the work status of patients after coronary artery bypass surgery. *Circulation* 66(Suppl III):43–49, 1982.
15. Hammermeister KE, DeRouen TA, English MT, et al: Effect of surgical versus medical therapy on return to work in patients with coronary artery disease. *Am J Cardiol* 44:105–111, 1979.
16. Barnes GK, Ray MJ, Oberman A, et al: Changes in working status of patients following coronary bypass surgery. *JAMA* 238:1259–1261, 1977.

Section 6
THE LATE PHASE: FOLLOW-UP

Chapter 31
LONG-TERM MANAGEMENT OF THE CORONARY ARTERY BYPASS GRAFT PATIENT

JAMES E. DALEN, M.D., M.P.H.

In some hospitals coronary artery bypass grafting (CABG) has become the most frequently performed major surgical procedure. It has become a low-risk, highly effective procedure for the treatment of coronary artery disease (CAD). Despite its efficacy, it must be made clear to the patient that it is not the "cure" for coronary artherosclerosis. It does not prevent progression of atherosclerosis in the native coronary circulation or in the bypass grafts. In some patients angina may persist or recur; myocardial infarction and sudden cardiac death are not prevented.

Although CABG is an almost routine procedure in some hospitals, it is not routine for the individual patient. For most patients, undergoing CABG is one of the most important events in their lives. It is, therefore, the ideal time for patients to change their life-styles with particular regard to risk factors for CAD. With the help of their physicians, patients who undergo CABG can modify their life-styles. Physicians caring for patients who undergo CABG must counsel them that their long-term prognosis is dependent on their own actions as well as the treatment prescribed by their physicians.

As shown in Table 31.1, the major risk factors for CAD—hypertension, cigarette smoking, and hypercholesterolemia—are present in a high percentage of patients who undergo CABG. In these data from the Coronary Artery Surgery Study (CASS) (1), it is also clear that those risk factors are essentially unchanged 5 years after CABG! This dismal record presents a critical challenge for physicians caring for patients who undergo CABG. It is far easier to prescribe drugs than it is to counsel patients about changes in life-style, but the dividends of changes in life-style are immense and justify the effort. The positive benefits are particularly great in young patients who undergo CABG.

CIGARETTE SMOKING

The fact that cigarette smoking is a risk factor for CAD is undisputed (2). The relative risk of CAD death in those smoking one pack a day or more is 2 times higher than in nonsmokers (3). The coronary event most clearly related to cigarette smoking is sudden cardiac death. In the Framingham study (4), the relative risk of sudden cardiac death in those smoking one pack

TABLE 31.1

PERSISTENCE OF RISK (A1) FACTORS 5 YEARS AFTER CABG[a]

Risk Factor	Before Surgery	5 Years after CABG
	%	%
Cholesterol ≥ 250 mg/dl	32	40
Cigarette smoking	39	31
Systolic pressure ≥ 160 mm Hg	6.7	11.2
Diastolic pressure ≥ 100 mm Hg	8.5	7.5
Overweight (≥115% age-, sex-, height-adjusted weight)	21	25

[a]Data from Coronary Artery Surgery Study (CASS): A randomized trial of coronary artery bypass surgery. *Circulation* 68:951–960,1983.

per day or more was 3 times higher than in nonsmokers.

Despite the wealth of data linking cigarette smoking to coronary artery disease, patients with documented CAD continue to smoke. In the CASS study of 14,517 patients with CAD documented by angiography between 1975 and 1977, 50% were current smokers, 30% had stopped smoking in the year prior to angiography, and only 20% had never smoked (5). Furthermore, more than 30% of patients continued to smoke 5 years after CABG.

The impact of continued cigarette smoking in patients with documented CAD is well established. In the CASS (5), the total mortality at 5 years was 15.7% in those who quit smoking after angiography, compared to 20.5% in those who continued to smoke (relative risk = 1.55, P < .001). Sudden cardiac death was nearly twice as frequent in those who continued to smoke.

Follow-up studies of patients who survive hospitalization for acute myocardial infarction (MI) or unstable angina have shown similar results. Daly and coworkers (6) followed 498 male smokers under age 60 who survived hospitlization for unstable angina or acute MI. At an average follow-up of 7.4 years, the mortality in those who quit smoking was 36%, compared to 82% in those who did not quit (relative risk = 2.4, P < .01).

Aberg and coworkers (7) followed 1,306 men after their first myocardial infarction. At the time of infarction 78% were smokers. Three months after infarction, 55% had stopped smoking, and 45% continued. At follow-up, after 10.5 years, the total mortality was 18% in those who quit, compared to 29% in those who continued to smoke (P < .001). The difference in mortality was most marked in men younger than 50 years, for whom the mortality was 10% in those who quit compared to 22% in those continuing to smoke (P < .02).

Although there are no randomized trials of the impact of quitting cigarette smoking after acute MI, these and other observational studies indicate that the relative risk of death in those who continue to smoke cigarettes after acute MI is approximately 2.0 (8). The IFSC Scientific Councils on Arteriosclerosis (9) estimate that the risk of fatal CAD in patients with a history of MI can be reduced by 20 to 50% by discontinuing cigarette smoking.

The benefits of smoking cessation in patients with established CAD may be due to an impact on the rate of progression of atherosclerosis in the native coronary circulation or in saphenous vein bypass grafts. The rapid onset of the decrease in risk of coronary death suggests that the benefits of smoking cessation may also be related to the impact of nicotine on coronary spasm, platelet function, and arrhythmias (8).

Physicians caring for patients undergoing CABG have an important obligation to counsel them with regard to smoking. It is important for the surgeon to explain that cessation of cigarette smoking is an important part of the treatment plan, and that continuing smoking will jeopardize the benefits of CABG. Physicians who intervene with smokers can have a very definite impact (10). Intervention must include counseling by the physician and should be supplemented by self-help booklets and, in some patients, treatment with nicotine-containing chewing gum. The cessation rates with nicotine-containing gum are doubled when physicians instruct patients on the use of the gum and provide follow-up counseling (11).

In patients who continue to smoke cigarettes

despite intensive intervention, it may be appropriate to advise a switch to pipe smoking. Hickey and coworkers (12) noted a better prognosis in survivors of acute MI who switched to a pipe than in those who continued to smoke cigarettes. In patients who switch from cigarettes to a pipe, it is important to monitor carboxyhemoglobin levels to make certain that the pipe smoke is not being inhaled (13).

Of all the potential interventions that might be prescribed for the patient who has undergone CABG, few have more benefit than cessation of cigarette smoking.

WEIGHT REDUCTION

In the eyes of many patients, being overweight is the most important risk factor for CAD. The evidence that obesity is an independent risk factor is minimal; however, obesity contributes to hypertension and hyperlipidemia and therefore indirectly contributes to an increased risk of CAD.

There are many reasons why CABG patients who are overweight should be counseled to lose weight. Weight reduction is the most visible sign of a change in life-style. Overweight patients who are successful in losing weight feel better, and may therefore be more successful in making other critical changes in their life-styles. Attention to their weight can help them to adhere to dietary changes aimed at reducing cholesterol levels. In hypertensive patients, weight reduction is a important part of their treatment that may reduce the need for antihypertensive medication.

In patients who are cigarette smokers, cessation of cigarette smoking should be given priority over weight reduction because of its more immediate impact on prognosis. Few patients can be successful at cessation of smoking and weight reduction at the same time. They should be counseled that first they must discontinue smoking, then weight reduction can be achieved even if they gain weight after stopping smoking.

Maintenance of ideal weight reinforces patients' confidence that they can make other changes in life-style that will have a positive impact on their future health.

LIPIDS

Epidemiologic studies performed over the past 3 decades have established that elevated serum cholesterol levels are associated with an increased risk of coronary atherosclerosis (14). More recent studies have demonstrated that the risk of CAD increases with increased levels of LDL cholesterol, but decreases as HDL cholesterol level increases and as the ratio of HDL to LDL or HDL to total cholesterol increases (15). Elevated cholesterol levels can be decreased by dietary intervention or by the use of a variety of lipid-lowering drugs.

Despite these facts, it has been difficult to demonstrate that lowering serum cholesterol levels in patients with established CAD decreases coronary heart disease mortality. May and coworkers (16) reviewed nine randomized trials with lipid-lowering drugs or diet or both in survivors of MI. The reduction in serum cholesterol levels in these trials ranged from 6.5 to 20%. Patients were not selected for these trials on the basis of elevated serum cholesterol. At an average follow-up of 5 years, no significant decreases in coronary or total mortality were noted. However, two recent trials in which patients were selected for intervention because of elevated lipid levels gave very positive results (17, 18).

The Lipid Research Clinics Coronary Primary Prevention Trial (LRC-CPPT) was the first randomized double-blind clinical trial to establish that lowering cholesterol levels reduces the risk of coronary heart disease (17). A total of 3806 asymptomatic men aged 35 to 59 with a plasma cholesterol of 265 mg/dl or greater were randomized to a lipid-lowering diet plus cholestyramine (24 gm/day) or diet plus placebo. They were followed for 7 to 10 years. The reduction in total cholesterol was 13.4% and the reduction in LDL cholesterol was 20.3% in the group treated with diet plus cholestyramine. In addition, there was a 2.4% increase in HDL cholesterol in the cholestyramine group. The cholestyramine group had a 19% reduction in the primary end point: definite coronary heart disease death or definite nonfatal MI (P < .05). In addition, the incidence of angina, coronary bypass surgery, and new positive exercise test were lower in patients treated with cholestyramine. There was no significant difference in the risk of death from all causes in the two groups. There were fewer deaths due to coronary heart disease in the cholestyramine-treated patients but a larger number of deaths due to accidents and violence. The number of cancer deaths was the same in the two groups. When the degree of reduction in total cholesterol in the cholestyramine group was compared to the incidence of coronary heart disease, it was determined that each 1% decrease in total cholesterol was accompanied by a 2% decrease in the incidence of coronary heart disease (19). This finding was consistent with earlier predictions based on epidemiologic observations (19). The LRC-CPPT trial makes it abundantly clear that reducing levels of total cholesterol and LDL cholesterol reduces the risk of fatal and nonfatal coronary heart disease.

In another major randomized clinical trial, the Helsinki Heart Study (18), aysmptomatic men aged 40 to 55 who had total non-HDL cholesterol levels 200 mg/dl or higher received gemfibrozil (600 mg/day) or a placebo for 5 years. Total cholesterol decreased by 8.5% from 270 mg/dl at baseline to 247 mg/dl in those treated by gemfibrozil. LDL cholesterol decreased by 8% and HDL increased by 8.7% over the 5 years of treatment. Since HDL cholesterol increased while LDL cholesterol decreased, the ratio of HDL cholesterol to total cholesterol increased from .18 to .21.

At the end of 5 years, the cumulative rate of fatal and nonfatal MI and cardiac death was 34% lower in the gemfibrozil group (P < .02). There was no significant difference in the total death rate in the two groups: 45 in the gemfibrozil, 42 in the placebo group. There were fewer (14 versus 19) cardiac deaths in the gemfibrozil group, but more deaths due to accidents and violence (10 in the gemfibrozil group versus 4 in the placebo group). The importance of the Helsinki Study is that it demonstrates that raising the levels of HDL cholesterol may have the same impact as lowering levels of LDL cholesterol. It is of note that the percentage increase in the ratio of HDL to total cholesterol increased by 17% in the Helinski Study (18) and

by 19% in the LRC-CPPT cholestyramine study (17).

The efficacy of a third cholesterol-lowering agent, niacin, has been reported by the Coronary Drug Project (CDP) Study Group (20). The CDP recruited 8341 male survivors of ECG-documented MI from 1966 to 1969. They were randomized to five treatment groups and a placebo group and were treated for an average of 6.2 years. When treatment was discontinued in 1975, there was no significant difference between total mortality in patients treated with niacin (3.0 gm/day) as compared to placebo. However, the patients treated with niacin had a lower rate of nonfatal MI than did the placebo group. The status of the participants in this trial was determined in 1983, nearly 9 years after the termination of the trial. The coronary heart disease mortality was 13% lower in the niacin group, and the total mortality was 11% lower than in the placebo group (P = .0004).

The relevance of these findings to patients undergoing CABG is quite clear. Campeau and coworkers (21) studied 82 patients 10 years after CABG. They found that the development of arteriosclerosis in saphenous vein bypass grafts and progression of disease in the native coronary circulation was related to lipid levels at baseline and at follow-up. As shown in Table 31.2, total cholesterol and LDL cholesterol levels were significantly higher (278 mg/dl versus 243 mg/dl) and the HDL levels were significantly lower (48 mg/dl versus 63 mg/dl) in patients who had progression of disease in the grafts and in the native coronary circulation.

TABLE 31.2

SERUM LIPID LEVELS 10 YEARS AFTER CABG[a]

Results of Follow-up Angiograms	No. of Patients	Total Cholesterol	LDL	HDL
		mg/dl	mg/dl	mg/dl
No new lesions	15	243	153	63
New lesions	67	278	190	48
	P value	.01	.005	.0001

[a]Data from The Lipid Research Clinics Program: The Lipid Research Clinics Coronary Primary Prevention Trial results. II. The relationship of reduction in incidence of coronary heart disease to cholesterol lowering. *JAMA* 251:365–374, 1984.

The beneficial effect of lowering cholesterol in survivors of CABG has been convincingly documented by Blankenhorn and coworkers (22). They performed a randomized trial in 162 non-smoking men aged 40 to 59 who had undergone CABG at least 3 months prior to randomization. The baseline lipid levels were: total cholesterol 244, LDL cholesterol 170, and HDL cholesterol 44 mg/dl. Both groups received dietary intervention. The treatment group received colestipol 30 gm and 3 to 12 gm of niacin daily. The response to drug treatment after 2 years was striking. Total cholesterol decreased by 26% in the drug treatment group as compared to 4% in the placebo group. LDL cholesterol decreased by 43% in the treatment group, as compared to 5% in the placebo group. HDL cholesterol increased by 37% in the drug group, 2% in the controls.

Coronary angiography was performed 2 years after treatment and compared to angiography performed at randomization. The follow-up angiograms demonstrated significantly less progression of disease in the drug treatment group. In the native vessels, the average number of lesions with increased stenosis was 1.0 in the drug treatment group and 1.4 in the placebo group (P = .03). In the grafts, the percentage of subjects with new lesions or new closures was 24% in the drug group and 39% in the placebo group (P = .03). As pointed out by Passamani (23), this study makes it clear that aggressive diet and drug therapy in survivors of CABG can lead to sustained large reductions in cholesterol levels and result in a reduced rate of development and progression of lesions in coronary arteries and saphenous vein bypass grafts.

These studies make it very clear that aggressive dietary and drug therapy in patients undergoing CABG can have a major impact on their prognosis. The past record of intervention in CABG patients is not admirable. In the CASS (1), the percentage of patients taking lipid-lowering drugs prior to CABG was 3.6. Five years after surgery, only 2.5% of the patients were taking lipid-lowering drugs. The percentage of patients with a serum cholesterol greater than 250 mg/dl prior to surgery was 32; 5 years after CABG, the percentage had increased to 40!

There are several potential explanations for this poor record. Physicians may feel unprepared to counsel patients with regard to diet, or they may be pessimistic with regard to its impact on patients with established coronary artery disease. Furthermore, the most commonly used lipid-lowering agents have multiple side effects that compromise patient compliance. In the past few years, several developments have increased the potential success rate of intervention in patients with elevated lipids. The public is far more interested in diet and its impact on cholesterol levels and on cardiovascular health. Americans are changing their dietary habits, and our society's cholesterol levels are decreasing. Physicians find patients far more receptive to dietary intervention than in the past. In addition, new, effective lipid-lowering drugs with fewer side effects are now available.

With this new public attitude toward dietary change, and with the availability of a wider array of effective drugs, the clinician is well-prepared to intervene on behalf of his or her patients. It would be difficult to find a group more appropriate for a lipid-lowering regimen than patients who have undergone CABG.

Intervention begins with diet. In some patients diet alone, without drugs, will be effective. The goal of intervention is to lower the total cholesterol to less than 200 mg/dl and LDL cholesterol to less than 130 mg/dl (24). There are no documented health hazards of maintaining a serum cholesterol level as low as 160 to 180 mg/dl (9).

The appropriate diet should restrict calories to maintain ideal weight. Saturated fat should be restricted to less than 10% of total calories, and daily cholesterol intake should be less than 250 to 300 mg/dl. A recent report from the Expert Panel on Detection, Evaluation and Treatment of High Blood Cholesterol in Adults (24) outlines a comprehensive approach to dietary intervention. In many cases, patients should be referred to a nutritionist for counseling. Follow-up cholesterol levels and reinforcement by the physician are critical.

In many cases, if not the majority, dietary intervention must be accompanied by drug therapy to reach a goal cholesterol level of less than

200 mg/dl. In selecting an appropriate lipid-lowering agent, the clinician must consider the risks as well as the benefits of the available drugs.

The bile acid–binding resins cholestyramine and colestipol have a well-established safety record. Given the fact that they are not absorbed into the systemic circulation, they are not associated with toxic systemic effects. However, these drugs have a very high incidence of GI side effects, including constipation, nausea, stomach discomfort, and heartburn. These side effects make it very difficult for patients to take the optimal dose of these agents (cholestyramine 24 gm/day, colestipol 30 gm/day). The dose must be gradually increased to optimal levels. Mineral oil is useful to prevent constipation (22). Since cholestyramine and colestipol can bind other drugs given orally, other drugs should be taken 1 hr before or 4 to 6 hr after cholestyramine or colestipol is taken. For patients who can tolerate optimal doses of these resins, total cholesterol may be lowered by 10 to 20%, LDL may be decreased by 20 to 30%, and an increase of 5% in HDL can be expected (19). These beneficial effects are well worth the extra time it takes the clinician to adjust the dose to avoid GI side effects.

Nicotinic acid (niacin) is an effective lipid-lowering agent that acts by inhibiting the production of VLDL, thereby lowering levels of VLDL and LDL cholesterol (25). It is contraindicated in patients with liver disease or active peptic ulcer disease. Its principal limitation is that it produces skin flushing and itching, which in many cases can be prevented with low-dose aspirin. To be effective, large doses of 3 to 6 gm/day are required. It should be given 3 times a day with meals. Therapy must begin with very low doses, 50 to 100 mg three times a day with gradual increases to the therapeutic dose. As with the bile acid–binding resins, it takes additional time to adjust the dose of nicotinic acid to avoid skin flushing and itching. In patients who can tolerate the optimal dose, total cholesterol and LDL cholesterol may be lowered by 15 to 30% and HDL may be increased by up to 23% (25). The combination of bile acid resins and nicotinic acid is an excellent regimen for lowering LDL and total cholesterol. In the study

reported by Blankenhorn and coworkers (22), the combination of diet, full-dose bile acid resins, and niacin lead to a decrease in total cholesterol of 26% and a decrease in LDL cholesterol of 43%.

Gemfibrozil is another lipid-lowering agent that was found to be effective in the Helsinki Study (18). In addition to lowering triglycerides by 43%, it caused a modest decrease in LDL (10%) and total cholesterol (11%). An additional beneficial effect is that it increases HDL cholesterol (10% increase in the Helsinki Study) (18), thereby increasing the HDL to total cholesterol ratio. It is contraindicated in patients with liver disease, gallbladder disease, and advanced renal disease. The optimal dose is 600 mg twice a day.

A new class of lipid-lowering agents, 3-hydroxy-3-methylglutaryl coenzyme A (HMG CoA) reductase inhibitors, inhibit cholesterol synthesis. The first of these agents to be released, lovastatin, has been shown to be extremely effective in lowering total cholesterol and LDL cholesterol at relatively low doses of 20 to 40 mg once or twice a day. In a multicenter trial, the reduction in LDL cholesterol in patients treated with lovastatin 20 mg twice a day was 32% and the reduction in total cholesterol was 27% with an increase in HDL of 9% (26).

If the clinician is willing to spend the necessary time with patients who have undergone CABG, the combination of dietary changes and the use of a variety of effective drugs can lead to a reduction in serum lipids to optimal levels (27).

HYPERTENSION

The presence of hypertension in patients undergoing CABG increases operative mortality and decreases long-term survival (28). In a series of 3479 consecutive patients having CABG, Jones and coworkers (28) defined hypertension as blood pressure elevated sufficiently to require antihypertensive medication at some time prior to CABG; they noted a prevalence of 36%. Hospital mortality for CABG in those with hypertension was 2.2% compared to 1.0% in those without hypertension ($P < .05$). In the CASS

(5) the prevalence of hypertension (defined as systolic pressure greater than 160 mm Hg or diastolic pressure greater than 100 mm Hg) prior to CABG was 7 to 9%. The incidence of hypertension 5 years after surgery was unchanged.

Randomized trials of treatment of hypertension after CABG have not been reported. However, it is clear that hypertension in patients with CAD needs to be treated just as in patients without CAD. In the Hypertension Detection and Follow-Up Program, there was a 20% reduction in total mortality in patients with a history of MI who had active treatment for hypertension (29).

In the absence of a contraindication, β-blockers are especially appropriate for the treatment of hypertension in patients with CAD because of their positive impact on prognosis (16). Calcium channel blockers are also useful, whereas diuretics are less appropriate because of their negative impact on serum lipid profiles (30). Exercise, weight reduction, and restriction of sodium and alcohol are also important aspects of the treatment for hypertension in the CABG patient (31).

EXERCISE

An increased risk of premature CAD in sedentary as opposed to physically active individuals has been demonstrated in many epidemiologic studies (32). Despite these studies, it is difficult to demonstrate a decrease in CAD mortality in randomized exercise trials (16). Randomized trials of exercise are difficult to perform because of dropouts and suboptimal compliance, and are difficult to interpret because of the potential impact of exercise on the other coronary risk factors: cigarette smoking, diet, blood pressure, and lipids. Furthermore, the reported trials have usually had a sample size too small to demonstrate a treatment effect. In a review of the reported exercise trials in CAD patients, Siegel and coworkers (33) reported a significant reduction in mortality in the pooled results.

Although it is difficult to document a decreased mortality in CAD patients who exercise regularly, the benefits to the individual patient are clear. Exercise has a positive impact on the mood of CAD patients; their sense of well-being is enhanced. The positive psychological benefits of regular exercise make it an ideal focal point in cardiac rehabilitation programs. Regular exercise helps the cardiac patient to deal with other needed behavioral changes—weight reduction, following a reduced lipid diet, and cessation of cigarette smoking.

Exercise for the patient undergoing CABG should begin with a phase I cardiac rehabilitation program in the early postoperative period (34). This supervised program permits assessment of an appropriate target heart rate. Following discharge, a phase II program should be continued on an outpatient basis for 8 to 16 weeks. This program consists of three to four sessions per week with exercise at 50 to 70% of functional aerobic capacity for 15 min progressing to 30 to 60 min per session.

A phase III exercise program of walking or bicycling is ideally performed in a supervised, monitored community center such as a YMCA or university campus. The eventual goal of an exercise program for the CABG patient is three to four sessions per week for 45 min at an intensity of 70 to 85% of functional capacity (34). After completion of the phase III program, the patient can continue the program on his or her own with follow-up by his or her physician.

The favorable impact of CABG can be markedly enhanced if patients can make changes in life-style that will modify CAD risk factors. With the help of their physicians, patients can make these changes and thereby greatly enhance their long-term prognoses.

References

1. Coronary Artery Surgery Study (CASS): A randomized trial of coronary artery bypass surgery. *Circulation* 68:951–960, 1983.
2. United States Public Health Service: *The Health Consequences of Smoking: A Reference Edition.* Atlanta, GA, Publication No. (CDC) 78:8357.
3. Kannel WB, McGee D, Gordon T: A general cardiovascular risk profile: the Framingham Study. *Am J Cardiol* 38:46, 1976.
4. Kannel WB, Thomas HE Jr: Sudden coronary death: the Framingham Study. *Ann NY Acad Sci* 382:3–21, 1982.
5. Vlietstra MB, Kronmal RA, Oberman A, et al:

Effect of cigarette smoking on survival of patients with angiographically documented coronary artery disease. *JAMA* 255:1023–1027, 1986.

6. Daly LE, Mulcahy R, Graham IM, et al: Long term effect on mortality of stopping smoking after unstable angina and myocardial infarction. *Br Med J* 287:324–326, 1983.

7. Aberg A, Bergstrand R, Johansson S, et al: Cessation of smoking after myocardial infarction—effects on mortality after 10 years. *Br Heart J* 49:416–422, 1983.

8. Mulcahy R: Influence of cigarette smoking on morbidity and mortality after myocardial infarction. *Br Heart J* 49:410–415, 1983.

9. Joint Recommendations by the ISFC Scientific Councils on Arteriosclerosis: Secondary prevention in myocardial infarction survivors. *Circulation* 65(I):216A–219A, 1982.

10. Ockene JK: Physician-delivered interventions for smoking cessation: strategies for increasing effectiveness. *Prev Med* 16:723–737, 1987.

11. Wilson D, Best A, Lindsay-McIntyre E, et al: Can training family practice physicians improve compliance with nicotine gum use? In Ockene JK (ed): *The Pharmacologic Treatment of Tobacco Dependence: Proceedings of the World Congress, Nov. 4–5, 1985.* Cambridge, MA, Institute for the Study of Smoking Behavior and Policy, 1986.

12. Hickey N, Risteard M, Daly L, et al: Cigar and pipe smoking related to four year survival of coronary patients. *Br Heart J* 49:423–426, 1983.

13. Ockene JK, Goldberg RJ, Dalen JE: Pipes, cigars and cardiovascular health. *Cardiovasc Med* 10:53–55, 1985.

14. The Pooling Project Research Group: Relationship of blood pressure, serum cholesterol, smoking habit, relative weight and ECG abnormalities to incidence of major coronary events: final report of the Pooling Project. *J Chron Dis* 31:201–306, 1978.

15. Gordon T, Castelli WP, Hjortland MC, et al: High density lipoprotein as a protective factor against coronary heart disease. *Am J Med* 62:707–714, 1977.

16. May GS, Eberlein KA, Furberg CD, et al: Secondary prevention after myocardial infarction: a review of long-term trials. *Prog Cardiovasc Dis* 24:331–350, 1982.

17. The Lipid Research Clinics Program: The Lipid Research Clinics Coronary Primary Prevention Trial results: I. Reduction in incidence of coronary heart disease. *JAMA* 251:351–364, 1984.

18. Frick MH, Elo O, Haapa K, et al: Helsinki Heart Study: primary-prevention trial with gemfibrozil in middle-aged men with dyslipidemia. *N Engl J Med* 317:1237–1245, 1987.

19. The Lipid Research Clinics Program: The Lipid Research Clinics Coronary Primary Prevention Trial results. II. The relationship of reduction in incidence of coronary heart disease to cholesterol lowering. *JAMA* 251:365–374, 1984.

20. Canner PL, Berge KG, Wenger NK, et al: Fifteen year mortality in Coronary Drug Project patients: Long-term benefit with niacin. *J Am Coll Cardiol* 8:1245–1255, 1986.

21. Campeau L, Enjalbert M, Lesperance J, et al: The relation of risk factors to the development of atherosclerosis in saphenous-vein bypass grafts and the progression of disease in the native circulation. *N Engl J Med* 311:1329–1332, 1984.

22. Blankenhorn DH, Nessim SA, Johnson RL, et al: Beneficial effects of combined colestipol-niacin therapy on coronary atherosclerosis and coronary venous bypass grafts. *JAMA* 257:3233–3240, 1987.

23. Passamani ER: Cholesterol reduction in coronary artery bypass patients. *JAMA* 257:3271–3272, 1987.

24. The Expert Panel: Report of the national cholesterol education program expert panel on detection, evaluation, and treatment of high blood cholesterol in adults. *Arch Intern Med* 148:36–69, 1988.

25. Shepherd J, Packard CJ, Patsch JR, et al: Effects of nicotinic acid therapy on plasma high density lipoprotein subfraction distribution and composition and on apolipoprotein A metabolism. *J Clin Invest* 63:858–867, 1979.

26. The Lovastatin Study Group III: A multicenter comparison of lovastatin and cholestyramine therapy for severe primary hypercholesterolemia. *JAMA* 260:359–366, 1988.

27. Dalen JE: Lowering serum cholesterol. *Arch Intern Med* 148:34–35, 1988.

28. Jones EL, Hurst JW, King SB III, et al: Clinical factors influencing survival and adequacy of revascularization after coronary bypass operation. *Int J Cardiol* 2:109–123, 1982.

29. Langford HG, Stamler J, Wassertheil-Smoller S, et al: All-cause mortality in the Hypertension Detection and Follow-Up Program: findings for the whole cohort and for persons with less severe hypertension, with and without other traits related to risk of mortality. *Prog Cardiovasc Dis* 29(1):29–54, 1986.

30. Johnson BF, Saunders R, Hickler R, et al: The effects of thiazide diuretics upon plasma lipoproteins. *J Hypertens* 4:235–239, 1986.

31. Stamler R, Stamler J, Grimm R, et al: Nutritional therapy for high blood pressure. *JAMA* 257:1484–1491, 1987.

32. Rippe JM, Ward A, Porcari JP, et al: Walking for health and fitness. *JAMA* 259:2720–2724, 1988.

33. Siegel D, Grady D, Browner WS, et al: Risk factor modification after myocardial infarction. *Ann Intern Med* 109:213–218, 1988.

34. Ward A, Malloy P, Rippe J: Exercise prescription guidelines for normal and cardiac populations. *Cardiol Clin* 5:197–210, 1987.

Chapter 32
FOLLOW-UP AFTER VALVE REPLACEMENT

STEVEN S. KHAN, M.D.
LAWRENCE S. C. CZER, M.D.

The replacement of an abnormal native valve with a prosthetic valve can be considered the substitution of one disease process for another. Instead of the patient's outcome being determined by the natural history of his or her valve disease (e.g., aortic stenosis), the patient assumes the risks of thromboembolism, anticoagulation-related hemorrhage, valve thrombosis, and mechanical valve failure associated with his or her valve. It is therefore important for the physician caring for patients with prosthetic valves to be familiar with specific problems associated with specific valves in addition to more general aspects of the care of patients after valve replacement. Thus, a change in heart sounds over the first few weeks after implantation may occur normally with one type of valve and may represent thrombosis of the valve with another. This section will discuss details of the clinical follow-up of patients with prosthetic valves and present guidelines for the use and interpretation of more invasive studies.

ROUTINE FOLLOW-UP OF PATIENTS FOLLOWING VALVE REPLACEMENT

Early Postoperative Follow-up

Patients should be seen by their primary physician between 7 and 10 days after surgery. The purpose of this initial visit is to ensure that the patient is continuing to do well, that his or her incisions are healing normally, and that all laboratory values are normal or are returning toward normal. The physician should therefore perform a brief history, a goal-directed physical examination, a chest x-ray, ECG, and routine laboratory studies (for example, electrolytes, creatinine, blood count, and, if the patient is receiving Coumadin, a prothrombin time). If the patient is receiving iron supplementation, it can be stopped at this visit if the hematocrit has returned to normal. Many patients will have a small or moderate pleural effusion at this visit that will require thoracentesis only if the patient is symptomatic or if the effusion is large (occupying more than one-third of the chest on a standard PA film), causes dyspnea, or results in hypoxemia.

If there are no problems at the first visit the patient is usually seen again at 4 to 6 weeks (with interim visits to check the prothrombin time as needed). At this second visit, the goal is to begin returning the patient to a normal life. If examination of the sternum reveals that it is healing properly, the patient is allowed to resume driving a car (barring other problems such as visual difficulties or arrhythmias test). The patient is encouraged to begin a regular exercise program, and a treadmill test may be performed to evaluate exercise tolerance, particularly if there is concomitant coronary artery disease. Digoxin or quinidine therapy can usually be stopped at this point if it was begun after surgery for perioperative atrial fibrillation or flutter. The patient should be advised to avoid lifting heavy weights (over 15 lb) and to avoid playing tennis or a full round of golf until 3 months after surgery. Avid golfers can usually begin putting and chipping at 6 weeks, however.

Chronic Follow-up

Frequency. It is impossible to make universal recommendations for the frequency of long-term follow-up since each patient has unique problems. As a general guideline, however, patients should be seen at least once every 3 to 4 months in the 1st year after surgery and at least every 6 months afterward (Table 32.1). Patients receiving Coumadin should have prothrombin times drawn monthly but do not have to be examined more frequently. Most patients can have their blood drawn at a laboratory and have their Coumadin doses adjusted by telephone. For patients who have received porcine valves the frequency of follow-up should increase as the patient nears the eighth anniversary of his or her valve replacement to at least one visit every 3 or 4 months.

History. The patient who is being seen for a routine follow-up should be questioned carefully about bleeding complications and symptoms of thromboemboli. Functional class should be determined by asking about specific tasks such as the number of stairs that can be climbed or the distance that can be walked without stopping. The Canadian Heart Association classification system provides more specific guidelines for determining a patient's functional class and therefore may be preferable to the New York Heart Association classification system for serial evaluation of patients.

If the patient is receiving Coumadin, he or she should be questioned about any particular bleeding complications such as blood in the urine or stool. Easy bruising is a common complaint, and, if the prothrombin time is within the recommended range, the patient should be simply reassured. Women of childbearing age who are receiving Coumadin should have a brief menstrual history taken, and, if pregnancy is suspected, Coumadin should be withheld pending the results of a pregnancy test. Coumadin is teratogenic and patients should be counseled that it is contraindicated in the 1st trimester of pregnancy. If a patient's prothrombin time is difficult to control, careful inquiry should be made about the patient's compliance with the prescribed Coumadin regimen. The patient's diet should also be investigated and any over-the-counter drug use determined. (Foods and medications that may interact with Coumadin are listed in Table 19.1.)

Classic symptoms of thromboemboli are significantly less frequent than the actual occurrence of emboli, and patients should therefore be questioned about unexplained episodes of dizziness, loss of memory, or the sudden occur-

TABLE 32.1

RECOMMENDATIONS FOR ROUTINE FOLLOW-UP AFTER VALVE REPLACEMENT

	Initial Postop Visit	Second Visit	First Visit	2nd to 8th Year	After 8th Year (Porcine Valves Only)
Timing of visits	7–10 days postop	2–4 weeks	Every 2–3 mo	Every 4–6 mo	Every 3–4 mo
History & physical	X	X	X	X	X
ECG	X			← ---------------Yearly --------------- →	
Chest x-ray	X			← ---------------Yearly --------------- →	
Laboratory tests[a]	X			← -----------Twice yearly ------------ →	
Echo/Doppler		X		← ---Yearly --- →	

[a]A minimum of CBC to evaluate for hemolysis, and electrolytes, BUN and creatinine if on diuretics. Other tests as appropriate. Prothrombin time should be tested monthly in patients on Coumadin.

rence of abdominal or peripheral pain and is-chemia, in addition to standard questions about episodes of unilateral loss of vision, amaurosis fugax, transient weakness or numbness in an extremity, or difficulty with speech. In the authors' experience with the St. Jude bileaflet valve, the majority (57%) of clinically evident thromboembolic events have been transient (1). In our series, valve location had no effect on the incidence of emboli, although several studies have suggested that other prosthetic valves have higher embolic rates when in the mitral position.

Physical Examination. The cardiac findings in patients with prosthetic valves will vary with the type and location of the valve. Although much has been written about the phonocardiographic findings in these patients, this discussion will focus on the findings evident to the clinician on auscultation.

Bioprosthetic valves produce heart sounds that are quite similar to those of normal valves. One-half to two-thirds of patients with mitral porcine valves will have a soft apical rumble (2) since most porcine valves are mildly to moderately stenotic. The diagnosis of stenosis of a porcine mitral valve is therefore dependent on a change in the quality of the diastolic murmur or the development of a new murmur in a patient previously known not to have one. Although normal porcine mitral valves are not associated with significant mitral regurgitation, patients can develop a normal systolic murmur after valve replacement, which has been attributed to the presence of the valve struts in the aortic outflow tract. Thus, in patients with a porcine mitral valve, the simple presence of either a systolic or a diastolic murmur does not indicate valve dysfunction; to reach this conclusion a change in the quality of a murmur or the development of a new murmur is required.

Porcine aortic valves also have opening and closing sounds that are similar to those of a normal valve. Since they are mildly to moderately stenotic, a systolic flow murmur will nearly always be present. However, since regurgitation does not occur with normal bioprosthetic valves, there should not be a diastolic murmur of aortic regurgitation. The finding of an apical blowing

diastolic murmur in these patients therefore requires investigation.

Ball valves, such as the Starr-Edwards valve, produce loud clicking heart sounds that can be audible in some patients from several feet away. Ball valves can be significantly obstructive and frequently produce loud murmurs in the aortic position, occasionally with an associated carotid shudder. These valves also should not produce significant regurgitation, and the presence of a diastolic murmur suggests paravalvular leak or significant valve dysfunction. In contrast to the frequent systolic flow murmur of aortic ball valves, mitral ball valves rarely produce diastolic rumbles. A mid-diastolic rumble in a patient with a mitral ball valve therefore suggests prosthetic valve stenosis. Another sign of prosthetic mitral valve stenosis is shortening of the interval between A2 and the mitral opening sound in a manner analogous to the shortening of the A2-OS interval in stenosis of native mitral valves. This is thought to be due to progressive elevation of left atrial pressure, resulting in earlier opening of the mitral valve relative to isovolumetric relaxation. A systolic murmur may also be heard in patients with mitral ball valves in the absence of mitral regurgitation and is thought to be due to aortic outflow tract obstruction by the struts of the valve.

The valve opening sounds in patients with standard disc valves (such as the Bjork-Shiley and the Medtronic-Hall valves) may be difficult to hear since the discs are lightweight and nonmetallic and do not strike any resonant structures during opening. In contrast to mitral ball valves, mitral disc valves frequently produce audible diastolic rumbles. The greater frequency of diastolic rumbles with disc valves is not due to higher gradients since recorded gradients are similar in both disc and ball valves. Instead, the preferential direction of flow through the major orifice of a disc valve may be more likely to produce audible sounds, whereas the more symmetric flow of ball valves may be less likely to produce an audible rumble. The mitral closing sound is usually easily audible with disc valves, and softening or absence of a mitral closing sound suggests that disc closure may be impaired by either thrombus or tissue ingrowth.

Aortic disc valves produce similar findings: a soft opening sound and prominent closing sounds. Softening of the closing sound of an aortic disc valve should also suggest valve dysfunction. A systolic flow murmur is virtually always present and does not indicate valve abnormality. Diastolic murmurs may occasionally be heard with normal aortic disc valves and do not mean that a paravalvular leak is present. The key to diagnosing aortic disc valve dysfunction on physical examination is therefore the detection of a change in the quality of a murmur or closing sound.

The St. Jude bileaflet valve may produce a unique spectrum of heart sounds. Early after valve replacement, the heart sounds may be difficult to distinguish from those of normal native valves. Over the ensuing week, however, the heart sounds tend to become sharper and the second heart sound in particular becomes more distinctly prosthetic. Although the normal St. Jude aortic valve is associated with mild regurgitation on Doppler examination, the murmur of aortic regurgitation is not normally audible. Since the St. Jude valve is substantially less obstructive than the Starr-Edwards valve, the systolic aortic outflow murmur is usually soft and may not be audible. The St. Jude valve in the mitral position produces a high-frequency closing click but infrequently produces a diastolic rumble. Multiple clicks may occasionally be heard and may be due to the valve leaflets drifting open in late diastole followed by reclosure as the left atrial and ventricular pressures equalize. Muffling of previously audible prosthetic closure or an increase in the intensity of a transprosthetic murmur suggests valve thrombosis (3).

Laboratory Follow-up

Patients seen in routine follow-up after valve replacement will require regular prothrombin times if they are receiving Coumadin. Prothrombin times can usually be safely evaluated once a month (every 4 to 6 weeks) after the patient's dosage has been stabilized. Patients should be instructed to report any new medications, whether obtained over the counter or by prescription from another doctor. If the pa-

tient reports that he or she is taking or will begin a new medicine, the prothrombin time may need to be evaluated more frequently. Table 19.1 lists medications that interact with Coumadin. If the patient is to begin taking a medication that has a significant interaction with Coumadin, it may be prudent to lower the Coumadin dosage before beginning the new medication. The patient should also be asked to avoid (or at least report) major dietary changes. If new medications are added that interact with Coumadin or if dietary changes have occurred that could affect vitamin K intake or metabolism (see Chapter 19) the prothrombin time should be checked within a week of the change. If the drug interaction is highly significant, the prothrombin time may need to be measured as frequently as every other or every 3rd day until the dosage has again stabilized.

The hematocrit should be checked if symptoms or signs suggestive of anemia develop, particularly since hemolysis may be an early sign of valve failure or paravalvular leak. If the hematocrit is found to have fallen, the primary differential is between occult blood loss and hemolysis. A Hemoccult test or stool guaiac should be done in the office to rule out subclinical gastrointestinal bleeding. If this is negative, laboratory tests should be done to evaluate the patient for hemolysis, including a serum LDH, a total and direct bilirubin, a reticulocyte count, a peripheral blood smear for schistocytes or other forms suggestive of a microangiopathic hemolytic anemia, and urine for hemosiderin (a breakdown product of hemoglobin). An elevated LDH or serum indirect bilirubin, the presence of hemosiderin in the urine, or the presence of schistocytes on the peripheral smear all suggest that hemolysis is present. If hemolysis is suspected on the basis of these tests, the valve should be carefully evaluated with Doppler examination, preferably color flow Doppler if available, while other factors that might be responsible for hemolysis are evaluated.

It should be noted that hemolysis due to a leaking or deteriorating valve does not require valve replacement per se. If the hemolysis does not result in significant anemia or can otherwise be controlled and the valve abnormality does not compromise the patient's hemodynamic status significantly, the patient can be watched closely and managed medically (i.e., with iron supplementation as needed).

Electrocardiograms. A routine electrocardiogram should be performed in the 1st month after valve replacement. In long-term follow-up, however, routine electrocardiograms are not essential. Their most cost-effective use is in diagnosing specific problems. It should be noted that patients who develop isolated left or right bundle-branch block postoperatively may have late resolution of this abnormality on follow-up electrocardiograms. If this is the case, it does not indicate that a new cardiac event has occurred. Resolution of AV block in patients with aortic valve disease may also occur after aortic valve replacement and appears to be more common in patients with aortic regurgitation. AV block is less likely to resolve in patients with calcific aortic stenosis. Patients who develop angina postoperatively should be evaluated with electrocardiograms. If simultaneous bypass surgery has been performed with the valve replacement, a treadmill test, possibly with thallium, should be performed. In patients without a preoperative history of coronary artery disease, the possibility of coronary emboli should be considered.

Chest x-Rays. The chest x-ray should be checked in the first 2 weeks after surgery to ensure that the usual postoperative pleural effusions have resolved. Infrequently, a patient will continue to have a large postoperative effusion several weeks after surgery, which will require thoracentesis. These effusions are usually bloody and, if they are larger than about one-third of the lung field on the PA chest film, should be removed to avoid the formation of a chronic fibrothorax. The postoperative chest film will always demonstrate sternal wires and possibly clips or rings at the origin of vein grafts. As with electrocardiograms, chest x-rays should be performed for specific indications or to answer specific questions; they provide little information when performed on a routine basis. Occasionally, a patient will be seen in follow-up without a record of the type of valve implanted. A simple PA chest x-ray can provide significant information about the type of valve

implanted and may allow precise identification. For example, if a patient has had a porcine valve implanted that has stents visible on the chest x-ray it is probably a Carpentier-Edwards valve. If stents are not visible it is probably a Hancock valve. Several atlases of the x-ray appearance of both common and uncommon valves have been published (4, 5). Photographs of some commonly implanted valves are shown in Figure 32.1.

Echocardiographic and Doppler Follow-up

The conventional echocardiographic assessment of prosthetic valves is frequently technically difficult, at least partially because of interference of the prosthetic valves with the echocardiographic signal. Metal and nontissue structures in the valve cause significant shadowing artifact on the two-dimensional echocardiogram and may preclude any specific diagnosis. In one study of 17 abnormal valves, two-dimensional echocardiography revealed no abnormalities in any of the 10 mechanical valves and was abnormal in only three of seven tissue valves (6). This suggests that two-dimensional echocardiographic evaluation alone has limitations even for evaluating bioprosthetic valves. If the quality of the image is good enough, however, the orifice area of bioprosthetic mitral valves can be determined by planimetry of the orifice as in native mitral stenosis. For porcine aortic valves, the two-dimensional echo provides little quantitative information in the evaluation of stenosis, although a rough idea can be obtained about the mobility of the valve leaflets and the presence of ventricular hypertrophy. For regurgitant lesions two-dimensional echo provides essentially no quantitative information, although chamber sizes can be determined and followed sequentially. A recent review has summarized M-mode and two-dimensional echocardiographic findings in normal and abnormal prosthetic valves (7).

The development of Doppler echocardiography has provided significantly better sensitivity in detecting prosthetic valve dysfunction than two-dimensional echocardiography (8). Doppler echocardiography measures the velocity of blood flowing through the chambers of the heart by measuring changes in the frequency of sound

FIGURE 32.1

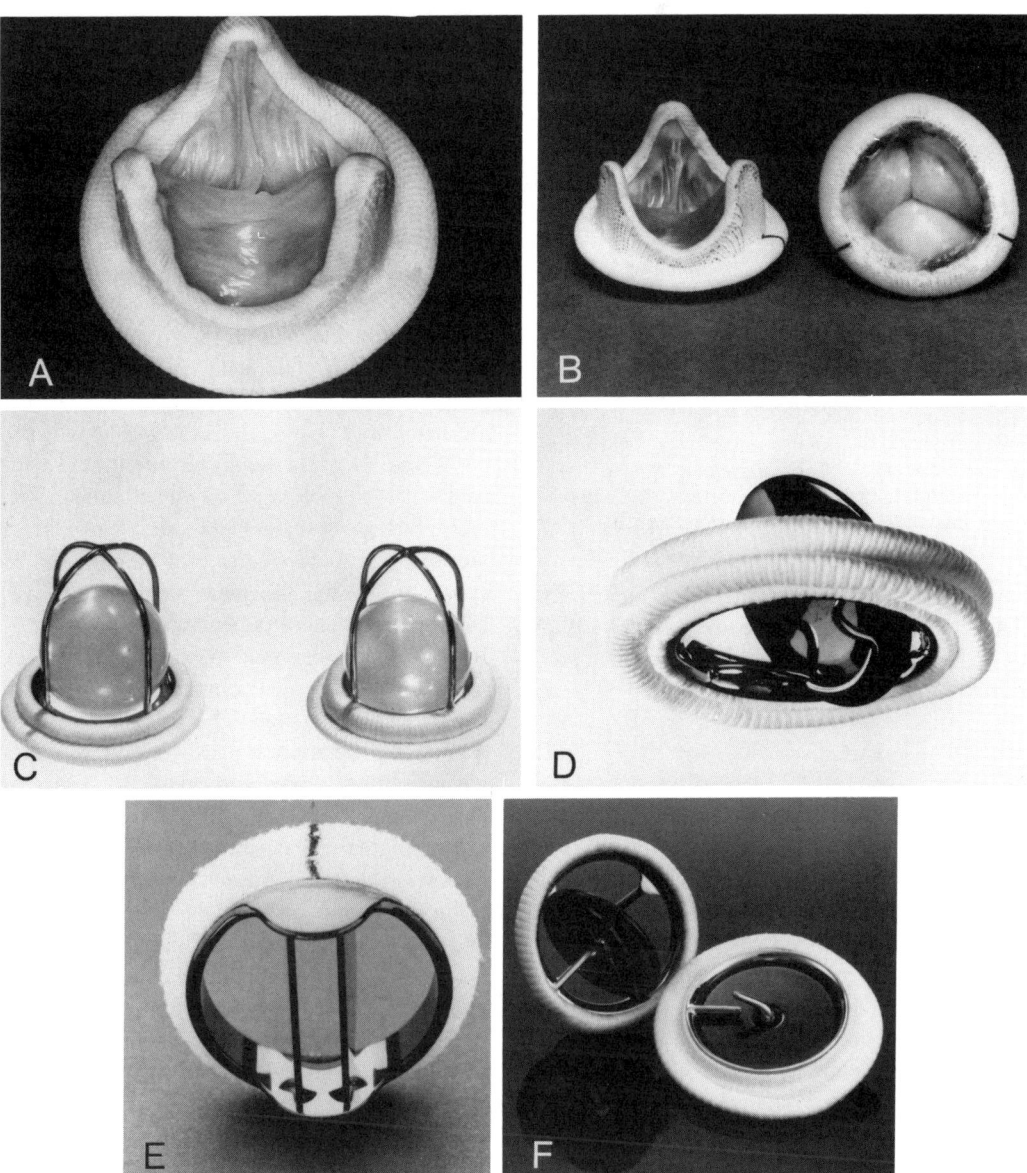

Photographs of commonly encountered valves. The top row shows the two most commonly implanted bioprosthetic valves, the Hancock II model 59 porcine bioprosthesis (**A**) and the Carpentier-Edwards bioprosthesis (**B**). These two valves can be distinguished on chest x-ray by the presence of radiopaque stents (the small metal projections supporting the leaflets) in the Carpentier-Edwards valve. The second row shows the two basic types of mechanical valve that are used—ball valves and disc valves: the Starr-Edwards ball valve (model 6000 on the left and 6120 on the right) (**C**) and the Bjork-Shiley disc valve (standard disc model) (**D**). The bottom row shows two of the newer generation disc valves, which appear to have superior hemodynamics compared to older models: the St. Jude dual disc valve (**E**) and the Medtronic-Hall disc valve. (**F**).

FIGURE 32.2

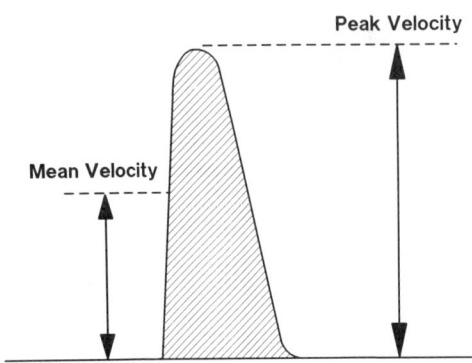

Mean versus peak Doppler velocities. This tracing is a schematic representation of a Doppler recording of flow across an aortic prosthesis. The Doppler tracing represents a record of the instantaneous flow velocity across the valve versus time. The *peak velocity* is measured as the height of the tracing. The *mean velocity* is the average area under the curve (the *shaded area*).

waves reflected from flowing blood (Fig. 32.2). The pressure gradient due to acceleration of flow across a prosthetic valve can calculated using the formula:

$$\text{Pressure gradient} = 4(V_2^2 - V_1^2) \quad (1)$$

where V_2 is velocity measured at the prosthetic orifice (position 2) and V_1 the velocity proximal to it (position 1). The velocity term V_1 may be ignored for mitral but not aortic prostheses (9).

Mean Doppler-derived gradients correlate well with mean gradients measured at separate times (10, 11) and during simultaneous catheterization (12). It is important to note, though, that many echocardiography laboratories report only the peak gradient. This may lead to misinterpretation since the instantaneous peak Doppler gradient will significantly overestimate the mean gradient and will also be higher than the peak-to-peak gradient measured at catheterization. Peak Doppler velocities as high as 4 m/second (corresponding to a peak gradient of 64 mm Hg) have been reported in normal prosthetic aortic valves (13). There is also evidence that the peak gradient from Doppler may overestimate the maximum instantaneous gradient in Starr-Edwards aortic valves (14), although these data are not from simultaneous measurements. In this study the overestimation by Doppler (mean, 22 mm Hg) persisted after correction for the left ventricle outflow tract velocity. In part, this may be due to the phenomenon of pressure recovery downstream to the prosthesis, which would lead to a lower gradient by catheter measurements than by Doppler. Thus, the peak gradient may be misleading and should not be used to judge prosthetic valve function; the mean gradient obtained is more reliable and correlates better with catheterization measurements for prosthetic valves. Normal values for both mean and peak gradients measured by continuous-wave Doppler are given by several authors (13, 15, 16). Normal Doppler for velocities for porcine, Bjork-Shiley, and St. Jude valves are listed in Table 32.2. As noted above, the peak gradient data should be interpreted with caution. It should be noted that the mean gradient has to be calculated using the correct method; specifically, it cannot be obtained by simply measuring the mean velocity and calculating the mean gradient using Equation 1. Instead Equation 1 must be calculated at each point on the Doppler tracing and the mean of these values calculated. This calculation is best done using the analysis packages on most Doppler machines, since hand calculation from paper tracings is tedious.

Valve area can be measured with a combination of Doppler and echo measurements by using the continuity equation (17, 18). In this calculation, the area and velocity are measured at a point distant from the valve and the velocity is measured at the valve itself. If there is no loss of blood between the two points, the flow (velocity times area) should be the same at both points. The area at the valve can therefore be calculated. In many echo laboratories this calculation is not done routinely but will usually be performed if asked for. Although there are several papers validating this method for native valves, it has not been applied systematically to prosthetic valves.

Another method to evaluate mitral valve area is calculation of the pressure half-time. This method has been very useful in the detection of native valve stenosis (19), and it has recently been applied to prosthetic valves (20, 21). The pressure half-time is the time it takes for the transmitral gradient to drop to half of its peak

TABLE 32.2

NORMAL DOPPLER VELOCITIES FOR PROSTHETIC VALVES

Valve	No. of Patients	Peak Doppler Velocity[a,b]	Peak Pressure Gradient[a]	Mean Pressure Gradient[a]	Percent Regurgitant[c]
Porcine valves					
Aortic					
Bhatia[d]	65	2.7 ± 0.7	31 ± 14	—	35
Literature[e]	—	3.2	41	—	
Alam[f]	56	2.1 ± 0.5	19 ± 9	11 ± 5	9
		(1.2–3.1)	(6–42)	(3–21)	
Panidis[g]	9	2.6 ± 0.6	30 ± 12	17 ± 10	44
		(1.8–3.6)	(12–53)	(5–36)	
Mitral					
Bhatia[d]	37	1.8 ± 0.4	13 ± 5	—	19
Literature[e]	—	1.8	13	—	
Alam[f]	105	1.5 ± 0.3	9.9 ± 3.4	4.8 ± 1.7	6
		(1.1–2.1)	(5–18)	(2–8)	
Panidis[g]	6	1.9 ± 0.3	15 ± 5	7 ± 1	0
		(1.6–2.3)	(10–23)	(5–8)	
Bjork-Shiley					
Aortic					
Bhatia[d]	20	2.6 ± 0.7	29 ± 15	—	35
Literature[e]	—	3.0	36	—	—
Panidis[g]	8	2.6 ± 0.5	27 ± 9	14 ± 6	62
		(1.8–3)	(13–36)	(6–23)	
Mitral					
Bhatia[d]	13	1.5 ± 0.3	10 ± 4	—	23
Literature[e]	—	1.9	14.4	—	—
Panidis[g]	8	1.6 ± 0.3	10 ± 3	5 ± 2	38
		(1.0–2.0)	(5–16)	(2–7)	
St. Jude					
Aortic					
Bhatia[d]	15	2.6 ± 0.7	30 ± 14	—	20
Literature[e]	—	2.9	33.6	—	—
Panidis[g]	38	2.3 ± 0.6	22 ± 12	12 ± 7	58
		(1–3.9)	(4–61)	(2–32)	
Mitral					
Bhatia[d]	17	1.5 ± 0.4	10 ± 4	—	6
Literature[e]	—	1.9	14.4	—	—
Panidis[g]	44	1.6 ± 0.3	11 ± 4	5 ± 2	32
		(1–2.5)	(4–24)	(1.8–5)	

[a]Values are presented as the mean ± standard deviation. Values in parentheses are the reported range of normal values.
[b]Doppler velocities are generally higher for the smaller valve sizes (see References 6, 13, 16a).
[c]The Percent Regurgitant column represents the percentage of normal valves found to be regurgitant in each study. The amount of valvular regurgitation found in these studies on normal valves has been mild or minimal.
[d]Data from Bhatia S, Moten M, Werner M, et al: Frequency of unusually high transvalvular doppler velocities in patients with normal prosthetic valves (abstract). *J. Am Coll Cardiol* 9:238A, 1987.
[e]Literature values are those quoted by Bhatia and coworkers as literature normal values ± 2 standard deviations.
[f]Data from Alam M, Rosman HS, Lakier JB, et al: Doppler and echocardiographic features of normal and dysfunctioning bioprosthetic valves. *J Am Coll Cardiol* 10:851–858, 1987.
[g]Data from Panidis IP, Ross J, Mintz GS: Normal and abnormal prosthetic valve function as assessed by Doppler echocardiography. *J Am Coll Cardiol* 8:317–326, 1986.

FIGURE 32.3

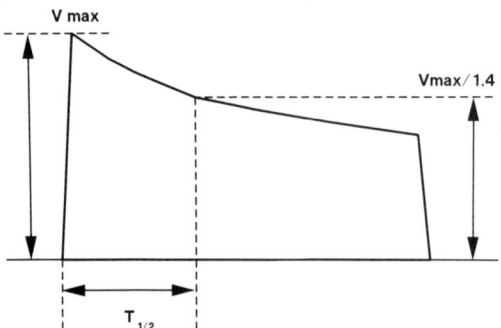

Calculation of pressure half-time. A schematic diagram of mitral flow in a patient with atrial fibrillation. The peak velocity (*Vmax*) is measured and this value is divided by 1.4 (the square root of 2). Next the time for the velocity to decay to Vmax/1.4 is found. This is the pressure half-time ($T_{1/2}$.) The mitral valve area can then be estimated as $220/T_{1/2}$.

value (Fig. 32.3). Mitral valve area has been empirically found to be equal to:

Mitral valve = 220 / (pressure half-time) (2)

It can be shown using Equation 1 that the pressure gradient will have dropped to half its peak value when the velocity has dropped to the peak velocity over the square root of 2 (peak velocity/1.4). The valve area calculated using this method has been reported to correlate well with catheterization-derived valve areas (8, 11, 20). Wilkins and coworkers however (10), reported poorer results, finding a correlation of only 0.65 between simultaneous Doppler- and catheterization-derived valve areas.

There are several limitations to be aware of when interpreting Doppler results. First, the quality of the data obtained depends heavily on the experience, skill, and patience of the echocardiographer. Second, the calculations discussed above were validated in specialized settings (usually university echocardiography laboratories), and results obtained in other laboratories with different techniques may not correlate as well with hemodynamic measurements. Third, Doppler energy is significantly attenuated by prosthetic valves as shown by Sprecher in vitro (22). This effect appears to be greatest for mechanical ball valves with only slight improvement in imaging flow behind disc valves. In

contrast, flow behind bioprosthetic valves appears to be well imaged. This limits the use of Doppler to imaging jets on the same side of mechanical valves as the transducer. For example, Doppler imaging of prosthetic mitral regurgitation will frequently be difficult from the standard (anterior) apical and parasternal views since the left atrium lies posteriorly behind the mitral valve. This has been confirmed by Azuma and coworkers (23), who reported that apical pulsed Doppler has only a 20% sensitivity in detecting bioprosthetic mitral valve regurgitation documented by left ventriculography. These difficulties can be overcome through the use of transesophageal echocardiography (discussed below). A fourth difficulty with pulsed and continuous-wave Doppler detection of regurgitation is that these methods can detect very small amounts of regurgitation, which may be caused by the process of normal valve closure without frank incompetence of the valve. Thus, Gibbs and coworkers (24) have reported that in patients with clinically normal mechanical valves, Doppler detects regurgitation in 18.4% of mitral and 42% of aortic valves. Table 32.2 summarizes the frequency of regurgitation in reported studies of porcine, Bjork-Shiley, and St. Jude valves. In conclusion, standard pulsed and continuous-wave Doppler echocardiography provides significant, clinically useful information on stenosis of prosthetic valves, particularly for mitral valves for which the pressure half-time method allows an estimate of valve area. These techniques do not provide optimum detection or quantitation of prosthetic valve regurgitation, however, particularly for mitral valves.

Color Doppler imaging is the newest modality of echocardiographic imaging that is helpful in evaluating prosthetic valves. Color flow Doppler has found its greatest use in the detection of valvular regurgitation and may allow the diagnosis of mitral paravalvular leaks (Fig. 32.4) (25). Two-dimensional patterns of blood flow are imaged using pulsed Doppler technology and are superimposed on a standard two-dimensional echocardiographic image of the heart. The direction and velocity of flow are coded in the color of the jets. In most systems, flow toward the transducer is colored red, flow away

FIGURE 32.4

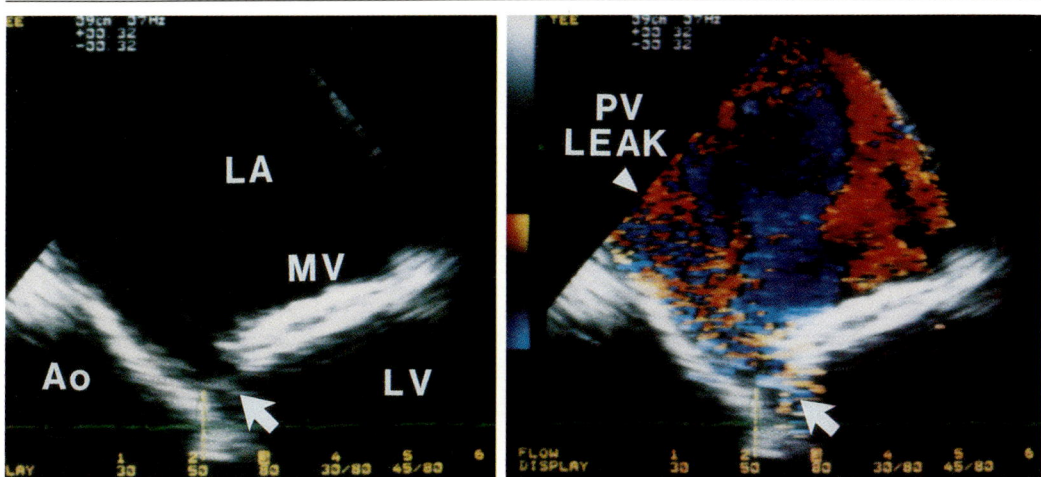

Transesophageal color Doppler diagnosis of a paravalvular leak. This is a transesophageal color-flow Doppler recording demonstrating a paravalvular regurgitant jet (*PV LEAK*) around a prosthetic mitral valve (*MV*). *Left*, The two-dimensional echocardiographic view without color flow imaging to demonstrate the anatomy. The left atrium (*LA*) is above, the left ventricle (*LV*) below, and the aortic outflow tract (*Ao*) is in the lower left corner of these figures. There is an echo-free space visible between the mitral valve and the anterior mitral annulus (*arrow*). Although suggestive of a paravalvular leak, this finding could also be due to echo dropout. *Right*, the color Doppler image of the same view. In this photograph, red represents flow toward and blue flow away from the transducer (which is located at the top of the image). The mosaic pattern of red and blue represents turbulent flow. The *arrows* identify the previously noted gap between the mitral valve and the anterior mitral annulus, and it is now clear that there is highly turbulent paravalvular flow in the gap, confirming the diagnosis of a paravalvular leak. The resultant jet swirls around the left atrium, resulting in vortices of blue and red flow. Transesophageal echocardiography can be safely performed both in patients undergoing surgery and in outpatients.

from the transducer is colored blue (although this may vary with the manufacturer of the equipment used), and turbulent flow is usually colored green.

Using color Doppler, the amount of regurgitation is judged semiquantitatively by estimating jet area and comparing it to chamber size (i.e., the ratio of jet area to left atrial area for mitral regurgitation) or by the distance that the regurgitant jet travels into the proximal chamber (graded simply on a scale of 1 to $4+$). Correlations with angiography have been good to excellent (26). When pulsed Doppler demonstrates valve regurgitation in normal valves, color flow Doppler can demonstrate that this is minimal or artifactitious (27). Severe or moderately severe regurgitation on color flow Doppler in a patient with symptoms suggestive of heart failure may be an indication for catheterization. In asymptomatic patients with moderate or severe regurgitation of a bioprosthetic

valve on color flow Doppler, the decision of when to perform catheterization needs to be individualized; possible indications might include development of left ventricular dysfunction, progressive dilation of the left ventricle, or development of pulmonary hypertension.

Transesophageal color Doppler can assess flow in the left atrium withoiut masking artifact, and is thus ideally suited for evaluation of prosthetic mitral regurgitation. Although minimally invasive and occasionally uncomfortable, transesophageal echocardiography and Doppler imaging can provide information on prosthetic mitral valve function that is otherwise unobtainable without cardiac catheterization. In an experienced laboratory this is a safe procedure and can be performed on an outpatient. Vandenberg and coworkers (28) have shown in an in vitro model of transesophageal imaging of prosthetic mitral valves that color flow Doppler imaging can reliably distinguish valvular and paravalvular leaks, and that regurgitant volume could be estimated for valvular leaks. In addition, transesophageal color Doppler has been found useful in assessing mitral and tricuspid valve repair and repair of aortic dissections (29).

Acoustic Techniques

Several techniques for evaluating valve function using analysis of the heart sounds have been proposed and at least two commercial devices have been marketed for this. Hylen and coworkers (3) first described the detection of aortic ball variance with special analysis of prosthetic valve opening and closing sounds, and similar analyses have been performed by Gordon and coworkers (31) with Smeloff-Cutter, Bjork-Shiley, and Starr-Edwards valves. Johnson and coworkers (32) have shown in patients with stenotic native aortic valves that patients with high aortic gradients also had a greater amplitude of higher-frequency sounds. It should be noted that these changes in the frequency content of the murmur did not correlate well with the valve area, only with the gradient. Patients with a low cardiac output and resultant low gradient despite severe aortic stenosis may therefore be missed.

One commercial device (the Klictrax manufactured by Medtronic) used spectral analysis to determine the frequencies and amplitudes of the valve opening and closing sounds. It was hoped that changes in the frequency content of the heart sounds would allow the diagnosis of valve dysfunction. This device is no longer being manufactured.

A more recent device, the Valve-Tracker (International Acoustics Inc.), uses a more complicated method of signal processing called deconvolution to obtain the "impact history" of the valve. Deconvolution is a mathematical technique that allows the separation of a complex waveform into its component waveforms (33). As implemented in the Valve-Tracker, this technique allows a precise determination of the timing of impacts of a disc or ball with the retaining structures of a valve. Changes in the timing of these impacts are used to diagnose abnormal valve function. The clinical utility of these techniques in evaluating valve function remains to be established, and there is as yet little or no literature documenting their sensitivity, specificity, or predictive accuracy in detecting valve dysfunction.

Cinefluoroscopy

Cineradiographic evaluation of prosthetic valves can provide two helpful clues to the presence of prosthetic valve dysfunction. The presence of rocking or tilting of the valve between systole and diastole can be a clue to the presence of paravalvular leaks. The normal Starr-Edwards aortic valve should rock less than 6° and the normal mitral Starr-Edwards less than 12° (34). The reliability of this measurement for the detection of paravalvular leaks is better for aortic valves than for mitral valves. Unfortunately, the absence of this degree of titling does not exclude the presence of dehiscence or paravalvular leak and, for the mitral valve, its presence does not necessarily indicate paravalvular leakage.

A second use of cinefluoroscopy is in the measurement of occluder motion and wear. Our cinefluoroscopic experience with the Harken caged-disc valve (35) demonstrated that measurement of the disc-to-sewing ring dimension can indicate the likelihood of excessive overall disc wear. Indentation or oblique flattening of the rounded poppet edge on its atrial aspect are additional cinefluoroscopic indications of excessive disc wear. Cinefluoroscopy of caged-ball valves may demonstrate poppet variance (swelling, shrinkage, wear) or escape. Reduced excursion or sticking of the poppet may occur due to ball variance or valve thrombosis.

Cinefluoroscopy is the imaging technique of choice when thrombus of a tilting-disc or bileaflet valve is suspected, because of the relative ease with which images can be obtained and the striking abnormalities produced by thrombosis. The normal ranges of opening angles of tilting disc valves have been published (36, 37), as well as the opening angles and opening and closing velocities of the bileaflet St. Jude valve (3). The St. Jude valve can be seen with standard cinefluoroscopy in the butterfly (tangential) view, but image enhancement by digital subtraction techniques allows imaging in oblique views and computerized calculation of leaflet separation and velocity (3).

Cardiac Catheterization

Evaluation of prosthetic valve function at cardiac catheterization can pose difficulties in both the collection and interpretation of data. Evaluation of prosthetic aortic valves may require transseptal catheterization, particularly with tilting-disc valves with which there is a risk that the catheter may enter the minor orifice of the valve and wedge against the upstream edge of the disc, preventing catheter removal. This can result in torrential aortic regurgitation and abrupt hemodynamic deterioration of the patient. Another risk is that a caged ball or disc valve may be pulled out of its cage when the catheter is withdrawn from the ventricle. This is a particular danger if the ball is reduced in size due to wear.

Although the valve area calculated with the Gorlin formula (38) has become the standard parameter for evaluating valve function, recent work has shown major flaws in its use for the evaluation of prosthetic valves. Several authors have noted that the Gorlin area appears to increase progressively as flow increases in prosthetic valves (39, 40). This may be due to differences between the pressure-flow relationship assumed by the Gorlin equation and the acutal pressure-flow behavior of valves (41, 42). Indeed, it has been shown that the Gorlin valve area inaccurately predicts actual prosthetic valve area for aortic Hancock and Bjork-Shiley valves when compared to identical valves studied in vitro (43). In view of the limitations of the Gorlin area several authors have proposed newer methods of evaluating prosthetic valve function using hemodynamic data obtained at catheterization. Cannon and coworkers have proposed an equation for the calculation of valve area using a linear relationship between pressure and flow that may be superior to the Gorlin equation (41); however, the use of this equation has not been validated with other sets of data. Data from the author's institution suggest that normal and stenotic valves cannot be reliably separated using the Gorlin formula (44) but that either the simple linear ratio of pressure to flow (the valve resistance) or Cannon's equation will allow reliable separation (45). Valve resistances (mean pressure gradient/mean flow rate $\times$ 1332)

of 80 dyn-cm/sec^{-4} or greater strongly suggest significant stenosis of bioprosthetic mitral valves; in our study this criteria allowed complete separation of normal from stenotic valves hemodynamically. The concept of a valve resistance is based on evidence that the relationship between pressure and flow in the normal mitral valve is linear (46, 47).

Philosophically, these newer approaches differ from the classic Gorlin equation in their attempts to use models of normal flow through valves to establish normal function. Abnormal valves are then defined as those that fall outside the normal range for a given valve. The Gorlin equation is instead based on a model of abnormal, stenotic flow and will have significant limitations when used to evaluate valves whose hemodynamic behavior does not fit this model.

PROBLEMS IN PATIENTS FOLLOWING VALVE REPLACEMENT

In addtion to the complications common to all types of prosthetic valves—thromboembolism, endocarditis, anticoagulant-related bleeding, and valve thrombosis—each type of prosthetic valve has specific complications associated with it depending on its design. Knowledge of the types of complications associated with different valve designs can be enormously beneficial when evaluating a patient with suspected valve dysfunction.

Thromboembolism

The incidence of thromboembolism is clearly related to the type of valve implanted and the anticoagulation status of the patient. Indications for anticoagulation and specific antithrombotic regimens for each type of valve are discussed in Chapter 19. Given optimal anticoagulation, the risk of thromboembolism for prosthetic valves should be about 0.5% per year. Reported thromboembolic rates for different types of valves are shown in Table 32.3. These thromboembolic rates are dramatically higher if patients are not maintained on anticoagulation. For the Starr-Edwards valve, for example, the rate of thromboembolism may be as high as 9% annually for patients off anticoagulants. In general, rates of thromboembolism appear to be

TABLE 32.3

THROMBOEMBOLIC RATES FOR PROSTHETIC VALVES[a]

	Aortic Position	Mitral Position
Starr-Edwards	3.97 (48)	5.87 (49)
Bjork-Shiley (spherical)	3.64 (50)	3.75 (50)
Medtronic-Hall	1.8 (51)	3.7 (51)
St. Jude Medical	2.44 (52–54)	2.89 (52, 54)
Omniscience	2.11 (55)	1.98 (55)
Porcine	1.49 (53, 56–58)	2.81 (56–59)
Ionescu-Shiley	—	0.39 (59)

[a]Adapted from Edmunds LH Jr: Complications of valve replacements. In Starek PJK (ed): *Heart Valve Replacement and Reconstruction*. Chicago, Year Book, 1987, p 318.

higher for mitral valves and higher for mechanical valves than for bioprosthetic valves. The risk of thromboembolism appears to diminish over time, although this has been disputed and may not be true for the St. Jude valve (1).

Valve Thrombosis

Thrombus usually develops at areas of stagnation of flow and is common at the junction between the prosthesis and the patient's tissues. In mechanical valves, the motion of the occluding device (ball or disc) may become restricted by thrombus and provide the first clues to its presence. Restricted motion of disc valves may be detected by measuring the opening angle of the disc (3, 36). If thrombus is present, fibrinolytic therapy may promote clot dissolution and avoid the need for valve replacement. Successful treatment of thrombosed aortic, mitral, and tricuspid valves has been reported (3, 60–66). We have successfully given intravenous streptokinase as an initial bolus of 250,000 units followed by a continuous infusion of 100,000 units/hr for 72 hr (3). Urokinase has also been reported to be effective for therapy of thrombosed valves (64).

Endocarditis

Although a full discussion of endocarditis complicating prosthetic valve replacement is beyond the scope of this chapter, several points need to be made. The best "treatment" for prosthetic valve endocarditis is clearly prevention. The American Heart Association has published

specific guidelines (67) for prophylaxis of patients undergoing various procedures (Table 32.4). Optimally, patients with prosthetic valves should receive parenteral regimens as prophylaxis. It has been our experience that it is uncommon that this recommendation is followed, possibly due to the logistics of administration. This is unfortunate, since parenteral antibiotics can be easily given in the physician's office or the patient can be given a prescription and have the antibiotics administered in an ambulatory care center or clinic at minimal charge. The inconvenience of this procedure is minimal when compared to the risks and consequences of prosthetic valve endocarditis.

If a patient develops endocarditis early after valve replacement (within 2 months) the most common organism is *Staphylococcus* (either *S. aureus* or *S. epidermidis*). These infections are believed to be related to operative contamination or infection immediately after surgery. Fungal and Gram-negative infections may also occur and have a high mortality. If endocarditis is suspected clinically, at least two sets of blood cultures (and preferably three or four) should *always* be obtained before beginning antibiotics. Empiric therapy should be directed against staphylococci pending the results of the blood cultures.

Infection of the valve occurring in the intermediate and late periods after surgery (several months to years postoperatively) more closely resembles classical subacute bacterial endocarditis of native valves both in the microbiology of the infecting organisms and in the clinical presentation. The most common organisms are streptococcal strains, and the aortic valve is more commonly involved than the mitral. Patients may develop new murmurs of valvular insufficiency or paravalvular leaks, embolic phenomena, heart failure, or heart block (suggestive of myocardial abscess). Echocardiography and Doppler studies are generally not useful in diagnosing prosthetic valve endocarditis, but can be helpful in evaluating sequelae such as paravalvular leaks, flail leaflets, and occasionally myocardial abscess formation.

Cinefluoroscopy is of little benefit in endocarditis unless large vegetations interfere with ball or disc opening or if valve dehiscence oc-

TABLE 32.4

PREVENTION OF BACTERIAL ENDOCARDITIS IN PATIENTS WITH PROSTHETIC VALVES[a]

Dental Procedures and Surgery
of the Upper Respiratory Tract

1. Ampicillin 1.0 to 2.0 gm plus gentamycin 1.5 gm/kg given i.m. or i.v. 30 min prior to the procedure, followed by 1 gm oral penicillin V 6 hours after initial dose.

2. In penicillin-allergic patients: Vancomycin 1 gm i.v. slowly over 1 hr.

Some patients with prosthetic valves in whom a high level of oral health is being maintained may be offered oral antibiotic prophylaxis for routine dental procedures. Parenteral antibiotics are recommended, however, for patients with prosthetic valves who require extensive dental procedures, especially extractions, or oral or gingival surgical procedures.

Genitourinary Tract and Gastrointestinal
Tract Surgery and Instrumentation

1. Ampicillin 2.0 gm i.m. or i.v. plus gentamycin 1.5 mg/kg i.m. or i.v. given 30 min prior to the procedure. The doses may be repeated 8 hr after the initial dose.

2. For patients allergic to penicillin: Vancomycin (1.0 gm given i.v. slowly over 1 hr, plus gentamycin 1.5 mg/kg i.m. or i.v. 1 hr prior to the procedure. These doses may be repeated 8 hr after the initial dose.

[a]Modified from Shulman ST, Amren DP, Bisno AL, et al: Prevention of bacterial endocarditis. *Circulation* 70:1123A–1127A, 1984.

curs with rocking of the valve. As with early postoperative endocarditis, antibiotic therapy should be begun only after several sets of blood cultures have been obtained and should be guided by the results of cultures. Serum antibiotic levels should be measured and confirmed to be bacteriocidal for the cultured organism. Valve replacement should be undertaken if the patient develops refractory heart failure or recurrent emboli, if the infection does not respond to antibiotics, or if significant hemodynamic deterioration occurs. Since surgery in an actively infected field is clearly undesirable, surgery should be delayed as long as possible (without endangering the patient) while intravenous antibiotics are administered.

Valvular and Paravalvular Regurgitation

Most mechanical valves have a normal amount of intrinsic regurgitation built into their design. The small amount of regurgitant flow present in the St. Jude valve, for example, is thought to allow microthrombi to be washed clear in areas where stagnation of flow may occur. Bioprosthetic valves are not regurgitant, however, and the presence of regurgitation in these valves should prompt further investigation. If large amounts of regurgitation occur with any valve, a cause should be sought. Regurgitation in these cases may be due to structural failure of the

valve or may be due to a paravalvular leak caused by partial detachment of the valve (Fig. 32.4). If paravalvular regurgitation occurs late after valve implantation, endocarditis should be suspected and blood cultures obtained even if there is no other evidence of infection.

Fluoroscopy may also be helpful in endocarditis in detecting rocking of the valve suggestive of detachment of the valve. In addition, wear of the poppet or leaflet may be detected by changes in their size on fluoroscopy. Color flow Doppler imaging has provided a significant advance in diagnosing regurgitation in prosthetic valves and can allow discrimination of valvular from paravalvular leaks in many cases. In addition, the amount of regurgitation can be estimated and serial comparisons made to determine if a paravalvular leak is worsening.

If significant rocking of the valve is found on cinefluoroscopy, urgent surgery is indicated. Similarly, if the amount of leakage is substantial and hemodynamically compromises the patient, surgery is indicated. Smaller degrees of paravalvular leakage without significant rocking of the valve can frequently be managed without reoperation, although many of these patients will have associated hemolysis. If the hematocrit can be maintained with iron supplementation the patient can be followed carefully without reoperation. If red cell destruction exceeds the patient's synthetic capability and a refractory severe anemia develops, however, surgery is indicated.

Structural Valve Failure

Strut fracture has been reported in several types of mechanical valves but has received greatest recent publicity in the Bjork-Shiley convex-concave valves. Strut fracture can be detected on PA chest x-rays or on cinefluoroscopy. Other valves in which strut fracture has been reported include the Beall valve (68, 69), the DeBakey valve (70), and certain models of the Bjork-Shiley valve (71, 72). Strut fracture may result in embolization of the disc or the strut and lead to acute hemodynamic deterioration.

A second mode of failure of mechanical valves is disc wear and ball variance. Both of these processes represent gradual deterioration of the occluding disc or ball over time due to wear. The poppet of ball valves may gradually shrink in diameter and can embolize acutely when the ball is smaller than the openings in the restraining cage. Models that have degenerated in this manner include the Starr-Edwards model 1200 valves (also susceptible to increases in size due to lipoid infiltration, cracking, and grooving), the Smeloff-Cutter valve, the Harken valve, the Braunwald-Cutter valve (73), and the SCDK-Cutter valves. We have seen the poppet of an aortic Smeloff-Cutter valve acutely embolize during cardiac catheterization when a catheter was withdrawn from the left ventricle. Subsequent examination of the poppet revealed significant ball variance. In general, ball variance is less common in mitral valves than in aortic valves.

Similarly, discs can wear and may embolize or seat improperly as their size decreases, leading to regurgitation. Excessive wear has been reported in the Beall 103 and 104 mitral valves and the caged-disc Hufnagel, Kay-Shiley, Kay-Suszuki, and Cross-Jones valves. Disc variance has not been a significant problem with newer disc valve models such as the St. Jude and Medtronic-Hall prostheses.

A few valves have had sufficient problems that they have required prophylactic replacement (that is, before clinical evidence of dys-function develops). Among these are early model caged-ball valves with Silastic poppets. Similarly, disc valves constructed with nontilting Silastic or Teflon discs have shown excessive wear, and the risk of acute embolization may warrant prophylactic removal of the valve. Another group of valves that may require prophylactic replacement is the early cloth-covered models of the Starr-Edwards and Braunwald-Cutter valves in which the cloth covering may separate from the valve cage, resulting in severe hemolysis.

Other Problems

When an aortic prosthesis is too large for the patient's aortic root, tissue ingrowth can occur and interfere with the valve opening or closure, resulting in either stenosis, regurgitation, or thrombus formation.

There are many reports of patients developing rupture of the left ventricle after mitral valve replacement (74–80), particularly with porcine heterografts. These tears may be due to the stents of the prosthesis lacerating the ventricular endocardium, and one reported case of rupture occurred during chest compression (81). Data at our institution suggest that ventricular rupture virtually always involves the posterior or posterolateral wall of the left ventricle and appears to be more frequent in patients with recent posterior myocardial infarction (82). This complication has a high fatality rate (6 of 7 died in our series).

Follow-up of Bioprosthetic Valves

Follow-up of bioprosthetic valves is initially simpler than follow-up of mechanical valves since patients are usually not receiving anticoagulants. However, after a period of 6 to 8 years the risk of valve degeneration begins to rise abruptly and requires careful observation of the patient. A baseline two-dimensional echocardiographic examination with Doppler evaluation of the valve for regurgitation and stenosis should be performed in the 1st year after implantation as a baseline study to evaluate the valve gradient, degree of regurgitation (if any), and chamber sizes. Yearly echo and Doppler evaluation should begin about 6 to 8 years after implantation. At 8 to 10 years after implantation, patients with bioprosthetic valves should be evaluated three to four times yearly or immediately if symptoms or signs suggestive of valve dysfunction develop.

It should be stressed that it is very uncommon for bioprosthetic valves to fail suddenly. Patients usually present with the gradual onset of symptoms that require adjustments in their lifestyle. In our experience, patients may become anxious about their valve failing abruptly as their valves reach the 8- to 10-year mark. When the physician begins to obtain yearly echocardiograms, patients should be reassured that failure, if it occurs, is virtually always a gradual process and that careful follow-up with their physician on a regular basis will allow ample time to detect the development of valve dysfunction.

References

1. Czer LSC, Matloff JM, Chaux A, et al: The St. Jude valve: analysis of thromboembolism, warfarin related hemorrhage and survival. *Am Heart J* 114: 389–397, 1987.
2. Smith ND, Raizada V, Abrams J: Auscultation of the normally functioning prosthetic valve. *Ann Int Med* 95:594–598, 1981.
3. Czer, LSC, Weiss M, Bateman TM, et al: Fibrinolytic therapy of St. Jude valve thrombosis under guidance of digital cinefluoroscopy. *J Am Coll Cardiol* 5: 1244–1249, 1985.
4. Morse D, Steiner RM: Cardiac valve identification atlas and guide. In Morse D, Steiner RM, Fernandez J (eds): *Guide to Prosthetic Cardiac Valves.* New York, Springer-Verlag, 1985, pp. 257–346.
5. Mehlman KJ, Resnekov L: A guide to the radiographic identification of prosthetic heart valves. *Circulation* 57:613–623, 1978.
6. Panidis IP, Ross J, Mintz GS: Normal and abnormal prosthetic valve function as assessed by Doppler echocardiography. *J Am Coll Cardiol* 8:317–326, 1986.
7. Kotler MN, Mintz GS, Panidis I, et al: Noninvasive evaluation of normal and abnormal prosthetic valve function. *J Am Coll Cardiol* 2:151–173, 1983.
8. Alam M, Rosman HS, Lakier JB, et al: Doppler and echocardiographic features of normal and dysfunctioning bioprosthetic valves. *J Am Coll Cardiol* 10:851–858, 1987.
9. Hatle L, Angelsen B: Diagnosis and assessment of various heart lesions. In Hatle L, Angelsen B (eds): *Doppler Ultrasound in Cardiology.* Philadelphia, Lea & Febiger, 1982, pp 196–204.
10. Wilkins GT, Gillam LD, Kritzer GL, et al: Validation of continuous-wave Doppler echocardiographic measurements of mitral and tricuspid prosthetic valve gradients: a simultaneous Doppler-catheter study. *Circulation* 74:786–795, 1986.
11. Sagar KB, Wann S, Paulsen WHJ, Romhilt DW: Doppler echocardiographic evaluation of Hancock and Bjork-Shiley prosthetic valves. *J Am Coll Cardiol* 7:681–687, 1986.
12. Holen J, Simonsen S, Froysaker T: An ultrasound Doppler technique for the noninvasive determination of the pressure gradient in the Bjork-Shiley mitral valve. *Circulation* 59:436–442, 1979.
13. Ramirez ML, Wong M, Sadler N, Shah PM: Doppler evaluation of bioprosthetic and mechanical aortic valves: data from four models in 107 stable, ambulatory patients. *Am Heart J* 115:418–425, 1988.
14. Rothbart RM, Smucker ML, Gibson RS: Overestimation by Doppler echocardiography of pressure gradients across Starr-Edwards prosthetic valves in the aortic position. *Am J Cardiol* 61:475–476, 1988.
15. Cooper DM, Stewart WJ, Schiavone WA, et al: Evaualtion of normal prosthetic valve function by Doppler echocardiography. *Am Heart J* 114:576–582, 1987.
16. Gibbs JL, Wharton GA, Williams GJ: Doppler echocardiographic characteristics of the Carpentier-Edwards xenograft. *Eur Heart J* 7:353–356, 1986.
16a. Williams GA, Labovitz AJ: Doppler hemodynamic evaluation of prosthetic (Starr-Edwards and Bjork-Shiley) and bioprosthetic (Hancock and Carpentier-Edwards) cardiac valves. *Am J Cardiol* 56:325–332, 1985.
17. Yoganathan AP, Cape EG, Sung HW, et al: Review of hydrodynamic principles for the cardiologist: application to the study of blood flow and jets by imaging techniques. *J. Am Coll Cardiol* 12:1344–1353, 1988.
18. Otto CM, Pearlman AS, Comess KA, et al: Determination of the stenotic aortic valve area in adults using Doppler echocardiography. *J Am Coll Cardiol* 7:509–517, 1986.
19. Hatle L, Angelsen B, Tromsdal A: Non-invasive assessment of atrioventricular pressure half-time by Doppler ultrasound. *Circulation* 60:1096–1104, 1969.
20. Fawzy ME, Halim M, Ziady G, et al: Hemo-

dynamic evaluation of porcine bioprostheses in the mitral position by Doppler echocardiography. *Am J Cardiol* 59:643–646, 1987.

21. Weinstein IR, Marbarger JP, Perez JE: Ultrasonic assessment of the St. Jude prosthetic valve: M mode, two-dimensional, and Doppler echocardiography.. *Circulation* 68:897–905, 1983.

22. Sprecher DL, Adamick R, Adams D, Kisslo J. In vitro color flow, pulsed and continuous wave Doppler ultrasound masking of flow by prosthetic valves. *J Am Coll Cardiol* 9:1306–1310, 1987.

23. Azuma SS, Abbasi AS, Fraser A, et al: Pulsed Doppler evaluation of regurgitation in mitral valve prostheses. *Cathet Cardiovasc Diagn* 14:243–247, 1988.

24. Gibbs JL, Wharton GA, Williams GJ: Doppler ultrasound of normally functioning mechanical mitral and aortic valve prostheses. *Int J Cardiol* 18:391–398, 1988.

25. Goyal RG, Kan MN, Soto B, et al: Color Doppler assessment of prosthetic valve function and its limitations (abstract). *Circulation* 74(Suppl II):389, 1986.

26. Helmcke F, Nanda HC, Hsiung MC, et al: Color Doppler assessment of mitral regurgitation with orthogonal planes. *Circulation* 75:175–183, 1987.

27. Dittrich H, Nicod P, Hoit B, et al: Evaluation of Bjork-Shiley prosthetic valves by real-time two-dimensional Doppler echocardiographic flow mapping. *Am Heart J* 115:133–138, 1988.

28. Vandenberg BF, Dellsperger KC, Chandran RB, et al: Detection, localization, and quantitation of bioprosthetic mitral valve regurgitation. *Circulation* 78:529–538, 1988.

29. Bolger A, Czer LS, Friedman AF, et al: Intraoperative transesophageal color Doppler imaging: advantages and limitations. *J Am Coll Cardiol* 11:217A, 1988.

30. Hylen JC, Kloster FE, Herr RH, et al: Sound spectrographic diagnosis of aortic ball variance. *Circulation* 39:849–858, 1969.

31. Gordon RF, Hajmi M, Kingsley B, et al: Spectroanalysis evaluation of aortic prosthetic valves. *Chest* 66:44–49, 1974.

32. Johnson GR, Adolph RJ, Campbell DJ: Estimation of the severity of aortic valve stenosis by frequency analysis of the murmur. *J Am Coll Cardiol* 1:1315–1323, 1983.

33. Ramirez RW: *The FFT, Fundamentals and concepts.* Englewood Cliffs, NJ, Prentice-Hall, 1985, p. 152.

34. White AF, Dinsmore RE, Buckley MJ: Cineradiographic evaluation of prosthetic cardiac valves. *Circulation* 48:882–890, 1973.

35. Gray RJ, Czer LSC, Chaux A, et al: Harken caged-disc mitral valve replacement, 1969–1975: analysis of late mortality, thromboembolism, and valve failure. *Texas Heart Inst J* 14:411–417, 1987.

36. Verdel G, Heethaar RM, Jambroes G, Van Der Werf T: Assessment of the opening angle of implanted Bjork-Shiley prosthetic valves. *Circulation* 68:355–359, 1983.

37. Czer LSC, Matloff J, Chaux A, et al: A 6 year experience with the St. Jude Medical Valve: hemodynamic performance, surgical results, biocompatibility and follow-up. *J Am Coll Cardiol* 6:904–912, 1985.

38. Gorlin R, Gorlin SG: Hydraulic formula for calculation of the area of the stenotic mitral valve, other cardiac valves and central circulatory shunts. *Am Heart J* 41:1–18, 1951.

39. Ubago JL, Figueroa A, Colman T, et al: Hemodynamic factors that affect calculated orifice areas in the mitral Hancock xenograft valve. *Circulation* 61:388–394, 1980.

40. Cosgrove DM, Lytle BW, Williams GW: Hemodynamic performance of the Carpentier-Edwards pericardial valve in the aortic position in vivo. *Circulation* 72(Suppl II):146–152, 1985.

41. Cannon SR, Richards KL, Crawford MH: Hydraulic estimation of stenotic orifice area: a correction of the Gorlin formula. *Circulation* 71:1170–1178, 1985.

42. Khan SS, Czer LSC, Gray RJ, et al: The Gorlin formula revisited: impact of the diastolic filling period on the pressure-flow relationship (abstract). *Circulation* 76(Suppl IV): 90, 1987.

43. Cannon SR, Richards KL, Crawford MH, et al: Inadequacy of the Gorlin formula for predicting prosthetic valve area. *Am J Cardiol* 62:113–116, 1988.

44. Czer LSC, Gray RJ, Bateman TM, et al: Hemodynamic differentiation of pathologic and physiologic stenosis in mitral porcine bioprostheses. *J Am Coll Cardiol* 7:284–294, 1986.

45. Khan SS, Czer LS, Gray RJ, Matloff JM: Use of the valve resistance in the separation of normal and stenotic Hancock mitral valves. *J Cardiac Surg* 3:241–246, 1988.

46. Yellin EL, Laniado S, Peskin S, et al: Analysis and interpretation of the normal mitral valve flow curve. In Kalmanson D (ed): *The Mitral Valve—A Pluridisciplinary Approach.* Acton MA, Publishing Sciences Group, 1976, p 163.

47. Jawad IA, Magdi HG, Brown RL, et al: Pressure-flow relations across the normal mitral valve. *Am J Cardiol* 59:915–918, 1987.

48. Miller DC, Oyer P, Mitchell R, et al: Performance characteristics of the Starr-Edwards model 1260 aortic valve prosthesis beyond 10 years. *J Thorac Cardiovasc Surg* 88:198–207, 1984.

49. Miller DC, Oyer P, Stinson E, et al: Ten to fifteen years reassessment of performance characteristics of the Starr-Edwards Model 6120 mitral valve prosthesis. *J Thorac Cardiovasc Surg* 85:1–20, 1983.

50. Karp RB, Cyrus RJ, Blackstone EH, et al: The Bjork-Shiley valve: intermediate term follow-up. *J Thorac Cardiovasc Surg* 81:602–614, 1981.

51. Starek PJK, Murray GF, Keagy BA, et al: Clinical experience with the Hall pivoting disc valve. *J Thorac Cardiovasc Surg* 31:66–68, 1983.

52. Burckhardt D, Hoffman A, Vogt S, et al: Clinical evaluation of the St. Jude Medical heart valve prosthesis. *J Thorac Cardiovasc Surg* 88;432–438, 1984.

53. Douglas PS, Hirshfield JW, Edie RN, et al: Clinical comparison of St. Jude and porcine aortic valve prostheses. *Circulation* 72(Suppl 2):135–139, 1985.

54. Lillehei CW: World-wide experience with the St. Jude Medical valve prosthesis: clinical and hemodynamic results. *Contemp Surg* 20:1–11, 1982.

55. DeWall R, Pelletier LC, Panebianco A, et al: Five-year clinical experience with the Omniscience cardiac valve. *Ann Thorac Surg* 38:275–280, 1984.

56. Jamieson WRE, Pelletier LC, Janusz MP, et al: A five year evaluation of the Carpentier-Edwards porcine bioprosthesis. *J Thorac Cardiovasc Surg* 88:324–333, 1984.

57. Magilligan DJ, Lewis JW, Tilley B, et al: The porcine bioprosthetic valve—twelve years later. *J Thorac Cardiovasc Surg* 89:499–507, 1985.

58. Oyer PE, Stinson EB, Reitz BA, et al: Long-term evaluation of the porcine xenograft bioprosthesis. *J Thorac Cardiovasc Surg* 78:343–350, 1979.

59. Gonzales-Lavin L, Tandon AP, Chi S, et al: The risk of thromboembolism and hemorrhage following mitral valve replacement. *J Thorac Cardiovasc Surg* 87:340–351.

60. Luluaga IT, Carrera D, d'Oliviera J, et al: Successful thrombolytic therapy after acute tricuspid valve obstruction (letter). *Lancet* 1:1067–1068, 1971.

61. Witchitz S, Veyrat C, Moisson P, et al: Fibrinolytic treatment of thrombus on prosthetic heart valves. *Br Heart J* 44:545–554, 1980.

62. Inberg MV, Havia T, Arstila M: Thrombolytic treatment for thrombotic complication for valve prosthesis after tricuspid valve replacement. *Scand J Thorac Cardiovasc Surg* 11:195–198, 1977.

63. Ledain L, Lorient-Roudaut MF, Gateau P, et al: Fibrinolytic treatment of thrombosis of prosthetic heart valves. *Eur Heart J* 3:371–381, 1982.

64. Joyce LD, Boucek M, McGough EC: Urokinase therapy for thrombosis of tricuspid prosthetic valves. *Eur Heart J* 3:371–381, 1982.

65. Gagnon RM, Beaudet R, Lemire J, et al: Streptokinase thrombolysis of a chronically thrombosed mitral prosthetic valve. *Cathet Cardiovasc Diagn* 10:5–10, 1984.

66. Draur RA: Successful streptokinase therapy of prosthetic aortic valve thrombosis. *Am Heart J* 108:605–606, 1984.

67. Shulman ST, Amren DP, Bisno AL, et al: Prevention of bacterial endocarditis. *Circulation* 70:1123A–1127A, 1984.

68. Carlson EB, Mintz GS, Bemis CE: Hemodynamic significance of normal and abnormal fluoroscopic patterns of disc motion in the Beall mitral valve prosthesis. *Radiology* 141:335–339, 1981.

69. Oliva PB, Johnson ML, Pomerantz M, Levene A: Dysfunction of the Beall mitral prosthesis and its detection by cinefluoroscopy and echocardiography. *Am J Cardiol* 31:393–395, 1973.

70. Zumbro GL, Cunder PE, Fishback ME, Galloway RF: Strut fracture in DeBakey valve. *J Thorac Cardiovasc Surg* 74:469–470, 1977.

71. Guit GL, van Voortuisen AE, Steiner RM: Outlet strut fracture of the Bjork-Shiley mitral prosthesis. *Radiology* 154:298–299, 1985.

72. Larrieu AJ, Puglia E, Allen P: Strut fracture and disc embolism of a Bjork-Shiley mitral valve prosthesis: localization of embolized disc by computerized axial tomography. *Ann Thorac Surg* 34:192–195, 1982.

73. Yakirevich V, Miller HI, Shapira I, et al: Intermittent poppet dislodgment in a Braunwald-Cutter prosthesis: non-invasive diagnosis and successful surgical treatment. *J Am Coll Cardiol* 3:442–446, 1984.

74. Bortolotti V, Thiene G, Casarotto D, et al: Left ventricular rupture following mitral valve replacement with a Hancock bioprosthesis. *Chest* 77:235–237, 1980.

75. Bjork VO, Henze A, Rodriguez L: Left ventricular rupture as a complication of mitral valve replacement: surgical experience with eight cases and a review of the literature. *J Thorac Cardiovasc Surg* 73:14–20, 1977.

76. Zacharias A, Groves LK, Cheanvechai C, et al: Rupture of the posterior wall of the left ventricle after mitral valve replacement. *J Thorac Cardiovasc Surg* 69:259–263, 1975.

77. Chi S, Beshore R, Gonzales-Lavin L: Left ventricular wall rupture after mitral valve replacement: report of successful repair in 2 patients. *Ann Thorac Surg* 22:380–382, 1976.

78. Nunez L, Gil-Aguado M, Cerron M, Celemin P: Delayed rupture of the left ventricle after mitral valve replacement with a bioprosthesis. *Ann Thorac Surg* 27:465–467, 1979.

79. Roberts WC: Complications of cardiac valve replacement: characteristic abnormalities of prostheses pertaining to any or specific site. *Am Heart J* 103:113–122, 1982.

80. Roberts WC, Morrow AG: Causes of early postoperative death following cardiac valve replacement: clinicopathologic correlations in 64 patients studied at necropsy. *J Thorac Cardiovasc Surg* 54:422–437, 1967.

81. Wild LM, Lajost Z, Lee AB, Wright J: Left ventricular laceration due to stented prosthesis. *Chest* 77:216–217, 1980.

82. Harold JG, Bateman TM, Czer LSC, et al: Mitral valve replacement early after myocardial infarction: attendant high risk of left ventricular rupture. *J Am Coll Cardiol* 9:277–282, 1987.

Chapter 33
LESSONS OF THE PAST AND PROMISES FOR THE FUTURE

JACK M. MATLOFF, M.D.
AURELIO CHAUX, M.D.

This book began with a review of the development of cardiac surgery, which has spanned nearly 100 years. Most of that evolution has occurred over the past 35 to 40 years. To give some sense of historical perspective, it should be appreciated that the first planned correction of a congenital extracardiac great vessel abnormality (closure of a patent ductus arteriosus) occurred just 50 years ago; correction of mitral stenosis by closed techniques became a reality 40 years ago; open-heart procedures using cross-circulation techniques and then heart-lung machines to divert blood from the heart while maintaining the systemic circulation were introduced 35 years ago; coronary angiography became a reality almost 30 years ago; total cardiac valve replacement was successfully accomplished only 27 years ago; and coronary artery bypass grafting and orthotopic allograft replacement of the heart has become a reality over the past 20 years.

In the interim, these procedures have become accepted surgical therapy and at the present time upwards of 250,000 open-heart operations are done each year, the vast majority in patients with coronary atherosclerosis. In addition, percutaneous coronary angioplasty, an invasive technique to control focal atherosclerotic obstructions, will probably be done in 300,000 patients this year; many of these will require some cardiac surgical involvement. Notwithstanding, cardiovascular disease is still the leading cause of death in western society. One and a half million Americans experience a heart attack and 750,000 die each year, 400,000 suddenly. Thus, invasive therapeutic technologies are being used only in approximately one-third of patients who might benefit from such therapy. However, these figures still represent progress: fewer people are dying each year from cardiac causes, and population studies indicate that more people are living longer than ever before. While there are no specific answers to explain exactly how this circumstance has come about, it is quite clear that cardiac surgery has contributed to this change.

CORONARY ARTERY BYPASS IN PERSPECTIVE

The earliest, objective postoperative studies that were done to evaulate the effects of coronary artery bypass included repeat coronary angiography. These demonstrated that such bypassed vessels did remain open in a predictable way. However, it was clear that the rate of success was not uniform between centers. Our own experience that patency rates of more than 90% could be anticipated was somewhat different from the 70% patency rates generally reported at that time. Time and experience have narrowed this difference and, while patency rates are still not uniform, there is more unanimity of opinion as to what this figure should be, especially when internal thoracic artery conduits are used. Today we know that these grafts also last longer than vein conduits, which are more susceptible to the atherosclerotic process. And this is true whether in situ or free internal thoracic artery conduits are used. Further research indicates that the reason for this may be an anatomic one, related to the integrity of the internal elastic membranes and of internal thoracic arteries as compared to other conduits.

Early patency rates of 90% or more appear to be standards to strive for. In retrospect, our early experience seems to have been achieved by a combination of factors, including appropriate selection of targets, exquisite attention to the details of technique, and the use of heparin postoperatively. The latter has now been replaced with the use of aspirin with or without persantine (1,2) to improve graft patency. Today heparin and aspirin, along with thrombolytic agents, have become cornerstones in the treatment of coronary artery disease, especially in its acute manifestations, for reasons that we did not appreciate in the beginning. Regardless, the lessons are clear: open grafts mean fewer symptoms, better ventricular function, fewer myocardial infarctions, and longer life. This is true even in patients who begin with compromised ventricular function; if they are free of ventricular arrhythmias and their grafts remain open they will survive, albeit occasionally with congestive heart failure that may have to be managed vigorously.

As to patency in the future, while the search for other more ideal and durable conduits continues, there is no other arterial substitute on the horizon that holds greater promise than what we already have. Ways are evolving to get the most advantageous use out of the internal thoracic artery, but initial long-term follow-up (3)

suggests that there is little advantage to the use of both internal thoracic arteries rather than one to the anterior descending. The use of magnification and finer monofilament sutures is becoming more widespread. The availability of intracoronary angioscopy (4) and, even more so, the promise of thermal coronary angiography (5) as an integral part of the technique of bypass point to a time when we will have a better understanding of the technical and anatomic factors that correlate with patency. Further progress in understanding the factors that are involved—intravascular clotting and lysis—and pharmacologic capability to prevent intravascular thrombosis while not interfering with extravascular clotting should bring us to a time when graft patency should approach 100%.

The experience with surgical therapy of coronary atherosclerosis has stimulated a number of other innovations. The need to protect the heart against ischemia during all forms of open-heart surgery has contributed to an improved understanding of the metabolic and biochemical consequences of ischemia and has resulted in the development of specific chemical solutions and hypothermia to retard but not truly arrest cardiac metabolism during cardiac surgery. Currently, these measures allow us to operate under more ideal circumstances, for longer periods of time, and on more damaged hearts that require more extensive surgery. Furthermore, more elderly, acutely ill patients can be operated on with greater safety, with less damage to the heart, and with greater anticipation of improved function after cardiac surgery. With some of the work that is being done with thrombolytic agents, free oxygen radical inhibitors, and reperfusion solutions, it is even appropriate to anticipate that the effects of a myocardial infarction will one day be fully reversible if therapy is begun early enough so that the goal of preserving ventricular function will be fully achievable.

It must be remembered that surgical therapy in coronary disease involves an invasive methodology to *bypass*, not reduce or remove, the intracoronary plaque or obstruction. Thus surgery always focuses on areas in the coronary arterial system that are away from the most diseased segments. Because of the magnitude of such procedures, cardiologists have been motivated to devise methods for attacking the plaque directly in a less invasive way. The best-known and most effective of these procedures is percutaneous transluminal coronary angioplasty (PTCA). Even though the primary success rate per vessel is less than that for coronary bypass, the recurrence rate is high (especially in the 1st year), and the completeness of revascularization is less, such therapy is a reality today. It has also been stated that the costs are less for PTCA; but even this is not clear because one has to factor in the costs for the surgical safety net that has to be in place, in one form or another, and the costs for the approximately 30 to 40% of patients who do not have a lasting therapeutic effect from the first procedure. Although it is still not entirely clear what the ultimate long-term result of PTCA will be, it is clear that this technique is still evolving and improving and is also spawning a number of newer, rather ingenious ways to attack the offending plaque directly. Early experience with an atherectomy catheter to "shave" down the plaque, by way of removing it, shows some promise for the future.

The best-publicized of these newer methodologies has involved the use of lasers. To date, these efforts have been limited by the problem of damage to normal tissue and the potential risk of excessive heat produced at the point of application. At Cedars-Sinai Medical Center, the use of an Excimer laser has been developed and investigated extensively for use in all types of vascular atherosclerotic lesions. Problems still exist in relation to steering the light energy directly to the plaque and being able to vaporize the entire plaque. In peripheral artery applications, totally occluded vessels are opened by application of laser energy, and then a balloon angioplasty catheter is used to accomplish angioplasty. Surprisingly, the preliminary results have been better in totally occluded vessels than in subtotally occluded vessels. Promising application to the coronary arteries has just begun clinically, and progress in "steering" the laser beam is being made. Such technology remains a promise for the intermediate future, perhaps over the next 5 years.

While all of these innovations hold the promise of extending life for even longer periods of time by preventing myocardial infarctions, the experience to date with invasive forms of therapy indicates that the basic disease process is not affected. While bypass does relieve symptoms, improve quality of life, and prolong life, at least in certain subsets of patients, it is still palliative therapy; and sooner or later, it can be anticipated that problems will recur and that second and even third reoperations may be in order, not only because the bypasses may become diseased but also because the disease may progress in the native arteries. Almost certainly, additional experience with PTCA will lead us to a similar conclusion. Clinically, it appears that the time frame over which these problems recur can be delayed depending on how well patients care for themselves; risk modification is a reality and each individual thus has responsibility for caring for his or her own health. *Bypass surgery offers a second chance that should not be squandered!* There are no insurance policies against future problems, except those that are paid for by the patient's own hard work. The most current report by Blankenhorn and coworkers (6) that the atherosclerotic process may be held stable and possibly even reversed in native coronary arteries and possibly in coronary bypasses by exquisite attention to the control of risk factors should provide motivation to control these factors.

The problem of later progression also seems to be related to the initial age at which coronary atherosclerosis manifests itself. The younger the patient is when there is need for initial invasive therapy, the sooner a problem is likely to reappear. This is especially apparent in those with strong family histories of coronary disease. When surgery is required in the mid-60s or later, a second operation is less likely to be needed. Such observations strongly support the concept that there are genetic factors that predispose to the development of atherosclerosis and, in fact, such research is actively ongoing, with the anticipation that therapeutic possibilities will be defined, if not in our lifetime then almost certainly in that of our children. At that time, the diagnosis of atherosclerosis, especially in the coronary arteries, should be made early enough that patients at risk for sudden death can be identified and their therapy will focus on prevention. Ultimately, therapy may even become curative in those patients in whom atherosclerotic plaques are already established.

VALVULAR HEART SURGERY IN PERSPECTIVE

While much has been accomplished to reduce the incidence of the streptococcal infections in childhood and early adolescence that cause rheumatic fever, there is still a significant population that suffers from the late sequela of rheumatic valvular disease. This is especially true in underdeveloped or Third World countries. Because the costs of valve substitutes is so dear to such patients there has always been a bias toward repair rather than replacement. However, it has been dissatisfaction with the long-term outcome of valve replacements in regard to function, longevity, the need for anticoagulation, and the combined incidence of thromboembolism and hemorrhage from excessive Coumadin that has been the primary stimulus to the development of reparative techniques. These have been so successfully pioneered by Dr. A. Carpentier of Paris, France, that his results with mitral valve repair have become the standard for all cardiac surgeons to emulate (7). Unfortunately, these techniques do not include the aortic valve. While tricuspid repairs are quite standard (8), since most of these lesions are regurgitant and can be modified by a ring annuloplasty, the results with mitral valve repair have been more difficult to achieve because experience plays such a large part in the application of these techniques. Therefore, an acceptable, standard result has been more difficult to achieve. Notwithstanding, Carpentier's work holds enormous promise for the future.

Although rheumatic valvular disease is a lesser problem in the United States, we are actually seeing more valve problems than previously, primarily because other causes of valvular heart diseases are manifesting themselves as our population ages. In addition to the congenital lesions, more forms of degenerative valvular disease are being seen, related to atherosclerosis, long-standing hypertension, infection, and simple "wear and tear." Clearly, the most significant increase in valvular disease is the result of atherosclerosis, which particularly affects the mitral valve, causing regurgitation, and, to a lesser extent, the aortic valve, which becomes calcified and stenotic. These problems are being seen in older, more acutely ill patients with complex anatomic problems.

Mitral Valve

As regards the mitral valve, concern has been expressed that removal of the valve, and especially division of the papillary muscles, adversely affects left ventricular function (9); other problems include the timing of a procedure, determining what procedure should be carried out, and how the success of the procedure should be evaulated. The ability to repair rather than replace the valve answers the first concern. Some of the remaining problems have been addressed by the application of color flow mapping in the operating room, either directly to the epicardium or via the esophagus (10, 11). Using this technique to evaluate leaflet function under varying physiologic conditions of afterload, it is possible to reproducibly evaluate mitral valve function after reparative procedures. Revascularization alone rarely improves mitral valve function (10, 12), but the additional application of an annuloplasty technique without the use of a ring, but with repair of chordae where indicated clearly gives excellent results. Furthermore, the result established at the time of surgery is predictive of the 1-year result. Thus, ischemic mitral regurgitation of moderate degrees is less of a problem than it has been in the past. In more advanced forms of ischemic-based mitral dysfunction, mitral valve replacement can be carried out, but the results are not ideal (13). This situation appears to be more an expression of advanced myocardial failure than of the procedure itself. Thus, the best hope for such patients would appear to be earlier diagnosis and therapy to prevent progression to such advanced states of ventricular dysfunction.

Aortic Valve

With regard to the calcific changes that occur in trileaflet aortic valves as a result of the rheumatic and atherosclerotic processes, aortic valve replacement has been the standard form of therapy. While both short- and long-term results have been good and have progressively improved, current attention is being directed to the development of means to débride the valve using ultrasonic energy. Such techniques may be particularly applicable where the disease process is not far advanced and surgery has been indicated primarily to accomplish revascularization. This addresses the problem of replacing the valve too early in the face of expected rapid progression to the need for replacement.

Valve Prostheses

Despite this emphasis on techniques to repair and preserve cardiac valves, the results of valve replacement surgery are excellent, even in patients who have complex problems requiring correction of mechanical lesions along with coronary bypass. When valve replacement is necessary, two generic types of valve substitute are available that have well-described and known clinical performance. These are tissue valves and prosthetic valves (14). Among the tissue valves, porcine valves are still the most commonly used. Although use of these valves usually avoids the need for Coumadin, hydraulic function is not ideal in smaller sizes, and durability beyond 10 years is questionable. Active research into methods of tissue preparation and preservation to achieve greater durability is continuing.

In addition, the use of homografts from cadaveric human sources is once again being advocated to achieve better function and greater longevity. These are currently used only for aortic valve replacement. As with mitral valve repair, excellent results with such procedures are more difficult to obtain because of the increased technical demands of implantation. Thus, the challenge for the future is to develop techniques for their implantation that are more easily accomplished by larger numbers of cardiac surgeons.

As for mechanical valves, 28 years of research have finally given us valve designs that allow for hemodynamic performance that approaches normal hydraulic function while still maintaining a low incidence of thromboembolism. With a few exceptions, these characteristics have been achieved without apparent adverse effect on durability. Currently, the most widely used valve of this type is the St. Jude Medical valve. It is bileaflet in design and fabricated from carbon (Pyrolyte) with proven durability. Unfortunately, anticoagulation with Coumadin is still necessary, but recent experiences suggest that very acceptable thromboembolic rates can be maintained with lower dosage levels of Coumadin assisted with adjunctive use of Persantine (15). The hope is that the future will define better pharmacologic agents to prevent thromboembolism, with virtually no threat of bleeding. If not, materials development and fabrication hold promise for the future evolution of an ideal valve substitute.

CARDIAC TRANSPLANTATION IN PERSPECTIVE

While we have stressed that there is almost no present cardiac disease for which there is not some form of palliative therapy, it is clear that there are *some* extremely complex congenital and far-advanced acquired degenerative cardiac lesions that cannot be effectively palliated. For these situations, it is safe to say that cardiac transplantation has become an acceptable alternative today. What has happened with in utero diagnosis of heart disease and with cardiac transplantation just after birth at Loma Linda University dramatically makes this point. This extension of the indications for transplantation and the expanding availability of these services highlight the need for adequate donor supply and how much we need a capability for prolonged preservation so that the donor supply can be international in scope.

Although significant progress is being made, the problems of rejection and modification of the immune system remain, as with all tissues and organs; but the real answer to consistently successful heart transplantation may very well lie within the realm of immunologic and genetic (including recombinant DNA) investigations. If and when these avenues of research are successful, the problems of donor organ availability may also be lessened by xenograft or cross-species transplants.

Thus, the current problems of cardiac transplantation are other than those of anatomic surgical techniques. They are problems that seem solvable by biochemical investigations. In addition to the critical issue of rejection there is much to be done with donor heart preservation. The importance of improved cardiac preservation has enormous implications for other forms of cardiac surgery as well. When these problems are resolved and a more satisfactory course can be achieved after transplantation, the indications for transplantation will be expanded, and currently acceptable forms of palliative therapy will be replaced by this more definitive form of therapy.

THE FUTURE

In many ways, concerns for the future of cardiac surgery are not so much surgical and medical as they are social and economic. As technologic advances are made, the population ages and patient expectations expand, ethical, legal, and financial issues come into more acute focus. As our capabilities expand, the costs of such therapy continue to increase; and this concurrence of forces creates an environment that is charged with the potential for social and political conflict. The issue may become not so much how patients with cardiac disease will be treated, but rather whether they will have access to such therapy. When one combines improved, earlier diagnostic techniques with the population trends that have been noted, the potential demands for such services could increase at least threefold, and potentially sixfold. Given the costs of invasive therapies, we will increasingly have to be aware of the hard questions that are sure to be asked. In an environment in which the biologic and medical barriers to improved cardiac health are being successfully confronted and overcome, it is ironic that we are rapidly moving away from the ethical issues that are concerned with *whether and to what extent we should be* testing the limits of life, to financial and social issues of *whether we can afford to.* There will be no easy answers for such questions; and we may soon find ourselves longing for the days when we simply had to decide whether and how we could accomplish an improvement in our patient's condition at an acceptable risk of morbidity postoperatively and of mortality.

References

1. Chesebro JH, Clements IP, Fuster V, et al: A platelet-inhibitor drug trial in coronary artery bypass operations: benefit of perioperative persantine and aspirin therapy on early postoperative vein-graft patency. N Engl J Med 307:73–78, 1982.
2. Goldman S, Copeland J, Moritz T, et al: Improvement in early saphenous vein graft patency after coronary artery bypass surgery with antiplatelet therapy: results of a Veterans Administration Cooperative Study. Circulation 77:1324–1332, 1988.
3. Loop FD, Lytle BW, Cosgrove DM, et al: Influence of the internal mammary artery graft on 10 year survival and other cardiac events. N Engl J Med 314:1–6, 1986.
4. Sherman CT, Litvack F, Grundfest WS, et al: Coronary angioscopy in patients with unstable angina pectoris. N Engl J Med 315:913–919, 1986.
5. Mohr FW, Matloff JM, Grundfest W, et al: Thermal coronary angiography. Ann Thorac Surg 45: 1988.
6. Blankenhorn DH, Nessim SA, Johnson RL, et al: Beneficial effects of combined colestipol-niacin therapy on coronary atherosclerosis and coronary venous bypass grafts. JAMA 257:3233–3240, 1987.
7. Carpentier A, Chauvaud S, Fabiani JN, et al: Reconstructive surgery of mitral valve incompetence. J Thorac Cardiovasc Surg 79:338, 1980.
8. Czer LSC, Maurer G, Bolger A, et al: Tricuspid valve repair: operative and follow-up evaluation by Doppler color flow mapping. J Thorac Cardiovasc Surg 98:101–111, 1989.
9. David TE, Uden DE, Strauss HD: The importance of the mitral apparatus in left ventricular function after correction of mitral regurgitation. Circulation 68(Suppl II):76, 1983.
10. Czer LSC, Maurer G, Bolger AF, et al: Intraoperative evaluation of mitral regurgitation by Doppler color flow mapping. Circulation 76(Suppl III):108–116, 1987.
11. Kleinman J, Czer LSC, DeRobertis M, Chaux A, Maurer G: A quantitative comparison of tranesophageal and epicardial color Doppler echocardiography in the intraoperative assessment of mitral regurgitation. Am J Cardiol 1989 (in press).
12. Czer LSC, Maurer G, Bolger A, et al: Ischemic mitral regurgitation: comparative evaluation of revascularization vs. repair by Doppler color flow mapping. Circulation 76(Suppl IV):389, 1987.
13. Czer LSC, Gray RJ, DeRobertis MA, et al: Mi-

tral valve replacement: impact of coronary artery disease and determinants of prognosis after revascularization. *Circulation* 70(Suppl I):198–207, 1984.

14. Czer LSC, Matloff JM, Chaux A, DeRobertis MA, Gray RJ: Comparative clinical experience with porcine bioprosthetic and St. Jude valve replacement. *Chest* 91:503–514, 1987.

15. Czer LSC, Matloff JM, Chaux A, et al: The St. Jude valve: analysis of thromboembolism, warfarin-related hemorrhage, and survival. *Am Heart J* 114:389–397, 1987.

INDEX

Page numbers in *italics* denote figures; those followed by "t" denote tables.

Dopamine
  circulatory effects of, 159–160
  contraindicated, 100
  for renal failure, 265
Doppler echocardiography
  for bioprosthetic valve evaluation, 348–349
  in valve replacement follow-up, 338–344
Double vessel disease, mortality rate for, 14
Duplex scanning, 28
Dyspnea, 237

Ebstein's anomaly, 22
ECG. *See* Electrocardiography
Echocardiography
  in mediastinal bleeding evaluation, 191
  for pericardial pain diagnosis, 241
  two-dimensional, 28
    for bioprosthetic valve evaluation, 348
    transesophageal, 96
  in valve replacement follow-up, 338–344
Edrophonium, 89, 102
Elderly
  clinical outcomes after surgery in, 31–34
  life expectancy of, 27
  nutritional status of, 30
  preoperative evaluation of, 27–31
  risk of in noncardiac surgery, 40
Electrocardiographic changes
  long-lasting pain and, 241
  postoperative, 140
  T-wave, 174
Electrocardiographic low voltage, 149
Electrocardiography, 69
  during CABG, 100
  intraoperative, 87
  in myocardial infarction diagnosis, 179–180
  signal-averaged, 215
  in valve replacement follow-up, 338
Electrolytes, in normal convalesence, 137–138
Embolic debris, 147–148
Emphysema, cardiac surgery and, 29
Endocarditis, 22, 245–246
  late, 23
  prevention of, 347*t*
  with prosthetic valves, 346–347
  surgical risk with, 41–42
  therapy for, 250
Endocrine system
  anesthesia effects on, 123–124
  postoperative dysfunction of, 151
Endoscopic retrograde cannulation, 273–274
Endoscopy, 272–273
Endotracheal intubation
  indications for, 99

trauma of, 142
Enflurane, 105
  arrhythmias with, 119
  endocrine effects of, 124
  hemodynamic effects and myocardial oxygen
    balance with, 120
Ephedrine, 93–94
Epicardial pacemaker electrodes, 219
Epinephrine
  circulatory effects of, 158
  elevated, 174
Erythrocyte sedimentation rate, 248–249
Esmolol, 89
  for atrial arrhythmias, 211
  intravenous, 90
Etomidate, 88, 123
Exercise
  benefits of, 331
  postsurgical program for, 306–309
  recommended frequency of, 314–315
  therapy, 312
    initiation of, 312–313
    lifetime, 317–318
    postdischarge program of, 316–317
    predischarge low-intensity, 315–316
    progressive in-hospital, 313–315
  tolerance of following valve replacement, 335
Exercise stress testing, 87
Exercise treadmill test (ETT), 14
Extracorporeal circulation
  arterial cannulation in, 59–60
  autotransfusion and blood conservation systems
    in, 61
  components and methodology of, 55–61
  concept of, 55
  in elderly, 31
  filters for, 59
  heat exchangers for, 59
  intrapericardial suction in, 61
  oxygenators in, 58–59
  priming solutions for, 60–61
  pumps for, 59
  tubing for, 56
  venous cannulation in, 56–57
  venting in, 60
Extracorporeal membrane oxygenation (ECMO),
  259

Factor VIII, 202
Family
  cardiac surgery effects on, 320–321
  preoperative fears of, 47
  preparation of for hospital environment, 49–50
  preparation of for surgery, 47–52